Globalisation of Addiction
A Study in Poverty of the Spirit

Praise for the hardback edition of *The Globalization of Addiction*

'For most of modern history, scientific investigations into the nature of addiction have been dominated either by pharmacological fundamentalism—the evil is caused by malevolent molecules—or by genetics and neuro-science, which situate addiction in the biology and brain of the individual. Yet despite decades of such research, a "cure" for addiction and even a comprehensive understanding of it have remained elusive. Bruce Alexander's *The Globalisation of Addiction* is a work of dazzling erudition that provides the missing pieces. It advances an emerging paradigm in which drug use and drug problems are understood in their full historical, cultural, and social-structural context. If we really want to know where our drug problems come from and what can be done about them, we have to move beyond a failed war on drugs and delve into the very nature of modern society. This great book shows us how to do that.'
Craig Reinarman, *Professor of Sociology and Legal Studies, University of California, Santa Cruz,* co-author of *Cocaine Changes: The Experience of Using and Quitting* and *Crack In America: Demon Drugs and Social Justice*

'This is a refreshing, iconoclastic view of addiction. It puts the subject within an unusually wide frame that includes the way society is structured and the world views that we all live by. It makes conventional views of addiction look narrow and inadequate. Not everyone will agree with Alexander's thesis, but everyone in the addiction field should read this book and have a position on it.'
Jim Orford, *Emeritus Professor of Clinical & Community Psychology, University of Birmingham, UK*

'Generously conceived and meticulously researched, *The Globalisation of Addiction* is an essential compendium of fact, theory, and analysis on the international malaise of drug addiction. Prof. Bruce Alexander's discussion of the history of addiction, its sources, characteristics, political and economic ramifications, and its potential resolutions is intellectually invigorating and serves as a forthright call to action. Everyone seriously interested in understanding the modern plague of substance dependence will benefit from reading this volume, a deeply original work that challenges the cherished assumptions of policy makers in London, Washington, Ottawa and in many capitals around the world.'
Gabor Maté M.D., author of *In the Realm of Hungry Ghosts: Close Encounters with Addiction*

'In *The Globalisation of Addiction*, Bruce Alexander has given us a remarkable gift. In addition to being extremely well written and erudite, it both organises an impossibly complex topic—addiction—and defines the cultural malaise (which Alexander labels "dislocation") that is at the root of what ails our modern world. Combining laboratory and clinical research with social and economic analysis, Alexander also delves into the lives of individual addicts, historical figures from St Augustine to Adolph Eichmann, and his own life and the lives of people in his social milieu. A recurrent major stop in this journey involves decisively illuminating forays into the city of Vancouver, its native and immigrant populations, and the artistic resurgence of its inner city. Bruce Alexander makes clear that the solution for the ever-spreading scourge of modern addiction lies not in the laboratory or the clinic, but in revolutionary change of the social and economic world we inhabit.'
Stanton Peele, *Senior Fellow, Drug Policy Alliance,* author of *Love and Addiction, 7 Tools to Beat Addiction,* and *Addiction-Proof Your Child*

'This fascinating, insightful, and scholarly book provides a unique and very personal overview of the "addiction field". Bruce Alexander has produced a panoramic perspective on "addiction" from his own extensive academic experience as a psychologist, together with the vast international literature on this expanding subject. As he notes, "addiction" includes a wide range of behaviours aside from the chronic use of legal and illegal mind-influencing drugs. Addiction is considered from a historical perspective and as a "societal" rather than an individual phenomenon. Nevertheless, the role of the individual, either as an "addict", therapist, or other actor in the addiction arena, is fully acknowledged. Much of the argument of this excellent book is presented from a global perspective. Even so, a sense of reality and immediacy is provided by discussion set in the city of Vancouver. This fills the role of a prototype or case study, illustrating some of the author's key general points about the historical development of addiction, together with the relevance of the global market in drugs and other addiction-related factors. He considers a wide range of issues underlying the worldwide spread of addictive behaviours. These include addiction as a response to social dislocation, the mythology of powerful "demon drugs", and the ideology of spiritual and other treatment approaches. He takes issue with many aspects of the "conventional wisdom" about addiction. Whether one agrees with him or not, this is challenging and thought-provoking.'
Martin Plant, *Professor of Addiction Studies, University of the West of England, Bristol, UK*
Moira Plant, *Professor of Alcohol Studies, University of the West of England, Bristol, UK*

Bruce Alexander is a psychologist and Professor Emeritus at Simon Fraser University, Canada, where he has worked since 1970. His primary research interest has been the psychology of addiction. He is best known in the UK and the USA for the 'Rat Park' experiments, which helped to demonstrate the falsity of the outworn belief that simple exposure to narcotic drugs can cause addiction. In Canada, he has been well known as a critic of the 'War on Drugs' for decades. His most recent work has been on the causes of the current worldwide proliferation of addiction, not only to drugs, but to a great variety of other habits and pursuits. Exploring this topic has required that he venture far beyond his training in psychology, particularly into the fields of history and anthropology. He is married, with four children and two grandchildren.

The Globalisation of Addiction

A Study in Poverty of the Spirit

Bruce K. Alexander
Department of Psychology
Simon Fraser University
Vancouver
British Columbia
Canada

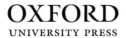
OXFORD
UNIVERSITY PRESS

OXFORD
UNIVERSITY PRESS

Great Clarendon Street, Oxford OX2 6DP

Oxford University Press is a department of the University of Oxford.
It furthers the University's objective of excellence in research, scholarship,
and education by publishing worldwide in

Oxford New York

Auckland   Cape Town   Dar es Salaam   Hong Kong   Karachi
Kuala Lumpur   Madrid   Melbourne   Mexico City   Nairobi
New Delhi   Shanghai   Taipei   Toronto
With offices in
Argentina   Austria   Brazil   Chile   Czech Republic   France   Greece
Guatemala   Hungary   Italy   Japan   South Korea   Poland   Portugal
Singapore   Switzerland   Thailand   Turkey   Ukraine   Vietnam

Oxford is a registered trade mark of Oxford University Press
in the UK and in certain other countries

Published in the United States
by Oxford University Press Inc., New York

ISBN 978-0-19-958871-8

Printed and bound in Great Britain by
CPI Antony Rowe, Chippenham and Eastbourne

Whilst every effort has been made to ensure that the contents of this book are as complete,
accurate and up-to-date as possible at the date of writing, Oxford University Press is not
able to give any guarantee or assurance that such is the case. Readers are urged to take
appropriately qualified medical advise in all cases. The information in this book is
intended to be useful to the general reader, but should not be used as a means of
self-diagnosis or for the prescription of medication.

To my four wonderful children, each of whom is finding a good path, in spite of all this. In order of appearance: Ben, Alexa, Paul, Dorian.

Acknowledgements

If it takes an entire village to raise a child, how many people does it take to write a book? This one was nourished and supported from conception by a multitude of thinkers. Some of these thinkers are professional scholars, some not. Some I know well, some I have only read. Some are long-dead historical figures. Those I encountered face-to-face often shared their personal stories with me, as well as their abstract ideas. These indispensable face-to-face collaborators included Benjamin Alexander, Paul Alexander, Nancy Alexander, Ethan Alexander-Davey, Kim Alscher, Barry Beyerstein, Jan Blomberg, Andrew Boden, Marilyn Bowman, John Bogardus, Paul Carter, Douglas Cameron, Roy Carlson, Charles Crawford, Harry Crosby, Phil Dalgarno, Earl Davey, Robert Derkson, Tana and George Dineen, Pat Erickson, Mary Etey, Harry Evans, Susan Evans, Rick Fence, Chaouac Ferron, Lorraine Fish, Rose-Hannah Gaskin, Kevin Gomes, Donald Gordon, Kathleen and Gordon Gray, David Hackley, Frank Harris, Ted Harrison, Amber Hui, Ivan Illich, Jangwon Kim, Sharon Kravitz, Michael Maraun, James Marcia, Ian Marcuse, Gabor Maté, Gary McCarron, Susan McCook, Teresa McInnes, Barry Morris, Bryan Nadeau, Dorian Alexander Nijdam, Stephen Ogden, Jim Orford, Eugene Oscapella, Stuart Parker, Terry Patten, Greg Placonouris, Ted Poole, Kevin Potvin, Mary Reid, Wyn Roberts, Ken Sailor, Ernesto Salvi, Dan Savard, Jeffrey Schaler, Anton Schweighofer, Stefa Shaler, Curt Shelton, Lauren Slater, Dan Small, Art Steinmann, Alexa Stone, Kerstin Stürzbecher, Sam Sullivan, Larry Tallman, Donald Todd, Arnold Trebach, Jon Tsou, Robert Underwood, Savannah Walling, Joan and Michael Wolfe, Linda Wong, Armine Yalnizyan, and Norman Zinberg. Members of my family and personal friends who appear on this list sustained the project with their encouragement and personal support, as well as their ideas.

Curt Shelton has helped with this book throughout. At the end, he organised the countless tasks required to bring the manuscript to completion and to get it to the publisher. He found a great burst of energy for this mountain of finishing work at a time when my own was running out.

This book was completed only because my wife, Patricia Holborn, treated the fragile gropings of my mind and the tumult of my enthusiasms with steadfast good humour, all the while keeping up with her own demanding professional responsibilities … and because she made the ever-fickle computer work when I could only curse … and because she maintained a degree of domestic order without which both manuscript and writer might have been submerged in the litter … and because in some other way that I do not fully comprehend, she breathed substance into the text. It is hers, too.

Also, a huge thank you to Inspiration Ledge.

Contents

Author's Note

Everything in this book is as factually accurate as I can possibly make it with one exception. Key details in biographical accounts of people who I know personally have been fictionalised to protect their identities. These fictions have been checked with the people involved to ensure that they do not distort the essential truth of their accounts, which have been approved by them for publication.

All quotations in the text are written in English. Where the original text was French, I translated the material myself with the guidance of my teacher and friend, Chaouac Ferron.

Introduction

Why are so many people dangerously addicted in the globalising world of the 21st century? Why does the range of addictions extend so far beyond drugs and alcohol to gambling, shopping, romantic love, video games, religious zealotry, television viewing, internet surfing, an emaciated body shape ... and on and on? Why has scientific medicine, a dazzling success in so many other domains, not brought addiction under control? These mysteries are best investigated by viewing addiction historically. A historical perspective affords an unhurried look at what addiction is, why it has always existed, why it appears to be spinning out of control just now, and what modern society can hope to do about it. Moreover, it provides a fresh view of certain aspects of the madness of today's world that might seem unrelated to addiction at first.

The value of a historical perspective seized my attention only a few years ago. Frustrated after decades of inconclusive research and marginally successful service in treatment and harm reduction, I changed my line of work permanently—or so I thought. I resolved to forget about addiction and to cultivate my interest in history instead, limiting my university teaching to the history of psychology for a few years. I read historians as well as others who could inform me about the past: anthropologists, political scientists, economists, ancient philosophers, and investigative journalists.[1] I deliberately avoided works concerning drugs or addiction, for my new interests were quite different. Without meaning to, however, I kept coming across insights into addiction that were more powerful than those I had encountered in the professional literature on addiction. I had been looking in the wrong place all along.

This book undertakes a fusion of the insights on addiction that arose from my historical interlude with the professional addiction literature. Even if this fusion-powered analysis has not generated a miracle cure, I am convinced that it constitutes a giant step forward.

Switching to a historical perspective on addiction is not as easy as it may appear, because conventional wisdom stands in the way. Today's conventional wisdom on addiction[2] was established in North America and Western Europe during the 19th and 20th centuries.[3] It is now disseminated everywhere on the world's information highways. Around the globe, people absorb it from childhood, quite unconsciously. Unfortunately, the conventional wisdom has led neither to a clear understanding nor to effective control of addiction during its long domination of public consciousness.[4] Well past its prime, it is overdue for an honourable retirement.

The conventional wisdom depicts addiction, most fundamentally, as an individual problem. Some individuals become addicted and others do not. An individual who becomes addicted must somehow be restored to normalcy. There is an odd dualism built into this individual-centred depiction: addiction is seen either as an illness or as a moral defect or—somehow—both at once.[5] Accordingly, addiction can be overcome by professional treatment or moral reformation of the afflicted individual, or both. Another fundamental assumption of the conventional wisdom is that drug and alcohol abuse are the prototypical addictions. If there are other types of addict, they will be recognised by what they have in common with alcoholics and 'junkies'.

The historical perspective of this book does not share these assumptions. Rather than an individual problem, the historical perspective views addiction as a societal problem. Addiction can be rare in a society for many centuries, but can become nearly universal when circumstances change—for example, when a cohesive tribal culture is crushed or an advanced civilisation collapses. From this perspective, addiction is not so much a problem of aberrant individuals as a latent human potential that expresses itself universally under particular social circumstances. Of course, the historical perspective does not deny that differences in vulnerability are built into each individual's genes, individual experience, and personal character, but it removes individual differences from the foreground of attention, because social determinants are more powerful.

Just as the historical perspective does not share the assumption that addiction is an individual problem, it does not share the assumption that drug addiction is the prototypical form of addiction. Throughout history, other kinds of addictive habits have been more widespread and just as devastating. I have written about drug and alcohol problems and the misbegotten 'War on Drugs' in past years,[6] but this book is about addiction per se, which, at the deepest level of analysis, has no necessary connection to drugs.

Although this book rejects the conventional perspective on addiction, it does not lay out its flaws one by one. That painstaking dissection has already been accomplished by many able scholars[7] whose works are cited here. Instead of continued embarrassment, the conventional perspective has earned its retirement. It has served honourably and, despite its flaws, it still provides a helpful and compassionate way to think about addiction in some treatment settings.[8]

I have, however, found it necessary to subject one particular part of the conventional wisdom to detailed analysis. The still widely held belief that addiction can be caused simply by consuming one of the 'addictive drugs' continues to obscure the field of addiction today. The evidence that refutes this belief has been known for decades, but, like a ghost that cannot rest in peace, the belief still haunts present-day discussions[9] with its dramatic images of irresistibly addictive drugs including heroin ('it's so good, don't even try it once'), crack cocaine ('the most addictive drug on earth'), and crystal methamphetamine ('more addictive than crack cocaine').

I have not allowed this ghostly belief to haunt the main text of this book, but have instead confined it to Chapter 8, which summarises the evidence for and against it in the case of heroin, the drug to which the belief has been applied with the greatest confidence for nearly a century. Trapped, and—for once—prevented from fleeing into the shadows when confronted, the belief can be critically re-examined by reviewing Chapter 8 any time that readers find its ghostly presence distracting them from the main argument. I recommend reading Chapter 8 under a strong reading lamp or outdoors, because ghosts lose their power in the light of day.

I have not discussed all of the other drugs that at one time or another have been presumed to instil addiction in all or most people who consume them because that would require too many chapters and because this book has a different purpose. Readers who feel haunted by the mythical addiction-causing properties of cocaine, crack, crystal methamphetamine, and so forth, will be referred in Chapter 8 to numerous other authors who are carrying out the necessary ghost-busting work brilliantly. None of this is meant to minimise the agonising reality of severe drug addiction, only to firmly assert the fact that it cannot be caused simply by exposure to a drug.

Whereas this book offers a historical perspective on addiction throughout the world, it begins and ends in the city of Vancouver, British Columbia, Canada. Vancouver provides an excellent case study of the spread of addiction on a globalising planet. It is a thoroughly modern city that was not founded until the late 19th century. It came into existence to fill a niche in the global economic system then maintained by the British Empire—the precursor of today's globalising civilisation.[10] There was little shared culture in early Vancouver to smooth the hard edges of its raw economic function. Despite its beauty, civility, and prosperity, Vancouver soon became known as the city with the biggest drug-addiction problem in Canada.[11] And Canada, peaceable and tidy as it is, has a world-class drug-addiction problem.[12] The United Nations Population Fund recently chose Vancouver as its example to prove that the social problems of 21st-century urbanisation strike rich cities as well as poor cities in the Third World.[13]

The history of Vancouver suggests, and a broader survey of history seems to confirm, that today's rising tide of addiction to drug use and a thousand other habits is the consequence of people, rich and poor alike, being torn from the close ties to family, culture, and traditional spirituality that constituted the normal fabric of life in pre-modern times. This worldwide rending of the social fabric ultimately results from the growing domination of all aspects of modern life by free-market economics, producing a lopsided kind of existence that will be called 'free-market society' in this book. Free-market society subjects people to unrelenting pressures towards individualism, competition, and rapid change, dislocating them from social life. People adapt to this dislocation by concocting the best substitutes that they can for a sustaining social, cultural, and spiritual wholeness, and addiction provides this substitute for more and more of us.

Please note: The cold war is over. The beautiful dream of a world founded on collective ownership of all means of production collapsed on itself in the USSR, China, and elsewhere in the 20th century. The ability of capitalism to produce the highest levels of innovation and productivity is undisputed. Although today's globalisation pits antagonistic regimes against each other, all of them, including China, India, Russia, Venezuela, and Vietnam, use market principles to organise at least some aspects of their economies and all are vulnerable to the depredations of hypercapitalism.[14] Capitalism does not necessarily produce excessive dislocation and addiction when it is kept in a healthy balance with the other institutions of society. Dislocation and addiction are, however, mass-produced by free-market society, which is a form of hypercapitalism that any regime can impose, whether it labels itself capitalist, neo-conservative, neo-liberal, market socialist, socialist, labour, or anything else. This book is not about resurrecting the dream of pure socialism, but it does confront the urgent necessity of *domesticating* modern capitalism in the end.

The analysis in this book could draw addiction scholars away from today's comfortably bounded professionalism towards a more intensely contested arena. However, their comfortable professionalism is already endangered, because the conventional wisdom upon which it is based has not prevented the carnage of addiction from expanding further and further beyond its old limits. Truly understanding addiction requires following wherever it leads, even into the darkest thickets of history, economics, and politics. In particular, understanding addiction now requires examining the continuing global advance of free-market society, even though this will still seem off-topic to some addiction professionals. Indeed, the global advance of free-market society exists in a distant semi-reality for many people in society at large. By contrast, historians and other social scientists recognise the advance of free-market society as one of the definitive and powerfully formative aspects of modern life. How could it fail to have a major impact on addiction or any other widespread human activity?

Adopting a global, historical perspective on addiction does not mean turning away from the valiant, individual struggles of addicted men and women and their families. Nor does it mean turning against the addiction professionals who have served the conventional wisdom with such compassion. It could mean, however, reorganising the practices of addiction professionals within a larger social project. In the end, I am a lifelong psychologist rather than a late convert to history. As a psychologist, I hope not only to analyse the human condition but also to improve it. I believe a global, historical perspective can reduce the burden of addiction in our times.

The subtitle of this book is meant to signal that its ambition extends well beyond the conventional limits of psychology and social science. To be fully comprehended, addiction must be analysed in spiritual as well as psychosocial terms. Although I am not a theist of any persuasion and do not believe in any kind of life after death, I am part of a civilisation that has been profoundly influenced by two millennia of Christian philosophy. As I dig deeper and deeper into the topic of addiction, I find it increasingly necessary to draw on the strengths of this Christian heritage, and of other spiritual traditions, as well as to point out their limitations.

This book has two parts. Part I (Chapters 1–8) is entitled *Roots of Addiction in Free-market Society*. The eight chapters of Part I define addiction and analyse why it is spreading so quickly as the world moves towards a global free-market society. This analysis is formalised as a 'dislocation theory of addiction'. Evidence supporting this theory is summarised at some length.

Part II (Chapters 9–15) is entitled *The Interaction of Addiction and Society*. It examines mass addiction not only as an *effect* of free-market society, but also as a *cause* of the structure and colour of the modern age and of two eras of Western civilisation's past when dislocation and addiction were also widespread. Part II argues that the destructive potential of addiction has not yet been fully appreciated, even now, in the era of a perpetual, ghastly war on drugs. In its final chapters, Part II proposes measures that can reduce the devastating spread of addiction in the modern world. Some of these proposals go far beyond the familiar measures on which the world has pinned its hopes of controlling addiction for more than a century.

This book has more endnotes and references than I would have liked. I did not amass these to overwhelm opposition, but rather to maintain my equilibrium when I reached conclusions that blatantly violated the conventional wisdom both of the addiction field and of mainstream political economics. I never seriously questioned either kind of conventional wisdom during the first half of my life, but now I believe they are both obsolete. Because I have drawn security from the shared wisdom of my society, however, I become dizzy when it falls away beneath my feet. Then I clutch at all the documentary support that I can reach.

Having relieved my vertigo, the massive documentation in this book went on to produce problems of its own. It generated so many citations and parenthetical elaborations that, in the interest of readability, they had to be removed from the text. However, because documentation is sometimes indispensable, this essential baggage has been consigned to about 1400 endnotes, some of them long. I trust that readers will pay no more attention to the superscripted endnote numerals that they find strewn throughout the text than they would to a litter of discarded baggage checks at a railway station—except at points where they feel the vertigo too and need to retrieve the evidence. Shorter versions of the analysis in this book, less cluttered with documentation but correspondingly more vulnerable to dispute, are available in several articles.[15]

Because this book is based upon a particular set of assumptions and values, I have made these explicit, although this might make members of my own profession squirm. There was a time in the 20th century when professional psychologists thought of themselves as 'pure scientists' and proudly described their research as 'value-free science'. Although admirable research grew from this resolute empiricism, most psychologists now recognise that the attempt to force all scholarship to conform to this empirical ideal was little more than academic machismo. Neither scientists nor psychologists can function unless their observations are structured by assumptions about the nature of reality. They draw these assumptions from their educational and cultural backgrounds and their own temperaments.[16] From professional psychology's beginnings in the 19th century, psychologists grounded their analyses of human behaviour on the assumptions and values of a burgeoning free-market society.[17] This was not a mistake, but a necessity at the time. If they had not, it is unlikely that they would have found the institutional support that they needed, or that anybody would have understood what they were talking about. On the other hand, I believe that psychology will be rebuilt on a different foundation in the future and that this will happen sooner rather than later.

For the present, mainstream psychology, like mainstream medicine, is inseparably wedded to the conventional wisdom on addiction. For this reason, it is not particularly useful on this topic. A glance at the bibliography of this book will reveal many fewer references to psychology and medicine than to history, social science, investigative journalism, and classic philosophy.

Endnotes

1   Although this may well be remembered as an era of trash journalism, excellent investigative journalism is still available and provides an important source of facts about the recent past. I have relied heavily on the *Globe and Mail* (a national Canadian newspaper published in Toronto) and *Le Monde diplomatique* (an international newsmagazine published in Paris). Both are considered 'elite' media because of the level of language that they use. Both are scrupulously accurate and they seldom disagree on the facts. The *Globe and Mail* unswervingly supports the expansion of free-market society, while *Le Monde diplomatique* unswervingly opposes it, but both do their work with intelligence and integrity. It is my hope that their countervailing editorial biases provide me with a reasonably accurate grasp of current affairs.

2   This conventional wisdom is frequently called the 'disease model of addiction' or the 'medical model of addiction' (Levine, 1978; Granfield and Cloud, 1999, Chapter 1; Schaler, 2000; Neve, 2005) or sometimes the 'biopsychosocial model' (Alcohol and Drug Services of British Columbia, 1996). I do not use these names for the conventional wisdom on addiction here because they imply that its origin is essentially medical, whereas it has a much broader social and religious foundation.

3   Meyer (1996).

4   See Reuter and Stevens (2007) for an authoritative study of the UK evidence that supports this conclusion. Older studies that reach the same conclusion include Musto (1987, esp. pp. 85–86) and Alexander (1990, Chapter 2). Further evidence is considered in detail in endnote 9 of Chapter 1.

5   Within the framework of the conventional wisdom, people argue endlessly over whether the basic cause is a medical problem or a moral error, but generally agree that it must be one of the other or both. Warburton *et al.* (2005, p. 2) characterised the dual character of the conventional wisdom concerning heroin thus: 'Media discussion of heroin use in particular is skilful at fusing the assumptions of the disease model with those of moral decadence, with purple metaphors of entrapment and enslavement.' Schaler (2000, p. 70) has pointed out that members of Alcoholics Anonymous support the concept of free will, which makes addiction a moral problem, but also support a concept of alcoholism as a disease that is out of control.

6   For example, Alexander (1990).

7   Each of the following works contradicts a major part of the conventional wisdom on the basis of empirical data and/or logical analysis: Brecher (1972); Ledain (1973); Peele and Brodsky (1975); Szasz (1975); Trebach (1982, 1987); Peele (1985, 1989); Peele *et al.* (1991); Alexander (1990, 1994); Erickson *et al.* (1994); J. B. Davies (1997); Reinarman and Levine (1997); Dineen (1998); Granfield and Cloud (1999); Schaler (2000); Klingemann et al. (2001); Orford (2001a, Chapter 13); S. R. Friedman (2002); Hammersley and Reid (2002); Sullum (2003); Shewan and Dalgarno (2005); Warburton *et al.* (2005); Dalrymple (2006a); DeGrandpre (2006). Of course, the scholars who have exposed the weakness of the conventional wisdom from so many directions disagree with each other on major points as well, and some will probably reject the historical perspective presented here.

8   For example, the conventional wisdom is built into many '12-step' programmes, which have helped countless addicted people. In a similar vein, Kuhn (1970) has pointed out that both Ptolemaic astronomy and Newtonian physics are still in use as engineering approximations, although the fundamental assumptions upon which they are based have been refuted by the newer disciplinary matrices of astronomy and physics.

9 Hammersley and Reid (2002).

10 K. Polanyi (1944); Saul (2005, Chapter 5).

11 E. Murphy (1922/1973, p. 138).

12 A comparison of quantitative studies of drug and alcohol abuse and dependence puts Canada in the same league with Australia, New Zealand, Great Britain, and Korea, although somewhat below the prevalence levels of the United States and well above those of Taiwan (Somers *et al.*, 2004).

13 Drake (2007); Leidl (2007).

14 Stiglitz (2002, pp. 217–218); Romero (2006).

15 Alexander (2000, 2001, 2004, 2006).

16 The clearest of modern thinkers have reached this conclusion, among them, William James (1907/1981, Lecture 1), Thomas Kuhn (1970), and much more recently Jon Tsou (2003).

17 N. Rose (1985); Danziger (1990); Martín-Baró (1994); Chrisjohn and Young (1997); Leahey (2001); Illouz (2007, pp. 1–25).

Part 1

Roots of Addiction in Free-market Society

Part I of this book, which comprises Chapters 1–8, is intended to identify the root cause of the current proliferation of addiction in the globalising world. The analysis is laid out in general terms in Chapter 1, using the history of Vancouver as an illustration.

The analysis cannot become more specific until Chapter 2 resolves a crucial semantic problem. A look around today's field of addictions (as it is sometimes called) will reveal a multitude of talented, compassionate people labouring in a fog of vague and conflicting definitions of the word 'addiction'. Because it is impossible to analyse addiction in all of these diverse senses of the word at once, this book focuses upon a single definition that encompasses the most destructive addictive problems in today's society. This definition is essentially the traditional meaning of the word 'addiction', as it appears in the *Oxford English Dictionary*.

Using this definition, Chapter 3 analyses the roots of addiction and the reason that it is now spreading so fast. This analysis is formalised as a 'dislocation theory of addiction'. The dislocation theory of addiction provides the theoretical basis for the rest of the book. Chapters 4–8, which constitute the remainder of Part I, summarise various types of evidence that support the dislocation theory. Although the greater part of this evidence is historical, some is drawn from quantitative research and clinical experience.

Chapter 1

Vancouver as Prototype

For over a century, aboriginal people scattered in little villages and camps around what is now called Burrard Inlet had seen European explorers, fur traders, and gold miners come and go.[1] They had tasted the dangers of trade whisky and had survived epidemics of European disease.[2] However, the British settlers who swarmed into the inlet after 1862 brought the full force of European civilisation to their land irrevocably, and it proved overwhelming[3]—both for better and for worse. Although some individual natives profited from trade and literacy in the decades that followed, their tribal cultures were devastated by the twin scourges of smallpox and alcoholism.[4] Meanwhile, the settlers' city flourished. The hodgepodge of crude plank shacks quickly grew into Canada's primary Pacific port, Vancouver.

The settlers struggled mightily against the smallpox and alcoholism that they had brought with them,[5] both for the sake of the 'Indians'[6] and for their own sake, because they were vulnerable too. These struggles enlisted the great institutions of modernity: science, state bureaucracy, free enterprise, and the reforming church. In the case of smallpox, science discovered vaccination and quarantine; state bureaucracy overcame political opposition and mandated mass treatment; free enterprise got the vaccine manufactured in a hurry and delivered it everywhere that trading vessels travelled along British Columbia's coastline and rivers; and the church encouraged the natives to abandon their own sacred healing practices in favour of others that had the blessing of their new, Christian God.[7] This struggle was a spectacular success. Smallpox and other infectious diseases are now rationally understood, preventable by public health measures, and, to some extent, treatable when they do occur. Endemic smallpox was eliminated from Canada by 1946.[8]

In the case of alcoholism, the struggle was an equally spectacular failure, in Vancouver as everywhere else. Despite enormous efforts, the same great institutions of modernity could not, and still cannot, prevent alcoholism and other forms of addiction from growing and spreading. Neither legal prohibition, moral medicine, scientific medicine, psychoanalysis, Alcoholics Anonymous, counselling, compassionate love, tough love, behavioural management, acupuncture, case management, therapeutic communities, civil commitment, eastern meditation, behavioural genetics, neuroscience, sophisticated advertising, antagonist drugs, psychedelic drugs, motivational interviewing, community reinforcement, treatment matching, harm reduction, nor any combination of these techniques has come close to overcoming alcoholism or any other type of addiction.[9] However, each approach can report genuine successes in some cases and each has sincere advocates who continue to hope that it can do the job on a larger scale, given enough time and public support.

Why were the institutions of modernity able to master smallpox and other communicable diseases, but not alcoholism and other addictions? When Vancouver's history is contemplated with this question in mind, a surprising conclusion rises to the surface. Alcoholism and other addictions continue to plague the modern city of Vancouver because they are unavoidable by-products of modernity itself.

At the heart of modernity lies free-market economics, which provides the economic structure for today's globalising world.[10] A society structured by free-market economics generates enormous material wealth and technical innovation and, at the same time, breaks down every traditional form of social cohesion and belief, creating a kind of dislocation or poverty of the spirit that draws people into addiction and other psychological problems. For this reason, a century of sophisticated and hugely expensive research has not been able to isolate the cause of addiction in the addicted individuals' childhood experiences, libidinal impulses, brains, or genes.

Vancouver is used in this book as the prototype of a modern city and a display case for an intractable addiction problem that is still spreading throughout the world.

Addiction in paradise

Today's Vancouver is a gleaming port city with suburbs extending many miles inland from the inlet where it was founded only one and a half centuries ago. Each year, it is again voted one of 'the most liveable cities in the world' by one or another international panel.[11] It has been designated the site of the winter Olympics in 2010. Nonetheless, thousands of ragged 'junkies'[12] in the notorious Hastings Corridor of Vancouver's Downtown Eastside[13] are dosing themselves with dangerous drugs every day that they can, and a few hundred will die before the end of the year from overdose, suicide, acquired immune deficiency syndrome (AIDS), hepatitis, violence, and other hazards of junkie life. Most of these addicted people are white, although a disproportionately large number are Canadian Native Indians.[14] Compared with the more publicised 'scene' in New York or Los Angeles, Vancouver's Hastings Corridor is less about stark racial contrast and hot violence than about sodden misery and slow death.

Impoverished drug users in the Hastings Corridor constitute only a fraction of Vancouver's addiction problem. Spreading in every direction from this epicentre is a vast, doleful tapestry of human beings struggling with other addictive miseries. There are drug addicts and alcoholics throughout the city,[15] gambling addicts in the casinos, money and power addicts in the financial district, video game addicts at their computers, television addicts on their couches, bulimics at the junk food stores, prescription drug addicts at the pharmacies, work addicts at their desks through the night, exercise freaks at the gyms, love addicts in other people's beds, tobacco addicts on the cancer wards, zealots hatching plots, and on and on. For the most serious of these addicts, whether they live in the Hastings Corridor or not, whether drugs are involved or not, addiction is a matter of life and death.[16]

Although they are the most notorious, the junkies of the Hastings Corridor in the Downtown Eastside are certainly not the most dangerous addicts in Vancouver. For example, some occupants of the city's boardrooms and management suites organise ruinous exploitation of the planet and its people, sometimes including their own shareholders.[17] Biographers of very rich people have shown that a large proportion of those who organise this kind of exploitation in Vancouver and elsewhere are manifesting severe addictions to power, wealth, sex, and work.[18] There are more immediate dangers as well. About 60 Vancouver prostitutes disappeared permanently over the past 20 years, probably as a consequence of another kind of dangerous addiction. A local man, Robert Pickton, has now been charged with the murders of 26 of the missing women on the basis of human remains that were laboriously sifted from the mud on his suburban pig farm. The accused is infamous for allegedly bringing prostitutes from down town for drunken and debauched parties regularly held on the farm site.[19] Is there a better way to understand this sort of hideous, repetitive crime than as addiction to debauchery and horror? Although it is too soon for this still-unfolding case to be analysed here, other serial killers and sexual predators have described the addictive nature of their own crimes in meticulous detail.[20]

Although people become dangerously addicted to a huge variety of activities, addiction is still generally understood in Vancouver as a drug problem. The City of Vancouver is currently implementing a 'Four Pillars Drug Strategy' with general approval from the public and major financial support from provincial and federal governments.[21] The four pillars envisioned in this approach are treatment of drug addicts, prevention of drug use, enforcement of drug laws, and reduction of harm for drug users. Of the four, harm reduction, although previously considered too radical, is now generating the most enthusiasm.[22] Its acceptance as a legitimate pillar was inspired by bold experimentation in Europe that entailed closer collaboration between medical, social, and police agencies, and testing of controversial harm-reduction methods, notably needle exchanges, safe injection sites, and opioid maintenance programmes. Civic leaders in Vancouver saw wisdom in this and brought it to public notice.[23]

Vancouver's Four Pillars approach has many virtues. It formalises a growing realisation that the War on Drugs of earlier decades did more harm than good.[24] It continuously monitors dangerous health problems, particularly AIDS, hepatitis, and overdose.[25] It engenders enthusiasm in the local media, compassion among the public, and financial support in legislatures. It supports novel experiments as well as time-tested methods.[26] It is being meticulously evaluated by a dedicated team of medical researchers, and the results made public. It evolved through open consultations among local groups—police, treatment agencies, citizen groups, and drug addicts—which had been at odds for decades. In my opinion, it represents the best face of Vancouver's compassionate pragmatism.

The past mayor and city council of Vancouver were elected in an electoral landslide in 2002, partly on a promise of implementing the Four Pillars approach. The 2005 election gave the city a new mayor with a renewed commitment to the Four Pillars approach. Reports on the Four Pillars approach have been generally encouraging.[27] It now seems reasonable to conclude that overdose death, new AIDS infections, and street crime are all down significantly from their peaks in the late 1990s, and that these changes correlate well with the dramatic increase in the number of Vancouver's addicts who are participating in methadone maintenance programmes and other harm-reduction measures.[28] There has also been a substantial increase in the quantity of decent, low-cost housing available to drug users in the Hastings Corridor of the Downtown Eastside.[29] Reports on the impact of the safe injection site are especially promising, if not yet conclusive.[30] A pilot project for prescribing heroin to street addicts opened in 2005 with good public support.[31] The current city government is striving to increase order in the city by cracking down on minor offences on the street while simultaneously expanding the number of drugs that can be obtained through maintenance programmes.[32]

Unfortunately, the intrinsic limitations of this admirable social experiment are becoming as obvious as its virtues. Some limitations are as follows. The Four Pillars approach addresses only a small corner of the addiction problem—illicit drugs. Even in the case of drug addiction, it lacks a clear analysis of root causes. In fact, the Four Pillars approach is based on the eclectic belief that the drug problem is best controlled through many different programmes, even if they conflict with each other in principle. Lacking a theoretical foundation,[33] the Four Pillars approach provides no way of assigning funding priorities to diverse agencies, all competing for scarce public dollars. These agencies sometimes seem to work at cross-purposes and to discount each other's accomplishments.[34] Moreover, all four 'pillars', including various forms of harm reduction, have been utilised extensively at various times in the 20th century in Canada, the United States, Europe, and China, both separately and in combination.[35] Despite their genuine successes as public health measures, their utilisation has not prevented the steady growth of addiction either to drugs or to innumerable other habits. This pattern is repeating in Vancouver, where there is no reason to believe that the prevalence of addiction to drugs or to anything else has decreased under the Four Pillars approach.

Moreover, problems associated with drug addiction persist: charges of police brutality against street addicts;[36] very high levels of property crime, much of which is carried out by drug addicts;[37] continuing difficulties in keeping more than a minority of needle-using addicts in methadone maintenance programmes;[38] and high levels of AIDS and hepatitis among street addicts.[39] To compound the city's problems, the provincial government of British Columbia has withdrawn some of the financial support promised by the previous government to redevelop the Hastings Corridor.[40] Homelessness is increasing and construction of subsidized housing units has diminished sharply.[41] Some of the political organisers working for the Provincial Government face possible criminal charges for allegedly using their administrative talents to organise drug trafficking and money laundering through their offices in the Provincial Parliament Building.[42] Paradoxically, Vancouver City Council has committed itself to raising money, some of which will support the Four Pillars approach, through expansion of the city's legalised gambling, particularly slot machines.[43] The Canadian federal government is threatening to close down the city's 'safe injection site' and needle exchanges and to move in the direction of an enforcement-oriented approach.[44] The wave of public optimism that the Four Pillars approach generated may be subsiding.[45] Highly publicised charges have been made that beggars and drug dealers on the streets in the downtown area are harming the local tourist industry, with the implication that the city must get tough again.[46] The current mayor intends to redirect the Four Pillars approach 'to ensure that public disorder becomes a main area of focus over the next 24 months'.[47] Most ominously of all, shrill calls by politicians for a new 'war' on methamphetamine made headlines in the city in 2005.[48]

All in all, the Four Pillars approach remains a model of compassionate pragmatism and indications are that it will be progressively improved. However, even dramatically improved, it will still be too limited in scope to have a major impact on addiction in Vancouver, or anywhere.[49] Therefore, the final chapters of this book will propose additional responses to addiction that go far beyond the Four Pillars approach.

Probable causes of addiction in Vancouver

Vancouver is celebrated for assiduous urban planning, good-humoured civility, and racial harmony, all framed by snow-capped mountain scenery.[50] Why, then, are so many of its citizens addicted to a multitude of less-than-lofty pursuits? The most obvious answer to this question is that, even more than most modern cities, life in Vancouver incessantly breaks down the cultural integrity of every segment of its population, a process that is called 'dislocation' in this book. The history of dislocation in Vancouver has followed different courses for people of aboriginal, Asian, and European origin, but the results are much the same and the process is still underway.

In Vancouver's first years, the aboriginal people suffered the most painfully obvious dislocation. From 1862 onwards, large numbers of settlers have been harvesting the local rainforest for the global lumber market and have been establishing other industries. As the city burgeoned, the space for its urban sprawl was acquired by confining the local native population to tiny reserves, thus destroying the territorial basis of their culture. Collectively owned native land, which had for countless centuries accommodated ornate communal houses, ancestral burial grounds, invisible spirits, and intertribal commerce, was transformed, almost overnight, into plots of 'real estate' for sale to the highest bidder on the free market.[51]

Many of the natives' traditional cultural practices were outlawed or mocked out of existence. The most famous example is their traditional potlatches, elaborate gifting ceremonies that redistributed aboriginal wealth, and sometimes ritually destroyed it, according to complex inherited obligations and kinship ties.[52] These ceremonies were the antitheses of the economic system that British civilisation demanded, in which goods must be sold in markets to the highest bidder, not given away ceremonially. Potlatches and another ritual, spirit dancing, were prohibited by law from 1884 until 1951 and people who were caught participating were often jailed.[53] Sometimes children found at a Potlatch were apprehended and taken from their parents.[54] The economic system that the British brought to Vancouver also dictated that aboriginal children must grow up speaking the language of commerce, which was English. It therefore seemed reasonable to the British, when the children would not conform, to beat the native languages out of them in the residential schools.

Although carried out with relatively little lethal violence, the dislocation imposed upon aboriginal people in British Columbia was arguably more severe than that in any other Canadian province.[55] British Columbia's Indians were dislocated physically from their land, socially from their culture and families, linguistically from their native tongues, economically from their livelihoods, and spiritually from their ceremonies, ancestors, and gods.

Laws have changed in the last few decades, but much of the complex aboriginal culture and many of the ancient languages may be gone forever. It is impossible to envision the future culture of the many native people who continue living in and around Vancouver. Treaties between the natives and the government have never been concluded for the majority of tribal groups. Even though the reserves were mostly established more than a century ago, the legal rights and responsibilities of the people who live there remain undecided, and the various government branches and the courts continue to contradict each other about what they are.[56]

Today, dislocatgied Indians are tragically overrepresented in the drug addict, prostitute, and AIDS populations of the Hastings Corridor and in the jails and alcoholism treatment centres throughout the province.[57] Only the colourful artefacts of once-vibrant native cultures remain to echo their former complexity and integration. Carvings and other objects speak silently of an elegant symmetry of the people, nature, guardian spirits, ritual words, ancestors, and indigenous wealth.[58] As an example, Figure 1.1 (here and in the colour section) shows a Coast Salish wooden 'spindle whorl', an everyday piece of equipment that was used by women to spin yarn from the wool of mountain goats.

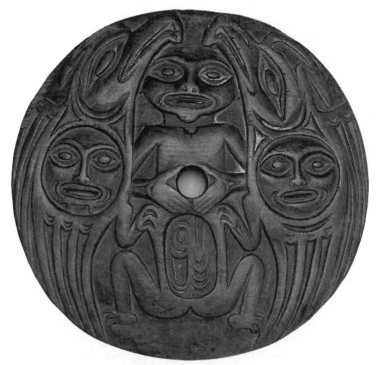

Figure 1.1 Spindle whorl, Northwest Coast Salish culture, wood, diameter 22 cm, early 19th century. (Private collection, courtesy of The Menil Collection, Houston, TX, USA. Photographer: Hickey-Robertson.)

Vancouver's Asian people have also suffered extreme dislocation. From its beginning to the present, Vancouver has been the landing point in Canada for a huge economic migration of East and South Asian workers, accelerating in the 1880s as shiploads of single Chinese men arrived to toil on the railroad and in the coal mines. Whereas Asian workers were always valued in the city's labour market, they were aliens to polite society until after World War II. In 1942, the entire Japanese–Canadian population of the city was stripped of its property, scattered into internment camps hundreds of miles from their homes, and not allowed to return until years after World War II had ended. In most cases, their property was not returned. Although Asians are currently the least drug-addicted of Vancouver's three main populations, opium addiction was a notorious problem of early Asian immigrants and many of their descendants today still struggle with deadly serious addictions, most conspicuously to gambling and work.[59]

Dislocation of Vancouver's white population has been almost as great as that of its native and Asian populations. With the completion of Canada's first transcontinental railway in 1886, Vancouver became a major terminus for the westward migration of people from their homes in Europe, eastern Canada, and the United States seeking prosperity in the wide-open free-market society of the new city. Members of all European religions and language groups, often refugees, were thrown together in the new city and province with good prospects for making a living, but scant hope of forming a stable and coherent community. The dislocation of Vancouver was mirrored in mining sites and mill towns across the province.

Whereas the dislocation imposed upon Vancouver's native and Asian populations was partly a manifestation of the ugly racism of an earlier era, the deepest motivations were probably economic rather than racial. White people who threatened the emerging free-market society were also subjected to harsh coercion and dislocation. For example, the Doukhobor people were a Russian Anabaptist sect that immigrated into eastern British Columbia just before World War I. Doukhobors lived and worked communally, refused any form of private ownership, and rejected all forms of materialism, especially the capitalist, materialistic values that were taught in the public schools. They were not politically Communists, but they rejected the fundamentals of free-market economics. Because their communities were non-violent and their communal farms and enterprises prospered, they earned the admiration of their neighbours. Although the Government of British Columbia was willing to exempt them from military service, it punished them financially for living and working communally, and it transported them in large numbers to Oakalla Prison in a Vancouver suburb for publicly protesting against materialism and for keeping their children out of the public schools.[60]

In response to government pressure and to the laxity of some of their Doukhobor neighbours, the 'Sons of Freedom' Doukhobor sect organised public protests (often naked to symbolise their extreme antimaterialism), burned some schools and public buildings, and even burned some of their own homes to demonstrate their renunciation of material values. When other governmental pressures failed to control the Sons of Freedom, the government seized 170 of their children and placed them in a residential school in New Denver, British Columbia, 'in an attempt to force the next generation to abandon their culture and assimilate. The children were cut off from their families'.[61] The school was maintained for 6 years. The children were not permitted to speak their own language and when parents were allowed to visit, they were kept apart from their children by a chain-link fence. Even today, the government of British Columbia refuses to fully repudiate the seizure of the children by issuing a formal apology, although it has expressed 'regret'. In 2004, the provincial Attorney General stated, 'We cannot fully understand or explain the motives for the government 50 years ago. We can recognise circumstances under which these events occurred and acknowledge how things might be done differently if we were doing it today.'[62]

The experience of the Doukhobors was atypical, but the message was for everybody. Nobody in British Columbia could stray very far outside the bounds of free-market orthodoxy. This was also made painfully obvious in Vancouver during the years of the Great Depression. Whereas the American depression government under Franklin Roosevelt relaxed the enforcement of strict free-market discipline during the financial crisis, Canadian federal and provincial governments did not. This eventually resulted in violently suppressed workers' protests, including Vancouver's 'Bloody Sunday' of 1938.[63]

While breaking down the cultures of immigrant groups, Vancouver did not evolve much local culture of its own, as have some of Canada's older eastern cities. By the time this became a possibility for Vancouver, the United States, only 50 km distant, had become an irrepressible exporter of prefabricated popular culture. Vancouver's potential for cultural evolution was drowned in infancy by a flood of imported music, movies, textbooks, magazines, experts, evangelists, and, more recently, television, professional sports, fast food, and video games. Immigrants from all over the world have come to Vancouver to find their place in Canadian society, but have instead found themselves adrift in 'Lotusland', a Canadian nickname for the city and the province.

Whereas dislocation is commonplace in modern cities, Vancouver's is extreme. No part of Vancouver's history is unified by a common religion, a single language, or a shared ancestry. From the beginning, the guiding lights in Vancouver and British Columbia politics were not religious or social leaders, but businessmen and property developers enlisted as politicians.[64] Traditional Vancouver occupations—mining, logging, fishing, and railway construction—separated working men from their families for months on end and moved them from place to place when resources were depleted. There has been too little time for many extended families or clans to become firmly established among the European settlers, although some have. Even today, it is frequently observed that the great majority of Vancouverites were born somewhere else.[65] Vancouver's image of itself is reflected in the city's first official 'crest', a woodcut print adopted in 1886.[66] Completely unlike the native carving that was made a few decades earlier, there are no symbols of nature, guardian spirits, ritual words, ancestors—and no symmetry; just fallen logs, engines of industry, and an expression of commercial optimism (see Figure 1.2).

Whereas Vancouver's history is one of severe dislocation, it is also one of affluence, energy, and optimism. Vancouver is prosperous and beautiful. It has never known invasion, bombing, revolution, famine, or plague. When the city was first incorporated and given its present name in 1886, little more than a century ago, its commercial

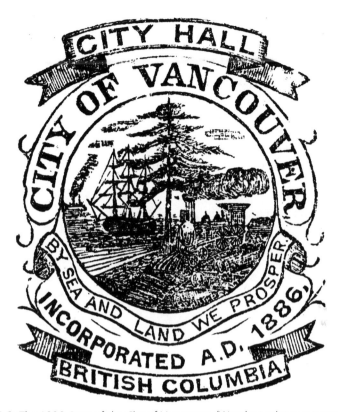

Figure 1.2 The 1886 Crest of the City of Vancouver. (Woodcut print courtesy of the City of Vancouver Archives.)

energy was sparked by access to free markets within the worldwide British Empire and by completion of the transcontinental railway. The scattered shanties, mills, and farms exploded into urbanity. Speculators rushed to buy land, the first newspaper was established, and an urban water system was planned. A shipload of tea—a million pounds—arrived from China, was loaded on railway cars, and rumbled over the mountains to the eastern Canadian markets. Global markets were open and growth was unstoppable, as the Great Fire proved. The entire city of 400 wooden buildings burnt to the ground with several fatalities, but it was resurveyed and mostly rebuilt, including a new city hall, electric streetlights, and a roller skating rink—all within the year 1886.[67]

Although it felt the full force of the Great Depression of 1929–1939,[68] Vancouver has been only lightly bruised by industrial blight, class struggle, slums, and organised crime.[69] Vancouverites complain most about the provincial government and the long rainy season, although the government is not violent and the climate is the most temperate in Canada.

If dislocation were the precursor to addiction, 'Lotusland' should also be 'Addiction City', despite all of its energy, prosperity, and conviviality. Alcohol and drug statistics indicate that it is. Throughout the 20th century and into the 21st, Vancouver has been Canada's most drug- and alcohol-addicted city and British Columbia its most drug- and alcohol-addicted province by a plethora of quantitative measures: per capita consumption of alcohol, death rate attributed to alcohol, prevalence of alcoholism, death rate due to heroin and cocaine overdose, prevalence of human immunodeficiency virus (HIV) infection and hepatitis C infection among injection drug users, availability of heroin and cocaine, self-reported use of all illicit drugs, arrest rates for drug crimes, costs of illicit drug use, and drug-related homicides.[70] Heroin statistics provide the most notorious example. British Columbia is one of ten provinces and three territories in Canada, yet in 1997, 61% of all heroin arrests in Canada occurred there.[71] Vancouver is the centre of a huge business in cultivation and exportation of marijuana whose annual value is measured in billions of dollars.[72] The 2004 Canadian Addiction Survey[73] reported higher per capita consumption of cannabis, cocaine, crack, and ecstasy in British Columbia than in any other province in Canada, and higher consumption of amphetamine and inhalants than in any other province except Quebec.[74] Addictions that do not involve alcohol and drugs are far more common in Vancouver than addictions that do.[75] Unfortunately, there is no adequate quantitative basis for comparing Vancouver with other cities on the prevalence of addictions not involving alcohol and drugs.

This chapter about Vancouver is intended to introduce two ideas, although, by itself, it cannot prove them. The first is that 'drug addiction' is merely a small corner of a larger addiction problem. The second is that large-scale dislocation, fostered by the continuing growth of free-market society, is the root cause of the current proliferation of addiction across the globalising world. The remainder of Part I formalises and develops these ideas. However, this cannot happen prior to a close examination of the word 'addiction', which has so many meanings that the issues have become badly confused.

Endnotes

1   The fur trade had a relatively minor impact on aboriginal life (Woodcock, 1977, pp. 21–22). British Columbia was in the pandemonium of a major gold rush in the 1860s (R. T. Wright, 1998, pp. 10–19), but it had little direct effect on the Vancouver area, which had the good fortune to possess no gold at all. The native population of Burrard Inlet in 1862 has been described by B. Macdonald (1992, pp. 10–11) and Barman (2005, Chapter 1).

2   Gibson (1982–1983); Fisher (1992, Chapters 1–3).

3   It was 'overwhelming' in part because of the sheer number of Europeans who appeared, in part because it was backed by irresistible military force, and in part because the trade goods that the British offered were irresistibly attractive to many aboriginal people, even though they found British culture abhorrent (Fisher, 1992, especially pp. ii–xxiv).

4   I have simplified this history for the purpose of using Vancouver as a manageably simple prototype. The fate of the Indians in what is now Vancouver is a part of a much larger drama of the Indians of Canada, and cannot be adequately understood in isolation from the larger history. The first smallpox epidemic preceded the arrival of British settlers in the Vancouver area by several decades, apparently having been spread along the early trade routes and from nearby British settlements in New Westminster, Fort Langley, and Victoria (see Carlson, 1997, Chapter 2). In addition, trade goods had arrived before the British settlers in Vancouver. Nonetheless, the settlements of the 1860s and onward imposed the

full, overwhelming force of European civilisation on the natives of the Vancouver area for the first time.

5 There are many credible claims that the colonial government initially and deliberately let the great smallpox epidemic of 1862 spread among the natives to reduce their population while vaccinating the white population (Warrior Publications, n.d.). Whether this is true or not, it is clear that the government eventually introduced large-scale vaccination in the native population, eliminating the disease.

6 It is no small task to decide what names to give the native people who occupied Vancouver before Europeans arrived. They were probably members of three different tribal groups, Musqueam, Squamish, and Tsleil'waututh, but were collectively called 'Indians' by the settlers and 'Coast Salish People' by anthropologists. There are arguments today for using the terms 'First Nations People', 'aboriginals', 'natives', and 'Indians'. I have used most of these terms in this book, including 'Indians'. For me, 'Indians' seems simple, unambiguous, and not in the least disrespectful, particularly because it is used so frequently by today's native people themselves. However, some people currently consider the word 'Indian' disrespectful.

7 Gibson (1982–1983); R. Boyd (1994, 1996, 1999); C. Harris (1994, 1997–1998).

8 Gibson (1982–1983); McIntyre and Houston (1999).

9 I summarised the evidence for this sweeping conclusion in an earlier book (Alexander, 1990). Reuter and Stevens (2007, Chapter 5) provided a recent review of evidence for the same conclusion in the UK. This endnote is intended to strengthen this conclusion by critically analysing some recent studies that could be taken to show that addiction treatment can have a major impact on the prevalence of addiction.

Treatment for alcoholism has been studied the most intensively. When the decades of results are examined carefully, some of the best-designed studies have negative outcomes, although there are many positive studies as well. Moreover, outcome studies frequently have inconsistent or uninterpretable results (W. R. Miller *et al.*, 1995). Despite loud claims to the contrary, the enormous American study of alcohol treatment, Project Match, did not provide any real evidence of the efficacy of treatment for alcoholism, as its designers confirm in the context of critical discussion (see Glaser *et al.*, 1999; Schaler, 2000, Chapter 9). Critical examination of newer data, collected as part of the National Epidemiologic Survey on Alcohol and Related Conditions, adds further reasons to believe that treatment cannot solve the problem of addiction (see D. A. Dawson *et al.*, 2005). Older, large-scale studies of treatment for drug addiction are similarly discouraging (Brecher, 1972, Chapter 10; LeDain, 1973, pp. 1005 1009; Musto, 1987, pp. 85 86; Alexander, 1990, Chapter 2) although loud claims that 'treatment works' are frequently heard.

The greatest current problem with reports of successful treatment is that the quantitative effects of treatment on a target measure, like number of days without drinking or average number of drinks per day, are usually used to demonstrate success. Such measures do show that well-delivered treatment can have a valuable effect in suppressing drinking or drug use for a time, but they show nothing about the effects of treatment on addiction itself. People who reduce their alcohol or drug consumption are often just as addicted as before, sometimes having switched to a legal or less physically damaging type of addiction. Alcoholics Anonymous (AA) and other 12-step organisations argue, rightly, that even completely eliminating alcohol consumption does not mean that a person is no longer addicted. Many members of AA continue to be alcoholics for the rest of their lives, although they no longer drink at all. The best-known example of ineffectiveness of 'successful' treatment might be the founder of AA himself, Bill W. His life and eventual death from emphysema caused by his tobacco addiction will be discussed in detail in Chapter 12 (see also Cheever, 2004).

Leading champions of treatment now argue that addiction is a chronic disease comparable to diabetes, hypertension, and asthma (Leshner, 1997; McLellan *et al.*, 2000). From this
point of view, treatment for addiction should not be expect to produce a cure, but should be
continued indefinitely, as for other chronic diseases. This position constitutes a reasonable
argument for publicly supported addiction treatment. However, in the context of this book,
it serves as confirmation—from the most prominent authorities—that addiction therapy
cannot come close to overcoming addiction.

The newest hope of a quantum jump in the effectiveness of addiction treatment comes
from the movement towards 'evidence-based treatment'. Whereas this administrative
innovation may well bring improvements, it cannot change the situation radically. After all,
evidence has been collected for a very long time, and most clinicians eagerly use it to
improve practice where they can. Imposing 'evidence-based practice' and 'best practices' on
clinicians who have other ideas is bound to have mixed results. Prominent advocates of
evidence-based treatment are correctly careful not to raise expectations too much, harken-
ing back to the argument that addiction is like an incurable chronic disease: 'In general,
our treatment interventions show small to moderate effects and repeated episodes of care
are the norm. Substance abuse treatment yields outcomes at least comparable with those for
other chronic conditions such as diabetes, asthma, and hypertension ... and there are no
magic bullets to cure addiction in one acute care episode' (Miller *et al.*, 2005).

The global harm-reduction movement has been the most heartening good-news story in
the field of addictions for the last two decades (Stimson, 2007). However, unlike treatment,
prevention, and law enforcement, harm reduction is not designed to reduce the incidence
of addiction. Drug use of all sorts, including addiction, has increased substantially in the
UK during a period of high public expenditure on harm-reduction measures. Apart
from HIV/AIDS, which has successfully been kept under control in the UK during this
period, the harms associated with drug use have not been reduced in any dramatic
way (McKeganey, 2006). This is not to diminish the important fact that harm reduction has
provided life-saving benefits and priceless encouragement to countless injection drug
addicts and prostitutes, but only to show that harm reduction cannot be expected to
control the increasing prevalence of addiction.

10 K. Polanyi (1944); Hobsbawm (1962, 1994); Berman (1982); J. Heath (2001); Saul (2004).

11 Fong (2005).

12 Some people consider the work 'junkie' as insulting to drug users. I find it unavoidable,
however, because it describes a well-known drug-using lifestyle to which a powerful
mystique is attached. Many regular drug users apply this word about themselves. Quite often
junkies look down on people who use heroin, but are considered mere 'skinpoppers' or
'chippers' rather than junkies. Many heroin users do not consider themselves junkies
and are not regarded as junkies by society.

13 There is no universally accepted name for the place I am calling the 'Hastings Corridor' in
the Downtown Eastside. In the half century since World War II, it has been variously known
as Skid Road, Hastings, Main and Hastings, or simply the Downtown Eastside (Sommers
and Blomley, 2002). In this book, it will be consistently called the Hastings Corridor. The
term 'Downtown Eastside' will be reserved for the much larger area of
low- and moderate-income dwellings and light industry on the waterfront of Burrard Inlet.
This area includes China Town, Victory Square, Strathcona, and Oppenheimer Park, and is
roughly bisected by the Hastings Corridor.

14 Craib *et al.* (2003).

15 See Priest (2003) for a recent journalistic account of middle-class drug addicts in Vancouver.

16 It is sometimes argued that using 'addiction' in this inclusive sense is unscientific or semantically sloppy, because the true meaning of addiction is more restrictive. The reasons that this is not so will be considered at length in Chapter 2. At this point, it should be sufficient to mention that numerous accounts of devastating, sometimes fatal, addictions that do not involve drugs have been published by addiction professionals over the past 30 years (Peele and Brodsky, 1975; Orford, 1985, 2001a, b; D. F. Jacobs, 1986; Alexander, 1990, Chapter 7; Killinger, 1991; Rabinor, 2002).

The ambiguity of the word 'addiction' is only a distraction here. The crucial issue in this book is the problem of dangerously compulsive lifestyles in general—any other name, originating in any language, would serve as well as addiction. The word 'addiction' is used throughout this book for consistency.

17 Ibbitson (2002a, b); Mitchell (2002); Sprague (2002); Thorsell (2002), R. Blackwell (2005). My apologies to Jimmy Pattison, Vancouver's home-grown billionaire. He is a driven, acquisitive person (Sutherland, 2004), but I do not think he fits the dark generalisations in this paragraph about some of his fellow businessmen.

18 P. C. Newman (1959; 1991, Chapter 17); P. Slater (1980); Pearson (1995); Barlow and Winter (1997, Chapter 1); Warde (2002); Lordon (2003, Chapter 2; 2004); R. Murphy (2004); Blackwell and Waldie (2005); Bower (2006).

19 Armstrong (2003c, d).

20 The Michael Briere case was the horror story of the hour in Canada as this was first written. In this case, a child-murderer and rapist described sex with a little girl as a 'lifelong yearning' that he kept fuelled with child pornography from the Internet (Blatchford, 2004). The infamous American mass murderer, Ted Bundy, gave a final interview to a psychologist hours before his execution as a mass murderer, after all appeals had failed (Dobson, 1995). Bundy attributed his serial killings of young women to a state of mind induced by his lifelong addiction to pornography, which he described in excruciating detail. However, his view of pornography as the *cause* of his addiction does not fit with the theory of addiction set forth in this book. A recent article on sex offenders in Vancouver (Armstrong, 2004c) describes others who prey on Vancouver's prostitutes in terms that strongly suggest addiction in a number of ways, including the fact that such people are quite often recognized as addicted to alcohol and drugs, and describe their compulsion to hurt women in much the same terms as they describe their compulsion to take drugs. In general, many serial killers describe their compulsions to kill and their subsequent revulsion at their own crimes in ways that are virtually identical to descriptions of inner conflict given by other types of addict, and many serial killers have the same kinds of early life experiences that severe addicts do. As a consequence, labels like 'addicted to violence' are often applied to serial killers in the professional literature (Gresswell and Hollin, 1997; Seltzer, 1998).

21 The logic and goals of Vancouver's Four Pillars Drug Strategy are summarized in a document first published in the year 2000 by the city's Drug Policy Coordinator, Donald MacPherson (2000, 2001).

22 Four Pillars Coalition (2005); PHS Community Services Society (2005).

23 Levy (2000); MacPherson (2000, 2001).

24 Alexander (1990).

25 Strathdee *et al.* (1997); Schechter *et al.* (1999).

26 Four Pillars Coalition (2005).

27 Armstrong (2003b, d); Kendall (2004).

29 Kendall (2004).

29 Four Pillars Coalition (2005).

30 E. Wood *et al.* (2004a); Kerr *et al.* (2005a).

31 M. Hume (2005b).

32 Boei (2006b).

33 This situation may be in the process of change, with the publication of a ground-breaking new city document devoted to the 'pillar' of prevention, which proposes a theoretical analysis that is quite similar to that proposed in this book (MacPherson *et al.*, 2005). How widespread this theoretical analysis will become within the Four Pillars Coalition remains to be seen.

34 E. Wood *et al.* (2003), E. Wood *et al.* (2004b).

35 See Musto (1987) for a comprehensive survey of the history of all four pillars in the United States from the beginning of the 20th century. See Dikötter *et al.* (2004) for the history of the four pillars in China prior to 1949.

   The existence of three of the four pillars probably needs no documentation, but it is less well known that harm reduction also has a very long history. Historical evidence appears in E. Murphy (1922/1973), Brecher (1972, Chapter 13), Ledain (1973), Trebach (1982), Musto (1987, Chapter 5), and Carstairs (2004, 2006). The long history of legal prescription of heroin to addicts in the UK is the best-known example (Trebach, 1982). The 1922 book by Emily Murphy is often cited now as an example of a sensationalized advocacy of harsher police methods. Although this is true, it also provides evidence of widespread prescription of narcotics to addicts, now classified as a harm-reduction measure, very early in 20th-century Canada. This was not legal in Canada, but it was widely tolerated (see also Carstairs, 2006, Chapter 5). The use of orally administered opium and morphine as replacement drugs for smoked opium in China has been documented by Dikötter *et al.* (2004, pp. 119–122).

36 Armstrong (2003b).

37 P. Sullivan (2003). The actual crime statistics are controversial, but this has not stood in the way of a growing public perception nurtured by local media that crime by drug addicts is out of control (Eurchuk, 2003).

38 Fischer *et al.* (2002); Kerr *et al.* (2005b).

39 E. Wood *et al.* (2005).

40 Armstrong (2004a); M. Hume (2004a).

41 Hume (2006a).

42 Culbert (2004a), M. Hume (2004c).

43 C. Johnson (2004).

44 A. Woods (2006); *Times-Colonist* (2006); Small (2007).

45 Theodore and Bisetty (2004); Carrigg (2004); Wente (2005).

46 Preston (2006). The current mayor, Sam Sullivan, maintains that harm reduction is the way to reduce this problem, but others disagree.

47 This quote ultimately comes from the Mayor's 'Project Civil City' report as quoted in a local newspaper (C. Smith, 2006b).

48 Harding (2005); Tierney (2005).

49 It is sometimes suggested that the Four Pillars approach could work better if it were combined with legalisation of currently prohibited drugs (Haden, 2006) or with alleviation of poverty (Carstairs, 2006, pp. 159–161). However, this provides little basis for optimism, as neither of these proposed adjuncts is likely to occur, and because the possibility that either would substantially enhance the effectiveness of the Four Pillars approach is not persuasive in view of the recent history of the UK (Newland, 2007).

50 Bula and Ward (2000); O'Brian (2004a); Fong (2005).

51 An apparent exception to this principle is 1000 acres of prime city land in downtown Vancouver that was set aside in 1888 and designated 'Stanley Park'. Barman (2005, Chapter 4) has shown how the park was envisioned from the very beginning as a civic showpiece and a tourist attraction, as well as a way of maintaining prices in the urban real estate by keeping the land off the market. The 100 or so residents of the new park, including some Indian families who had lived there for generations with the burial sites of their ancestors, were evicted to make the park seem like pristine wilderness. A few of the families managed to maintain their homes within the park for decades by virtue of their stubbornness and ability to defend themselves legally. Thus, Stanley Park also functioned as an agent of dislocation in service of free-market society.

52 Woodcock (1977, Introduction).

53 Tennant (1990); Alfred (1999, pp. 7–20). See also Jilek (1981) for a description of the banning of 'spirit dancing'.

54 Spalding *et al.* (2006).

55 Compared with Indians in the other provinces where Europeans arrived earlier, British Columbian Indians were given much smaller reserves, making it more difficult or impossible for them to continue their aboriginal style of life. Moreover, unlike other Canadian Indians, most British Columbian Indian tribal groups were not given the opportunity to sign formal treaties, which would have formally guaranteed their tenure on their tiny allotments of reserve land and implicitly acknowledged the status of their aboriginal nations. From 1927 to 1951, British Columbian Indians were prohibited from seeking redress for these injustices in court (Tennant, 1990, Chapter 8). Lacking legal guarantees, the British Columbia reserves were gradually reduced in size as various parcels of land became desirable to settlers. On the other hand, it has been claimed that these severe dislocations were partially offset by 'the special political tradition of the coastal peoples':

> More developed before contact than the political traditions in the interior of the province (or in most parts of the United States), the coastal traditions had an easier time surviving contact. Indeed, they proved able to evolve and adapt within the new political regime, even when that regime outlawed Indian claims activity.

Tenant (1990, p. 70).

56 Mickleburgh (2003a).

57 MacPherson (2001, p. 40); Edgar (2003a); Pynn (2003).

58 Holm and Reid (1975, pp. 58–61); Suttles (1983).

59 This generalisation is based on personal communications with Vancouverites of Chinese descent. Some anthropological support for this generalisation has been reported in other cities with a large Chinese immigrant population (Papineau, 2005).

60 Janzen (1990); Kolesnikoff (2000).

61 Matas (2004, p. A8).

62 The quote is from Matas (2004). See also Willcocks (2004).

63 Berton (1990).

64 S. Hume (2003b); Barman (2005, pp. 85–93).

65 Almost half of the adults in Vancouver were born outside of Canada, and many of the rest have come to Vancouver from eastern Canada (Ramsey, 2003). See also Mahoney (2005b).

66 B. MacDonald (1992, p. 22).

67 Pethick (1984).

68 Berton (1990).

69 McDonald and Barman (1986).

70 E. Murphy (1922/1973, p. 138); Smart and Ogborne (1996, p. 72); Tremblay (1999); MacPherson (2001, pp. 20–21); Culbert (2004b); Desjardins and Hotton (2004); Carstairs (2006, p. 11). Although British Columbia is Canada's most drug-addicted province, it is usually surpassed in this regard by Canada's arctic territories (i.e. the Yukon, the Northwest Territories, and Nunavut). In the 2002 statistics, one of 25 Canadian cities, Thunder Bay, had a higher drug offence rate than Vancouver. These exceptions, however, fit easily with the theoretical analysis that will follow.

71 Tremblay (1999, p. 10).

72 Hardy (2003).

73 Canadian Centre on Substance Abuse (2004).

74 Canadian Centre on Substance Abuse (2004, p. 3). In this survey, British Columbia did not, however, score at the top of the provinces in measures of alcohol consumption that might be indicative of alcoholism.

75 Alexander and Schweighofer (1988).

Chapter 2

Addiction$_1$, Addiction$_2$, Addiction$_3$, Addiction$_4$ ...

Addiction is not a promising conversational topic. When an everyday conversation goes there, it is time to anticipate misunderstanding and hard feelings, partly because people use the word 'addiction' in such different ways. The semantic problems that undermine everyday conversations also undermine scholarly discourse. Scholars, like everybody else, use different definitions for 'addiction' and sometimes change definitions as the conversation proceeds. I have learned by hard experience that there can be no productive interchange about addiction unless people can agree on exactly what the central word in the discussion means.

This chapter summarises the history of the word 'addiction', beginning with its traditional meaning in the English language. Four contemporary descendants of the traditional meaning are then described and are designated addiction$_1$, addiction$_2$, addiction$_3$, and addiction$_4$. Although each of these contemporary meanings of addiction can be used properly in everyday language and in academic discussions, this book is about addiction in the sense of addiction$_3$. This chapter will show why addiction$_3$ best encompasses the most dangerous addiction problems of the globalising world and why it is best suited for precise analysis. The chapter will also show why the other three definitions are so hard to ignore.[1] At the end, it will show how confused definitions of addiction have, in some cases, contributed to large-scale suffering and death.

Although hanging subscripts below the word addiction—while simultaneously floating superscripts above other words to designate endnotes—might make reading this chapter taxing, all this numeralising is intended to serve the vital function of making the meaning of 'addiction' in this book crystal clear. And, once this short stretch of semantic forced labour has been endured, later chapters can proceed with a lighter, but surer, step.

Traditional meaning of the word 'addiction'

For most of its long history in the English language, the word 'addiction' was not a conversation-stopper. Prior to the mid 19th century, it had a simple two-part definition that came into the language before the time of Shakespeare. This traditional definition was remarkably similar to the ancient use of the Latin noun *addictionem* and the verb form, *addicere*.[2]

The traditional English definition appeared in the first 'fascicule' of the authoritative dictionary of the English language, the *Oxford English Dictionary*, published in 1884. It reappeared, essentially unchanged, in all subsequent editions.[3] A quite different definition (addiction$_1$) eventually grew out of the traditional definition, first appearing in the 1933 *Supplement* to the dictionary and finally being added to the main text in 1989. This adjunct definition will be discussed later in this chapter. Here is the traditional definition as it appeared from 1884 to the current edition:[4]

> **Addiction** ... [ad. L. *addiction-em*, n. of action f. *addīc-ĕre*; see ADDICT.]
> 1. *Rom. Law.* A formal giving over or delivery by sentence of court. Hence, a surrender, or dedication, of any one to a master.
> 2. The state of being (self-) addicted or given *to* a habit or pursuit; devotion.[5]

Part 1 of this traditional definition refers to the judicial action of legally sentencing a person to be a bond slave. The word 'addiction', in this sense, is still an essential vocabulary item for historians because judicial enslavement was once a common practice. Part 1 of the definition remains important in modern times because it deepens the understanding of part 2.

Part 2 refers to a similar state of servitude, not to a slave-master but to a 'habit or pursuit'. Part 2 does not refer to any form of external coercion, but rather to being '(self-) addicted'. The examples of usage over the centuries that are provided by the dictionary show that addiction, thus defined, may or may not be destructive to the addicted individual and to society. Addiction to alcohol or vice can, of course, have tragic consequences. On the other hand, strong devotion (i.e. addiction) to a worthy cause or a benevolent god can be the foundation of a positive, fulfilling life.

Part 2 of the traditional definition of addiction is schematised in Figure 2.1 as a single circle representing a multitude of 'habits or pursuits' to which a person may become addicted. This circle can be sliced like a pie into any number of segments, because the number of possible habits or pursuits to which a person can be addicted is unlimited. The only important categorical division between segments is that some addictions have destructive consequences (these are represented by the darker segments on the left side of the circle) and some do not (these are represented by the lighter segments on the right). Destructive addiction to drugs or alcohol is one of many darker segments, and is neither more nor less important than any of the others.

Both in its destructive and non-destructive forms, 'addiction' could be a weighty word in its traditional meaning.[6] Shakespeare, for example, used it with gravity in *The Life of King Henry the Fifth*, written around 1600 AD. In a tense moment at the start of the play, the Archbishop of Canterbury describes Henry V as a great sovereign and intellectual, adding that this is 'a wonder' because, as a younger man:

> ... his addiction was to courses vain,
> His companies unlettered, rude, and shallow,
> His hours filled up with riots, banquets, sports;
> And never noted in him any study,
> Any retirement, and sequestration,
> From open haunts and popularity.[7]

As the play unfolds, knowledge of Henry V's youthful addiction to wild living to the detriment of his kingly studies gives unwise confidence to his arch-enemy,

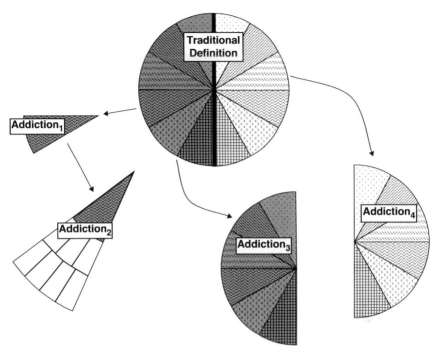

Addiction₁: Overwhelming involvement with drugs or alcohol that is harmful to the addicted person, to society, or to both.

Addiction₂: Encompasses addiction₁ and non-overwhelming involvements with drugs or alcohol that are problematic to the addicted person, society, or both.

Addiction₃: Overwhelming involvement with any pursuit whatsoever (including, but not limited to, drugs or alcohol) that is harmful to the addicted person, to society, or to both.

Addiction₄: Overwhelming involvement with any pursuit whatsoever that is not harmful to the addicted person or to society.

Figure 2.1 Four contemporary ways of using the word 'addiction' derived from the traditional definition.

the Dauphin of France.[8] It is not until King Henry has proven invincible in battle and magnanimous in victory that his youthful addiction is forgotten, in the final act of the play.

The weight that the word 'addiction' can have when used in a positive sense is seen in the King James Version of the Christian Bible, originally published in 1611. This was the standard Bible for English-speaking Protestants until the mid-20th century. The word 'addicted' appears in I Corinthians, originally a letter from St Paul the Apostle to the early Christian community at Corinth written in 59 AD. In this letter, Paul chastises Corinthian Christians for moral laxity, finding it necessary to address them as children rather than as 'mature Christians'. Towards the end of the letter, he urges them to emulate the members of the family Stephanas, whom he praises *for their addiction*, as follows:

> 16:15 I beseech you, brethren, (ye know the house of Stephanas, that it is the firstfruits of Achaia and *that* they have addicted themselves to the ministry of the saints,)
> 16:16 That ye submit yourselves unto such, and to every one that helpeth with *us*, and laboureth.[9]

In Paul's eyes, the fact that the members of the Stephanas family were addicted to the 'ministry of the saints' made them ideal role models for the wayward Corinthians. More recent translations[10] of these verses make the same point, although they do not use the word 'addicted', which by the 19th century had begun to evoke images of sordid drunkenness and drug use that would confuse Paul's meaning. 'Addiction' is still a literally correct term to use for deeply committed Christians according to the *Oxford English Dictionary*, but it has become safer to avoid it.

Beyond Shakespeare and the learned translators of the King James Bible, David Hume, Jane Austen, Charles Dickens, and countless other masters of the English language used the word 'addiction' in the inclusive, traditional way.[11] The idea that the concept should be pared down to a disease of drug or alcohol use had little currency before the 19th century.[12] Like the *Oxford English Dictionary*, *Webster's American Dictionary* defined addiction only in the traditional way from its earliest edition in 1806 at least through to the 1902 edition.[13]

The traditional meaning of addiction, in both the destructive and the positive forms, remains in widespread use today outside the literature on drug addiction. In this traditional meaning, 'addiction' is an indispensable word, because it gives a name to a basic fact of human psychology: human beings often undergo full psychological metamorphoses by becoming so involved with a new habit or pursuit that their involvement is comparable to voluntary slavery. Beyond providing a name for this overwhelming involvement, the traditional meaning of addiction naturally provokes two important questions. First, why would people ever put themselves into a state of voluntarily servitude to a habit or pursuit? Secondly, how can this state of voluntary servitude be destructive and shameful in some instances and not destructive—even admirable—in others? Because the definition of addiction used in this book, addiction$_3$, is very close to the traditional definition, these questions remain built into it. A major purpose of this book is to answer them.

Addiction$_1$

The traditional definition of 'addiction' was gradually obscured in the 19th and early 20th centuries[14] during a period of intense public alarm over excessive drinking and, later, drug taking. During this period, the meaning of the word 'addiction' was simultaneously narrowed, moralised, and medicalised for many people.

Beginning early in the 19th century, a powerful mass movement in North America and Europe proclaimed that alcohol, which they characterised as 'ardent spirits', 'hard liquor', or 'demon rum',[15] was a serious menace. At first, temperance activists preached moderation as the solution, but as the century wore on, they became convinced that universal abstinence was the only way. As the temperance movement gained confidence, its rhetoric gained flamboyance. In 1919, for example, on the eve of national alcohol prohibition in the United States, preacher Billy Sunday announced on a coast-to-coast radio hook-up that:

> The reign of tears is over. The slums will soon be a memory. We will turn our prisons into factories, our jails into storehouses and corncribs. Men will walk upright now, women will smile and the children will laugh. Hell will be forever for rent.[16]

Despite the temperance leaders' pious hyperbole, their concerns were well-founded—more and more men and women of the 19th century were falling into the liquor-centred, socially abhorrent, and personally destructive lifestyles that the movement described, and many still are.[17] A variety of names for excessive drinking were used in the temperance movement, although the word 'addiction' eventually became a preferred term along with 'alcoholism'.[18] Although the overwhelming involvement with alcohol that the temperance crusaders increasingly called 'addiction' fits within the traditional definition of addiction, it fundamentally narrows the traditional definition because it was limited to drinkers, it was always morally reprehensible, and it was akin to a progressive disease. This grim and restrictive way of using the word is called 'addiction$_1$' in this book. The subscript '1' is not meant to suggest that it corresponds to part 1 of the traditional definition—which it does not—but that it became the dominant image of addiction in Western society during the 19th and 20th centuries and remains so for many people today.

The material and social harm of addiction$_1$ can be horrendous, yet the spiritually minded temperance activists perceived—correctly I believe—an even more nightmarish feature: addicted$_1$ people seemed to have lost their *souls* to alcohol. In non-religious terms, those who became addicted$_1$ were so overwhelmingly involved with drinking that they became different people, alien to their own society and to their own previous identities. Many temperance activists thought this nightmare metamorphosis was caused by alcohol itself.[19] Why, apart from a kind of possession by 'demon rum', would anyone give themselves over to the horrors of life as an alcoholic? Secular scholars have been trying ever since to agree upon a solution for this mystery that is more credible than the capture of an incautious soul by a liquid demon. My dream is that this book will finally provide an adequate answer.

The stigma of addiction$_1$ was originally applied to drinkers, but it was not confined to them for long. By the end of the 19th century, the sensational images of the temperance movement had become fearsome archetypes for new anti-drug movements, including the 19th-century anti-opium movement and later movements bent on ridding the planet of cocaine, heroin, marijuana, LSD, barbiturates, amphetamine, ecstasy, methamphetamine, etc. Like the temperance movement, the various anti-drug movements conflated all drug users with the worst addicts$_1$, ignoring the fact that the majority of drug users were not addicted$_1$ and that the majority of actual addictions$_1$ to drugs were not permanent. All drug users were perceived to be on the verge of becoming permanently 'hooked' by their drug, and of turning against the truly important aspects of life: family, work, community, self-respect, and religion. All drug addicts were said to be dishonest and ruthless in the single-minded pursuit of their drug, somehow becoming criminal masterminds despite the profound brain damage that the drugs inevitably produced. People hooked on drugs were given labels like 'drug fiends', 'junkies', 'opium drunkards', and 'hopheads', as well as drug addicts. Such people were often understood to be possessed by a demonic intoxicant, and to be 'lost', 'hopeless', 'ruined', or 'doomed'—as, indeed, the worst of them were. Simultaneously, they were said to suffer from the medical disease of addiction and to be in urgent need of medical treatment.

The imagery of the temperance and anti-drug movements was powerfully visual. Fearsome pictures of addicts$_1$ were engraved in public consciousness by the new photographic newspapers of the 19th century[20] and the electronic media of the 20th. The images of the ruined alcoholic and the diseased junkie became cultural arche-types, known throughout the world. In North America, these images were most often associated with opium in the decades around World War I,[21] heroin in the decades before and after World War II,[22] 'crack' cocaine in the 1990s,[23] and at the beginning of the 21st century with the stimulant drug methyl amphetamine, often shortened to 'crystal meth', 'methamphetamine', 'crystal', or 'ice'.[24]

The word 'addiction' has come to evoke these powerful images reflexively. Even in scholarly settings where 'addiction' can be carefully defined at the beginning of a dis-cussion, cultural conditioning often prevails and many people's understanding of the word reverts to the dramatic images of addiction$_1$ by the end.

When the definition of addiction$_1$ finally appeared in the main text of the *Oxford English Dictionary* in 1989 (after its debut in the *Supplement* of 1933), it was appended as '2b' to part 2 of the traditional definition. The original part 2 was renumbered '2a'. Definition 2b reads as follows:[25]

> 2. b. The, or a, state of being addicted to a drug (see ADDICTED *ppl a. 3b*); a compulsion and need to continue taking a drug as a result of taking it in the past. *Cf.* drug-addiction s.v. DRUG sb.[1] I b.

The new definition corresponds to addiction$_1$. It entails overwhelming involvement with drug habits, but with no other habits or pursuits. Both its medical and its moral-istic qualities become evident when the definition above is closely examined, along with the text citations and cross-references that it contains. The new definition is *moral* because there is no possibility that addiction, as redefined, could be anything but an evil. No benign words like 'devotion' appear in this definition, and the word 'drug-addiction', which is cross-referenced with this definition, is explained with a variety of moralistic terms, including 'drug evil' and 'drug-fiends'.[26] The new defini-tion is *medical* because, unlike the traditional definition, it has the qualities of a med-ical diagnosis: it is a 'compulsion' that has a specific cause—taking a drug—and is accompanied by 'withdrawal symptoms'. ('Withdrawal symptoms' are mentioned in definition 3b of the word 'addicted', which is cross-referenced within the new defini-tion of 'addiction'.) Although it can be traced back to the traditional definition histor-ically, addiction$_1$ marks off only a small segment of the traditional definition's inclusive meaning.

The text in Figure 2.1 contains a brief definition of addiction$_1$, as well as the other three descendants of the traditional meaning. The arrows in Figure 2.1 show how addiction₁ and the others have been historically derived from the traditional definition. Figure 2.1 and the remainder of this book utilise Jerome Jaffe's apt two-word description of addiction as 'overwhelming involvement', to encapsulate part 2 of the traditional definition.[27]

Addiction₂

During the early and mid-20th century, the usage of 'addiction' gradually expanded its scope beyond addiction₁, but not back towards the traditional definition. More and more people began using 'addiction' to encompass all socially unacceptable uses of alcohol or drugs, including, but not limited to, the overwhelming involvement that is the essential component of both addiction₁ and the traditional definition. Some of the ways of using drugs that were labelled addiction in this looser sense *did* cause serious physical, psychological, or social harm, although they did not entail overwhelming involvement. Others caused no discernible harm other than breaking drug laws or provoking the distaste of polite society.[28]

Some people found themselves labelled 'addicted', in this loose sense, simply because they used a drug from time to time that had been labelled 'addictive' by their society, which seemed to imply that all users must be addicted. Others were labelled addicted in this loose sense because they sometimes used drugs or alcohol as a way of emboldening themselves to criminality or flamboyant sexuality, but without the overwhelming drug involvement that defines addiction₁. Some acquired the label by using drugs without medical approval to control chronic pain or anxiety. Non-Western people sometimes found that their use of a drug, like home-grown opium, although completely normal and traditional within their own culture, had been labelled 'addiction' by outsiders whose understanding of the drug derived from a different world.[29]

This looser meaning of addiction will be designated 'addiction₂' in this book. I have not found addiction₂ in any dictionary. It is not a precisely definable term, but rather a grab-bag usage. It is best understood as the usage of a society that is preoccupied with drug problems, and loosely symbolises this heterogeneous collection of problems with the word 'addiction'. Although addiction₂ is often called simply 'addiction' or 'the addiction problem' in everyday language, it is also frequently called 'drug abuse' or 'substance abuse'.

The relationship of addiction₁ and addiction₂ to the traditional definition is represented in Figure 2.1. The arrows show the lines of descent of addiction₁ and addiction₂ from the traditional definition, and the graphical representation illustrates that addiction₂ includes a mélange of problems that lie outside the traditional definition of addiction. On the other hand, addiction₂ (like addiction₁) leaves out overwhelming involvements with most of the habits or pursuits that fall within the traditional definition.

Although the diverse set of problems that comprise addiction₂ are rarely listed together as a formal definition of 'addiction', the word 'addiction' is often used to denote them in the professional literature[30] as well as in public discourse. For example, the highly publicised *Canadian Addiction Survey*, published in November 2004 by the Canadian Centre on Substance Abuse, primarily documents the extent of alcohol and drug *use* in Canada. As well as reporting their frequencies of drug use, the survey informants were asked to elaborate on various 'harms' arising from their drug use, but only a few data were reported that would provide any indication of the prevalence of addiction₁ among those included in this 'addiction survey'.[31] Similarly, the definition of 'substance dependence' in the DSM-IV (the standard American classification system for mental disorders[32]), which is widely taken to be equivalent to 'addiction', corresponds more closely to addiction₂ than to addiction₁, because it is possible to be classified as substance dependent without showing any signs of overwhelming involvement at all.[33] Although addiction₂ includes a very broad set of problems and although it overlaps only slightly with the traditional dictionary definition of 'addiction', using the word 'addiction' in this broad sense is not illogical. However, terms like 'drug misuse', 'the drug and alcohol problem', or 'excessive appetites'[34] seem more suitable than 'addiction' for this heterogeneous domain of problematic drug use.

Although the traditional meaning of addiction remains established in the current dictionary and throughout English literature, 'addiction' is almost always used in the sense of addiction₁ and addiction₂ in medical and political discussions. In fact, some authorities in the addictions field insist with solemn authority that applying the word 'addiction' to anything beyond alcohol or drug use is merely metaphorical.[35] In apparent opposition to the *Oxford English Dictionary*, the *Oxford Dictionary of Psychology* defines 'addiction' exclusively as drug addiction.[36]

Thus compressed, confused, and contested, the word 'addiction' has fallen into a labyrinth of tedious expert dispute[37] that has endured from the 20th century into the 21st. Many authorities on drug addiction have striven to establish a consensus on the meaning of the word, with no lasting success. On the other hand, the authoritative international classification systems for mental diseases,[38] the DSM and the ICD,[39] tried to expunge the word 'addiction' from scholarly discourse, replacing it with 'substance dependence', 'substance abuse', and 'dependence syndrome'. The proposed replacements have joined the semantic clutter in the labyrinth because their definitions are not clear enough and because cultural differences make it difficult to agree on what kinds of drug use are problematic.[40]

Leaving addiction₁ and addiction₂ behind, along with the DSM-IV and ICD definitions, this book will use 'addiction' in a way that is much more closely linked to the traditional English language definition. This definition of 'addiction' will be labelled addiction₃.

Addiction₃

The existence of a well-established, professional field of addictions that focused its attention on addiction₁ and addiction₂ for most of the 20th century has created a widespread impression that, strictly speaking, 'addiction' is limited to the use of alcohol and drugs, but this is not the case.

During the last decades of the 20th century, many people recognised the similarity between addiction problems that did not involve drugs and the highly publicised miseries of alcoholics and junkies. Moreover, landmark research showed convincingly that seriously compulsive love relationships and gambling habits had the same psychological dynamics as addiction$_1$; could be every bit as overwhelming, intractable, and dangerous; and could be treated with the same type of therapy.[41] More recent research suggests that addictions that do not involve drugs have the same underlying neurochemistry as drug addictions.[42] The set of overwhelmingly involving, destructive addictions that includes, but goes far beyond, drugs and alcohol is designated addiction$_3$ in this book.

Addiction$_3$ may be viewed as an expansion of addiction$_1$, but it is better understood as a reassertion of the traditional definition because it is not limited to drug or alcohol use or to any other habit and because it does not have the derogatory overtones of addiction$_1$. The overlapping relationships between these three ways of using the word 'addiction' and their lines of descent are schematised in Figure 2.1.

The late 20th-century recognition of serious addictions$_3$ in which drugs play no major part was not so much a discovery as a *rediscovery* of a fact that had been known throughout history but had been lost in the glare of terrifying images of alcohol and drug addiction that burst forth in the 19th century. Overwhelming involvements with habits other than alcohol or drug use fit the traditional definition of addiction perfectly. Moreover, detailed descriptions of overwhelming, abhorrent, sometimes life-threatening addictions that do not necessarily involve alcohol or drugs can be found in the literature of Western civilisation from the time of Plato and Aristotle[43] onward. Some of these ancient descriptions convey the same horrified recognition that surfaced in the 19th-century temperance literature—severe addiction$_3$ entails not merely a destructive habit, but a kind of slavery, even the loss of a soul. When people become severely addicted$_3$, they not only change what they do, but who they are.

Like addiction$_1$ and the traditional definition, addiction$_3$ does not refer to an ordinary habit, but to an overwhelming involvement. Gambling, love, power-seeking, religious or political zeal, work, food, video game playing, Internet surfing, pornography viewing, and so forth can take up every aspect of a severely addicted$_3$ person's life—conscious, unconscious, intellectual, emotional, behavioural, social, and spiritual—just as severe drug and alcohol addiction can. Such overwhelming involvements often entail a startling blindness to the harm that the addiction$_3$ is doing, which is aptly called 'denial'. Many instances of addiction$_3$ do not involve a single habit, but rather an 'addictive complex' of several habits that constitute a single addictive lifestyle.

There is a continuum of severity for addiction$_3$. At the mild end of the continuum, addiction$_3$ only occasionally overwhelms a person's life, a common problem that can be handled with humour and aplomb. Mild forms of addiction$_3$ may be short-lived (e.g. a short, but all-consuming affair with a lover, cult, or drug), situational (e.g. gamblers who do not lose their money if they stay away from the race track), socially acceptable (e.g. a lucrative work addiction$_3$), episodic (in the case of a 'binger'), or simply less than fully overwhelming. In the middle of the continuum, addicted$_3$ people strive to maintain a 'double life', which produces the appearance of normal psychosocial integration more or less successfully.[44] At the severe end of the continuum, addiction$_3$ can be totally overwhelming and unconcealable. The addicted$_3$ person's previous lifestyle can be destroyed. Irrevocable harm can be inflicted on other people. The overwhelming involvement of addiction$_3$ can reach an unrelenting, hellish intensity, and may have fatal consequences.

Like the traditional definition of addiction, addiction$_3$ does not refer to a medical condition. It is not a pathological invasion of an otherwise healthy person. Rather, it is a state of a person as a whole. Unlike a disease, there is no diagnostic rule that separates mild instances from severe ones that warrant intervention.[45]

Addiction$_3$ is parallel to addiction$_1$ in several important ways. Just as most people consume alcohol and drugs without becoming addicted$_1$, most people engage in all of the activities that can be objects of addiction$_3$ without becoming addicted$_3$. Just as addiction$_1$ can be treated with modest success by alcohol and drug counsellors and by self-help groups, all forms of addiction$_3$ can be treated in a similar manner with the same modest success. Just as many problems surround alcohol and drug use that cannot be called addiction$_1$ because they do not entail overwhelming involvement—although they may reasonably be called addiction$_2$—many problems surround frequent gambling, sex, shopping, television, computers, or a million other habits and pursuits that cannot be called addiction$_3$.[46] These could quite reasonably be called 'addiction$_5$', if there were the slightest need to invent any additional ways of subscripting the word 'addiction'.

Addiction$_4$

Addiction$_3$ is equivalent to the traditional meaning of addiction in every respect but one. The traditional meaning also encompasses overwhelming involvements that are not destructive. These kinds of addiction are often seen as admirable, as illustrated by the biblical quotation earlier in this chapter. Non-destructive addictions will be called addiction$_4$ in this book. Addiction$_4$ designates overwhelming involvements with any habit or pursuit whatsoever when such involvements are not destructive either to the addicted person or his or her society. Therefore, the traditional definition is a combination of addiction$_3$ and addiction$_4$.

Today, the word 'addiction' is not used as commonly in the positive sense of addiction$_4$ as it was in the past, probably because the word reflexively evokes scandalous images of addiction$_1$. Nonetheless, it is occasionally used in the sense of addiction$_4$ in the professional addiction literature,[47] more often in other fields of scholarship,[48] and perhaps most often in contemporary Christian writing where there are favourable references to 'addiction to Jesus' and 'addiction to Bible reading'.[49] When the word 'addiction' is left out of the picture, the concept of an overwhelming involvement that is admirable or even saintly is commonplace. The lives of Martin Luther King and Mother Teresa are contemporary examples. Outside the logical analysis of this book, however, there is no reason that lives like these should be labelled 'addiction$_4$'— 'addiction' is no longer a comfortable term to apply to great people, no matter what subscript is hung beneath it. Religion and romantic love are examples of familiar pursuits for which both addiction$_3$ and addiction$_4$ are well known. Figure 2.1 represents addiction$_4$ as a mirror image of addiction$_3$, at least hypothetically providing a positive counterpoint for every addiction$_3$.[50]

Addiction$_4$ is less common than addiction$_3$, but it is not a fiction. Many of the saintly and heroic role models of Western civilisation exemplify addiction$_4$. I have been privileged to know several people involved in various forms of social activism, religion, and other compassionate causes whose lives have approached addiction$_4$ for some extended periods.[51] Moving biographies have been written about people whose entire adult lives were apparently dominated by addiction$_4$ in the most positive sense.[52] Possible exemplars of addiction$_4$ who will be discussed at some length later in this book include St Augustine and the co-founder of Alcoholics Anonymous (AA), best known as 'Bill W'.

A full understanding of the relationship between addiction$_3$ and addiction$_4$ might finally fulfil the unredeemed promise of psychology to comprehend the entire spectrum of human motivation, from the horrors of compulsion to the triumphs of faith and love. I am not yet confident, however, that I fully understand addiction$_4$. This book focuses on explaining addiction$_3$ and reducing the devastation that it causes. Nevertheless, addiction$_4$ will be considered in the later chapters because it must be included for a full discussion of addiction$_3$. The pressing issue of this chapter is establishing that addiction$_3$ is the most useful way of looking at the addiction problems of the globalising world.

The significance of addiction$_3$ in the 21st century

Addiction$_3$ entails a destructive transformation of a person's life and identity. When severe, it can cause great harm to individuals and to society. Because the prevalence of addiction$_3$ is increasing around the world, it poses a substantial and growing danger at the beginning of the 21st century.

It may still be hard to appreciate the full extent of the danger arising from addiction$_3$ when it does not involve drugs and alcohol, partly because the field of addiction assumed for decades that the only serious addictions were to drugs and alcohol. Moreover, whereas today's popular media terrify us with images of the most dangerous drug addictions$_3$, they usually reassure us with good humoured portrayals of addictions$_3$ to food, consumer goods, sex, religion, television, video games, and so on.[53]

However, addictions$_3$ that do not have drugs or alcohol as their objects are more prevalent than drug addictions and just as dangerous in severe cases. Stanton Peele and others who see beyond the conventional wisdom on addiction have long been aware that the majority of severe addictions$_3$ are to habits other than drug use.[54] Anton Schweighofer and I carried out some quantitative research in the late 1980s that confirmed this conclusion for university students. We assessed the relative frequencies of severe addiction$_3$ to drugs and alcohol as opposed to other habits and pursuits with a self-report interview that used exactly the same definition for all kinds of addiction. Alcohol or drug addictions comprised only 19.3% of the most severe instances of addiction$_3$.[55] The most frequent severe addictions$_3$ for our sample of university students were to romantic love and to eating (or dieting). The students described a great variety of other severe non-drug addictions$_3$ including sports, work, and socialising.

Many forms of addiction$_3$, in addition to those involving drugs, can cause death in severe instances. There are suicides among addicted gamblers,[56] murders and suicides carried out by addicted lovers when they are thwarted,[57] fatal cases of diabetes caused by prolonged, addictive overeating,[58] fatal accidents of people addicted to extreme sports and other forms of risk-taking, and so on. Beyond actual fatalities, severe addiction$_3$ can become a kind of living death, supplanting the full lives that addicted people had hoped to live and that their society had anticipated for them. Severely addicted$_3$ people sometimes feel out of control and possessed by the object of their addiction. The desperate struggle to support an addictive$_3$ lifestyle can provoke actions that cause self-loathing at the time or years later·

People who fail to maintain their addicted$_3$ lifestyle (e.g. gamblers who have lost all their money) often live on the verge of depression, violence, or suicide. However, people who succeed in maintaining their addiction$_3$ often feel guilty or empty nonetheless. Just as 'junkies' are not otherwise happy and well-integrated people who happen to want some heroin every few hours,[59] severe gambling, food, sex, and work addicts$_3$ are not otherwise happy, well-integrated people who happen to overindulge regularly.[60] People who are severely addicted$_3$ have a tragic, engulfing problem, whether or not their addiction involves drugs or alcohol and whether or not it causes bodily damage.

The prevalence of addiction$_3$ of all sorts is very large, and growing. The indications of increasing prevalence of addiction$_3$ to drugs and alcohol are best known. The growth is visible geographically in the apparently inexorable spread of the intravenous drug-using population in the Hastings Corridor area of Vancouver's Downtown Eastside. Statistical evidence generally indicates expanding addictive use of heroin, cocaine, amphetamines, and alcohol throughout the world.[61] The phenomenal growth of heroin use in the UK since the 1950s and in China since 1990 are among the most dramatic instances.[62] Alcohol addiction$_3$ also appears to be increasing substantially in the UK, especially among women, although addiction$_3$ is only a portion of a national drinking trend loosely called 'binge drinking'.[63] The list of legal drugs that are sometimes used for addictive purposes around the world, including many familiar pharmaceuticals, has grown very long.[64] Scandals involving drug and alcohol addiction fill the media, such as the downfall of the famous American media personality and political commentator Rush Limbaugh, who, like many other respectable people, became severely addicted to a legal pharmaceutical.[65]

The prevalence of addictions in which drug use plays no important role is growing as fast as or faster than the prevalence of drug addiction$_3$, although the evidence is neither so well quantified nor so highly publicised. Addiction professionals have published a mountain of literature on devastating, occasionally fatal, addictions$_3$ that do not involve drugs.[66] Investigative journalists, biographers, and autobiographers also provide a large number of accounts.[67]

In addition to stories of addiction, there is a huge literature of 'recovery stories', many of them written by people who have joined Alcoholics Anonymous or any of the '12-step' organisations that have derived from it. Twelve-step programmes have spread from alcoholism to myriad other addictions, creating an alphabet-full of active organisations modelled on Alcoholics Anonymous (AA), including BA (Bloggers Anonymous), CA (Cocaine Anonymous), DA (Debtors Anonymous), EA (Emotions Anonymous), FA (Fundamentalists Anonymous), GA (Gamblers Anonymous and Gamers Anonymous), and onward through the alphabet.[68] Many other 12-step programmes are not so easily recognised by their name. The Augustine Fellowship (also known as Sex and Love Addicts Anonymous) publishes a directory of 900 groups that hold weekly meetings, of which 720 are in the United States. There are also online meetings everyday. The Augustine Fellowship is not the only organisation of its type. Its materials on the Internet[69] are very similar to those more recognisable 12-step organisations such as Sexaholics Anonymous and Sex Addicts Anonymous.

There is also a vast literature of inspirational books, self-help books, and websites advocating different methods of 'recovery' from addiction$_3$ to a broad spectrum of habits and pursuits, although the word 'addiction' is not applied in some cases.[70] Very large numbers of people who watch television and play video games—including many children—are addicted to the point of causing serious life problems, such as failing in school, living in isolation, weight loss, losing jobs, and divorce.[71] Finally, there is literature on controlling relatively mild forms of addiction$_3$. For example, the famous 'Atkins diet' is understood by its author and millions of readers as a way of dealing with addictive overeating, even in cases where obesity is not severe.[72]

Many quantitative studies have attempted to measure the prevalence of addictions$_3$ that do not involve drugs or alcohol.[73] However, this literature is unsatisfactory because there are too many different operational definitions of addiction and because the cut-off points that determine which addictions$_3$ are serious enough to count are entirely arbitrary. Moreover, such studies usually attempt to measure only one form of addiction$_3$, most often gambling, whereas to know the prevalence of addiction$_3$, it is necessary to know how many people have any addiction$_3$ whatsoever. This is made even harder because many addictions do not have a single identifiable object but rather form an addictive complex with many objects.

Although the lack of an adequate operational definition for addiction$_3$ precludes large-scale quantitative surveys, there is no end to the indirect indications that the prevalence of addiction$_3$ is growing fast. In a famous book entitled *Bowling Alone*,[74] Robert Putnam showed that the community and religious affiliations of people in the United States, notably neighbourhood bowling leagues, are declining precipitously. Concurrently, however, AA and many of the other 12-step groups for addicted$_3$ people are growing rapidly.[75] Beyond self-help groups, addiction$_3$ treatment has become a growth industry. For example, a shocking number of profit-making enterprises cater for people who are obese or bulimic.[76] Forty-three different kinds of treatment for alcoholism have been the subject of quantitative evaluation research.[77]

The newest frontier for addiction is the computer. The phenomenal rise in popularity of computer games and of game companies with billions of dollars in annual revenues has been followed by a wave of accounts of gaming addiction.[78] 'Gamers Anonymous' appears to be a rapidly growing organisation, with, ironically, an online website. GA is far from the only self-help website for game addicts and their relatives.[79] Because of the accessibility of computers, the creative brilliance of the game programmers, and the billion-dollar profits that game companies can earn, it is safe to predict that overwhelming involvement with these games will very soon replace drugs as the most feared addictions for children, and that chat room, blogging, gaming, and web-surfing addictions will move far up the list of dangerous addictions for adults.

Three decades ago, when I began giving public lectures on my experiences working with heroin addicts in Vancouver, a few audience members would surprise me by confiding that, apart from the issue of illegality, their own lives included addictions that were very much the same as those of the junkies I was describing. These people discretely labelled themselves addicted to consumer spending, dysfunctional love relationships, smoking tobacco, and so forth, rather than heroin. This has changed over the years. When I speak publicly now, people identify themselves as addicts quite openly, and nobody seems at all surprised by such confessions, as if what had once been shocking has grown commonplace.

An indirect indication of the growth of addiction is the astronomical increase in the prevalence of clinical depression and a great variety of other vaguely defined psychological states with depressive components, like chronic anxiety and chronic fatigue syndrome.[80] Depression and addiction are closely intertwined problems—people who suffer from one of them very often suffer from the other.[81] The reasons that they are intertwined will be discussed in the next chapter.

As the spread of addiction₃ batters the world like a hurricane, side streams of turbulence flow in every direction. For example, corporations have learned to analyse and systematically cultivate addictive propensities of their customers behind the scenes. This has been documented most spectacularly in the manipulation of nicotine levels of tobacco by cigarette manufacturers,[82] but it has been documented in other industries as well, for example, among purveyors of automobile accessories and airline points.[83]

Another side stream is that addiction has been made to seem 'cool' in advertisements, creating consternation among those, including myself, who are convinced that it isn't. In fashionable advertisements, clothing is sometimes modelled by people who deliberately affect the attitudes of junkies in a style that, at its most recent peak of popularity, was called 'junkie chic' or 'heroin chic'.[84] Goods are sometimes successfully marketed by direct appeal to images of heroin addiction, notably the perfumes 'Opium' and Dior's 'Addict' and 'Euphoria'.[85]

Fashionable use of heroin, the drug that universally symbolises addiction, began early in the 20th century in the rich and 'wild' sectors of society[86] and continues today. Large and growing numbers of young working adults use heroin from time to time, provocatively daring society to label them as addicts.[87] Fashionably funny accounts of mild forms of addiction₃ are more and more a topic of popular entertainment.[88] Entertainment media fascinate us with the often painful and rarely funny addictions₃ of stars such as Elvis Presley, Michael Jackson, Robert Downey Jr, and Britney Spears.[89] A growing genre of 'underground' writing celebrates the benefits of addiction₃, while ignoring the harms.[90] Among the cleverest of these is the series of humorous books celebrating the life of 'Couch Potatoes' (i.e. people who devote themselves to watching particularly vacuous television programming for great amounts of time).[91] The newest addictive chic is anorexia among the starlets at the same time that anorexia is coming to be understood as addiction to starvation.[92] There are 'Pro-Ana' websites where anorexic girls display glamour photographs of emaciated celebrities as well as their own starved bodies and offer each other encouragement on losing more weight.[93]

All sorts of products are promoted for their addicting qualities. Advertising for video games frequently extols their addictive qualities, as if these were shining virtues.

Purveyors of other kinds of entertainment also tout their products' addictive features. Here are a few lines from a sophisticated advertising campaign for a book on the puzzle game Sudoku, written in the form of a letter:

> Dear Sudoku Enthusiast:
>
> My name is… and I just have to get this off my chest before I explode… **'I am *Proud* To Be a Compulsive Sudoku Addict Completely Beyond all Hope and Reason!'**[94]

Having flaunted his addiction to Sudoku, the author of the book goes on to assure his readers that they too will be proud to be 'compulsive Sudoku players', once he explains himself. He then explains the rewards of Sudoku, many of which have an unmistakably addictive character: solving Sudoku puzzles puts people in a 'meditative state' of 'ecstatic experience'; Sudoku produces a powerful sense of self-satisfaction, which is what got the author 'hooked'; 'Sudoku World' is 'a wonderful, peaceful place where everything always works out fine if you can just solve the puzzle!' When a person cannot solve the puzzle, however, Sudoku World is said to become a hell of 'masochistic torture'. Fortunately, a book now available for only US$17 will make every single puzzle solvable. The author describes how his family learned to play Sudoku together, fostering warm spousal and intergenerational relationships. Moreover, his wife no longer watches her irritating television shows compulsively. These family benefits of Sudoku are not explicitly claimed for all players, although their universal application is implied. Once the author's book is purchased, there will be only the benefits of Sudoku addiction, and no further costs.

Like stereotyped drug pushers, such advertisers discount the harm that results from severe addiction₃, making sport of those who believe—as I do—that it is tragic. The harm done by addiction₃ extends beyond the normal purview of secular psychology. The temperance and anti-drug movements saw a spiritual as well as secular tragedy in the hopeless drunk and the ruined junkie. They eventually concluded that society could only be saved from this menace by the complete prohibition of alcohol and drugs. I cannot dismiss their analysis merely because it overemphasised drugs, misjudged the benefits of prohibition, and advocated a kind of Christian theocracy. The spiritual harm produced by addiction₃ is absolutely real, whether or not drugs are involved. It can be described in the languages of many secular and spiritual traditions. In this book, it will be described in the psychological language of Erik Erikson, the social science language of Karl Polanyi, the rationalist language of Socrates, and the Buddhist language of Vipassana meditation, as well as the Christian language of St Augustine and St Paul.

Although the harm that addiction₃ causes addicted individuals can be great, the social harm can be greater. As a single example, political and religious fanatics (i.e. people who are addicted₃ to simplistic doctrines and creeds) are working serious destruction upon today's world as this is being written. Part II of this book elaborates on the social consequences of addiction₃, showing why society cannot embrace addiction₃ with good-humoured complacency, even when no drugs are involved.

Some people believe that today's growing concern about addiction is overblown. The apparent surge in addiction is sometimes dismissed as a trendy way of describing personal idiosyncrasies, a convenient excuse for criminality, or a way to generate business for treatment professionals. This perception is reinforced when lawyers and expert witnesses hold forth on addiction$_3$ in courtrooms with the most pretentious psychobabble and neurochemical puffery. A few opportunistic lawyers have had clients exonerated on the defence that their crime was caused by the disease of addiction.[95] But the spread of addiction$_3$ has done far too much harm to be discredited by those who exploit it for vanity or profit.

For all these reasons, a comprehensive understanding of the causes and effects of addiction$_3$ is extremely important to the emerging global society of the 21st century. The attempt to outline the causes and effects of addiction$_3$ begins in the next chapter. First, however, a final aspect of the definition problem must be examined more fully: addiction$_3$ is frequently conflated with addiction$_2$, making precise analysis impossible and sometimes causing human suffering on a massive scale.

The importance of distinguishing addiction$_2$ from addiction$_3$

Although some dangerous forms of addiction$_2$ call for social intervention, addiction$_2$ usually needs to be understood and treated quite differently from addiction$_3$. The consequences of overlooking this distinction can be grave. For example, adolescents who are caught using illegal drugs recreationally are sometimes forced into addiction treatment by their parents, although there is no reason to think that they are addicted$_3$. In the United States, the consequences of this ill-considered treatment of adolescents have sometimes been tragic when 'boot camp' treatment agencies have employed brutal forms of 'therapy'.[96] As a second example, people who have car accidents when their blood alcohol levels exceed the legal limits in Canada and the United States have been forced into AA or treatment centres modelled on its philosophy. These intensive treatments were specifically designed for people who are alcoholics or, in the terminology of this book, addicted$_3$ to alcohol. Although some of those arrested for drunken driving are indeed alcoholic, many are not. Rather, they are guilty of a serious error of judgement or of criminal neglect and should be treated accordingly.[97] Perhaps worst of all, throughout the 20th century, people in severe pain who cried out for strong pain-killing drugs were often mistakenly labelled as addicted$_3$ by their doctors and nurses. Many patients have been inadvertently tortured by well-meaning practitioners, who took it as their professional responsibility never to give drugs to addicts and never to prescribe enough 'addictive drugs' to cause addiction$_3$.[98] Millions of cancer, HIV, and burn patients still die in agonising pain for this reason, especially in poor countries.[99] This widespread problem is sometimes called 'pseudoaddiction' within the medical profession.[100] None of this is to say that the various forms of addiction$_2$ should be ignored. But this book is about the globalisation of addiction$_3$—addiction$_2$ encompasses a set of problems that extends beyond addiction$_3$ in a variety of directions, calling for quite different interventions.

A nameless form of addiction$_2$

One form of addiction$_2$ causes particular confusion when conflated with addiction$_3$, causing untold misery and making serious analysis impossible. This relatively common way of using drugs once had a perfectly good name in the English language, but its name was, in a sense, kidnapped. This semantic kidnapping has remained an unsolved crime for too long, causing great confusion. The next few pages are intended to solve the mystery.

Consider all of the people who regularly use one of the currently illegal or socially disapproved drugs and who, in addition, suffer from side effects, cannot be persuaded to quit, obtain their drugs illegally if they must, and continue their regular drug use for a prolonged period, even an entire lifetime. All of these people would be labelled 'addicted' within the conventional wisdom. Most would fit the definition of 'substance dependent' in the DSM-IV. Some of these people would also fit the definition of addiction$_3$ in its most destructive form. However, others of them are very far from being addicted$_3$. In fact, their drug use is, in a crucially important way, the opposite to addiction$_3$, although it can be classified as addiction$_2$.

These regular, but non-addicted$_3$ drug users rely on their drugs to keep themselves performing in normal, socially acceptable ways. They are definitely not addicted$_3$, because they do not have an overwhelming involvement with their drug use, which does not alter their normal personality or alienate them from society, although it may injure their health. Quite the contrary, people who use drugs in this way are dedicated to living stable, socially approved lives. Their drug use gives them pain relief, energy, or composure that they find indispensable for coping with the obstacles that they must face in their normal lives—although they must often endure harmful side effects.

Although a few people who use drugs in these ways lapse into addiction$_3$,[101] there are a great many fully documented instances where even a lifetime of regular use of marijuana, heroin, morphine, opium, cocaine, amphetamine or tobacco has been compatible with a reasonably happy, productive, socially acceptable life and has not led to addiction$_3$, even after many decades.[102] For example, some people use marijuana regularly to control glaucoma, or to endure the nausea of chemotherapy during treatment for cancer, or simply to get a good night's sleep, even when chronic bronchitis is a result. Some use heroin, morphine, or another opioid to keep their minds off chronic bodily pain or incipient depression, because other painkillers do not work for them and because the side effects of the opioid, which may include tolerance and withdrawal symptoms, are less debilitating than chronic pain. Some smoke cigarettes to get through the day without being crippled by anxiety, even though they are aware that they may be shortening their lives by smoking. Some use stimulants like cocaine or methamphetamine as anti-depressants to enable them to meet their obligations, despite side effects like insomnia and chronic nervousness. One well-documented example is Dr William Halsted, a brilliant American surgeon and medical school professor, who injected a minimum of 180 mg of morphine daily during most of his long and distinguished career. This fact was known only to his very closest friends and only became public knowledge after his death. His life story, including his reliance on morphine, was published in the *Journal of the American Medical Association* 50 years after his death.[103] Dr Halsted may properly be called 'addicted$_2$' in the terminology of this book, but he was not addicted$_3$. On the other hand, it is possible to become ruinously addicted$_3$ on 180 mg of morphine per day, or less.

This form of addiction$_2$ could be labelled 'self-medication', although this term is too narrow because not all of these drug users have a medical disease. It is also sometimes called 'functional addiction', but this term is not widely accepted either. The term 'self-medication' will be temporarily used in the next few paragraphs. Then I will daringly attempt to snatch the precise name of this way of using drugs from its kidnappers.

'Self-medicators' take pains not to alienate their families with their drug use. Sometimes their families and closest friends are unaware that they smoke marijuana every night, or take a painkiller like heroin from time to time through the day, or need daily stimulants or anti-depressants to keep functioning, or sneak away for cigarettes more than once each hour, and so on. More often, their family and friends are vaguely aware of their regular drug use, but 'look the other way', treating it with the same restraint that they would apply to other unwelcome but tolerable habits. It could be said that whereas 'self-medication' threatens people's health and strains their family life, it does not threaten their souls, as does addiction$_3$.

Naturally, 'self-medicators' use as little of their socially disapproved drug as they can in order to keep their lives together. However, this minimum is often much larger than the amount used by recreational users and may be as large as the amounts used by some people who are truly addicted$_3$ to these same drugs. 'Self-medicators' stop using their drug promptly if the pain or other distress that it serves to control subsides, just as a person with a broken leg stops using crutches as soon as he or she can walk properly without them.

'Self-medicators' are indistinguishable in every way—except in the symbolic meaning of their drug—from millions of other people who regularly use a multitude of legal drugs, such as SSRI (selective serotonin reuptake inhibitors) anti-depressants to control incapacitating depression or multiple cups of coffee to endure the boredom of their work. The well-documented side effects include loss of sexual function and occasional risk of suicide (SSRI anti-depressants) and a heightened risk of bladder cancer (coffee). In the case of SSRI anti-depressants, these side effects have been denied by the drug manufacturers, but they have been documented in carefully controlled research and the evidence has stood up in court.[104] Like the illegal drug habits described above, these legal drug habits can be called addiction$_2$, but not addiction$_3$. Lauren Slater has recently published a fascinating description of a depressed person who finds herself addicted$_2$ to *both* SSRI anti-depressants and a legally prescribed opioid drug that she would be unable to purchase on the street without violating the narcotic laws.[105] It is clear from her description that both drugs are being used in the same way, for the same purpose.

Throughout the 20th century, many conscientious doctors and addiction researchers have spoken out on the importance of distinguishing self-medicating addiction$_2$ from addiction$_3$. However, the distinction is often ignored or denied, despite the mountain of documentation that has built up.[106] It has come to seem odd that a person could use a drug whose side effects may shorten his or her life without being labelled 'addicted' in the strongest sense of the word. However, there is nothing odd about it outside the conventional wisdom on addiction. Non-addicted people do many things regularly to enhance their well-being, some of which may shorten their lives, without being labelled 'addictions'. Regular, risky activities carried out by non-addicted people include 'extreme sports' as well as ordinary body-crunching sports like football or hockey, hazardous occupations like mining, fighting in wars, or simply driving an automobile. Physicians routinely prescribe drugs that have extremely harmful side effects, because they believe that the benefits will outweigh the costs for their patients. In addition to anti-depressants, some of the drugs that are currently being used to control arthritis, acne, and psychosis come with a risk of seriously damaging side effects, including incurable brain damage (tardive dyskinesia) in the case of some anti-psychotic drugs.[107] Yet millions of patients and doctors—quite reasonably—accept the risks in order to reduce the even more devastating consequences of serious diseases. 'Self-medicators' make the same kind of reasoned decision in their drug use as these medical patients.

Authorities have long struggled to decide on a generally acceptable name for this form of addiction$_2$, but no agreement has been reached.[108] However, the solution is obvious outside the conventional wisdom on addiction. This form of addiction$_2$ is simply 'dependence' in the normal English meaning of the word.[109] Many people are 'dependent', in this sense, upon their jobs, their families, their recreational sports, their cars, their times of prayer or meditation, or on one or more drugs in order to carry out their lives in successful ways. Many non-drug dependencies entail serious risks and side effects—those associated with driving a car are the most obvious. Dependencies on drugs are susceptible to a characteristic set of harmful effects, which may include withdrawal symptoms and alienation of friends and relatives if the drug is socially abhorred. When dependencies on drugs have one of these effects, they can reasonably be labelled addiction$_2$. Addiction$_2$ sometimes causes very serious problems, but it is qualitatively different from addiction$_3$.

This form of regular drug use cannot be called 'dependence' within the conventional wisdom on addiction, because the word 'dependence' has been kidnapped[110] from its normal meaning and is now frequently used as a synonym for addiction$_1$ thus blurring the distinction between addiction$_2$ and addiction$_3$. The kidnapped word is usually disguised in a composite form, such as 'drug dependence' or 'substance dependence'. The equation of 'dependence' with addiction$_1$ is a part of the specialised language of the conventional wisdom on addiction, since none of the definitions of 'dependence' in the *Oxford English Dictionary* (1989) could be considered equivalent to addiction$_1$. None of them carries the implication of overwhelming involvement or of giving oneself over to servitude. None mentions drugs or alcohol, either in the definitions or the text examples that the dictionary provides. Because this book leaves the conventional wisdom behind, the form of addiction$_2$ that was temporarily called 'self-medication' here will consistently be called by its normal English name, 'dependence', from this point on. I hope this will become part of a concerted campaign to free the English language from the confusions that have been imposed upon it by the conventional wisdom on addiction.

It is important to distinguish dependence from addiction$_1$ for very practical reasons. The most obvious one is that it is cruel not to prescribe drugs to dependent patients who cannot live normal, productive lives without them.[111] This distinction is recognised in the logic of methadone maintenance programmes, which have been traditionally designed to provide methadone to heroin users who can stabilise their lives by becoming dependent on methadone, but to withhold it from heroin users who may simply sell the methadone or use it to supplement their addiction$_1$. Many general practitioners find themselves in an agonising conflict when they recognise that they can perform an important service by regularly providing restricted drugs to patients who are dependent on drugs other than opioids, although this practice is generally illegal.[112] I have personally known a few courageous Canadian GPs who have conscientiously broken laws that prevented them from caring for their dependent patients in this way. There may be times when it is desirable to prescribe these drugs to people who are addicted$_3$ as well, as is currently being proposed by mayor Sam Sullivan of Vancouver,[113] but the outcome of this is harder to predict.

Although dependence on drugs in the normal English meaning of the term 'dependence' is essentially different from addiction$_1$ and addiction$_3$, some people manage to combine elements of both. In such cases, drug use serves to maintain a socially acceptable lifestyle, but the dependent people also have a strong sense of their lifestyle as not fully authentic, and of themselves as addicted.[114] Lauren Slater has published a valuable self-analysis by a person who saw herself in this borderline position in her use of a prescribed anti-depressant medication.[115] In other instances, a person's doctor or family may correctly perceive that his or her dependent drug use is drifting towards addiction$_3$, whereas the person does not. In the past, some people have been pushed from stable drug dependence to drug addiction$_3$ by the imposition of harsh prohibition laws. By creating an artificial scarcity, these laws forced those people to devote their lives to obtaining the drug upon which they depended.[116] However, under most conditions, drug dependence is a stable condition that lasts as long as there is a need that can be controlled pharmacologically, often for a short period, sometimes for a lifetime. Whereas some people do drift from dependence to addiction$_3$,[117] others drift from addiction$_3$ to dependence, the most familiar example being those heroin users who establish stable and socially acceptable lives while still taking methadone every day.

Prospects for theoretical analysis

The mysterious transformation of ordinary people into drug addicts$_1$ urgently requires explanation. Fortunately, addiction$_1$ is well suited to theoretical analysis because it refers to a single recognisable phenomenon, whatever drug is involved, including alcohol. Unfortunately, however, analysis of addiction$_1$ is hindered by the secretiveness of addicts, because drug addictions are socially abhorrent or illegal. People in this situation have many reasons to lie to authorities. It is perhaps for this reason that theories of addiction$_1$ are so often drawn from research on laboratory rats, an aspect of current scholarship that—I predict—future generations will find hilarious.

Addiction$_2$ is such a diverse group of problems that it will be difficult to analyse with any single theory, although eclectic conceptual models are being articulated to guide practice and social policy by Jim Orford[118] and others. In fact, there is little real need for a theoretical explanation of addiction$_2$. Generally speaking, people acquire the label of addicted$_2$ either because they stubbornly insist on the recreational use of drugs that their society finds offensive, or because they get drunk or stoned and make a serious error of judgement, or because they are dependent on drugs that keep their lives together much as other people are dependent on some other type of 'crutch'. No special theoretical explanation is required in any of these cases. For the most part, addiction$_2$ can be understood in the same ordinary way as most other human actions. Addiction$_2$, however, partly overlaps with addiction$_3$, which does require theoretical analysis.

Theoretical analysis of addiction$_3$ is sorely needed, for the same reason that theoretical analysis of addiction$_1$ is. In its most severe instances, addiction$_3$ entails a mysterious personality metamorphosis that can be extremely harmful, whether drugs are involved or not. This harmful metamorphosis is a spreading menace in the globalising world. Addiction$_3$ is easier to study than addiction$_1$ because people are generally willing—in fact, eager—to discuss their own experiences with legal addictions. It is better suited for theoretical analysis than addiction$_2$ because it refers to a single state of overwhelming involvement that is likely to have the same underlying cause whatever habits or pursuits are its object.

Addiction$_4$ also entails a personality metamorphosis and requires theoretical analysis to provide a full account of human motivation, but that is not the primary task of this book.

As the remainder of this book is primarily about addiction$_3$, there will be less need for subscripts after this chapter. However, they will still pop up once in a while—just often enough, I hope, to keep the analysis from going adrift.

Summary and anchor

This is the only boxed summary in this book. My hope is that a weighty concrete block of text can function as an anchor that will keep the book centred on the definitions that have been introduced, despite the distraction of more forceful images that abound in popular culture. I hope that readers who feel the slightest sense of drift in their conception of what addiction means in this book will return here to be reminded.

1 In plain English, this book is about harmful addictions, whether or not alcohol or drugs are involved.

2 In the more precise terminology that is necessary to make certain key distinctions, this book is about the globalisation of addiction$_3$. Addiction$_3$ is overwhelming involvement with any pursuit whatsoever that is harmful to the addicted person and his or her society.

3 Addiction$_1$ is only of concern in this book for historical reasons and inasmuch as it is a subset of addiction$_3$ that is restricted to alcohol and drugs. Addiction$_2$, a heterogeneous collection of harmful drug and alcohol problems that includes, but is not limited to, addiction$_1$, is not a central topic in this book except as it is essential to distinguish addiction$_3$ from addiction$_2$ at several points. Addiction$_4$—overwhelming involvement that is *not* harmful—will be considered in Part II, but only incidentally.

4 Addiction$_3$, the main topic of this book, does not necessarily entail drug use, withdrawal symptoms, pharmacological tolerance, endorphin deficiency, or any variety of dopamine insufficiency. Of course, addiction$_3$ does have a physiological substrate, as every human activity does, but this book analyses it at the psychosocial level.

5 The word 'dependence' will be used only in its normal English dictionary meaning in this book, rather than in its conventional use in the drug addiction field as a synonym for addiction$_1$ (in phrases like 'drug dependence' and 'substance dependence'). In the language of this book, some people are dependent upon regular use of drugs, including illegal ones, to help cope with the exigencies of their normal lives. Such people are no more addicted$_3$ than people who are dependent on automobiles or vigorous physical exercise for the same reason or than people who break their leg and are dependent on crutches for a time. People who are dependent on drugs in this sense fit the definition of 'addicted$_2$', however.

6 Phrases like 'addictive drugs' are not used in this book, because such phrases designate drugs that are said to cause addiction in people who use them a few times. The next chapter addresses the crucial issue of what causes addiction$_3$. The answer is *not* drugs.

Endnotes

1 Other meanings exist as well. For example, the casual use of 'addiction' to describe a simple habit—'I'm addicted to my morning walk'– is a harmless pleasantry. Another example is that, until a few decades ago, most psychologists agreed that a person was addicted if they experienced pharmacological tolerance for their drug of choice and withdrawal symptoms when they stopped using it. This definition largely disappeared when it became clear that cocaine addiction did not produce any powerful form of withdrawal symptoms.

The set of four definitions, addiction₁, addiction₂, addiction₃, and addiction₄, will be used consistently throughout this book, but this is at best an ephemeral solution of the semantic problem of organising all of the current definitions of addiction. As it is impossible for me to write unambiguously about addiction without using subscripts, I am searching for new words in other languages to replace the now hopelessly ambiguous English word 'addiction'. My current choice as a replacement is the French *l'asservissement*, although it is not perfect because it suggests a state of involuntary servitude rather than one that entails some an act of choice on the part of the addict. The French verb *s'adonner* seems more appropriate, but I do not think there is a noun form in proper French (i.e. *l'adonnement'*). Other possibilities that have been brought to my attention are the German *die Sucht*, the Dutch *verslaving*, the Swedish *hemfallenhet*, and the Finnish *riippuvuus*.

2 Like the English, the Latin word was used in both a legal and a psychological sense. In Roman law, for example, an *addictus* (past participle of the verb *addicere*) was a person legally given over as a bond slave to his creditor. However, *addicere* could also be used to describe strong devotion, which could be either destructive or admirable. The admirable sense of the word is illustrated in the phrases *senatus, cui me semper addixi* ('the senate to which I am always devoted') and *agros omnes addixit deae* ('he devoted the fields entirely to the goddess') (C.T. Lewis & Short, 1879).

3 The *Oxford English Dictionary* (1933, 1989) is the authoritative dictionary of the English language. An enormous work, it required over half a century to assemble and publish (Burchfield, 1972, Introduction; Winchester, 2003). The original edition came out in separate 'fascicules' that were published at different times over a span of many years. The wording of the traditional definition of addiction is the same in all editions including the current online edition launched in 2000.

4 Italics and uppercase in original. Part of this definition, which the dictionary had already designated as obsolete in 1884, is omitted for simplicity. It reads as follows: †3. The way in which one is addicted; inclination, bent, leaning, *penchant*. Also in *pl. Obs.* (Note: † is the symbol used in the *Oxford English Dictionary* to denote an obsolete usage.)

5 In the 1989 and 2000 editions, definition '2' is numbered '2.a'.

6 The word can be lightened with qualifiers, however. It is correct English to speak of being 'a little addicted'.

7 Shakespeare (*c.* 1600/1984, Act I, Scene I).

8 Shakespeare (c. 1600/1984, Act I, Scene II; Act II, Scene IV).

9 *Holy Bible, Authorized (King James) Version* (1611/1956, I Corinthians 16:15–16, italics in original).

10 *Holy Bible, New Living Translation* (1996), *New American Bible* (2002).

11 Use of the word by Austin, Dickens, and countless others can be documented by word searches of electronic versions of their texts for the stem 'addict'. For example, David Hume (1739/1888, p. 551) saw 'addiction' as the way that a person can instil in himself the all-important 'general rules' for acquisition of knowledge in *A Treatise of Human Nature*.

12 It is sometimes argued that the idea of addiction was a new social construction or a 'fetish' that grew out of the economic tensions of the 19th century (see Levine, 1978; Reith, 2004, p. 290). This certainly could be true of the sensationalized image of the alcoholic and the junkie that became popular at that time. However, the use of the word 'addiction' to describe destructive lifestyles centred on alcohol goes back much farther than the 19th century (Jessica Warner, 1994) in accordance with the traditional definition of addiction. It is the *exclusive* use of the word to describe overwhelming involvement with alcohol and drugs that was new in the 19th century.

13 See Jessica Warner (1994) for Webster's 1806 definition. See also *Webster's International Dictionary of the English Language* (1902).

14 Paradoxically, the last two centuries during which the term 'addiction' became muddled saw the emergence of clear, accepted understandings of many diseases that had confused meanings for millennia: smallpox, tuberculosis, cholera, appendicitis, and so on (Starr, 1982). Along with clear definitions of these problems came accepted causal theories and effective means of control.

15 'Spirits' were distilled alcohol, in the form of whisky, gin, brandy, etc. At first, the temperance movement regarded wine and beer as acceptable alternatives to spirits, but this changed over the decades.

16 Cited in Levine (1984, p. 110).

17 Charles Dickens (1833–1835/1994), writing as a reporter under the pseudonym Boz, wrote a composite description in his article *The Drunkard's Death*. Some of the autobiographical descriptions of contemporary Canadian alcoholics in a recent book by Crozier and Lane (2001) seem to me quite similar.

18 The more common terms at first were 'inebriates', 'drunkards', 'sots', and the like, but 'addicts' gradually took their place and was used to describe the same people (Aaron and Musto, 1981, pp. 138–139). The word 'addiction' became the word to describe a degraded lifestyle in the temperance rhetoric at the same time that it was being accepted as the name of a disease by the medical profession. Alcoholism later became another name for the same disease.

19 Aaron and Musto (1981, pp. 145–157) point out that in the early American temperance movement there was considerable attention given to social causes as well, but as the 19th century proceeded, alcohol was more and more represented as the cause of all evil, and other social causes were ignored in the simplistic rhetoric of the National Prohibition Party and the Anti-Saloon League, which gained control of the temperance movement.

20 E. Murphy (1922/1973); Silver and Aldrich (1979).

21 E. Murphy (1922/1973); Carstairs (2006, Chapters 1 and 2).

22 Alexander (1990, Chapter 4); Carstairs (2006, Chapter 3).

23 Reinarman and Levine (1997, Chapter 1).

24 Armstrong (2004b); G. Smith (2004b); Hawthorn (2005).

25 Italics and uppercase in original.

26 The term 'drug-addiction' in this moralistic sense does not appear in the 1884 fascicule or in the main text of the 1928 edition. A form of it does appear in the 1933 *Supplement*.

27 Jaffe elaborated the phrase 'overwhelming involvement' as follows:

Addiction is thus viewed as an extreme on a continuum of involvement and refers ... to the degree to which drug use pervades the total life activity of the user and to the range of circumstances in which drug use controls his behavior.

Jaffe (1985, p. 533).

Although Jaffe, writing a chapter on 'drug addiction and drug abuse', clearly intended to limit addiction to overwhelming involvement with drugs, the phrase 'overwhelming involvement' is applied much more broadly in this book, in accordance with the traditional definition. Other modern authors have used similar language. For example, Chein *et al.* (1964, p. 26) used the phrase 'total personal involvement' in their classic study of heroin addiction.

28 P. Cohen (2004).

29 Coomber and South (2004).

30 See Felitti (2003) and Ganguly (2004) for recent examples.

31 I base this characterisation of the Canadian Addiction Survey on the 'Highlights' published in November 2004, which presented some data and contained a summary of the 'key objectives' of the survey on p. 2 (Canadian Centre on Substance Abuse, 2004). Further data in future reports may require that my characterisation be revised. However, the survey highlights were publicized, and no question was raised about the implicit definition of addiction (i.e. addiction$_2$) that was thus established. The alcohol use disorders identification test (AUDIT), is a ten-items subtest included in the Canadian Addiction Survey. Three of the ten items of this subtest could reasonably be judged as indicative of addiction$_1$. However, these three items were not reported separately. The AUDIT data were reported in terms of the percentage of subjects classified as passing the threshold for 'hazardous drinking', a threshold that could easily be passed without positive answers to any of the three items that are indicative of addiction$_1$.

32 Room (1998). DSM stands for the *Diagnostic and Statistical Manual of the Mental Disorders* (American Psychiatric Association, 1994, 2000).

33 The formal diagnostic algorithm in this document (American Psychiatric Association, 2000, p. 197) would probably apply the label of 'substance dependence' to most people who were addicted$_1$ to a drug (these people would probably fit criteria 5, 6, and 7) and to a great many more people who fit the definition of addiction$_2$ but not addiction$_1$. 'Substance abuse' as defined by DSM-IV would be applied to many people who fit the definition of addiction$_2$, but to none who fit the definition of addiction$_1$.

34 Orford (2001a) has made a good case for the term 'excessive appetites'.

35 See O'Brien (2001) and Reuters (2007). While not agreeing that addiction$_1$ is the only valid definition, Orford (2001a, Chapters 1–6) shows how the fear of using the term 'addiction' metaphorically still haunts the academic literature and also how definitions of addiction have been burdened by the expectation that they include something comparable to pharmacological tolerance and withdrawal symptoms. See also M.B. Walker (1992, pp. 171–189).

36 Coleman (2001).

37 Orford (2001a) provides an excellent summary of many conflicting definitions of addiction and of the issues that make the definitions appear irreconcilable.

38 The words 'disease' and 'disorder' are often contested in this context. However, that dispute is beyond the boundaries of this book.

39 ICD is shorthand for *The International Statistical Classification of Diseases and Related Health Problems* published by the World Health Organisation (2007). Unlike the ICD, the DSM is concerned only with mental disorders.

40 Room (1998). The unclarity the DSM-IV definition is obvious, even though the language is studiously crafted by expert committees. In solemn bureaucratese, the DSM-IV states, 'The essential feature of Substance Dependence is a cluster of cognitive, behavioural and physiological *symptoms* indicating that the individual continues use of the substance despite significant substance-related *problems*' (American Psychiatric Association, 2000,

p. 92, emphasis added). By itself, this cannot be adequate because many people act in ways that others label as 'symptoms' and use many substances despite 'significant problems'. Specifically what cluster of symptoms and what substance-related problems constitute addiction? The DSM-IV goes on to say that people can be formally diagnosed as 'substance dependent' if they meet any three of seven quite diverse criteria. In other words, one distressed drug user could be diagnosed as 'substance dependent' on the basis of three of the criteria, and a second could be so diagnosed on the basis of three entirely different ones. What would the two distressed drug users have in common that would make them 'substance dependent'? This kind of definition has an administrative utility, making it possible to define people as substance dependent or not according to an apparently impartial rule. However, it is impossible to extract a clear sense of what 'substance dependence' actually is from it.

41 Peele and Brodsky (1975) did the classic study on love addiction. See Orford (2001a, pp. 38 *et seq.*) for a review of the literature that established gambling as a treatable addiction in the decades following World War II. In the same book, Orford provides a valuable review of the literature on addiction to love and sex in this period (Chapter 6). Later studies amply confirmed the essential similarity of addiction to drug use on one hand and a great variety of pursuits that do not involve drugs on the other. See, as examples, Alexander and Schweighofer (1988); Shaffer *et al.* (1989); Alexander (1990); Lau (2001); Wiebe *et al.* (2001); Rabinor (2002); Fish (2004); and Faiola (2006).

Some people still believe, despite overwhelming evidence to the contrary, that addiction$_1$ is more dangerous than addictions$_3$ that do not involve alcohol or drugs because of the unique addictive potency of drugs like heroin, cocaine, and alcohol. Some of the evidence against this residual belief in demonic addictiveness of drugs is reviewed in Chapter 8 of this book.

42 Maté (2008, Chapter 20).

43 See, for example, Plato's description of 'the tyrannical personality' in the *Republic* (*c.* 360 BC/1987, Book 9), Aristotle's descriptions of 'incontinence' and 'vice' in the *Nichomachean Ethics* (*c.* 330 BC/1925, Book 7), or, eight centuries later, St Augustine's introspections on his own addictive sexuality in the *Confessions* (397 AD/1963). I have not studied aboriginal mythology or Asian classics, but I am told that both contain powerful images of addiction without reference to drugs. Such images are found in the 'Wendigo' myth of the Cree people and in classic works of the Indian subcontinent, the Mahabharata and the Ramayana (Savannah Walling, personal communication).

44 Blomqvist (2004, pp. 150–151).

45 Orford (2001a) has shown how the search for such dividing lines has only led to confusion.

46 For example, computer use provides many new opportunities for addiction$_3$ and the hopefully never-to-be-invented addiction$_5$. Full-blown cases of addiction$_3$ have come to light in which people have been lost to their families and to society because of their full-time commitment to computing activities including programming, computer games, pornography, Internet browsing, and blogging. These addicted$_3$ people are served by a new generation of addiction treatment centres and self-help groups that cater to their hi-tech addictions (Hafner, 2004; Kershaw, 2005). There are many other kinds of problems as well. For example, some people must spend such long hours working at the keyboard that they suffer from stress injuries.

Some people use the computer regularly to relieve the stains of non-cybernetic reality, and feel guilty about it. Problems like these are quite reasonably labelled an 'excessive appetite' because of their side effects, but not addiction$_3$ because they do not supplant a person's normal life.

47 Rather than addiction$_4$, Schaler (2000, pp. 5–6), for example, uses the phrase 'positive addiction' as I have in an earlier book (Alexander, 1990, Chapter 3). However, 'positive addiction' is more often used in a quite different sense to differentiate addictions that are said (wrongly) to be invariably beneficial, like running, from addictions that are said (wrongly) to be invariably harmful, like drug use.

48 Land (1971).

49 See the Christian webpage *Addicted to Jesus* (www.dokimos.org/addicted.html). A Google™ search of the words 'addicted to Jesus' will reveal other similar sites. On some Christian sites, the injunction to be addicted to Jesus does not use the actual word, although the meaning is evident. For example, some of these sites quote St Paul in saying: '*Be not drunk with wine, wherein is excess; but be filled with the Spirit*' (Ephesians 5:18).

50 This leads to the interesting question of whether or not addiction$_4$ to drugs is possible. It is not necessary to resolve this complex issue in this book, which is about addiction$_3$. However, I think addiction$_4$ to drugs does occur, although probably rarely. I have provided an example of addiction$_4$ to opium in an earlier publication (Alexander, 1990, p. 121; see also Westermeyer, 1982, pp. 140–144).

51 Alexander (2003a, b).

52 Csillag (2003); Hawthorn (2003).

53 For example, compare G. Smith (2004b) with Richer (2004). These two articles on the utterly vile consequences of becoming addicted to crystal meth and the delightful consequences of becoming addicted to an iPod both appeared in the same day's edition of the *Globe and Mail* newspaper.

54 Peele (1976).

55 Alexander and Schweighofer (1988).

56 Bailey and Elliot (2003); Thank Ha (2004); Picard (2005a).

57 Dobson (1995); Mickleburgh (2003b, c, d, e); Blatchford (2004). The four articles by Mickleburgh are reports of a recent murder trial in which a British Columbian man killed his six children and then attempted suicide in front of his wife who had been in the process of leaving him. All testimony indicated that he loved his wife and children deeply, but possessively and jealously. A great variety of psychological jargon was introduced in the courtroom testimony. In the context of this book, the term 'addiction' fits well. I have no desire to argue against the other psychological terms that were applied, however. My hope is to go beyond issues of jargon.

58 Picard (2002, 2004a); Kirkey (2007).

59 Zinberg (1984, p. 76).

60 D.F. Jacobs (1986), Bailey and Elliot (2003), Renzetti (2005b), Kirkey (2007), Maté (2008, Chapter 21).

61 National Institute on Drug Abuse (2002), Orford (2001a, pp. 68–74), Canadian Centre on Substance Abuse (2004, pp. 10–11), Volkow (2005). The use of tobacco in the Third World is expanding rapidly, although it has contracted somewhat in the developed world.

62 UK statistics analysed by De-Angelis *et al.* (2004), Dalrymple (2006a, p. 16), and Reuter and Stevens (2007, p.7). The number of registered drug users in China increased from 70,000 in 1990 to 1.16 million in 2005 (S. G. Sullivan & Wu, 2007). Most of the statistics do not separate out heroin users who are addicted from those who are not. However, a substantial proportion of heroin users in every country are likely to be addicted, because heroin is used everywhere as a drug of addiction.

63 Plant and Plant (2006, Chapter 2). Although it is impossible to know how many binge drinkers are actually alcohol addicts₃, the fact that alcohol-related liver disease, mortality, and psychiatric problems are all increasing rapidly (Plant & Plant, 2006, pp. 37, 69–70) suggests that many are. See also Newland (2007).

64 Shewan and Dalgarno (2005); Fischer *et al.* (2006).

65 Barron (2003); Meier (2007).

66 Peele and Brodsky (1975); Hatterer (1980); Orford (1985, 2001a); Alexander (1982; 1990, Chapter 7); Woodman (1982); D.F. Jacobs (1986); Arterburn and Felton (1991); Killinger (1991); Dobson (1995); Hodge *et al.* (1997); Greenfield (1999); Maté (2000; 2008, Chapters 9 and 10); Rabinor (2002); Young (2004); Kirkey (2007). In addition to case studies, Hatterer (1980) provides an extensive bibliography of scholarly and popular works on addictive use of food, sex, work, and gambling that were published before 1980.

67 Pearson (1995); Lau (2001); deGraaf *et al.* (2002, Chapter 13); S.A. Miller (2002); Priest (2002); Armstrong (2003a); Chaker (2003); Gartner (2003); Harmon (2003); Spears (2003); Vermond (2003); Anderssen (2004a); Hafner (2004); Valpy (2004a); I. Brown (2005b); Kershaw (2005); Renzetti (2005b); Sutherland (2005); Mickleburgh (2006b); C. Reynolds (2006); Schick (2007).

68 At least one serious 12-step organisation is Google™-able for most letters of the alphabet. See Wikipedia for an incomplete list of 49 different organisations (http://en.wikipedia.org/wiki/List_of_Twelve-Step_groups). Some websites devoted to blogging addiction are meant to be humorous, but some are quite serious and are based on the same 12-step model as AA.

69 http://www.slaacincinnati.org/characteristics.htm

70 Overcoming addictions that do or do not involve drugs is the main topic of the following books: B. Perkins (1991); LeVert and McClain (1998); LeSourd (2002); J. Wright (2003). There is another type of book that provides methods for recovery from a large variety of personal problems, of which addiction is explicitly mentioned as one; for example Vanier (1998, p. 113) and T. Moore (1992).

71 Becker (2007); Kubey and Csikszentmihalyi (2002); Young (2004); Thorsen (2005); C. Reynolds (2006); EverQuest Widows (2007).

72 Das (1998); Atkins (2002). Dr Atkins shows how people's eating fits the definition of addiction₃. He proposes a metabolic explanation for the addiction that seems to me as plausible as the neurochemical explanations for heroin and cocaine addiction that are briefly discussed in Chapter 8 of this book (see Atkins, 2002, pp. 200–201).

73 Alexander and Schweighofer (1988); M.B. Walker (1992); Orford (2001a, pp. 48–53); Wiebe *et al.* (2001); Papineau (2005).

74 Putnam (2000).

75 Lieberman and Snowdon (1993); Putnam (2000).

76 Orford (2001a, Chapter 5).

77 W.R. Miller *et al.* (1995).

78 References appear in endnote 71 in this chapter.

79 On-Line Gamers Anonymous (2007). EverQuest Widows (2007) is one of many other self-help sites. Its users are wives of players of a single popular game.

80 For the increasing prevalence of depression see M. Wilson *et al.* (2000), Dufour (2003a, pp. 110–112), Galloway (2004), Galt (2004a) and Homer-Dixon (2006). It is hard to measure the rate of growth of depression accurately, notwithstanding the existence of excellent quantitative studies (Cross-National Collaborative Group, 1992). The real growth rate is augmented by the highly successful, often unscrupulous, marketing campaign for

anti-depressants, especially after the release of SSRIs in the 1980s (see Breggin, 1994; Healy, 2003). Although there are some quantitative studies that purport to show that the prevalence of depression is actually not increasing (J. Murphy *et al.*, 2000), I am convinced by friends and relatives that most people who are diagnosed as depressed are not victims of seductive marketing. I have not used anti-depressant medication myself, but several close friends or relatives have used it and plan to continue (four use SSRI anti-depressants daily, one uses marijuana daily for the same purpose). All of these people are admirably independent thinkers, who would never fall victim to seductive advertising. All detest being dependent on a drug and being implicitly labelled as having a form of mental illness. Yet all have told me of reaching points in their lives where they could not continue to function without going on an anti-depressant regime. The alternative would have been incapacitating despair or suicide. For the overlap between depression and chronic fatigue syndrome, see Center for Disease Control and Prevention (2005).

81 As examples, see Mays (1999) and Wild *et al.* (2005).

82 Kessler (2001); DeGrandpre (2006, Chapter 3).

83 McArthur and Pitts (2003); Snyder (2003); Timson (2003).

84 Clinton (1997); Steel and Trieu (1997).

85 Malhotra-Singh (2002); Jong-Fast (2006).

86 Jonnes (2002).

87 Shewan and Dalgarno (2005); Warburton *et al.* (2005).

88 My favourite example is the American cartoon 'Cathy', by Cathy Guisewite.

89 Goldman (1981); B. Woodward (1984); Crosbie (2003a, b); Williamson (2003); *Globe and Mail* (2004a).

90 Issachar (2001); *Modern Drunkard Magazine Online* (n.d.).

91 Mingo *et al.* (1985); Fenwick (2004).

92 Rabinor (2002).

93 Norris *et al.* (2006); Shimo (2006).

94 Intelm (2006). Extraordinary capitalisation and punctuation in original text.

95 Dineen (1998); Peele and Butler (2006).

96 Trebach (1987); Alexander (1990, pp. 72–73); Schaler (2000, pp. 41–44); Szalavitz (2007).

97 Peele (1989).

98 Alsop (1974), Health and Welfare Canada (1984), Musto (1987, Chapter 1), D.E. Weissman and Haddox (1989).

99 This is notoriously true in developing countries where 'Pain relief hasn't been given as much attention as the War on Drugs has' (McNeil, 2007).

100 D.E. Weissman and Haddox (1989); Porter-Williamson *et al.* (2003).

101 Brown-Bowers (2007).

102 Zinberg and Lewis (1964); Lindesmith (1968, Chapter 3); Penfield (1969); Brecher (1972); McLellan and Weisner (1996); Sullum (2003, pp. 42–46); Warburton *et al.* (2005); DeGrandpre (2006, Chapters 3 and 4); Gzoski (2006). Westermeyer (1982, pp. 140–144) has provided a particularly poignant example of a lifetime of non-addicted₃ opium use.

103 Penfield (1969).

104 DeGrandpre (2006, Chapter 1).

105 L. Slater (2007).

106 Chein *et al.* (1964, pp. 22–29); Lindesmith (1968, Chapter 3); E. H. Kaplan and Wieder (1974, pp. 45–46); Jaffe (1985, pp. 532–533); Musto (1987, pp. 123–124, 318 note 3);

Alexander (1990, Chapter 3), P. Hoffman (1998); Shewan and Dalgarno (2005); Warburton *et al.* (2005); DeGrandpre (2006, Chapters 3 and 4).

107 DeGrandpre (1999); Alexander and Tsou (2001); T. Clark (2004); Kolata (2004); Picard (2004b, 2005e); Abraham (2005); Ubelacker (2005b).

108 Lindesmith (1968, Chapter 3) and Jaffe (1985, pp. 532–533) discuss some of the names that have been proposed.

109 *Oxford English Dictionary* (1989). See definition 2 for the word 'dependence'.

110 A similar radical change in meaning is currently underway with the word 'binge' (Plant & Plant, 2006, pp. viii–xii). When people are comfortable with a well-established meaning of a word that is abruptly changed by professional fiat or political enthusiasm, the charge of 'kidnapping' does not seem to me too strong.

111 Alexander and Tsou (2001); McNeil (2007).

112 Brecher (1972); Musto (1987, Chapter 6); Carstairs (2006, Chapter 5). In many cases, the drugs that doctors have been prosecuted for prescribing are not the most infamous prohibited drugs (e.g. cocaine), but others that are pharmacologically equivalent (e.g. Ritalin®, generically methylphenidate) and are also prohibited (Beyerstein & Alexander, 1985; Libby, 2005).

113 *Vancouver Sun* (2007).

114 See Davidson (1964) for a beautifully written case study.

115 L. Slater (1998, esp. pp. 177–200).

116 Brecher (1972).

117 Brown-Bowers (2007).

118 It seems possible to me that addiction$_2$ can be encompassed within a 'model' of 'excessive appetites' that incorporates a variety of processes. Such a model has been proposed by Orford (2001a, b) who also extends the range of addiction$_1$ and addiction$_2$ beyond alcohol and drugs to gambling, sexuality, eating, and exercising, but rules out most of the other addictions that I have included in addiction$_3$.

Chapter 3

The Dislocation Theory of Addiction

The nightmarish transformation of a familiar person into the slave of a destructive habit cries out for explanation. However, no consensus on the cause of the continuing spread of addiction₁ or addiction₃ has grown out of the conventional wisdom on addiction, even though hundreds of explanatory theories have been proposed by talented therapists and researchers during the past two centuries and by theologians and philosophers in the centuries before that.[1] These theories or 'models' of addiction conflict in every imaginable way,[2] and yet they all threaten to live forever, since they can be neither proved nor disproved. Moreover, none of them has generated an effective method of preventing the continuing spread of addiction or of treating individual cases successfully. This impasse does not prevent some true believers from trumpeting that their theory alone is 'scientific' or 'evidence-based'. Meanwhile, the problem of addiction continues to expand globally. We stand individually adamant but collectively flummoxed.

Under these conditions, theoretical discussions of addiction often feel less like scholarly collaboration than holy wars between champions of diverse philosophical, scientific, and spiritual assumptions that underlie the conflicting theories.[3] Some of the underlying assumptions will be examined in Part II of this book. For now, it is enough to acknowledge that it is foolhardy for anybody, myself included, to claim objectivity. Some scholars avoid the holy wars by arguing that all of the logically conflicting theories can be true at the same time, but this good-natured eclecticism can never generate a concise and coherent explanation of addiction.

This situation is muddled and chaotic, but it is not hopeless. Standing apart from the theoretical mêlée in the field of addictions, historians quite often agree on the cause of addiction when they encounter it in a particular historical context. In fact, historical scholarship seems to lead naturally and easily to a promising understanding of addiction in the modern world, which—I dare to hope—may become the basis for consensus in the 21st century. Therefore, this chapter formalises the insights that have emerged from historical research in the form of a compact 'dislocation theory of addiction'.

The dislocation theory of addiction

Why are so many people dangerously addicted to destructive habits in the globalising world of the 21st century? Why does the range of addictions now extend far beyond alcohol and drug use to gambling, shopping, dysfunctional love relationships, video gaming, religious zealotry, television viewing, Internet surfing, maintaining an emaciated body shape, and so on? Why has scientific medicine, a dazzling success in so many domains, made so little progress with addiction? These questions, and many others, can be answered on the basis of three principles that emerge from a historical perspective. All three principles are explained briefly in this chapter in order to present the entire theory in a compact form. A fuller explanation of each principle and its supporting evidence follows in Chapters 4–8.

Psychosocial integration is a necessity

'Psychosocial integration' is a profound interdependence between individual and society that normally grows and develops throughout each person's lifespan. Psychosocial integration reconciles people's vital needs for social belonging with their equally vital needs for individual autonomy and achievement. Psychosocial integration is as much an inward experience of identity and meaning as a set of outward social relationships. An enduring lack of psychosocial integration, which is called 'dislocation' in this book, is both individually painful and socially destructive.

Human beings are not psychologically self-sufficient. From early childhood until old age, individuals in every culture devote themselves to establishing and maintaining a place in their society. In a complementary manner, society's subgroups and institutions, starting with the family, open their doors to maturing individuals at appropriate stages of development. These subgroups give as much latitude as they can to individuals' unique preferences and needs for autonomy, but always within limits that allow each subgroup to carry out its essential economic and social functions. Following Erik Erikson,[4] this complex, ever-changing state of interdependence is called 'psychosocial integration' in this book.[5]

Although psychosocial integration denotes interdependence between a person and a society, it is experienced on several other levels as well. Psychosocial integration is experienced as a sense of identity, because stable social relationships provide people with a set of duties and privileges that define who they are in their own minds. It is experienced as a sense of oneness with nature, because members of viable societies share and reinforce a conceptualisation of their society's place in the natural world. It is quite often experienced as connection with the divine, because members of viable societies usually share a way of understanding the unseen world beyond mundane space and time that surrounds their social world.[6]

The use of the word 'soul' has been banned from the social sciences because it implies immortality in Christian theology. Yet 'soul' has a way of doggedly creeping back into the conversation. For example, Karl Polanyi pointed out that, 'The discovery of the individual soul is the discovery of community ... Each is implied by the other.'[7] Polanyi, an economic historian, recognised that the individual's soul is as essential part of the experience of psychosocial integration of individuals in their communities. The word 'soul' is used in this psychosocial sense in the remainder of this book, without implying anything whatsoever about immortality.

Erik Erikson and Karl Polanyi were not alone in recognising the necessity of integrating social belonging and individual autonomy for the achievement of human wholeness. This central fact of human nature has been recognised by countless other great thinkers as well, notably Plato,[8] Charles Darwin,[9] Peter Kropotkin,[10] Alfred Adler,[11] and Erich Fromm.[12] The importance of this fact is acknowledged by many contemporary social scientists[13] who use a great variety of alternate names for psychosocial integration, such as 'belonging', 'community', 'wholeness', 'social cohesion', or simply 'culture'. Most of these terms could be used interchangeably with 'psychosocial integration'.[14]

In today's Vancouver, the subgroups and institutions that provide the bases for psychosocial integration typically include nuclear families, children's play groups, schools, employment groups, sports teams, informal friendship groups, and various neighbourhood, recreational, ethnic, religious, or nationalistic organisations. These subgroups and institutions often have short lives and conflicting values, making psychosocial integration a difficult, often precarious, achievement. In the aboriginal culture that existed only 150 years earlier where Vancouver now stands, the list of subgroups was quite different. As well as nuclear families, it included long-dead ancestors, a large extended family, the village of birth, aboriginal social classes, gender groups, and clans that extended beyond the village and family. Because the subgroups all grew from a relatively stable and internally consistent aboriginal tradition, attaining psychosocial integration was far less difficult.[15]

Apart from these differences, the process of achieving psychosocial integration would be fundamentally the same in contemporary and traditional cultures[16] and equally essential in both. Establishing the delicate interpenetration of person and society enables each person to satisfy simultaneously both individualistic needs and needs for community—to be free and still belong. It enables society to benefit simultaneously from the diverse, creative abilities of its individual members and still maintain order and collective purpose.[17] Psychosocial integration makes human life bearable, and even joyful at its peaks.[18] Moreover, it is a key to the success of the human species, which flourished by simultaneously evolving close cooperation and individual creativity.

Lack or loss of psychosocial integration was called 'dislocation' by Karl Polanyi. Dislocation, in this broad sense of the word, does not necessarily imply geographic separation. Rather, it denotes psychological and social separation from one's society, which can befall people who never leave home, as well as those who have been geographically displaced.[19] Like psychosocial integration, dislocation has been given many names,[20] perhaps the most familiar being 'alienation' or 'disconnection'. However, in this book, the term 'dislocation' is used exclusively. It refers to an enduring lack of psychosocial integration, no matter how it comes about.

People can endure dislocation for a time. However, severe, prolonged dislocation eventually leads to unbearable despair, shame, emotional anguish, boredom, and bewilderment. It regularly precipitates suicide[21] and less direct forms of self-destruction.[22] This is why forced dislocation, in the form of ostracism, excommunication, exile, and solitary confinement, has been a dreaded punishment from ancient times until the present. Solitary confinement is an essential part of the most sophisticated modern technologies of torture.[23]

Material poverty frequently accompanies dislocation, but they are definitely not the same thing. Although material poverty can crush the spirit of isolated individuals and families, it can be borne with dignity by people who face it together as an integrated society. On the other hand, people who have lost their psychosocial integration are demoralised and degraded even if they are not materially poor. Neither food, nor shelter, nor the attainment of wealth can restore them to well-being. Only psychosocial integration itself can do that.[24] In contrast to material poverty, dislocation could be called 'poverty of the spirit'.[25] This phrase is suggested by Jesus' words in the Beatitudes, 'Blessed are the poor in spirit, for theirs is the kingdom of heaven.'[26] These words did not promise material wealth to the demoralised and degraded Galilean subjects of the brutal Roman empire, but rather a spiritual community to which they could truly belong, for it is 'theirs'. (This understanding of the Beatitudes is shared by many contemporary Christians,[27] although, like most biblical phrases, this one is subject to a variety of interpretations.)

Dislocation can have many causes. For example, it can arise from an earthquake that destroys a village or from an individual idiosyncrasy that a society cannot tolerate. It can be inflicted violently by abusing a child, ostracising an adult, or destroying a culture. It can be inflicted with the best of intentions, by inculcating an unrealistic sense of superiority that makes a child insufferable to others or by flooding a local society with cheap manufactured products that destroy its economic basis. It can be chosen voluntarily if a person is drawn from social life into the single-minded pursuit of wealth in a 'gold rush' or a 'window of opportunity'. Most importantly for this book, dislocation can become the norm if a society systematically curtails psychosocial integration in all of its members. If the dislocation theory of addiction is correct, there are billions of severely dislocated people in today's world, because dislocation is inseparable from the free-market society that is being globalised.

Globalising free-market society undermines psychosocial integration

Whereas individual people can become dislocated by misfortunes in any society, including tribal, feudal, and socialist ones, and whereas the downfall of any society produces mass dislocation, only free-market society produces mass dislocation as part of its normal functioning even during periods of prosperity. Along with dazzling benefits in innovation and productivity, globalisation of free-market society has produced an unprecedented, worldwide collapse of psychosocial integration.

A free-market society is a social system in which virtually every aspect of human existence is embedded within, and shaped by, minimally regulated competitive markets. This sort of social system would have been inconceivable a few centuries ago,[28] but it is fast becoming a planetary standard.

The fundamental promise of free-market economics is that free markets based on intense, unrelenting individual competition maximise everybody's well-being in the long run, multiplying individual happiness and the 'wealth of nations'.[29] The ideal that gradually emerged from this promise is that free, competitive markets must dominate every possible aspect of human life and that the only really important functions of government are to maintain the efficiency of markets and to help them grow. Laws should function, for example, to protect private ownership and enforce the fulfilment of contracts, but not to provide a safety net for those who become ill or cannot find employment. Public expenditure is necessary to provide the infrastructure for economic development, but not to maintain communities that are torn apart by market forces. Although this free-market ideal has proven to be only partly attainable, and although there have been halts, reversals, and powerful countercurrents,[30] the free-market imperative has been expanding and consolidating its hold on every aspect of people's lives around the globe for the last few centuries while the corporations that dominate the markets have grown ever larger and less subject to local restraints.[31] Globalisation involves much more than an economic system of course, but free-market economics is at the heart of it.[32]

Along with its dazzling benefits, the global movement towards free-market society has costs, one of which is the destruction of psychosocial integration. The destruction of psychosocial integration is shockingly obvious in the homeless, the physically violated, and the destitute, but this book will show that it affects the protected, safe, and wealthy with a similar force. To the degree that labour, land, credit, goods, education, medicine, entertainment, etc. are traded in free, competitive markets, dislocation becomes inevitable for everybody. This is because competitive free markets work efficiently only if each buyer and seller takes the role of an individual economic actor, pursuing his or her individual enrichment—however he or she individually defines it—competitively and acquisitively. This economic individualism allows the law of supply and demand to work its magic. Adam Smith's 'invisible hand' will bring the beneficence of the market to all, but only if they remember that 'business is business' and that they must always 'think for themselves'. People can only be this individualistic when they are unencumbered by loyalties to their family, friends, traditional obligations, customs, trade unions, or guilds. Acting on traditional loyalties is criminal or unethical in free-market society because it constitutes nepotism, favouritism, or discrimination. Nor can people in a free-market society be encumbered by the transcendental values of a religion, culture, ethnic group, or nation.[33] As a single, classic example, the free market in labour, in its original form, used the threat of starvation to force masses of people into tedious, meaningless toil in factories. Forms of society that guaranteed that whatever food there was would be shared by all had to be destroyed so that the market could supply the labour needs of the free-market society.[34] In a similar way, traditional sources of psychosocial integration in every type of society came to be identified as 'market distortions' that had to be eliminated.[35]

For these reasons, the ideal form of free-market society would inevitably create universal dislocation.[36] Although today's global society falls glaringly short of the ideal form of free-market society in many ways,[37] none of the deviations from the free-market ideal, including government subsidies and bailouts, corporate collusion, vast transnational conglomerates, non-compete agreements, or widespread corruption decrease the dislocation that globalising society imposes on most people most of the time. Even where supposed free-market society falls scandalously short of the free-market ideal, governments and corporation leaders strive to impose 'market discipline' on their underlings—and sometimes on themselves—in the name of the ideal.[38]

To the degree that Western civilisation approximates a free-market society, dislocation is not the pathological state of a few but the general condition. Because the expanding reach of free-market economics engulfs ever more aspects of life, dislocation is increasing. Because dislocation makes parents desperate and families dysfunctional in Western society, it affects children as much as it affects adults who participate directly in commerce. Because Western free-market society provides the model for globalisation, dislocation is being globalised along with the Internet, the English language, and Mickey Mouse.[39]

The complex history of dislocation and addiction in former socialist societies like China and the USSR provide crucial cases for the dislocation theory of addiction to explain, and they will be discussed in Chapter 6. However, the dislocation theory primarily concerns the way that free-market society generates mass dislocation, without intending to deny that other kinds of society engender problems of their own.

Addiction$_3$ is a way of adapting to sustained dislocation

However dislocation comes about, it provokes a desperate response. Dislocated people struggle valiantly to establish or restore psychosocial integration—to somehow 'get a life', to 'figure out who they are', or to 'build community'. Many eventually achieve a sufficient degree of psychosocial integration. However, those who do not often adapt to the anguish of sustained dislocation by devoting themselves to narrow lifestyles that function as substitutes for psychosocial integration. Individually, these substitute lifestyles have distinct names: junkie, miser, shopaholic, workaholic, crackhead, alcoholic, religious zealot, anorexic, bulimic, etc. Collectively, they make up addiction$_3$. Addiction$_3$ is neither a disease nor a moral failure, but a narrowly focused lifestyle that functions as a meagre substitute for people who desperately lack psychosocial integration.

Even the most harmful[40] addictions serve a vital adaptive function for dislocated individuals. For example, the barren pleasures of a junkie—membership of a drug-injecting subculture with a powerful mystique, transient relief from pain, the excitement of petty crime—are more sustaining than the unrelenting torment of social exclusion and aimlessness.[41] At the other end of the social hierarchy, endlessly amassing expensive merchandise and organising it for display and consumption provides an equally narrow sense of meaning for affluent North Americans bereft of richer purposes, reaching grotesque 'shopaholic' proportions in some of them.[42] Religious or political fanaticism provides a sense of belonging and purity for people whose sacred traditions have been profaned beyond recovery.[43] 'Co-dependent relationships' and addictive ties to 'dysfunctional families' provide emotionally captivating substitutes for a network of healthy relationships.[44] Devotion to a violent youth gang, harmful as it is to society and, often, to the gang member's own values, is more endurable for many school dropouts than no identity at all.[45] Addictions$_3$ often serve other functions simultaneously, but their *raison d'être* is to substitute for psychosocial integration.

Addictions may endure for days, for years, or for a lifetime, but they are not sufficiently close, stable, or complex to afford a complete substitute for psychosocial integration. Nevertheless, people for whom addiction is the most achievable substitute for psychosocial integration cling to their addictions with grim resolution, despite the harm that follows. Often they flatly deny the harm, despite the most obvious evidence. Often they appear insatiable. Without their addictions, they would have terrifyingly little reason to live.

To say that an addiction is 'adaptive' is not to imply that it is *desirable*, either for the addicted person or for society, but only that, as a lesser evil, it may buffer a person against the greater evil of unbearable dislocation. Addictions₃ do not have the depth or breadth to produce 'wholeness' (a term Erikson used interchangeably with psychosocial integration) and so addicted people do not find the contentment they are seeking. In their futile attempts to achieve psychosocial integration by narrowing their lives, addicted people often exacerbate their own dislocation; for example, by stigmatising themselves, by ruining their health, or by irrevocably alienating the people who care most about them.

It is possible to dream that society will benefit from the insatiability that comes with addiction through the brilliant achievements of addictively competitive Chief Executive Officers (CEOs),[46] the economic stimulus of addictively spending consumers, and huge government revenues from those who pour their livelihoods into slot machines and lotteries. However, such dreams pale in the face of the long-range costs of corporate and government corruption, stress diseases, family devastation, environmental destruction, and so on. Nevertheless, corporations compete by systematically encouraging addictive consumption in their customers and addictive work habits in their employees, thus acting as 'pushers' for the most common addictive habits of our times. Their incessant advertising lulls us in our pallid dream.

At best, addictions can be narrowly creative and marginally socially acceptable, as in the case of some bohemian artists, high-tech wizards, or brilliant mathematicians.[47] More usually, however, addictions are banal and harmful, as in the case of a thieving street junkie; an irresponsible alcoholic; a youth ready to kill or be killed for his gang; a driven, ruthless CEO; a compulsive 'consumer' who bankrupts his or her family and depletes irreplaceable resources; or a religious or political fanatic, willing to kill indiscriminately for the cause. Often addicted people concoct unique combinations of addictive pursuits, far more complex than the familiar ones described here.

Only chronically and severely dislocated people are vulnerable to addiction.[48] Why would anybody who was not suffering from an agonising lack of psychosocial integration ever devote his or her life to a narrow, dangerous, offensive lifestyle?[49]

The question above expresses one of the psychological assumptions upon which this book is based. People generally behave adaptively, both in an evolutionary sense and in a psychological sense. In an evolutionary sense, this assumption means that people act in ways that have promoted inclusive fitness during the long evolutionary history of the human species. These ways of acting are likely to be beneficial in the present as well. In a psychological sense, this assumption means that people generally act both in their own personal interest and in the interest of the other people that they care about. There are exceptions, but, at least for biologists, the burden of proof is always upon those who claim that a behaviour that is widespread throughout a species is maladaptive,[50] since this is not the normal expectation.

Since the 19th century, however, the conventional wisdom has consistently viewed addiction as maladaptive and explained it with malign hidden causes like loss of will power to 'addictive drugs', unconscious fixations of the libido, deficiencies in the brain reward system,[51] neural sensitisation to the reinforcing effects of drugs,[52] and genes for addiction[53]—or some combination of these. But theories based on these hidden causes have failed to generate either a generally believable account of addiction or anything more than marginally effective forms of therapy.[54] A reasonable conclusion after more than a century of frustrated searching for the hidden underlying disorder is that it does not exist. Addiction is, in fact, *not* maladaptive for growing numbers of people under the dislocating conditions of our era. *There is no underlying disorder.*

Although only dislocated people become addicted, many severely dislocated people live and die in ways that cannot be called 'addiction' without stretching the word too thin. Many of them 'get by' by dint of admirable resolution and a little help from their friends. Others may become depressed, suicidal, apathetic, murderous, or mentally erratic, rather than addicted.[55] Thus, dislocation is a necessary, but not sufficient, cause of addiction.

As a person in any society can become dislocated, addiction can occur anywhere and at any time in history. For example, descriptions of the scandalous addictions of some Roman emperors document the presence of addiction throughout the Roman empire, centuries before its collapse.[56] However, the only accounts of addiction$_3$ as a universal condition that I have found prior to the era of free-market society were written by Plato[57] during the collapse of the Athenian Empire and St Augustine[58] during the collapse of the western Roman Empire. In both cases, the collapsing empire was demoralised and chaotic, producing universal dislocation. Both Plato's and St Augustine's accounts will be described in Part II of this book.

As psychosocial integration is a fundamental human need, and free-market society, by its nature, produces mass dislocation at all times (not just during times of collapse), and as addiction is the predominant way of adapting to dislocation, addiction is endemic and spreading fast. Free-market society can no more be addiction-free than it can be free of intense competition, income disparity, environmental destruction, unequal access to life-saving medical care, or dishonest business practices.[59] There can be no 'technical fix' or 'market solution' for problems that are built into the structure of society itself. Instead, today's society must either modify its free-market structure enough to keep its side effects under control or watch these side effects continue to spread.[60]

Society obviously is not going to revert to tribalism or embrace socialism in the 21st century. My aim is not to reverse the course of time, but to describe the origins of the present proliferation of addiction in the globalisation of free-market society. I hope to show by the end of this book that this knowledge can point society towards effective ways of dealing with addiction in the future on personal, professional, and social levels.

The dislocation theory in historical context

Although some of the theories of addiction that grew out of the conventional wisdom on addiction during the last couple of centuries have stirred up public enthusiasm for a time, none of them has led to a settled, consensual understanding of addiction, or to an effective means of controlling its spread. The dislocation theory is intended to replace most of them. When conventional wisdom in any field proves unfruitful over an extended period, paradigms must shift.[61]

Beyond spawning a throng of ineffectual theories, the conventional wisdom rests on dubious assumptions drawn from scientific medicine and Christian theology. One major assumption is that the cause of addiction lies most fundamentally within the addicted individual—addiction is either a disease of excessive drug consumption or a sinful form of drug consumption, or both.[62] Addiction can only be remedied by restoring the addicted individual, medically or morally, or both,[63] with care always taken to avoid the error of blaming society for the person's illness or weakness. Another major assumption of the conventional wisdom is that drug addiction is the prototypical addiction, with alcohol being one of the so-called addictive drugs. Simultaneously with individual interventions and scientific research, the conventional wisdom envisions a perpetual war on drug traffickers, because intrinsically addictive drugs are a menace to civilisation and because traffickers are the most corrupt type of human beings. The historical perspective from which the dislocation theory is derived contradicts this conventional perspective in every regard.

Although the dislocation theory shares none of these conventional assumptions, it is not new. Rather, it is a formalisation of some ideas rooted in the classical philosophy of Western civilisation,[64] but previously recognised only by a small number of writers on addiction.[65] The most important classical source is Plato's *Republic* (to be discussed in Chapter 13). The most important sources within contemporary social science theory are Erik Erikson's anthropological psychology and Karl Polanyi's political economics, both of which were developed in the mid-20th century. Primary 20th century sources in the addiction literature are *The Road to H*, a study of young heroin addicts in New York City by Isidor Chein and his colleagues,[66] *Love and Addiction* by Stanton Peele and Archie Brodsky,[67] and *Excessive Appetites* by Jim Orford.[68] The central ideas of the dislocation theory can also be traced back to the temperance movement early in the 1800s, before temperance ideology was reduced to the simplistic proposition that alcohol was the only important cause of alcohol addiction.[69]

Erikson's cross-cultural and psychoanalytic research is the single most important predecessor to this book. Erikson did not use the word 'addiction' in the way this book does, because he wrote in the psychoanalytic vocabulary of half a century ago when the word 'addiction' meant addiction$_1$. As a neo-Freudian, Erikson was obliged to discuss the then-conventional psychoanalytic idea that addiction$_1$ is the outcome of incomplete resolution of the tensions of the oral stage of development, but he gave the distinct impression of not taking this idea seriously.[70] On the other hand, Erikson was quite serious in his discussion of the relationship between prolonged failure of psychosocial integration among adolescents and what he called 'negative identity', which is essentially the same thing as addiction$_3$. For example:

> Youth sometimes prefers to be nothing, and that totally, rather than remain a contradictory bundle of identity fragments ... an almost wilful *Umschaltung* to a negative identity ... prevails in the delinquent (addictive ...[71]) youth of our larger cities, where conditions of economic, ethnic, and religious marginality provide poor bases for any kind of positive identity.[72]

Although this quotation concerns 'youth', Erikson's theory is not limited to problems of the teenage years. Instead, it describes the continuing challenges to psychosocial integration or the progress of ego development that begin in early childhood and persist until old age.[73] Dislocation can occur at any time during the life cycle and therefore addiction can become a substitute for psychosocial integration at almost any age. A number of scholars have used Erikson's analysis as the basis of their own understandings of addiction, which are generally in accord with the dislocation theory.[74]

The dislocation theory is not confined to the academic literature. Outside the received economics of free-market society and the conventional wisdom on addiction, variations of the idea have a role in everyday discussions and written culture, particularly through the books of popular sociologists and historians[75] and some books on 'pop psychology'.[76]

Boundaries of the dislocation theory

All theories have a limited domain of application. The dislocation theory is less limited than many theories of addiction, however, because it applies to any addiction whatsoever, from alcohol to zealotry. Moreover, it is not limited by the assumption that drug addiction is the prototypical form, and that addiction must, therefore, involve some type of withdrawal symptoms, tolerance, or dopamine depletion. As it does not medicalise addiction, it is not limited to addictions that have crossed a nebulous line between those that are socially acceptable and those that seem to require treatment. Finally, although it pays special attention to the role of free-market society as a cause of dislocation in the globalising world, it is a theory that can be applied anywhere that addiction is found.

On the other hand, the dislocation theory is bounded in several ways. Most importantly, it is only a theory of addiction$_3$ (and, secondarily addiction$_1$). The dislocation theory is not intended to explain most recreational, cultural, ritualistic, or therapeutic use of psychoactive drugs. People use drugs for pleasure and to cope with stress of all sorts, but it is only that minority of drug users who become overwhelmingly involved with their drugs in a destructive way who are included within the scope of the dislocation theory. Because the dislocation theory is not a theory of addiction$_2$, it does not address the 'drug problem', but, rather, the 'addiction problem'. And, because the dislocation theory is not a theory of addiction$_4$, it does not explain the lives of heroes or saints, although it may offer some insights into them.

Another boundary is that the dislocation theory does not explain why some dislocated people become addicted$_3$ to a particular habit or pursuit, whereas other equally dislocated people regard that habit with revulsion while becoming addicted to a different one. The dislocation theory cannot solve this riddle because the answer does not appear to lie in a difference in kind or degree of dislocation.

Part of the solution may be that people who are drowning in a flood of dislocation clutch desperately at any bit of flotsam that will save their life. They would be expected to hold on for dear life to the first addiction that will keep them afloat, ignoring all others. However, this primacy explanation for people's choice of addictions is not fully adequate, because many affluent people in free-market society have an opportunity to select among many addictive possibilities, for example between gambling, overeating, drugs, alcohol, computer games, and dysfunctional love relationships. Having chosen, they have time and opportunity to experiment freely and to change their mind and choose a different one. Yet, they tend to make consistent choices, often angrily disdaining other people's addictions, just as others disdain theirs. Such people's addictive choices seem somehow to fit their personalities, rather than resulting from fixations upon whatever happens to pass by in a desperately dislocated moment.

Erik Erikson provided a more complete explanation of the choice of addictions in an article first published in 1946.[77] In the diagnostic language of that era, he described his patients' 'compulsions' and 'neurotic fixations',[78] many of which comprised addiction$_3$ in the language of this book. In many cases, he traced the origins of the addiction to the *fragmentation of identity* (one aspect of dislocation in the language of this book) that came from immigration of European refugees to the United States before and after World War II, and the subsequent conflict between the powerful identities of European, American, and Jewish cultures. He traced the particular 'compulsions' that individual patients adopted to particular elements of the old culture that had to be repressed or thwarted in that person's attempt to achieve psychosocial integration in the new world. The repressed elements of cultural identity that re-emerged in addictive form were sometimes inculcated by experience in childhood in the 'old country', and sometimes inculcated unconsciously by parents from the old country as they struggled to raise their children in the new world.

Erikson's complex insights would suggest that Sigmund Freud may deserve the last word here. Why a dislocated person becomes addicted to a particular habit and not to some other can perhaps best be determined by searching the dark recesses of his or her unconscious and applying the abstruse symbolic equations of psychoanalytic theory.

The greatest limitation of the dislocation theory is that it cannot explain why one dislocated person becomes addicted and eventually meets a tragic end whereas another similarly dislocated person gradually overcomes his or her handicaps and builds a stable, satisfying life of psychosocial integration and lives to share it with his or her grandchildren. My experience of watching people grow up is that reaching, or failing to reach, the invisible threshold that begins a stable life of psychosocial integration is a matter of scant inches, even though the consequences are immense. Predicting which of a group of children with similar backgrounds will reach this threshold is as difficult as predicting which of a group of university students will accumulate a high enough grade point average to enter medical school and which ones will miss this goal by a point or two and have entirely different lives as a consequence. The difference between those who reach the threshold and those who do not is tiny, like the difference between people who fall off a cliff and people who teeter on the edge but manage to recover their balance. People in free-market society who become severely addicted are, in this sense, scarcely different from those who do not.

The historical perspective and the dislocation theory illuminate this mystery to the extent of showing that a person's society has a major influence on the probability that psychosocial integration will be achieved, and that sustained lack of psychosocial integration is a necessary precursor of addiction. It leads to very practical considerations of how society must be changed when addiction threatens to go out of control. But finding the formula that predicts which particular person will succeed or fail in constructing adequate psychosocial integration out of their unique allotment of talents, opportunities, and challenges lies beyond its reach. A kind word at the right moment, a minor genetic advantage, a microgram of dopamine, a tiny flash of insight can be the seeds of destiny for individual human beings.

A junkyard of false dichotomies

The dislocation theory of addiction flatly contradicts the conventional wisdom that underpins most current theories of addiction. Opposition between the dislocation theory and the conventional wisdom cannot be resolved empirically, since the competing positions are built on fundamentally different assumptions and different definitions of key terms. As Thomas Kuhn has shown, this situation has existed often in the history of science and is typically resolved by the rise to prominence of a community of scholars devoted to a particular paradigm or 'disciplinary matrix', rather than by empirical evidence or logical debate. I believe that the conventional wisdom on addiction constitutes something akin to a Kuhnian paradigm that has reached the end of its serviceability and is about to be replaced by a new one.[79]

One sign that a paradigm is crumbling is that it cannot resolve old questions and move on to new ones. Therefore, it gets bogged down in irresolvable debates that dissipate intellectual energy, hindering progress towards the paradigm shift that is needed. In the case of the conventional wisdom on addiction, several of these irresolvable debates can now be recognised as false dichotomies. Exposing these false dichotomies built into the conventional wisdom can not only hasten its dissolution, but can also serve to highlight the key ways in which the dislocation theory stands totally apart from it.

False dichotomy 1: 'medical problem' or 'criminal problem'?

There have been decades of futile debate about whether drug addiction is a medical problem that falls in the domain of health professionals or a criminal problem that belongs to the domain of the police and the courts. This dichotomy grew naturally from the dual origins of the conventional wisdom in scientific medicine and in temperance moralism. In the recent past, the criminal view has lost ground, and it is now widely assumed that addiction is a medical problem or, more broadly, a health problem. But the debate is not really over. The 'criminal problem' view remains embedded in the conventional wisdom and can regain its ascendancy in any future period when, frustrated by the inability of treatment and harm reduction to do much about the continuing increase in addiction,[80] people again turn to punishment as the primary remedy. For example, Theodore Dalrymple argued flamboyantly for a rejection of the medical view of addiction and subtly suggested—if I understand him correctly—a reinstatement of the criminal view,[81] thus perpetuating the eternal, irresolvable argument. However, the dislocation theory can dispel this false dichotomy.

The medical–criminal dichotomy is false because addiction is neither a medical nor a criminal problem. Addicted people are neither suffering from a disease that can be cured nor engaging in criminal behaviour that should be punished. Rather, they are *adapting*, as well as they are able, to the rising tide of dislocation that threatens to engulf them. Adaptation is neither a disease nor a criminal act, but this does not mean that it is not a problem.

In free-market society, addiction is best understood as a *political* problem, rather than a medical or criminal one. If the political process does not find new wellsprings of social meaning and membership to replace those that have been paved over by globalising free-market society, ever more people will become addicted, ever more severely with terrible consequences for society. Saying that addiction is a political problem does not make it solely the domain of professional politicians, however. Citizens, who collectively hold the ultimate political power, must exercise it for the common good when politicians do not, if society is to address its deepest problems.

False dichotomy 2: 'out of control' or 'acting of their own free will'?

Many people regard loss of self-control as the definitive quality of addiction. For example, Alcoholics Anonymous (AA) requires its members to admit that they are *powerless* to control their drinking (i.e. out of control). Other people take the opposite point of view. For example, Jeffrey Schaler in his important book, *Addiction is a Choice*,[82] argues eloquently that people choose to be addicted of their own free will.

Unfortunately for addicts' beleaguered self-esteem, the forced choice between seeing themselves as either out of control or in control creates a nightmarish dilemma. If they are out of control, they have lost their souls, for the soul is usually seen as the seat of free choice. If they are in control, they have lost their social acceptability, since a person who is wilfully doing evil is reprehensible. Both alternatives provided by this dichotomy are equally cruel and—fortunately—equally false.

This false dichotomy arises from the dual origins of the conventional wisdom on addiction. Medical problems are traditionally understood to be out of the individual patient's control, requiring medical attention. By contrast, criminal problems result from the wrongdoer's wilful choice in the tradition of Christian moralism. The dichotomy is also built into the aetiology of the English word 'addiction', which, as shown in Chapter 2, builds the definition of addiction on the imagery of voluntary enslavement. Voluntary enslavement is a self-contradictory idea, because voluntary slaves would at the same time be enslaved and be enforcing slavery upon themselves. As both slave and master, they would be both out of control and in control at the same time.

At first glance, several facts would appear to make addicted people seem out of control. They often quite sincerely feel unable to control their lives and their families feel unable to control *them*. Actively persuading addicted people that they are out of control has proven therapeutically valuable in AA. Being out of control is sometimes included in formal diagnostic criteria, including the DSM-IV.[83] Moreover, the idea of being out of control is built into one of the oldest (although sometimes contested[84]) working rules of addiction treatment that 'you can't help somebody until they want to be helped'. The addict who does not 'want to be helped' is implicitly judged to be beyond control of any intervention that society could possibly offer.

Upon a second glance, however, other facts make addiction seem to be under the addicted person's control. Some severely addicted people do not feel out of control, and will explain at length the purposes that their addictive life serves for them.[85] Other addicted people are inconsistent in this regard, feeling out of control at some times and in control at others. Many people who have genuinely benefited from membership in AA report that they never felt quite honest about their public affirmations that they were out of control. In addition, many motives have come to light that could account for people attributing their addictive behaviours to the control of 'addictive' drugs.[86] These will be discussed in Chapter 8. Logically, the fact that certain addicted people are beyond the control of their parents does not mean that they are out of their own control. They may be fully in control of themselves, no matter how disobedient they are. Some therapists work hard to persuade their clients that they are not in the least out of control.[87] Sometimes therapy based on this principle succeeds.

Within the conventional wisdom on addiction, there is no way out of the quagmire created by these conflicting facts. Moreover, the dichotomy about whether addiction is out of or in the addicted person's control is only a special case of the ancient conundrum of determinism and free will that has drawn scholars into endless loops of futile argumentation from the early days of Western philosophy.[88] Philosophers can argue forever about whether any behaviour whatsoever—not just addiction—is or is not under the control of a person's free will.

From the standpoint of the dislocation theory, this long-standing debate about whether addicts are out of control or in control is another false dichotomy. It is pointless to classify addicted people as *either* out of control or in control. The dislocation theory bypasses this hopeless quagmire by shifting to an adaptive level of analysis in which control is not an issue. Dislocation is dangerous and painful in the extreme, and dislocated people adapt to it as well as they can. Some of them adapt by taking up an addictive lifestyle. Behavioural adaptation is a process common to all living things, and there is no reason to speak of it as either out of control or in control. Adaptations are understood in terms of the functions they serve, rather than whether they are voluntary or not. From an interior view, complex behavioural adaptations of human beings generally have both voluntary and involuntary aspects. Addicted people experience the same impenetrable mishmash of feeling out of control and in control as everybody else.

False dichotomy 3: 'psychological' or 'physical' addiction?

It is common for people to argue that a particular addiction should be classified as essentially psychological or, on the other hand, essentially physiological. But this is another false dichotomy. Addiction$_3$, whether to heroin, alcohol, love, gambling, or any other sort of habit, is a comprehensive way of living that can be described both in psychological terms (such as 'suffering from dislocation') and physical terms (such as 'withdrawal symptoms'). Naturally, psychological aspects of addiction all have physiological correlates that can be discovered if sufficient research is undertaken. It is equally true, however, that the physiological aspects of addiction have what may be called psychological correlates (i.e. they can be experienced, directly or indirectly).[89]

Decades of work with heroin addicts have convinced me that it is superficial to think that their addictions are essentially physical. It is true that many of them suffer from withdrawal symptoms and have developed tolerance to their drugs, but their addictions generally also entail very low self-esteem, psychological identification as a junkie, and a characteristic emotional blunting. It is similarly superficial to think of addictions that do not involve drugs, addiction to romantic love for example, as essentially psychological and thus disconnected from physiology. Such thinking ignores the addicted lovers' long periods of autonomic distress, not to mention the electrochemical discharge of neurons that subtends every one of their most tender longings.

False dichotomy 4: drug prohibition or legalisation?

Many people passionately believe that prohibiting drugs helps to control the problems of addiction, whereas others believe, just as passionately, that legalising the prohibited drugs would eliminate many or most of these problems. The passions on both sides of the argument are easily comprehensible. People who believe in drug prohibition have often witnessed the horrors of severe drug or alcohol addiction first hand and have been assured by the highest authorities that this dire fate awaits their own children if drugs are not totally banned. People who favour legalisation, on the other hand, know that drugs laws have terrorised drug addicts as well as non-addicted drug users and Third World peasant farmers for much of the 20th century and into the 21st. They also know that unenforceable drug laws foster government corruption. They see prohibition as a central aspect of a cruel and futile War on Drugs.

Discussions about addiction are often disrupted by passions over prohibition and legalisation. Some people seem to fear that the drugs they want to prohibit will be legalised if they do not condemn them incessantly in the most extreme language, regardless of the literal truth. Other people turn every discussion of addiction towards the issue of replacing stringent drug prohibition with 'legalisation', 'decriminalisation', or the sale of drugs in a 'regulated market', as if one of these could substantially reduce the problem of addiction. (Although there are differences between legalisation, decriminalisation, and a regulated market, all three entail making currently prohibited drugs much more accessible. For convenience, I will refer to all three alternatives collectively as 'legalisation' here. 'Legalising' drugs in this book means simply making them legally available to consumers in a prudent way.)

The passionate arguments on both sides of this prohibition versus legalisation debate have become predictable with long repetition that extends back at least to the 1960s. I have participated in heated public debates on this topic myself, supercharged with my own youthful vehemence. However, this debate has little relevance to the problem of addiction, which is the topic of this book.

In the unlikely event that either prohibition or legalisation of drugs could be wholeheartedly embraced as public policy, or that public policy were to shift radically from one to the other, the addiction problem would remain about the same as before. Only a small proportion of serious addictions are drug addictions and these occur only in people who are severely dislocated. Moreover, legal prohibition has very little effect on the availability of drugs to those who are determined to use them. It has proved impossible to enforce drug prohibition even in prisons! If the dislocation theory of addiction is correct, neither experimenting with drugs nor occasionally being prevented from experimenting by futile efforts to enforce prohibition could have much effect on the likelihood that a person becomes addicted.

Simple social justice requires ending the ghastly War on Drugs, because of the cruel and outrageous way that drug laws have been enforced throughout the 20th century and are still being enforced in many countries today.[90] However, the effect of ending drug prohibition may be neither as simple nor as predicable as anti-prohibitionists believe. For example, the loosening of prohibitions on gambling in Canada, which has taken place during my lifetime, probably has eliminated some forms of injustice, but it has certainly not decreased gambling addiction, which has become a major problem. Moreover, legalising some forms of gambling has introduced a serious, unforeseen form of injustice. Governments have become dependent on gambling revenue to keep taxes down, giving citizens who do not gamble a vested interest in licensing lottery ticket vendors and gambling machines in public places, thereby increasing the addictive misery of some of their own neighbours.[91] Whereas there is nothing to be gained by going back to gambling prohibition, there is no reason to think that legalising gambling has done much, if anything, to increase overall social justice or quality of life or to reduce addiction.

The problem of drug law will be taken up again later. The final chapter of this book will argue that whereas current drug laws urgently need to be changed, changing them does not have to force a dichotomous choice between more stringent national prohibition laws on the one hand and national legalisation on the other. A promising alternative that leaves this false dichotomy behind will be discussed at that point.

Evidence for the dislocation theory

Chapters 4–8 summarise the evidence for the dislocation theory of addiction. This evidence will be organised around the three principles of the theory, showing that: (i) psychosocial integration is a necessity (Chapter 4), (ii) free-market society undermines psychosocial integration (Chapter 5), and (iii) addiction is a way of adapting to dislocation (Chapters 6–8).

Endnotes

1   American physician Benjamin Rush (1790) provided the earliest analysis of alcoholism in modern medical terms. Many more medical analyses, some quite technical, were added in the 19th and 20th centuries. Some major reviews and collections of theories of addiction (or 'models' or 'research perspectives') include Lindesmith (1968, Chapter 7), Lettieri *et al.* (1980), Musto (1987, Chapter 4), Peele (1988), Alexander (1990), Walker (1992), W. R. Miller and Hester (1995), Lowman *et al.* (2000), Orford (2001a), and R. West (2001). Theological explanations have existed since the time of St Augustine and Buddha. Philosophical explanations have existed from the time of Plato and Aristotle.

2   There are theories of addiction based on the assumptions of psychoanalysis, behavioural psychology, behavioural genetics, humanistic psychology, neurochemistry, economics, sociology, evolutionary biology, immunology, and theology. There are theories that attempt to explain the causes of addiction$_1$, addiction$_2$, or addiction$_3$, as well as theories that do not

explain addiction at all, but only recovery. There are theories that seek to identify a material cause, efficient cause, final cause, or formal cause of addiction, as well as theories that reject causal analysis in favour of actuarial prediction. Some competing theories are based on diametrically opposite metaphysical assumptions; as examples, determinism or free will, material monism or mind-body dualism, positivism or social construction.

3   Lindesmith (1968, p. 158) reached a similar conclusion.

4   Students of Erikson will know that he typically patterned his discussion of psychosocial integration after Freud's sequential stages of psychosexual development (Erikson, 1963). However, in the interest of an overall picture, I have folded Erikson's sequential stages into a single general process. Erikson too follows that simplifying strategy at some points in his writing (see Erikson, 1959, pp. 113–114, Section III).

5   Although Erikson used a great variety of other words, such as 'wholeness' or 'healthy personality', more frequently than he used 'psychosocial integration', this book will doggedly stick to 'psychosocial integration'. Although this bit of jargon is decidedly less lyrical than some of Erikson's synonyms, it conveys the essential idea with greater specificity.

Although psychosocial integration is a more specific term than the others, Erikson did not provide a compact or operational definition for it. It may be possible to define this essential concept more precisely than Erikson did, but for the moment, I prefer a more lengthy definition, hoping that people will recognize what it refers to from their own experience. Many essential words cannot be reduced to a compact definition, for example, 'science', 'art', 'cause', and 'self'. To insist on a compact definition for a concept that is better explained in a more lengthy way is, in my view, self-defeating.

6   K. Polanyi (1944). See also Glendinning (1994). Although the author of this fascinating book of popular psychology speaks of living in a 'primal matrix' more often in environmental and spiritual than in social terms, this seems to me primarily a difference in emphasis. The meaning of 'psychosocial integration' and Glendinning's 'primal matrix' are, I believe, quite close. Dufour (2005, esp. pp. 117–120) speaks of human identity as founded more on a relationship to some sort of god than to society. However, I think this is also just a difference in emphasis, since he says that a relationship with God can only be achieved in conjunction with other people who help to socially construct the deity (see pp. 121–124 and 213) and, conversely, enduring relationships with other people can only become established when people share an understanding of transcendent reality (pp. 132–133 and 277–278). Moreover, Dufour's (2003a, pp. 230–231) concept of *la première domination (ontologique)* could serve as the framework for a secular description of the transcendent component of psychosocial integration. See also O'Meara (2004, pp. 50–51, endnote 44, pp. 99–102). J. Jacobs (1961) has pointed out that membership in neighbourhood and district groups within large cities can easily accommodate religious and ethnic pluralism, but even in the most pluralistic society, the basis of spiritual identity is in subgroups.

By contrast, some forms of popular psychology and spiritualism advocate a radical individualism in which a person establishes a relationship with the cosmos by intense introspection and by muting their social and cultural attachments. (The film *What the Bleep do we know?* and a book by Candace Pert (1997) illustrate this kind of popular psychology.) I believe that this spiritual individualism is better understood as an aspect of dislocation.

7   K. Polanyi (1935, p. 370).

8   Plato's and Socrates' version of this idea will be explained in Chapter 13.

9   Many people interpret Darwin's most famous book, *The Origin of Species* (1859/1958a), as pointing in the opposite direction, to a biological world in which each individual struggles for survival in constant competition with others of his species. But *The Origin of Species* says

virtually nothing about the human species. In his later book on human psychology, *The Descent of Man, and Selection in Relation to Sex* (1871/1981), Darwin states clearly that the social instinct is the strongest of human drives. This is discussed at length in Chapter 4.

10 Kropotkin (1914/1972).

11 Adler (1934/1954). See also Ansbacher (1999).

12 Fromm (1941).

13 P. Slater (1976); Berman (1982); Cushman (1995); Kawachi *et al.* (1997); O'Meara (2004, pp. 63–64); Dufour (2005).

14 There are, however, some terms currently used by social scientists that carry too much baggage from free-market ideology to capture the essential idea of psychosocial integration. For example, in some current social science literature, the term 'social capital' is used interchangeably with terms like 'social cohesion', 'community', 'social ties', and so forth (Kawachi *et al.*, 1997; Putnam, 1993, 2000; Granfield and Cloud, 2002; Kushner and Sterk, 2005). However, these authors give 'social capital' a qualitatively different meaning than psychosocial integration, as defined here. The most basic difference is that, like other kinds of capital, social capital can be exchanged for other kinds of wealth and can be used to create material wealth (Illouz, 2007, pp. 62–67). Of course, some kinds of cooperation and trust do contribute to wealth creation (Putnam, 1993) and these can reasonably be called social capital. Full psychosocial integration, however, quite often interferes with the economic functioning of free-market society. It is possible to have a great deal of social capital and to be very good at networking, but still be completely lacking in psychosocial integration.

Psychosocial integration differs from capital in other ways as well. For example, many forms of capital, including stock shares, real estate, tools, and coal, are all interconvertible with money, but psychosocial integration is not. Lack of psychosocial integration is as much a problem of capital-rich societies as of poor ones in the contemporary world. Unlike capital, psychosocial integration cannot be bought or sold, given away, divided, or stolen, although it can be destroyed. This is not to say that psychosocial integration is intrinsically unquantifiable, only that the kinds of measures that have been used to operationalize social capital are not encompassing enough. Another difference between psychosocial integration and capital is that capital is the domain of professionals, like bankers. We cannot go to our neighbours for finance capital, because they probably neither have much nor understand how to invest it. On the other hand, psychosocial integration is something that neighbours understand culturally and instinctively, although they probably have a different word for it. We are better off avoiding professionals in this domain. Finally, B. Edwards and Foley (1998) have argued that the term 'social capital' is a structural economic parameter that should not be used as a psychological property of an individual. Yet it is clear that, in a dislocated society, some people manage to achieve satisfactory psychosocial integration, whereas others do not.

15 Erikson expressed the idea this way:

> However, many of the mechanisms of adjustment which once made for evolutionary adaptation, tribal integration, national or class coherence, are at loose ends in a world of universally expanding identities. Education for an ego identity which receives strength from changing historical conditions demands a conscious acceptance of historical heterogeneity on the part of adults, combined with an enlightened effort to provide human childhood anywhere with a new fund of meaningful continuity.

Erikson (1959, p. 40).

16 It would be fundamentally the same because it would be structured by the same stages of psychosexual development and would entail the same kinds of tensions and sensitive accommodations in both cultures.

17 J. Jacobs (1961).

18 Erikson makes this same crucial point, although he restricts himself to language that is more professional. For example:

> We know that when this [i.e. psychosocial integration] is achieved, play becomes freer, health radiant, sex more adult, and work more meaningful. Having applied psychoanalytic concepts to group problems we feel that a clearer understanding of the mutual complementation of ego synthesis and social organisation may help us to appraise therapeutically a psychological middle range, the expansion and cultivation of which on ever higher levels of human organisation is the aim of all therapeutic endeavour, social and individual.

Erikson (1959, p. 26).

19 This usage is concordant with normal English usage (see the *Oxford English Dictionary*, 1989: 'dislocation', definition 2, and 'dislocate', definition 2). I have adopted 'dislocation' for this purpose following K. Polanyi (1944). For example, Polanyi (p. 33) introduces his discussion of the industrial revolution thus: 'At the heart of the Industrial Revolution of the eighteenth century there was an almost miraculous improvement in the tools of production, which was accompanied by a catastrophic dislocation of the lives of the common people.'

20 Other terms that are given approximately the same meaning include: 'anomie' or 'anomy' (Tennant, 1990, p. 72), 'identity diffusion', 'alienation', 'disembedding' (Giddens, 1990), the 'empty self' (Cushman, 1995, pp. 245–248), 'loneliness' (Vanier, 1998), loss of 'social capital' (Putnam, 2000; Granfield and Cloud, 2002), 'les désarrois de l'individu-sujet' (Dufour, 2001), 'désaffiliation' (Castel, 1999, as cited in Bonelli, 2003), 'destruction des solidarités locales' (Champagne, 2003), and 'la mort sociale' (Bourdieu, 1981/2003). The term 'disconnection' might be the most frequently used in the everyday English language of my city. Of these terms, only 'loss of social capital' seems to me problematic as an alternative for dislocation for reasons explained in endnote 16 of this chapter.

21 Durkheim (1897/1951) argued that the primary cause of suicide in 19th century Europe was the failure of people to achieve or maintain integration with their society. His conclusion was based on minute analysis of suicide statistics, which showed that suicide was less frequent at times and in places that favoured psychosocial integration. This conclusion has been challenged in the more recent literature (Kushner and Sterk, 2005). M. J. Chandler and colleagues carried out quantitative studies of suicide among aboriginal children in British Columbia over two time periods, 1987–1992 and 1997–2000. These studies showed that the relative frequency of suicide was much higher among aboriginal children whose bands were more estranged from their traditional culture than those whose bands were less estranged. In both studies, bands that had a positive rating on all seven of the 'cultural continuity variables' had no suicides at all, whereas those bands with a positive score on none of the cultural continuity variables had child suicide rates of 137.5 and 61 per 100,000 of the population (M. J. Chandler and Lalonde, 1998; M. J. Chandler *et al.* 2003).

22 See Bourdieu (1981/2003); Glendinning (1994, Chapter 6); Gosline (2007); Rayner (2007).

23 Klein (2007, Chapter 1).

24 For example, this has been the tragic experience of many tribal groups of Canadian Indians who were given substantial amounts of money in payment for the land and resources that

had been the backbone of a healthy culture and their psychosocial integration. This will be documented with the recent example of Davis Inlet in Chapter 6. The same principle had been abundantly documented in the world anthropology literature half a century ago (K. Polanyi, 1944, pp. 99, 153–161, 291–293).

25 See K. Polanyi (1944, p. 157). deGraaf et al. (2002, Chapter 9) reached a similar conclusion in their study of 'affluenza'.

26 *Holy Bible, Authorized (King James) Version* (1611/1956, Matthew 5:3).

27 Naturally, the Christian interpretation is often stated in more theological language, which I have not used because I am not a Christian. See Chappell (2006) for an example.

28 This is documented in Chapter 5. See especially endnote 5 in that chapter.

29 Adam Smith (1776/1991) popularised this idea in his classic work, *An Inquiry into the Nature and Causes of the Wealth of Nations.*

30 Among the reversals were the Speenhamland period in England (1795–1832; see K. Polanyi, 1944) and the 'welfare state' period in Western Europe and North America in the 30 years following World War II. See also Bayly (2004, e.g. pp. 295–300) for a description of various forms of resistance to the spread of Western economics throughout the long 19th century. See Stiglitz (2002) and Klein (2007) for failures and reversals precipitated by the International Monetary Fund in the 1990s. The most successful reversals in the 21st century have been in numerous Latin American countries that have retreated from extreme forms of free trade and privatisation (Ramonet, 2006–2007; Klein, 2007, pp. 543–549).

31 Tawney (1926/1947, Chapter 5); M. Friedman and Friedman (1979); Fukuyama (1989); Soros (1997); Saul (2004); Batan (2004); J. Jacobs (2000); J. Heath (2001); Lordon (2003, 2004); Homer-Dixon (2006, pp. 203–204); Clerc (2007); Klein (2007). K. Polanyi (1944) believed that the 19th century civilisation, dominated by free-market society, had finally collapsed by the end of World War II. Whereas some aspects had permanently collapsed, such as the gold standard and the domination of world power by the European nations, free-market society rose from the rubble of war and renewed its worldwide hegemony in the late 20th century and the beginning of the 21st.

32 Bayly's (2004) influential history of the modern world stresses the importance of a variety of economic and non-economic factors in the genesis of modernity, in contrast to the stricter economic determinism of the scholars whose work is more central in this book including Tawney, K. Polanyi, J. Hill, Prebble, Hobsbawm, Berman, Ramonet, and Dufour. Nevertheless, Bayly (2004, pp. 3–5, 290–292, 473–475) explicitly acknowledges the definitive role of capitalism in shaping the modern world and provides abundant examples of its fundamental importance throughout his account. Whereas I lean towards a stronger form of economic determinism than Bayly's, the dislocation theory of addiction would stand whether the economic system is seen as the single fundamental cause of modern dislocation or as only one of the major causes.

33 K. Polanyi (1944); M. Friedman and Friedman (1979); J. Heath (2001, pp. 24–26, 124–125); McQuaig (2001); Dufour (2003a, b); Bayly (2004, pp. 290–292); O'Meara (2004, pp. 63–64); *Globe and Mail* (2007a); Luciw (2007); Galt (2007); Ramonet (2007). Dufour has expressed this as follows:

> … nothing, neither social life nor culture, can resist the requirements of the market. This goes to the point that a society which is ideally subordinated to the market cannot function without destroying a large portion of its industrial, social, and cultural fabric so that it can organise itself to provide for intense flow and instant re-organisation. This is because capital goods must be received and then sent off again as quickly as they

came … As far as possible, it becomes necessary in peacetime to reorganise large sectors of society in the manner that would be found in a refugee camp.

Dufour (2003b, pp. 97–98).

J. Heath says it even more bluntly:

One of the perverse features of living in a capitalist society is that not only does acting in your self-interest often lead to beneficial consequences for society as a whole, but the flip side is also true—often not acting in your own self-interest generates harmful effects.

J. Heath (2001, p. 124).

34 K. Polanyi (1944, pp. 163–165).
35 For an example of the application of this principle in modern times, see Cordonnier (2006) on the logic of the campaign of the OECD against the European welfare state.
36 This realisation has been recognised in diverse ways by countless thinkers. As examples: J. Heath (2001) characterised Canada as an idealized version of free-market society and argues that making the market system function efficiently is the basis of human well-being. He poignantly described some of the loss of psychosocial integration that this would entail, but considers this inevitable. For example:

Welcome to the culture of efficiency. It's not perfect, but it's not so bad either. This is the compromise at the heart of our society. The world we live in clearly fails to satisfy many of our deeper needs and impulses. And yet, any serious attempt to change it seems to entail even greater sacrifice. We may be as close to utopia as we can get…

J. Heath (2001, p. 2).

French economist Frédéric Lordon has commented on the futility of expecting that improvement in the conditions of life will follow if corporate administrators can be convinced to behave in a more socially responsible way. He urged people to:

… stop expecting corporate management to be able to do anything other than that which the system of structural constraints that they work within almost inevitably requires of them. Rather than expecting administrators to become socially responsible and virtuous as if by intervention of the Holy Spirit, people must look towards the areas of real power, namely those areas that design and re-design the economic structures, make and remake the international regulations that determine all the rest.

Lordon (2004, p. 23).

37 Saul (1995, especially Chapter 4); Soros (1997); Stiglitz (2002, 2006).
38 This endnote briefly describes six ways in which the reality of globalising free-market society differs from the ideal, showing in each case how the potential to cause mass dislocation remains essentially intact nonetheless:
   a. Although current 'free-market' societies allow economic freedom in some domains, they offer nothing like the full range of economic freedom that free-market ideology claims.
      Free markets do not arise freely, but are imposed and entrenched by whatever amounts of administrative and military force are required. This has been occurring for centuries and continues today, most visibly in the countries of Africa, as well as Afghanistan, Iraq, and Cuba (K. Polanyi, 1944; Prebble, 1963; McMurtry, 1998, pp. 259–296; E. M. Wood, 1999; Stiglitz, 2002; P. Adams, 2003; Ghafour, 2003; Achcar, 2004; Warde, 2004; Caplan, 2005; Beder, 2006). Rebellions against free-market economics are only allowed to last for

a short period before being suppressed, if possible, by national or international military force. Attempts to suppress rebellions against free-market society include the unsuccessful military incursions in communist Russia in the decades following World War I and in Cuba and Venezuela more recently. There were successful interventions late in the 20th century against elected governments in Chile and Nicaragua (Klein, 2007, Chapters 2 and 3).

Once entrenched, free-market societies do not allow the complete freedom to buy and sell, which is, in theory, their essential feature. In international markets, the greatest free-trading nations in Europe and North America impose crippling tariffs on farm produce from the Third World for domestic political reasons (Stiglitz, 2002, p. 61; N. Reynolds, 2005).

National markets are similarly distant from the free-trade ideal. Even in the current phase of intense 'deregulating' in order to facilitate corporate profit making (Klinenberg, 2003), businesses are tightly regulated—and subsidized—by governments to buffer natural boom-and-bust cycles, to prevent disastrous collapses of individual corporations or sectors (K. Polanyi, 1944; Drohan, 2003b; J. Saunders, 2003a; J. Simpson, 2003; Campbell et al., 2004; Tuck, 2004; McCarthy, 2005a), to prevent market crashes (D. Smith, 2001), to protect corporations from legal liability for their losses and their own dishonesty (Salutin, 2002; B. McKenna, 2002b), to prevent the accumulation of capital by political enemies (Partridge, 2001), to achieve military and geopolitical objectives camouflaged as economic objectives (British American Security Information Council, 2006), and to induce corporations to move to particular localities (Keenan, 2003; Tuck, 2003).

Buying and selling is not allowed in free markets if it deviates too far from the ideology of those who control the markets. This is illustrated by the struggle of a Vancouver magazine, *Adbusters*, to buy advertising time from commercial stations for high-quality television commercials that criticized television itself and other aspects of free-market economics (Friesen, 2004). The *Adbusters* case is highly publicized, but only because the editors of the magazine, zealous activists, were able to marshal the resources to continue that case over a decade.

However, despite intense regulation of 'deregulated' markets, massive public subsidies for 'private' business, and so on, 'market discipline' prevails in the lives of most individuals most of the time, such as when people are seeking a job, buying a house, or recovering from a personal disaster. Society does not generally interfere with the free play of the market to reduce dislocation, although it interferes copiously to entrench and protect the market itself. Moreover, the most onerous losses to the public are justified by reiterating the necessity of universal application of ideal (but illusory) free-market principles. A recent illustration is the rhetoric surrounding the sell-off of a Crown Corporation in British Columbia that the public wanted to remain under public control (Jang, 2003). Thus, dislocation remains great in a so-called 'free-market' society, even though the 'freedom' is greatly exaggerated.

b. Another deviation from the ideal is sometimes called 'monopoly capitalism'. As capitalism evolved in the 19th century, more and more corporations ceased to function in the interest of their own individual profit, coalesced into highly integrated monopolies, cartels, and transnational corporations, and colluded under informal arrangements and formal contracts created specifically to reduce competition (Lenin, 1916/1966; von Hayek, 1944, Chapter 4; Heilbroner, 1961, Chapters 10 and 11; Baran and Sweezy, 1966; Dobbin, 1998; B. McKenna, 2002a; Berger, 2003; Reguly, 2003; McFarland, 2004; Yakabuski, 2004). The emergence of monopoly was accelerated by privatisation of government services in the Third World and the former USSR at the end of the 20th century, where this form of monopoly creation was enforced by the financial power of the International Monetary Fund and the United States (Stiglitz, 2002). However, even those advocates of free-market economics who acknowledge its dilution with monopoly capitalism from the late 19th century onward (e.g. von Hayek, 1944, Chapter 4) continue to refer to the era of monopoly and transnational capitalism as a 'free-market' system, and to assert that any step to regulate it, other than to facilitate competition, is a step along the 'road to serfdom'. Whereas the transition from Adam Smith's world of individual entrepreneurs to the world of monopoly capitalism did greatly dilute the literal meaning of 'free markets' at the corporate and intercorporate level, it did not reduce the dislocation arising from personal competition at the level of individual workers and customers (Heilbroner, 1961, pp. 269, 282–283).

c. A further difference between the reality and the ideology of 'free-market society' concerns the pragmatic commercial honesty that is supposed to prevail within markets and the supposed ability of the government to police dishonest corporations for the sake of efficiency of the market and the long-term public interest. The illusion of honesty is being dispelled by overwhelming evidence of corporate and government collusion and corruption. Corporations have huge political power through their official and unofficial lobbyists (Milner, 2003a; *New York Times*, 2005). Sometimes, corporate leaders and government officials are 'in bed with each other', and sometimes no bed is required because they are the very same people serving their conflicting institutions in their own interest. This has become infamously obvious in the case of the current American Vice President, Dick Cheney, and former American National Security Advisor, Richard Perle, although there have been many other less widely publicized cases (see Stiglitz, 2002, pp. 173–178; Frank and Cherney, 2003, 2004; Milner, 2003b; R. Blackwell, 2004; Dizard, 2004; J. Saunders, 2004; Warde, 2004; Krugman, 2005). Whereas corporate control of government is most conspicuous in the United States, Canada is catching up fast (Dobbin, 2003, Chapters 4 and 6). Corporations have proven able to circumvent government regulations in cases where maintaining the public good would reduce corporate profits (D. Saunders, 2003). This is particularly evident in recent litigation involving American weapons manufacturers, but there are many other sectors in which it occurs (Dobbin, 2003, Chapters 4 and 6; McFarland, 2003; B. McKenna, 2003; Wayne, 2005; Weiner, 2005). Governments have also failed to prevent the elite of free-market society from preying on the stockowners and consumers that are the presumed beneficiaries of the free-market system. High-level administrators often loot companies of immense sums to maintain lavish lifestyles (Associated Press, 2003; R. Blackwell, 2003b, c; Pitts, 2003; Galloni and Mollenkamp, 2004; Howlett *et al.*, 2004) or bring well-established companies to ruin through irresponsible speculation motivated by their personal addictions to wealth and power (Lordon, 2003, 2004). There is a long history in Africa of corporations from free-market societies financing private armies to slaughter civilians who stand in the way of their profit-making (Buckner, 2003; Drohan, 2003a). International free-trade agreements are routinely violated by governments hoping to keep the favour of key corporations and industries (Milner, 2003a).

Although these forms of dishonesty and corruption reduce the conformity of free-market society to its own ideals, they do not really reduce the dislocation produced by free-market society for most people (Lordon, 2003, p. 40). Rather, they increase it by restoring the law-of-the-jungle quality that was envisaged by some of the most avid defenders of market freedom like Herbert Spencer and Ayn Rand.

It might be hoped that the clean-up of corporate corruption that appears to be underway in the United States could serve to mitigate some of the harm produced by free-market society. It now seems more likely that, although the clean-up will provide some economic benefits for defrauded shareholders, it will serve ultimately to further entrench free-market economics in the modern world. This view has been stated eloquently in a discussion of the conviction of businesswoman Martha Stewart in the *Globe and Mail* business section:

> This was the beauty of American capitalism. Problems arose and were fixed in a hurry, before investors decided the stock markets were a fool's game only... Some of Ms. Stewart's many defenders say [the American department of] Justice turned her into a showcase because she was a celebrity. Another way of looking at it is that the government couldn't ignore her just because she was a celebrity. If it had, it would have been slaughtered by the rabble for unequal treatment—one law for the rich, another for the poor. The Justice department did the right thing.

Reguly (2004, p. B2).

d. Another gap between the reality and the form of free-market society is documented by Canadian scholar John Ralston Saul (2004). Saul argued that the era of 'globalism' (i.e. the spread of unregulated free trade though the entire world) has reached an end to be followed by a period of recrudescent nationalism. Even if this is so, it is clear that the new national powers that may set the tone for the next few decades are all committed to free-market ideology within major segments of their own economies, even if they refuse to be subservient to international free-market conventions.

e. The logic of free-market economics holds that people will best satisfy their pre-existing needs in a free and open market. But it is now standard practice to imbue people with needs artificially through the use of highly sophisticated advertising techniques (e.g. Langreth and Harper, 2006). Naturally, the needs that are thus created are the most profitable ones that can be imagined by the corporations that pay to create them. Yet even this gap between the ideal and the reality of free-market society has not spared consumers from dislocation. Rather, it increases the dislocation they must endure by creating expensive needs that require them to work all the harder, at the expense of family and culture.

f. The 'third way' philosophy of the present British government (Giddens, 1998) promises more regulations on the free market in the public interest. However, this only increases the constraints within which markets operate. It does nothing to relieve the unrelenting competition between individualized participants that causes dislocation. Mass dislocation and addiction are clearly not decreasing under the regime of the 'third way' in today's UK (Renzetti, 2005a; Dalrymple, 2006a, p. 16; Jenkins, 2006; Plant and Plant, 2006; Newland, 2007).

Thus, in spite of all of the qualifications that the term 'free-market society' requires, the current globalising society nonetheless exerts overwhelmingly powerful pressure on individuals to function in their own personal economic interest and in disregard for the family and cultural associations with others that might otherwise afford them psychosocial integration. In fact, the potential for dislocation is probably greater under 21st-century capitalism than in previous centuries, because earlier forms of free-market society maintained a certain brutal honesty, whereas modern free-market governments conceal its nature, in part by promulgating the ideology of ideal (but illusory) free markets, and in part by speaking in lofty terms of social justice and environmental concern. This mass deception destroys people's contact with reality and thus further reduces the possibility of psychosocial integration with the real world.

39 Although the causal relationship between globalising Western free-market society and dislocation is the mainstream view among social scientists, the influential political scientist Samuel Huntington maintains a rather different view, namely that the historical roots of contemporary dislocation is a technical 'modernisation' that proceeded separately from Western culture, leaving modernised non-Western civilisations still essentially non-Western (Huntington, 1996, Chapter 3). I will not challenge Huntington's position here (although I think the world has become much more uniform that he supposes) as it does not contradict the essential fact that modernisation (in Huntington's language) is inevitable in the contemporary world and that it inevitably leads to dislocation of individuals, as Huntington himself confirms (pp. 76, 97–98).

40 I believe that the four addictions mentioned in this paragraph are among the most harmful, both socially and individually. This may seem surprising in the case of 'shopaholism', but, when its environmental implications and its increasingly global prevalence are fully explored, I believe that it may prove to be the most dangerous of all (e.g. Suzuki and McConnell, 1997; Dobbin, 1998; Klein, 2000; Chase, 2002). The argument is explained in more detail in Chapter 10.

41 Chein *et al.* (1964, Chapter 9, p. 216); Gay *et al.* (1974); Granfield and Cloud (1999, Chapter 2); Pryor (2003); Dalrymple (2006a, Chapter 2).

42 Naomi Klein (2000) has described this brilliantly for the youth culture and the 'branded' merchandise of the late 20th century. See also deGraaf *et al.* (2002), McInnis (2003), Homer-Dixon (2006, pp. 197–198) and Bower (2006).

43 This will be documented in detail in Chapter 10.

44 Alexander and Dibb (1975).

45 Bourgois (1997).

46 For example, Bailey and Elliot (2003). French economist Frédéric Lordon (2003) provides an especially apt description of 'addictively overworking CEOs'. For example, his descriptions of the higher-level executives of the failed French corporation Moulinex lays out both the harm that such people do and the addictive basis for it in detail:

> … they are swept into the game of competition where they invest themselves that much more deeply because the game has become the basis of their personal identity. Workers must not be allowed to be valued more than things, because if they did the capitalists would not be able to live out their competitive passion with full intensity. And they addict themselves to the powerful emotions of the struggle to the death with that much more excitement… because it is never them who has to die!

Lordon (2003, Chapter 2, p. 23).

47 James M. Barrie, the author of *Peter Pan*, provides an example. His life is discussed at length in Chapter 9. See also the account of the extraordinary addiction of American 'Civil War re-enactor', Robert Lee Ogden (Horowitz, 1999). A useful description of the creative addiction of mathematician Paul Erdös is provided by P. Hoffman (1998).

48 This statement flies in the face of the conventional wisdom in the field of addiction. Evidence that supports it appears in Chapters 4–8 of this book. Peele *et al.* (1991, p. 43 *et seq.*) developed a similar idea.

49 The claim that dislocation is a necessary precursor of addiction can be viewed as a tautology. This does not seem like a serious problem to me, partly because the hypothesis fits the historical evidence so well. The dislocation theory of addiction is really meant to be a

paradigm for the study of addiction, and tautologies are frequently built into successful paradigms (Kuhn, 1970).

50 Darwin (1871/1981, p. 381); Symons (1979, p. 46); W. J. Bock (1980); Mayr (1982, p. 132).

51 K. Blum *et al.* (1996).

52 T. E. Robinson and Berridge (2001).

53 K. Blum *et al.* (1996).

54 There is a great deal of evidence supporting the point that therapy for addiction is only marginally effective. I have summarized some of it in Chapter 1, endnote 9 of this book.

55 See Durkheim (1897/1951), Bourdieu (1981/2003) and Homer-Dixon (2006, p. 198). A recent epidemic of school 'shooters' in North America can be traced back to painful isolation of teenagers (K. Newman, 2006). A startling analysis of the causes of homicidal mania and business catastrophe (Duclos, 2002) implicates dislocation as the ultimate cause.

56 Suetonius (*c.* 100 AD/1957); Gibbon (1776/1974).

57 Plato (*c.* 360 BC/1987).

58 St Augustine (397 AD/1963, 426 AD/2000).

59 Many people have shown logically or empirically that the woes enumerated in this paragraph cannot be eliminated in free-market society (Lenin, 1916/1966; Rivière, 2003; Velásquez, 2003; B. McKenna, 2004a, c). There is a comfortable Canadian belief that Canada has avoided the corporate corruption that has been exposed elsewhere, but this is just a vanity (Drohan, 2004a, b). The remainder of Part I of this book is intended to show that addiction should be added to the list of unavoidable consequences of free-market society.

60 This crucial point is made eloquently by Velásquez (2003) and by Peele *et al.* (1991, pp. 374–378).

61 Kuhn (1970).

62 Alexander (1990); Alexander *et al.* (1998).

63 S. R. Friedman (2002).

64 Specifically, Plato's concept of the 'tyrannical personality' in *The Republic* (*c.* 360 BC/1987, Book 9, lines 571–576) and St Augustine's analysis of a beggar's chronic drunkenness in the *Confessions* (397 AD/1963, Book VI, Chapter 6).

65 See explanations of addiction proposed by Freud (1929), Adler (1934/1954), R. K. Merton (1957), Cloward and Ohlin (1960), Chein *et al.* (1964), Erikson (1968), Khantzian *et al.* (1974), Peele and Brodsky (1975), Peele (1985), Wurmser (1978), Marlatt (1985a), D. F. Jacobs (1986), Orford (1985, 2001a), and Homer-Dixon (2006, pp. 197–198).

66 Chein *et al.* (1964).

67 Peele and Brodsky (1975).

68 Orford (1985, 2001a).

69 Aaron and Musto (1981, pp. 145–157).

70 He said, for example:

> A related problem is the belief (reflected in much of contemporary obstetric and pediatric concern with the methods of child care) that the establishment of a basic sense of trust in earliest childhood makes adult individuals less dependent on mild or malignant forms of addiction, on self-delusion, and on avaricious appropriation. Of this, little is known…
>
> Erikson (1959, pp. 62–63).

71 The word that I have elided here from Erikson's text is 'homosexual'. Its inclusion could divert attention from the main point here into a discussion of homosexuality, a vast topic on which I have no expertise. It is important to remember that Erikson was writing half a century ago and that a revolution in sexual attitudes has occurred between then and now.

72 Erikson (1968, p. 88). See also Erikson (1959, pp. 129–133) and E. L. Burke (1978).

73 See Erikson (1959, p. 113, Section III).

74 E. L. Burke (1978), Mijuskovic (1988), and Glendinning (1994) have written accounts of addiction similar to the dislocation theory based on Erikson's terminology.

75 Granfield and Cloud (1999, Chapter 5) have summarized several contemporary sociological analyses, particularly those of Anthony Giddens (1991), which are very similar to the dislocation theory. See also R. K. Merton (1957), Chein *et al.* (1964), Peele (1985, p. 129), S. R. Friedman (2002), Dufour (2003a, p. 27), Eckersley (2005), and Fish (2006). Historians who used this idea will be cited in Chapter 6.

76 'Pop psychology' is a derogatory term that academic psychologists apply to psychology books that sell to a wider audience than their own. However, the pop psychology literature, often written by professional practitioners who do not choose to write in an academic style, often seems more informative than the conventional wisdom that professional psychologists usually embrace. My current favourite pop psychology authors on the topic of addiction are Gabor Maté (2000, 2005a, b) and Chellis Glendinning (1994). Fish (2006) provides an excellent review of this enormous literature.

77 Erikson (1946, republished in Erikson, 1959, pp. 18–49).

78 More often he simply called these 'neuroses'; however, he uses the phrase 'neurotic fixation' as well (e.g. Erikson, 1959, p. 40). This is not to say that all the neuroses he described could be characterized as addictions, but many could.

79 Kuhn (1970). Neither the conventional wisdom nor the dislocation theory fulfils all of the criteria of a Kuhnian paradigm in the history of physical science. Yet Kuhn's analysis seems to fit the situation in a broad sense. Kuhn (1970) clearly intended that his historical analysis be applied to psychological as well as physical science.

80 Some of the evidence for this inability is documented in Chapter 1, endnote 9.

81 Dalrymple (2006a, pp. 109–110, 114). See also Mason (2006).

82 Schaler (2000). See also Dalrymple (2006a).

83 American Psychiatric Association (1994, p. 161). DSM-IV (*Diagnostic and Statistical Manual of the Mental Disorders*) is the standard American classification system for mental disorders.

84 W. R. Miller (1989) contests the rule and proposes to alter people's motivation with 'motivational interviewing'.

85 This is often apparent both in the records of clinicians and accounts by addicts themselves (e.g. Chein *et al.*, 1964, Chapter 9; Khantzian *et al.* 1974; Gresswell and Hollin, 1997; Granfield and Cloud, 1999, esp. p. 109; Crozier and Lane, 2001; Pryor, 2003).

86 See J. B. Davies (1992, 1997) and Dalrymple (2006a).

87 Schaler (2000, esp. pp. 141–146).

88 James (1907/1981, pp. 54–57); Rorty (1979). Schaler (2000, p. 69) has argued, wrongly, I believe, that 'a determinist could accept the free-will model'.

89 The complementarity of psychological and physiological descriptions is argued eloquently by Wilber (1996, Chapter 5).

90 Alexander (1990, Chapter 2); McNeil (2007).

91 Picard (2006).

Chapter 4

Psychosocial Integration is a Necessity

The first principle of the dislocation theory of addiction is that psychosocial integration is an essential part of human well-being, and that dislocation—the sustained absence of psychosocial integration—is excruciatingly painful. The strongest evidence for this principle comes from evolutionary and anthropological observations made in the 19th and 20th centuries.[1]

The 19th and early 20th centuries were the golden age for research on aboriginal culture and traditional peasant life, both of which were being overrun by colonisation and industrial revolution.[2] Sensing the vulnerability of traditional human societies to the approaching steamroller, scholars of that day wanted to study them before they were crushed. One of the 19th century scholars was Charles Darwin.

Darwin's evolutionary anthropology

On the surface, Charles Darwin would seem the worst possible source for a testimonial that psychosocial integration is necessary for human well-being. Darwin's theory of evolution is often viewed as a scenario of unrelenting individual competition for survival and reproductive success.[3] Even his name has been appropriated as a synonym for ruthless individual competition, which is said to be 'Darwinian'. Although this single-minded view of evolution is still held today by many people who think of themselves as 'Darwinists',[4] Charles Darwin's own view of evolution was considerably more complex.

Darwin studied the social life of aboriginal people first-hand during his voyage around the world on the *Beagle* and second-hand through his wide correspondence with European explorers and anthropologists. Whereas Darwin's most famous book on evolution, *The Origin of Species*, does depict evolution largely as the product of ruthless individual competition for survival and reproductive success, it says nothing specifically about the evolutionary descent of the human species. Two decades later, Darwin published two books that were more directly concerned with human evolution and psychology, *The Descent of Man* and *The Expression of the Emotions in Man and Animals*. When these books are taken into account along with *The Origin of Species*, it becomes evident that Darwin had a much more complex view of human evolutionary psychology than most of the Darwinists who currently speak for him. In fact, Darwin laid a solid theoretical foundation in evolutionary biology for the necessity of psychosocial integration to human well-being.

There is no contradiction between *The Origin of Species* and Darwin's later writings that specifically concerned human evolution. His ideas on human evolution had been worked out long before *The Origin of Species* was published and are fully in accord with it.[5] *The Origin of Species* describes evolution in a very general sense that must be made more specific to describe the enormously diverse selective pressures and adaptations that comprise the evolutionary histories of various species.[6]

In *The Descent of Man*, Darwin described the innate drive towards social contact, which he called the 'social instinct', as one of the most conspicuous adaptations of *Homo sapiens* and of other animal species that form long-lasting social groups. He argued that human beings are not only powerfully drawn to the company of their own community by the social instinct, but are also innately inclined to feel 'sympathy' for them, and innately predisposed towards cooperative behaviour and selfless sacrifice within their tribal societies. He called this predisposition the 'moral sense'. He described the psychological importance of the social instinct and the moral sense in *Homo sapiens* unambiguously:

> I fully subscribe to the judgement of those writers who maintain that of all the differences between man and the lower animals, the moral sense or conscience is by far the most important .... It is the most noble of all the attributes of man, leading him without a moment's hesitation to risk his life for that of a fellow-creature; or after due deliberation, impelled simply by the deep feeling of right or duty, to sacrifice it in some great cause.[7]

In Darwin's view, the moral sense was not acquired primarily through culture or education, although these played a role. More fundamentally, the moral sense was an adaptation of the human species that was inherited as a consequence of organic evolution:

> ... it can hardly be disputed that the social feelings are instinctive or innate in the lower animals; and why should they not be so in man? [Various British psychologists] believe that the moral sense is acquired by each individual during his lifetime. On the general theory of evolution this is at least extremely improbable.[8]

Darwin did not see the social instinct and the moral sense as mechanical drives or blind reflexes, but as deeply felt human needs that gave people great pleasure when they were satisfied. He commented on this in his autobiography, written in the last 6 years of his life, as follows:

> A man who has no assured and ever present belief in the existence of a personal God or of a future existence with retribution and reward, can have for his rule of life, as far as I can see, only to follow those impulses and instincts which are the strongest or which seem to him the best ones. A dog acts in this manner, but he does so blindly. A man on the other hand looks forwards and backwards, and compares his various feelings, desires, and recollections. He then finds, in accordance with the verdict of all the wisest men that the highest satisfaction is derived from following certain impulses, namely the social instincts. If he acts for the good of others, he will receive the approbation of his fellow men and gain the love of those with whom he lives; and this latter gain undoubtedly is the highest pleasure on this earth. By degrees it will become intolerable to obey his sensuous passions rather than his higher impulses.[9]

Darwin was no romantic: he understood that human beings, like all animals, are motivated to compete aggressively for individual survival and reproductive success. He believed that the same social instinct that inclines people to altruism towards their own group or tribe also predisposes them to ruthless aggression towards members of competing tribal groups.[10] He recognised that some people would be inclined to exploit others in the most cooperative groups by cheating, and recognised the necessity for groups to exert strong social controls against this threat.[11] However, he maintained that the success of the tribe in intertribal warfare depended upon the governing of life within tribal communities by adaptations other than direct competition, most especially cooperativeness and self-sacrifice.

Darwin emphasised that organic evolution in general took place through a variety of different processes, of which the natural selection of competing individuals (i.e. the 'survival of the fittest') *was only one*. Darwin argued that a different process, natural selection between incessantly warring tribal groups, explained how the social instinct and the moral sense had arisen through the course of evolution. This evolutionary process has more recently been called 'group selection' by biologists, although Darwin described it simply as one aspect of natural selection:

> When two tribes of primitive man, living in the same country, came into competition, if the one tribe included (other circumstances being equal) a greater number of courageous, sympathetic, and faithful members, who were always ready to warn each other of danger, to aid and defend each other, this tribe would without doubt succeed best and conquer the other.... Thus the social and moral qualities would tend slowly to advance and be diffused throughout the world.[12]

> In however complex a manner [the feeling of sympathy] may have originated, as it is one of high importance to all those animals which aid and defend each other, it will have been increased, *through natural selection*; for those communities, which included the greatest number of the most sympathetic members, would flourish best and rear the greatest number of offspring.[13]

Darwin recognised that the qualities that would evolve through the natural selection of groups would be different from, and sometimes conflict with, those that would evolve through natural selection of individuals. Specifically, he saw that whereas the natural selection of individuals would not favour the 'moral sense', natural selection of groups would. He saw that both kinds of evolutionary processes (and other evolutionary processes as well) could take place at the same time and that for some kinds of traits the influence of group selection would prevail over the influence of individual selection. As Darwin put it:

> It must not be forgotten that although a high standard of morality gives but a slight or no advantage to each individual man and his children over the other men of the same tribe, yet that an advancement in the standard or morality and an increase in the number of well endowed men will certainly give an immense advantage to one tribe over another. There can be no doubt that a tribe including many members who, from possessing in a high degree the spirit of patriotism, fidelity, obedience, courage, and sympathy, were always ready to give aid to each other and to sacrifice themselves for the common good,

would be victorious over most other tribes; *and this would be natural selection.* At all times throughout the world tribes have supplanted other tribes; and as morality is one element in their success, the standard of morality and the number of well-endowed men will thus everywhere tend to rise and increase.[14]

Another way to say this is that the urge for social belonging is just as essential to human well-being as the urge to individual competition, and the two instinctive, but conflicting, motives exist for the same reason—evolution. It follows that individuals must always experience a conflict between one set of motives that impels them towards individual competition and another that impels them towards social integration and cooperation. In my opinion, all psychological thinking will be greatly advanced when the implications of Darwin's dual view of human motivation[15] are fully recognised, but this book restricts itself to the topic of addiction.

Darwin's analysis of human psychology depicts human beings as locked in an inescapable inner conflict between individual survival needs and social needs, a conflict that can be traced to both individual selection and group selection operating simultaneously, producing conflicting motives. Thus, Darwin established a biological basis for precisely the conflict between the individual and social needs that Erikson saw being meticulously reconciled in the process of psychosocial integration. Darwin's theory serves well to explain why little children, with their intensely powerful individual needs, so readily accept the multitude of restraints they must endure so that other people will know that they are 'good'. It also explains why adolescents are so desperate for acceptance by their peers. Finally, Darwin's theory can also explain why politics is so often a wrestling match between the relative importance of 'individual rights' and of 'group rights'.[16] Both values are expressions of powerful, innate human needs. Both can inflame passions. Both are essential to human well-being.

Darwin's reliance on group selection as an explanatory device for the evolution of human cooperativeness and sympathy has been the subject of bitter controversy, as group selection has been scorned as unscientific by many contemporary biologists over the last few decades.[17] On the other hand, there have always been influential biologists who agreed with Darwin about the role of group selection and the importance of the 'social instinct'. Currently, the tide appears to be turning in Darwin's favour. The evidence for Darwin's view has been powerfully argued by many scholars,[18] notably David Wilson and Elliot Sober. Wilson and Sober extended Darwin's general ideas on this topic into a 'multilevel selection theory' and cited evidence from biology as well as anthropology that human beings are adapted by evolution to live in communal and egalitarian communities.[19] The disdainful rejection of group selection by the majority of biologists in the recent past is probably better explained by the political climate than by the weight of evidence. Group selection does not fit with the dominant free-market ideology. Free-market ideology portrays unceasing individual competition as the path to universal wealth, progress, and happiness,[20] and therefore regards individual gratification as the singular basis of all human motivation. The individualistic competition that Darwin described in *The Origin of Species* has been a matter of great importance to free-market ideologists since the book was first published in 1859, as Darwin himself was well aware because of his family connections to the British Whig Party.[21]

Kropotkin's anthropology

Another famous student of 19th century anthropology was the Russian geographer and, later, revolutionary anarchist,[22] Prince Peter Kropotkin. Kropotkin's book on this topic, *Mutual aid: A Factor of Evolution*, first appeared in 1902. Summarising his own observations of tribespeople carried out incidentally during his early geographical research in Siberia, together with other 18th-and 19th-century studies of tribal people, Kropotkin wrote as follows:

> … primitive man has one quality, elaborated and maintained by the very necessities of his hard struggle for life—he identifies his own existence with that of his tribe; and without that quality mankind never would have attained the level it has attained now.
>
> Primitive folk… so much identify their lives with that of the tribe, that each of their acts, however insignificant, is considered as a tribal affair. Their whole behaviour is regulated by an infinite series of unwritten rules of propriety which are the fruit of their common experience as to what is good or bad—that is, beneficial or harmful for their own tribe… [23]

Kropotkin was not arguing for the existence of a 'noble savage'. He was not a student of Rousseau, but a resolute Darwinist. He recognised that most tribal people practised infanticide as a means of population control, that tribal life entailed frequent, cruel warfare against other tribes, and that evolution had produced strong drives towards individual ascendancy as well as group cooperation. However, he observed over and over that the preferred undertakings of most people, most of the time were carrying out co-operative tasks prescribed and regulated by the complex multi-layered social organisation of their own society.

Kropotkin also studied the social life of European and Asian peasants, relying on ancient and contemporary social historians. He concluded that the primary loyalties of agricultural human beings were to their villages, with lesser ties to individual families. In the complex multi-layered social structures that developed in agricultural villages, people's loyalties were all-important, leaving little room for individual competition.[24]

In support of his conclusion that the strongest peasant motivations were communal, Kropotkin cited the long history of determined peasant resistance to the destruction of village communes, a destruction that had been instituted all over Europe with the rise of modern nation states and industrial agriculture. The true 'tragedy of the commons' was not that commons-based farming broke down because individual peasants grabbed more than their fair share (as has been claimed[25]) but that the commons lands were relentlessly destroyed by administrative and military force in order to provide land and people for the free markets in real estate and labour. Late in the 19th century, when some states, notably France, Germany, and Russia, relaxed the laws in a way that allowed peasants to own their land in common again, large numbers of people who had been forced previously to live in a market society in which land was individually owned re-pooled their land to reinstitute communal agriculture. Kropotkin also found support for his observation of the naturally communal psychology of modern agricultural people in the various Anabaptist sects, such as

Mennonites and Hutterites, which endured violent persecution and fled en masse from place to place in order to retain their communal way of life.[26]

Although the great mass of people in the middle ages were peasants, a considerable number lived in 'free cities' that were the home of artisans and the great medieval guilds. Medieval free cities were built around social ties of the citizens to their villages of origin and to the guilds that regulated their economic activity. The markets of medieval cities were regulated by complex social obligations for the benefit of the entire community and had no similarity with the free-market ideal described by Adam Smith.[27] The overused word 'free' has very different meanings for different people. In this instance, the idea of 'free cities' is antithetical to the idea of 'free markets'.

Polanyi's economic anthropology

More recent evidence for the universality of socialised production and the virtual absence of free-market-style bartering and individual competition in primitive societies was reviewed by Karl Polanyi (1944) in his famous book, *The Great Transformation*. Anthropological studies of Melanesian Islanders and many other primitive peoples led Polanyi to this generalisation:

> The outstanding discovery of recent historical and anthropological research is that man's economy, as a rule, is submerged in his social relationships.... Take the case of a tribal society. The individual's economic interest is rarely paramount, for the community keeps all its members from starving unless it is itself borne down by catastrophe, in which case interests are again threatened collectively, not individually. The maintenance of social ties, on the other hand is crucial. First, because by disregarding the accepted code of honour, or generosity, the individual cuts himself off from the community and becomes an outcast; second, because, in the long run, all social obligations are reciprocal, and their fulfilment serves also the individual's give-and-take interests best. Such a situation must exert a continuous pressure on the individual to eliminate economic self-interest from his consciousness to the point of making him unable, in many cases (but by no means all) even to comprehend the implications of his own actions in terms of such an interest. This attitude is reinforced by the frequency of communal activities such as partaking of food from the common catch or sharing in the results of some far-flung and dangerous tribal expedition. The premium set on generosity is so great when measured in terms of social prestige as to make any other behaviour than that of utter self-forgetfulness simply not pay. Personal character has little to do with the matter. Man can be as good or evil, as social or asocial, jealous or generous, in respect to one set of values as in respect to another. Not to allow anybody reason for jealousy is, indeed, an accepted principle of ceremonial distribution... The human passions, good or bad, are merely directed towards non-economic ends. Ceremonial display serves to spur emulation to the utmost and the custom of communal labor tends to screw up both quantitative and qualitative standards to the highest pitch. The performance of all acts of exchange as free gifts that are expected to be reciprocated though not necessarily by the same individuals—a procedure minutely articulated and perfectly safeguarded by elaborate methods of publicity, by magic rites, and by the establishment of 'dualities' in which groups are linked in mutual obligations— should in itself explain the absence of the notion of gain or even of wealth other than that consisting of objects traditionally enhancing social prestige.[28]

Polanyi pointed out that the profound demoralization caused by colonialisation of primitive people was not due primarily to economic exploitation, for the demoralisation was as great in cases where the colonized people realized a net economic gain. Rather, the demoralization arose from the destruction of their cultures, without which people were individually, as well as collectively, shattered. Without their societies, primitive people are everywhere seen 'dying of boredom… or wasting their lives and substance in dissipation'.[29]

Nor did free-market societies form any part of the ancient Western world, although it was a settled agricultural civilisation with highly sophisticated economic activity. There was no hint of free markets in Plato's idealised *Republic*.[30] Athens' famous free market in food, the *agora*, may well have been the beginning of free-market culture in Western civilisation, but it was a rare exception in its day.[31] Aristotle made it clear in his *Politics* that subsistence farming (a so-called 'householding economy') is the normal way for people to live and that production for individual gain is 'not natural to man'.[32] The period of Rome's predominance:

> … in spite of its highly developed trade, represented no break in this respect; it was characterized by the grand scale on which redistribution of grain was practiced by the Roman administration in an otherwise householding economy, and it formed no exception to the rule that up to the end of the Middle Ages, markets played no important part in the economic system; other institutional patterns prevailed.[33]

Even the 'mercantile system' that prevailed in England between the 1500s and the 1700s remained one full step away from a free-market system. Every aspect of commercial organisation was subject to control of the monarch and parliament. Governments of the day freely ruled against free-market economics when they took it to be in the national interest to erect barriers against free trade or to regulate prices. Polanyi summarised the nature of the mercantile system as follows:

> The 'freeing' of trade performed by mercantilism merely liberated trade from particularism, but at the same time extended the scope of regulation. The economic system was submerged in general social relations; markets were merely an accessory feature of an institutional setting controlled and regulated more than ever by social authority.[34]

Adam Smith's *An Inquiry into the Nature and Causes of the Wealth of Nations,* published in 1776,[35] was a call to replace the waning mercantile system with a closer approximation of a free-market society. When free-market society removed most individual economic activity from the rubric of social control, the result was a burst of economic growth accompanied by mass dislocation. The psychological results of the dislocation that Polanyi perceived were catastrophic:

> … robbed of the protective covering of cultural institutions, human beings would perish from the effects of social exposure; they would die as the victims of acute social dislocation through vice, perversion, crime, and starvation.[36]

Erikson's anthropological psychology

Erik Erikson, who coined the term 'psychosocial integration', was a mid-20th-century student of history and anthropology as well as psychoanalysis. He established the universal necessity of psychosocial integration through direct observations of middle-class American children of the 1930s and 1940s, direct observation and anthropological studies of native Indians living on reservations in the United States, and historical studies of Martin Luther and George Bernard Shaw. His most famous book, *Childhood and Society*, includes comparative studies of the development of psychosocial integration in middle-class American children and members of two American Indian tribes, the Dakotas of the American plains and the Yurok of the American west coast. In these developmental studies, Erikson described the specific conflicts of individual needs and social accommodation that must be reconciled at each stage for psychosocial integration to be successfully established and maintained. He emphasised that, from the earliest stages onwards, developing human beings need the opportunity to express their individuality and feel 'free' as well as the opportunity to belong and feel that they are 'good'.

Erikson's language is seldom dramatic, but he strongly conveys the point that achieving psychosocial integration is essential both to individuals and to their societies. He makes the necessity of psychosocial integration most explicit when discussing adolescents and young adults, for whom he calls the experience of psychosocial integration 'ego identity':[37]

> ... in the social jungle of human existence, there is no feeling of being alive without a sense of ego identity. To understand this would be to understand the trouble of adolescents better, especially the trouble of all those who cannot just be 'nice' boys and girls, but are desperately seeking for a satisfactory sense of belonging... [38]

> ... many a late adolescent, if faced with continuing diffusion, would rather be nobody or somebody bad, or indeed, dead—and this totally, and by free choice—than be not-quite-somebody.[39]

Other support

The anthropological observations of Darwin, Kropotkin, Polanyi, and Erikson find strong support in more contemporary anthropology.[40] Perhaps the single best-known contemporary description of the comprehensive and essential nature of psychosocial integration in a pre-modern society comes from a study of the 'water temple system' of Bali.[41] In addition, the native people of western Canada, whose subjugation was not completed until the 20th century, have been particularly well placed for contemporary anthropological research.[42] The social life of these Canadian aboriginal people will be discussed more extensively in Chapter 6.

The evidence that people's well-being is dependent upon membership in cohesive groups and the observation that the absence of this membership leads to psychological problems have found professional advocates outside anthropology in the last few decades. The 'liberation psychology' of Ignacio Martín-Baró takes this position explicitly.[43] The subdiscipline of community psychology is committed to 'fostering community' on the grounds that community breakdown is a major cause of mental health problems.[44] Many sociologists and public health professionals have undertaken the task of measuring and raising the level of various indices of 'social capital' in communities, in the expectation of improvement in a variety of health parameters, including addiction. Some results of these interventions will be discussed briefly in Chapter 7.

Beyond academia, there is the testimony of the existentialist writers of the 19th and 20th centuries who have meticulously explored the anxiety and dread of modern Western people. The existentialists could achieve neither rational nor religious certainty, nor a sense of meaning in the absurd and pointless social world into which they had been thrown. While celebrating the power and responsibility of each person to create his or her own meaning, the existentialists documented their own drift towards neurosis, madness, suicide, and sexual deviance,[45] thus providing detailed introspective accounts of the anguish and misery of dislocation.

The influence of existentialism is evident in descriptions of the pain of dislocation that is the topic of many contemporary novels and biographies, some of which enjoy great popularity.[46] Whereas existential descriptions of the absurdity of modern society and the anguish of dislocation accord well with the dislocation theory of addiction, the existentialists' hope that individuals can produce adequate meaning by their own individual efforts does not. Meaning has a social basis in the dislocation theory.

Some of the greatest thinkers of the recent past have made a point of the harsh consequences that befall a society, like our own, that seems determined to ignore psychosocial integration. One of the most concise and lucid statements of this point was written by Albert Einstein in an amazing article that appeared in an American magazine in 1949. After tactfully explaining why economists did not have any exclusive claim to 'scientific' expertise about the nature of human society, Einstein wrote his own analysis of the malaise of the society of his day, based in part on his own reading of anthropology.

He blamed the malaise partly on economic injustice, but stressed that the greater problem was the 'crippling of social consciousness' that modern capitalism inevitably produced. Einstein started his argument with an explanation of the human innate need for social life and a description of what is called 'psychosocial integration' in this book:

> Man is, at one and the same time, a solitary being and a social being. As a solitary being, he attempts to protect his own existence and that of those who are closest to him, to satisfy his personal desires, and to develop his innate abilities. As a social being, he seeks to gain the recognition and affection of his fellow human beings, to share in their pleasures, to comfort them in their sorrows, and to improve their conditions of life. Only the existence of these varied, frequently conflicting, strivings accounts for the special character of a man, and their specific combination determines the extent to which an individual can achieve an inner equilibrium and can contribute to the well-being of society.[47]

Einstein continued by characterising extreme individualism as the 'crisis of our time' and arguing that this crisis is caused by what is called 'free-market society' in this book.

> ... the essence of the crisis of our time... concerns the relationship of the individual to society. The individual has become more conscious than ever of his dependence

upon society. But he does not experience this dependence as a positive asset, as an organic tie, as a protective force, but rather as a threat to his natural rights, or even to his economic existence. Moreover, his position in society is such that the egotistical drives of his make-up are constantly being accentuated, while his social drives, which are by nature weaker, progressively deteriorate. All human beings, whatever their position in society, are suffering from this process of deterioration. Unknowingly prisoners of their own egotism, they feel insecure, lonely, and deprived of the naive, simple, and unsophisticated enjoyment of life…

The economic anarchy of capitalist society as it exists today is, in my opinion, the real source of the evil. We see before us a huge community of producers the members of which are unceasingly striving to deprive each other of the fruits of their collective labor—not by force, but on the whole in faithful compliance with legally established rules.[48]

As a consequence of this and other articles written in the post-World War II period, Einstein, who then lived in the United States, was investigated by one of the American federal police forces. The Federal Bureau of Investigation accumulated an 1800 page dossier on him, with the intention of publicly exposing him as an anarchist, communist, and traitor.[49]

Recently, another prominent scientist, Canadian geneticist and environmentalist, David Suzuki, made a point that is similar to Einstein's:

We met people striving to find solutions, and as they talked about the way they lived and their most fundamental visions for the future, we had to reflect on what had brought each of us the most personal happiness in the past. This exercise made us realize that, beyond very basic levels, our separate experiences of satisfaction, contentment and joy had very little to do with material consumption and comforts. They had more to do with connecting with others, with feeling useful and, amazingly enough, with sharing everything—from food and feelings to ideas and beliefs.[50]

Influential Christian leader Jean Vanier has described the misery of extreme dislocation[51] in particularly eloquent terms. He has also described the conflict that people feel between the need for group belonging and the need for individual accomplishment—the conflict that grows out of Darwin's two levels of human evolution:

So here is the paradox: as humans we are caught between competing drives, the drive to belong, to fit in and to be a part of something bigger than ourselves, and the drive to let our deepest selves rise up, to walk alone, to refuse the accepted and the comfortable… [52]

However, it is not the observations of great scientists, anthropologists, or theologians that finally convince me that psychosocial integration is as essential condition of human well-being, because such evidence is always arguable. Rather it is face-to-face accounts given by my own friends and family—people I personally know and trust—of the emotional anguish that arises from the loneliness and fragmentation of lives in free-market society. These same relatives and friends also speak enthusiastically of their individual achievement and their taste for competition. All people who I know well seem to feel both sets of needs strongly, although they do not usually feel both of them at the same time, for one is antithetical to the other.

When I speak on this topic professionally, members of the audience are often eager to add their own testimony on the lack of psychosocial integration that they feel and the anguish that it causes. I also see the anguish of dislocation leading otherwise critical people to uncritical wishful thinking; for example, responding with poignant eagerness to dubious opportunities to 'build community' that are available on 1,450,000 sites that can be Googled on the Internet as this is being written. Beyond this, the reflections of my own later years have revealed, to my surprise, that psychosocial integration has been just as essential a need in my own life as individual accomplishment. The experience of sustained mutual recognition and belonging has proven essential for me to feel contentment in life. I wish I had understood this sooner.

It now seems obvious that the greatest single political division of the past two centuries, the division between capitalism and socialism, has been built on a false dichotomy. Extreme capitalists have claimed, falsely, that human beings need only individual autonomy, achievement, and the products of the market. If people could not feel satisfied in Margaret Thatcher's or Ronald Reagan's free-market society,[53] it must be because their needs for individual freedom and material wealth are *insatiable*, and they must be provided with more of them through the free play of market forces.[54] Extreme socialists have claimed, just as falsely, that human beings need nothing more than the support and guidance of their society to prosper psychologically. If people could not feel satisfied in Mao's China, it must be that they needed more diligent re-education in social theory from their comrades. Both of these extreme ideologies are caricatures of human nature.[55]

Human beings must satisfy *both* their need for individual autonomy and their need for social belonging. There is no adequate substitute for either one. This is why Chairman Mao, in his period of immense popularity and power, was unable to purge China of individualism. This is also why the United States, in a century of military and political dominance, was unable to purge South America of communism. One current reminder of this duality in human motivation is the strong and persistent ambivalence of the citizens of the former East Germany, who lived under a collectivist regime for half a century, and, having rejected it, were warmly welcomed into the free-market society of West Germany in 1990. Poignant accounts of their nostalgia[56] for the unfree, unproductive, but stable social life of East Germany—as well as their appreciation of the new freedoms and opportunities in the west—illustrate the complexity of human motivation.[57] Perhaps the least welcome reminder of this duality in human motivation is the current resurgence of fervent ethnic and racial nationalism in Europe, supported by vigorous political parties and an erudite group of intellectuals.[58] Society has been lightning-quick to recognise, correctly, the potential for violence that inheres in this kind of nationalism. However, it has been too slow to perceive that popular nationalism is the natural expression of an irrevocable human need for a feeling of belonging in one's own country that can be eroded by mass immigration. It is unlikely that society will be able to devise ways of controlling popular nationalism until it is willing to understand its origins.

The genius of a successful culture is that it provides adequately for individual autonomy and social belonging at the same time—a balancing act of the greatest virtuosity, since the needs often conflict with each other.[59] The crucial flaw of globalising free-market society is that the balance has shifted so far in favour of individualism that it is now extremely difficult to recover equilibrium because of the catastrophic damage—environmental, social, psychological, and spiritual—that this imbalance has already caused. The remedy for this imbalance is not a shift to the other extreme of all-encompassing collectivism, but re-establishment of the balance, if this is still possible.

Perhaps the vacuous and simplistic nature of contemporary political rhetoric reflects a loss of faith that the essential balancing act can be achieved. Imagine a pair of circus acrobats who have just tripped and fallen off a high wire in the middle of their performance, one on the left side of the wire and the other on the right side. As they hurtle downward, they can be heard bombastically arguing about whether it is more intelligent and graceful to be on the right or the left of the wire. In reality, of course, only the act of balancing itself has any intelligence and grace. The absurdity of the dispute becomes more and more evident as the disputants approach the ground.

Endnotes

1 There is another biological line of argument, based on the concept of 'neoteny', which will not be discussed in this book. Ancient scholars and modern biologists have noted that human beings lack the morphological and behavioural adaptations that allow individual members of other mammalian species to survive outside groups (see the myth of Prometheus, as recounted by Plato, c. 388 BC/1956; S. J. Gould, 1977; Dufour, 2005). Other primates are better adapted for survival in isolation, although they, like human beings, normally live a social existence. Human beings are said to be 'paedomorphic' or 'neotenous' relative to other primates, meaning that the adult form retains many juvenile features, including those that make it vulnerable to the physical environment and to predators outside a social group. Because of this, human beings can only survive in a condition of close social integration, which requires the social construction of a god or gods and a consequent reduction in the individually competitive nature that evolution might otherwise favour.

2 The worldwide destruction of aboriginal people is described by Bayly (2004, Chapter 12).

3 Dawkins (1989); J. Jacobs (2000); N. Reynolds (2006b).

4 Perhaps most famously by Dawkins (1989), but by many others as well.

5 Desmond and Moore (1991, p. 262); Darwin (1887/1958b, pp. 130–131).

6 Darwin (1859/1958a).

7 Darwin (1871/1981, pp. 70–71).

8 Darwin (1871/1981, p. 71).

9 Darwin (1887/1958b, p. 93, see also p. 89).

10 Darwin (1871/1981, pp. 85, 94–95).

11 Darwin (1871/1981, pp. 92, 163–165).

12 Darwin (1871/1981, p. 162–163).

13 Darwin (1871/1981, p. 82, italics added).

14 Darwin (1871/1981, p. 166, italics added).

15 See D. S. Wilson and Sober (1994) and D. S. Wilson (2002, Chapter 1). In the broadest terms, it seems to me that a society that ignores either of these two fundamental motivations is unfit for habitation by human beings. This would apply to extreme forms of

communism, which allow no room for individual competition, and to extreme forms of individualism, which threaten to engulf today's free-market society.

16 Alfred (1999); Ignatieff (2000).

17 D. S. Wilson (2002).

18 Henderson (2005).

19 For example, D. S. Wilson and Sober (1994), Sober and Wilson (1998), and D.S. Wilson (2002). Although D. S. Wilson and Sober do not explicitly postulate a psychological need of human beings to experience social belonging, as Darwin did with his concept of the 'social instinct', I think that this conclusion follows inevitably from the analysis that they have made.

20 For example, T. Friedman (2000).

21 Desmond and Moore (1991).

22 It might seem as if Kropotkin's anthropology grew from his political views, but in fact his anthropology was developed long before his radical politics (Todes, 1987, p. 547).

23 Kropotkin (1914/1972, pp. 109–110).

24 Kropotkin (1914/1972, Chapter 4).

25 The phrase 'tragedy of the commons' and the widely circulated idea that the commons failed because of uncontrollable individual greed come from a famous article by Hardin (1968). Actual historical evidence flatly contradicts Hardin's theoretical argument that commons must inevitably fail (McKibben, 2007, p. 199).

26 Kropotkin (1914/1972, Chapter 7).

27 Kropotkin (1914/1972, Chapter 5).

28 K. Polanyi (1944, pp. 46–47).

29 K. Polanyi (1944, p. 158).

30 Plato (c. 360 BC/1987).

31 K. Polanyi (1957).

32 Cited in K. Polanyi (1944, p. 54).

33 K. Polanyi (1944, p. 55).

34 K. Polanyi (1944, p. 67).

35 Adam Smith (1776/1991).

36 K. Polanyi (1944, p. 73).

37 Ego identity has its origin in psychosocial integration, and is experienced not only as a sense of social solidarity, but also as a sense of assured, developing individuality (Erikson, 1959, p. 102). Erikson repeatedly reminds his readers that, whereas the crisis of ego identity peaks in adolescence, the more general problem of identity formation and maintenance is a life-long process (e.g. Erikson, 1959, p. 113, Section III).

38 Erikson (1959, p. 90).

39 Erikson (1959, p. 132).

40 See review by D. S. Wilson (2002). See also a remarkable book by J. Jacobs (1961, esp. Chapters 1–6) that can be viewed as an anthropological study of people living in large American cities prior to about 1960.

41 Lansing (1991).

42 Sproat (1868/1987); McFeat (1966); Tennant (1990); K. T. Carlson (1997).

43 Martín-Baró (1994).

44 Sarason (1974); Jason and Kobayashi (1995); Moane (2003).

45 Sartre (1938/1969); Genet (1943/1963); Tillich (1952, pp. 71–74).

46 See S. Martin (2003) for a review of the popular Canadian author David Adams Richards, whose novels depict the anguished lives of 'outsiders' in Canada and their proclivity for addiction to alcohol, drugs, and tobacco. Richards' autobiographical writing tells a similar story about his own life (Richards, 2001). See also Patrick Lane's memoir, *There is a Season* (2004), and Canadian novels by B. Morgan (1994), Clarke (1997), MacLeod (1999), Sweatman (2001), Flood (2002), Cruise and Griffiths (2003), Lansens (2003), Kogawa (2003), A.-M. MacDonald (2003), A. York (2003), Sakamoto (2004), and Coupland (2006). See also D. Bock (2006).

47 Einstein (1949/1998, p. 3).

48 Einstein (1949/1998, p. 5).

49 Larousserie (2005).

50 Suzuki and Dressel (2002, p. 2).

51 Vanier uses the word 'loneliness' rather than dislocation, but his descriptions make it clear that he is giving it a very similar meaning (Vanier, 1998, Chapter 1).

52 Vanier (1998, Chapter 1, p. 18).

53 Homer-Dixon (2006, pp. 192–193).

54 J. Heath (2001, pp. 248–249, 305); Morris and Sayre (2004, p. 20); Anderssen (2004a). Most psychological research views human and animal motivation as homeostatic rather than insatiable. 'Insatiability' is normally linked to particular types of psychological disorder, like compulsion, and particular types of personality like Cushman's (1995) 'empty self'.

55 Although this caricatural dichotomy was conspicuous in the competing ideologies of the 'Cold War', it played an equally fundamental role in World War II. K. Polanyi (1935) showed that the philosophical essence of fascism lay in abhorrence of individual freedom and equality, seen as modern abominations that blocked the way to a statist, *Volk* utopia. German fascists identified free-market capitalism and Christianity as the embodiments of this abomination and, in contrast to more recent ideology, regarded socialism as a repugnant offshoot of capitalism that espoused both individualism, equality, and—the ultimate horror—withering away of the state in favour of a universal, racially inclusive domination of human kind by the working class (K. Polanyi, 1935).

56 This nostalgia is sometimes referred to as 'ostalgia' because *Ost* is the German word for east.

57 Vidal *et al.* (2004). Economic issues often loom just as large in 'ostalgia' as psychological ones, because many East Germans have been impoverished financially as well as psychosocially by the regime change. I am not emphasising these economic issues here because they are not relevant to the theoretical issues at hand.

58 O'Meara (2004) has written extensively about the intellectual movement, the *Groupement de Recherche et d'Etude pour la Civilisation Européenne*. See also Alexander-Davey (2005).

59 Tawney (1926/1947); K. Polanyi (1944, pp. 254–258B); Wilber (1996, p. 296); Dufour (2005, pp. 345–346).

Chapter 5

Free-market Society Undermines Psychosocial Integration

The second principle of the dislocation theory of addiction is that globalisation of free-market society produces a general breakdown of psychosocial integration, spreading dislocation everywhere. After defining free-market society, this chapter reviews historical and contemporary evidence that free-market society is spreading irrepressibly, producing mass dislocation in every stratum of world society.

A free-market society is one in which virtually every human activity is structured by competitive markets that are only regulated to the extent necessary to maintain their economic efficiency. Polanyi explained that a free-market society:

> … must comprise all elements of industry, including labor, land, and money…. But labor and land are no other than the human beings themselves of which every society consists and the natural surroundings in which it exists. To include them in the market mechanism means to subordinate the substance of society itself to the laws of the market.[1]

Thus, within free-market society, the competitive marketplace becomes the matrix of human existence. As free-market society expands, its scope becomes ever more engulfing and its corporations become multinational Goliaths. Activities that formerly fell outside the market become gradually commercialised, while objects that formerly existed outside the market are gradually commoditised and capitalised. Public information media ceaselessly promote the ideology of free-market society and advertise its glittering products. The ideal of free-market society, stated in language derived from Friedrich von Hayek, Milton Friedman, Margaret Thatcher, and the so-called 'Washington Consensus', is built into globalisation as it is understood in today's world.[2]

Today, people in my city worry because their medical care, education, and hydroelectric power, previously understood as government services assured to all at minimum cost, are inexorably being 'privatised' (i.e. being drawn into the free market). People worry because housing prices have become so high and so volatile that having a secure home is impossible except for the rich. In my university, professors worry that intellectual community is being eroded as ideas are drawn into the market as 'intellectual property' or 'proprietary knowledge'. People often associate these problems with the current government or a particular jurisdiction, but this view is too narrow. These problems are elements of the global advance of free-market society that has been underway for the last few centuries.

Some aspects of the spread of free-market society, like the conquest of the globe by McDonald's and Wal-Mart and the adoption of radical free-market economics in

Eastern Europe, are highly publicised and celebrated. However, many structural movements towards free-market society occur without fanfare or even acknowledgement. For example, governments often sign 'free trade' agreements without any real public discussion. After the agreements come into force, it becomes clear that they include a legal infrastructure that prevents communities from functioning in any way that might interfere with domestic or foreign business profits. Such free trade agreements often make it difficult for people to enact safety and environmental regulations through their governments, to run cooperatives and collectives that would compete with multinational corporations, or to preserve land that is publicly owned for environmental, agricultural, or cultural purposes.[3]

Although the public is often unaware of the global march of free-market society, it shapes our lives. Historians and social scientists do not overlook it, although they often disagree sharply about its costs and benefits.[4] I am convinced that practitioners in the field of addiction cannot overlook the globalisation of free-market society either, because the current irrepressible spread of addiction cannot be adequately comprehended unless the dislocation produced by the ever-expanding free-market society is taken into account.

It is important to emphasise again that the second principle of the dislocation theory does not mean that dislocation occurs *only* in free-market society. Individual misfortunes can dislocate any person, anywhere, at any time. Tribal, feudal, and socialist societies often dislocate certain individuals and groups in the course of local conflicts. The catastrophic collapse of any society inevitably produces mass dislocation. However, only free-market society inexorably destroys psychosocial integration everywhere, even at the best of times.

This chapter next describes the spread of mass dislocation in the early centuries of free-market society. It goes on to describe the continuing growth of dislocation as the globalisation of free-market society advances into the 21st century.

The birth of free-market society

Although human beings have always bartered and competed for individual advantage *on some occasions*, historians and economists agree that people never formed free-market societies before the modern era. Markets in pre-modern Europe, for example, were never the primary organising institution of society. Even where markets had an important role, they were definitely not 'free'. Markets everywhere were subordinated to the larger concerns of society and religion.[5] In pre-modern Europe, both prices and the nature of goods that could be sold were tightly regulated to maintain peace and stability among the groups that used the market for their mutual advantage. This was particularly true in the money markets. Loans that were seen to be unfair to the borrower, broadly defined as 'usury' or 'avarice', were punished severely.

The Bavarian Beer Purity Law of 1516 provides a currently familiar example of the subordination of markets to the needs of society. This law set maximum retail prices for a stein of beer and restricted the ingredients in beer to the three that were then known in Bavaria: water, hops, and barley. (Yeast was added to this list after its role in the chemistry of brewing was better understood.) There were at least three purposes to the law: preserving product quality for the consumer; protecting the consumer from excessive prices; and protecting the valuable stocks of certain grains, particularly wheat and rye, from being used for purposes other than food.[6] Although this law obviously violates the ideal of a market regulated only by the laws of supply and demand, the portion of it restricting ingredients in beer was ensconced in German law for more than four centuries. This law was finally quashed by the European Court of Justice in 1987 on the grounds that it created a trade barrier and thus constituted illegal protectionism (i.e. it contravened the goal of a global free market in beer). Because of protests of this decision by German beer drinkers, however, a weakened form of the law is still enforced in Germany.[7] As a result of the popular appeal of the law among beer drinkers, the concept is still used to market beer. One popular Canadian beer is brand-named '1516 Bavarian Lager'.

It was not only products that were regulated prior to free-market society, but also customers. Markets were definitely not open to everybody who wanted to buy or sell. Participation was restricted in ways that benefited and stabilised local communities of producers and consumers.[8] The forms of regulation varied locally, but markets everywhere were embedded in larger social systems and were strictly controlled to benefit society.

This is not to idealise pre-modern Europe as a blissful economic collective with cheap bread and beer. A highly structured class system and a corrupt church often engaged in large-scale economic exploitation. The protections built into local markets by law and tradition were often subverted by sharp practice, leading to lawsuits and rebellions. Fierce capitalistic competition sometimes broke out in commercial cities spread all over Europe, notably Florence and Flanders. However, in theory and in action, the accepted guiding principles of social life for the overwhelming majority of people did not derive from free-market principles but rather from regimes that held piety and community well-being as their highest values.[9]

The route towards the modern practice of embedding social life in the structure of the market, rather than the other way around, has been most thoroughly documented in England. This economic evolution was not uniquely English by any means, but England eventually set the pace and style for the rest of the modernising world[10] and dominated the world in the 19th century because it made the system work most effectively. In the 20th century, the United States assumed the leading role. For this reason, the current language of globalisation is English and the uniform of globalisation is the American version of the English business suit. Fortunately, the cuisine of globalisation is more varied.

In the late 1400s, England had a rural, manorial economy that was just a few steps removed from feudalism. The legal status of serfdom had not yet completely disappeared from English law.[11] Ordinary people did not speak of free markets or capitalism—they had never heard of such a thing. Three centuries later, in 1776, Adam Smith described an emerging British economy in which the free market was the prototypical form of trade. He provided a justification for free markets that became the bedrock of today's economic orthodoxy. Prices will reach optimum levels only if they are set by the interplay of supply and demand in a minimally regulated market. Optimum prices will insure that the market distributes goods and services with the greatest possible benefits to the greatest number of people. Between the late 1400s and 1776, recognisable free markets, but still no fully fledged free-market society, had come into existence. The gains in economic vitality were obvious to all. The human suffering of this transition period and the industrial revolution that followed is most usually depicted by historians in terms of poverty, starvation, war, and injustice, but in this book the destruction of psychosocial integration is more important and will be highlighted in what follows.

In retrospect, the first concrete steps[12] towards free-market society and the dislocation that followed it can be recognised in the agricultural 'enclosure movement' that first became evident in the late 1400s.[13] Landlords and prosperous yeoman farmers were increasingly attracted by continental European buyers who sought high-quality goods and were prepared to pay with silver from the New World. Systematic 'enclosures' and evictions of small, subsistence farmers in England created large tracts of land to pasture the sheep whose wool sustained an expanding export trade in English broadcloth. Evictions of the small farmers broke down the local structure of neighbourhoods, hamlets, and the 'commons', from which the 'commoners' drew their name. Early on, the enclosure movement drew strong condemnation from church and state, notably from the great Catholic humanist, Thomas More, in his book *Utopia*, published in 1516.[14] Condemnation notwithstanding, large-scale, forced displacement of long-settled populations proved unstoppable, although some English monarchs successfully slowed this process in the interest of social stability.[15] As time passed, minds changed and the enclosure movement was able to draw more and more legitimacy from the throne, political power from parliament, and sanctity from English Protestantism.[16]

Additional steps moved English agriculture, previously structured by custom, local regulation, and by powerful ideals of Christian charity and secular neighbourliness,[17] further and further towards free markets in commodities, land, and farm labour.[18] These additional steps included a steep rise in prices and rents; the sale of land that had been seized from Catholic monasteries and churches for commercial farming; the 'engrossment' of small farms into larger ones that could produce surpluses for regional and international markets; the adoption of powerful methods of increasing production, including the extensive use of manure and other fertilisers; and specialisation of different regions of the countryside for modes of production that were dictated by shifting market imperatives. All of these brought individual wealth to the larger farmers at the expense of traditional ways of doing things,[19] increasing both dislocation and destitution of the smaller farmers. Although many large farmers grew wealthier, they too experienced the loss of social relations and traditions that had previously bolstered their own psychosocial integration.

In the mid-1600s, England was riven by bloody strife and revolution. There were many reasons for this strife, some of which were economic. Although some people saw the economic change that had begun in the previous century as a great and exciting opportunity, others were horrified by the dislocation, poverty, and repression that resulted and were willing to fight to defend their way of life. It was the stately role of King and Parliament to mediate between these two groups. As time passed, the state came down more and more on the side of free markets. Lethal force was applied to the degree necessary to suppress rebellions and protests of the poor. The decisive role of military and civil coercion by the British government in establishing a domestic free-market system has been documented by many economic historians.[20]

Spreading from the agricultural sector, a manufacturing-based market economy, including substantial iron and coal industries, had begun by the 1600s, continued to expand through the 1700s, and exploded into the industrial revolution in the 1800s. The industrial labour that was needed came from massive migration of the rural poor from their farms, hamlets, and commons as more and more of the land was enclosed and people were absorbed into urban slums and foreign colonies. Many forms of dislocation that did not necessarily entail geographical displacement were also imposed by governments and the courts in support of the burgeoning free-market society. These included forced apprenticeship of children of the poor, suppression of voluntary associations of working people that strove to introduce collective rather than individual bargaining, elimination of local charity, which had sustained the 'undeserving poor' thereby keeping some people out of the labour market, and confinement of vagrants and the destitute in houses of correction where lessons on the new realities were underscored with whips and branding irons.[21]

This enormous structural change in English society had both benefits and costs. Free-market society was very good for the bank accounts of English landowners with an eye for business and of the most entrepreneurial commoners who rose to positions of wealth and power in the flourishing middle class.[22] It was very good for the geopolitical stature of England, which expanded into a global power called 'Great Britain', because free-market economics provided an ideal financial and social structure for dominance, not only in global trade but also in global warfare.[23] It was good for the incomes of British traders and colonists who employed free-market principles to extract great wealth from the rest of the world.

Free-market society was very bad, however, for the lower strata of the English working class and worse still for colonial labourers and slaves. Although the sun never set on the global British Empire, it set far too early on these workers and their children who toiled arduously for bare subsistence—when they had the good fortune to find work and could muster the strength to carry it out.[24] Their privations were both psychosocial and material. Amidst desperate poverty, there was little hope of developing stable new social customs and ties to replace those traditional forms of psychosocial integration that had been ruptured.

The necessary connection between the new economics and human misery was recognised both by intellectuals who were infatuated with free-market capitalism, like William Townsend and Herbert Spencer, and by those who were horrified by the suffering it produced, like Robert Owen and Karl Marx.[25] In the late 1800s, a strong countermovement of British working-class unions and humanitarians within the middle and upper classes finally gained real power and the cruelties of free-marketisation were reduced in Great Britain itself. However, they continued to increase around the globe.

From England, the movement towards English-style free-market society spread like wildfire in all directions, becoming truly global within a few centuries.[26] A few decades after Adam Smith wrote *The Wealth of Nations*, Ricardo's law of comparative advantage extended the faith in benign optimisation to the effects of free trade between rich and poor nations. Growing industrial development provided the basis for indomitable English military and naval power based on modern finance, technology, and mass production of strategic supplies. Businessmen and soldiers carried the principles of free-market society from England to the rest of the British Isles and to the British colonies abroad, where English unions and humanitarians had little to say about it. Particularly visible instances of dislocation acquired their own names, such as the 'slave trade' that carried millions of blacks from African villages to the cane and cotton fields of the New World,[27] 'clearances' of the clan society from the Scottish highlands,[28] 'transportation' of thousands of convict labourers from England to settle in Australia,[29] and the *grand dérangement* of the Acadian population of maritime Canada.[30] Around the world, British settlers, traders, and colonial administrations reproduced their own dislocation by devastating aboriginal and other pre-modern societies everywhere—including Canada—and harnessing the energy of the dislocated 'coloured' people as producers and consumers in the global free markets. This process degraded stable pre-modern societies around the globe into what is now called 'the Third World'.[31]

Increasing British economic and military power hastened the growth of free-market society in continental Europe, where its spread was enthusiastically accelerated in France by Napoleon I and his successors after the revolution of 1789 and was propagated across the continent during the brief period of French imperial domination.[32] It was impossible to stand up to the British without adopting the economic system that was the foundation of their economic and military strength.[33] There was no resisting the spread of free-market economics. As A. C. Bayly put it, 'The elaborate system of commercial and trade regulation of the eighteenth century was abolished by consent in northwestern Europe. It was blown apart by British and French gunboats in China and the Ottoman Empire and North Africa.'[34] Whereas the European empires eventually fell apart, the expansion of free-market society continued, providing the economic structure for what is now called globalisation.

In the 20th century, globalisation was slowed by two world wars, an economic depression, and a 'cold war'. However, it regained full stride with the collapse of the Soviet Union and raced into the 21st century. Something close to a worldwide free-market society had been achieved by the end of the 20th century. John Ralston Saul described it as follows:

> Never before had the great nations so explicitly and single-mindedly organised their core relationship around naked, commercial self-interest, without the positive and negative counterweights of social standards, human rights, political systems, dynasties, formal religions, and, at the negative extreme, supposed racial destinies.[35]

It is not only left-leaning intellectuals like John Ralston Saul, R. H. Tawney,[36] and Karl Polanyi[37] who recognise the establishment of a worldwide free-market society. Economists and historians across the political spectrum do as well. George Soros, billionaire financier and economist, acknowledges 'the untrammelled intensification of laissez-faire capitalism and the spread of market values into all areas of life'.[38]

In some cases, such as the United States in the late 1800s and today's Singapore and China, the movement towards free-market society brought many people the benefits of affluence, modern medicine, science, and national pride, although it was always mixed with protests by the poor and excluded that had to be violently suppressed. In other cases, like today's Nigeria and Angola, only foreign investors and the very richest local opportunists benefited, while the great mass of people received starvation and oppression for their portion.[39] *In every case*, however, movement towards free-market society brought mass dislocation.

As time passes, the ravages of dislocation are becoming more and more evident among rich nations as well as the poor ones, entrepreneurs as well as subsistence workers, libertarians as well as socialists. Free-market society exploits human cultures in the same relentless way that it exploits the earth's minerals, eventually leaving behind only low-grade ore and depleted tailings. Even the people who benefit the most from free-market society cannot escape the feeling that something fundamental is missing from their lives of affluence, longevity, and independence. Moreover, many of the compensations that free-market society provides for dislocated people are eminently suitable as objects of addiction. Some earliest items of international trade in the new global markets—opium, tobacco, and rum—quickly became infamous for their capacity to provide addictive solace on a mass scale.[40] Other major trade items turn out to facilitate addiction in ways that took longer to become apparent. For example, relatively cheap sugar, furs, and cotton fabrics enable addictive consumption of food and fashions.

The clearances of the Scottish highlands afford a more detailed case study of how free-market society imposed mass dislocation on older forms of society. Later sections of this chapter provide examples from the 20th and 21st centuries.

The Highlands clearances (c. 1750–1850)

For many centuries before the modern era, people of the highlands and islands of northwestern Scotland all belonged to one of the many 'clans'[41] that divided the territory among them. Clan members were expected to support their clan chief with the produce from their little family plots of land and with their valour on the battlefield. In return, the clan chief used his power to preserve his people's rights to their tiny farms in perpetuity. Members of a clan quite often had the same family name as the clan chief. Even those who were not related by blood were expected to think of the other clan members as relatives and of the clan chief as their ritual father. Interclan battles, often provoked by boundary disputes or cattle theft, were frequent, bloody, and gallant. These little wars were ritualised with the flash of tartans, the skirl of bagpipes, and stories of the great heroes of the past whose spirits were said to live forever in the mountains and glens. The clans could be united, but only when they rose in opposition to invasions from the south or the east.

In everyday life, the clan members were hunters, cattle herders, and part-time subsistence farmers. The ideal of a clansman was to be fearless and violent in battle and gentle with women and children at home. The aged were cared for in the houses of their children. There was little need to export or import goods and little use for money. Highlands society was viewed with wistful admiration by romantics, but with disdain by those who hungered for 'progress' and 'improvement' on its sprawling territory.[42]

Repeated English invasions had civilised the lowlands of eastern and southern Scotland, and some aspects of English society had spilled over into the highlands. Some clans sold cattle in the lowlands to raise money.[43] However, until the second half of the 1700s, the greater part of the highlands had not experienced the blessings of English civilisation, and the great majority of highlanders preferred it that way.[44] English remained a foreign language; all levels of society spoke Gaelic. Although earlier encroachments had somewhat changed the traditional clan structure, most highlanders still retained a strong sense of clan identity and felt a deeply ingrained sense of loyalty to the clan chief.[45] Common people lived in stable families and occupied well-defined social strata either within communal townships based on 'runrig' farming or within communities of 'crofters'.[46] Although highland society suffered from famine in poor years, it offered psychosocial integration to even its poorest members, and emigration was uncommon.

After the last mass uprising of the clans against English domination was defeated at the Battle of Culloden in 1746, the British government undertook the destruction of highland society once and for all. The traditional bearing of arms was prohibited, as were the symbols of the old life, including tartan, kilt, and bagpipe. The hereditary powers of the chiefs were abrogated and some of their lands were confiscated and sold, along with their inhabitants, to lowland Scots or English gentry. Clan chiefs who retained land were admitted into English society, but only if they transformed themselves from Gaelic-speaking chiefs to English-speaking landlords.

The free market took up the work of cultural destruction where the military left off.[47] In an era of international war and population explosion, England needed more meat and wool than it could produce, and newly minted landlords of the spacious highlands had the opportunity to sell these commodities at unprecedented profits in a huge market. At the same time that the Scottish landlords were losing their traditional status in highland society, they learned to covet the prestige that the export market could bring: homes in London, city wives with worldly *repartée* and *décolletage*, English peerages, continental food and art.

The highlands had always produced cattle and grain, but had consumed most of it locally. However, it was quickly discovered that a landlord's wealth could be multiplied by replacing the cattle with new breeds of hardy sheep and reducing the human population from many settled families to a few perambulatory shepherds. Most of the clansmen, now redefined as agricultural workers subject to the laws of supply and demand in the labour market, remained a warrior race in their own minds and would have nothing to do with running sheep, especially on the lands of evicted comrades and kinsmen. It became evident that either the free market was to be thwarted by highland tradition or the highlanders had to be evicted. The evictions that ensued were so vast in scope that they became known as 'clearances'.

Legal eviction notices procured by former clan chiefs or imported landlords usually allowed highland families a few months to voluntarily pull down their houses and leave. Many refused and saw their homes burnt to the ground by the sheriff. In lieu of their ancestral land, the families were sometimes offered less arable land, where they might subsist by growing potatoes, or a house site on the coast along with the opportunity to join the herring fishery or to work as miners. The dislocation and starvation that resulted were described as both inevitable and just within the free-market logic of the day, and these arguments were upheld in Scottish courts.[48]

A few chiefs, mindful of their hereditary obligations, strove to resist the economic pressure towards clearances or to create viable economic alternatives for dispossessed clansmen, but the 'market forces' of the day swept these into bankruptcy and their people were cleared anyway.[49] For thousands of ordinary people, the only options were to flee to the slums of Glasgow or to emigrate in disease-ridden boats for Canada or other destinations at their own expense.

Sporadic rebellions against the clearances by disarmed highlanders were quelled by regular troops from Scottish regiments, dispatched by the English king at the request of local chiefs or English landlords. The legality of this military coercion was upheld in court on free-market principles. Justifications for the clearances written for the public stressed the improved productivity of the land, which was true; the poverty of the cotters under the traditional system, which was true enough; and the happiness of the evicted people, which was an outrageous lie.[50] The pitiless cruelty of the burnings and subsequent exile, including deaths by exposure, starvation, and infectious disease, were documented by first-hand witnesses.[51] The enduring despair of the survivors over the loss of their way of life was documented in a mournful folk literature, mostly written in Gaelic.[52]

Highlanders who were not evicted or starved were deliberately stripped of their cultural memory. The life of James Loch, a famous highlands administrator, has been described thus:

> ... for the rest of his life, he worked to complete the clearance of the interior, to carve the emptied lands into great sheep farms, to build harbours, bridge rivers, turn cattle-tracks into macadam roads, and to so mould and control the lives of 'the ignorant and credulous people' that at one time the young among them had to go to his agents for permission to marry. 'In a few years,' he wrote, before a quarter of his long service was run, 'the character of the whole of this population will be completely changed.... The children of those who are removed from the hills will lose all recollection of the habits and customs of their fathers.[53]

As sheep replaced people and hamlets, the highlands became far more productive of exportable wealth than they had been before. A few of those who were not exiled prospered, primarily chiefs who had transformed themselves into British gentry and their overseers. English entrepreneurs who acquired highland estates became immensely wealthy. Some of those driven off the land were lost in the growing army of day labourers that filled the slums of industrial Great Britain. A few became great soldiers, wealthy traders, and captains of industry, playing a major role in Scotland's domination of the world's ship building, tobacco trading, and other enterprises.[54]

Canada benefited from the clearances, which forced tens of thousands of hardworking settlers to Nova Scotia, to Lower and Upper Canada, and to the Red River settlement in the wilderness beyond. Some overcame their dislocation by establishing new colonies of Scots that survived and prospered in Canada.[55] Some established more independent lives as traders, farmers, and miners in the free-market environment. Others flowed into a rising tide of dislocated, addicted vagrants. Many helped to impose the dislocation that they had earlier experienced themselves upon the Canadian Indians, Inuit, and Métis.[56]

The English appear to have established alcoholism in the highlands without actually supplying the alcohol. Distilled spirits had been brought to Scotland by Christian monks a thousand years before the clearances. The use of distilled spirits and ale was always an integrated aspect of clan life. Heavy ceremonial drinking was part of occasional clan rituals, particularly among the men. At such ritual events, drinking was accompanied by conversations, song, story telling, and improvised poetry.[57] I have found no mention, however, of alcoholism or other forms of addiction by historians of the clan era.[58] On the contrary, even English historians, who looked at the highlanders as fearsome enemies, noted that both men and women were unusually healthy and hardy.[59] In the aftermath of the clearances, however, alcoholism became a significant trouble for many, and many others found drinking troublesome enough that they became abstainers.[60] It is difficult to make a definitive statement about why drinking became a problem just at this time, in part because Scottish historian Robert Mathieson attributed it more to malnutrition than dislocation, although he had much to say about other psychological reactions to dislocation, such as 'passivity'.[61] However, other historical cases in which the connection between dislocation and addiction are more certain will be discussed in the next chapter.

Because free-market society now dominates the globe,[62] the dislocation of human beings has spread to an unprecedented extent. But it has not finished spreading. The remainder of this chapter is devoted to examples of its continuing expansion in the Third World, among the working people in the developed world, and among the affluent of the richest countries. As with its earlier expansion, the dislocating effects of free-market society have been recognised as such by those who support globalisation and by those who oppose it.[63] Jeanne J. Kirkpatrick, former United States Ambassador to the United Nations and outspoken neoliberal, has been quoted as follows: 'Modernity's final stage is globalisation. Globalisation threatens the annihilation of traditional society. Globalisation is the future.'[64] Nobody has made the point with more flair and certainty than free-market society's great icon, Margaret Thatcher, when she said, '... there's no such thing as society. There are individual men and women and there are families.'[65]

Continuing dislocation in today's Third World

As early as the 1600s, England began imposing free-market economic structure, along with military control and material exploitation, on indigenous people in its colonies. The early fur trade between the Hudson's Bay Company (chartered in 1670) and Canadian native people began a continuing history of colonialism in Canada that will be discussed in Chapter 6. By the 1800s, most other European nations were also imposing free-market economics on their colonies—by force when necessary—producing unprecedented wealth and innovation for the colonisers, along with mass dislocation and dire poverty for most colonial subjects.[66] This practice has continued, both in its classic form and in newer forms, into the post-colonial period of the late 20th and early 21st centuries.[67]

In the classic form, Third-World people are still being brutalised and dispossessed, and their cultures are still being destroyed to accommodate multinational corporations with interests in agribusiness, oil, and tourism (including, ironically, 'ecotourism').[68]

As well as being driven from traditional societies, people may be lured from them by the prospects of fabulous wealth in new markets.[69] Often the destruction of the natural environment in the Third World leads to local violence and wars as people fight each other over remnants of their natural resources.[70] Third-World rulers are no longer compelled by imperial armies to permit this exploitation of their own people, but are vulnerable to flattery, bribery, and, when all else fails, to assassination by foreign agents working in the interests of foreign powers and corporations.[71] Newer engines of dislocation are emerging in the Third World as well, a few of which are described below.

International financial aid

Beginning in the last decades of the 20th century, the International Monetary Fund (IMF), the World Bank, and other international lending agencies have used their desperately needed loans to the Third World to impose ultra-orthodox free-market 'structural adjustments' on many countries, with further mass dislocation and devastating poverty among the results.[72] Although the effects of this pernicious 'aid' have been decried by left-wing economists for many years,[73] today's best-known description comes from an insider, Joseph Stiglitz, former Chief Economist of the World Bank and winner of the 2001 Nobel Prize in Economics.

Stiglitz has recounted in detail how the imposition of orthodox free-market principles by the international lending agencies caused economic disaster and personal dislocation in Argentina, Thailand, Russia, and many other countries. These principles included wholesale privatisation of government enterprises, whether they were functioning efficiently or not; removal of tariff protections for industry, including industries that were vital for local employment and stability; elimination of food subsidies for the poor, even when mass starvation was the foreseeable result; stripping countries of the political power to protect their own economies, thus leaving them at the mercy of 'market forces'; forcing elementary schools to collect 'cost recovery' fees, even when it meant that huge numbers of children could not attend; closing local banks or subjecting them to ruinous competition by foreign banks; and forcing balanced budgets on governments at all points in their economic cycles. Each of these structural adjustments has caused severe hardships, including large-scale starvation and disease in some countries, as well as local rebellions that had to be suppressed by military force.[74]

Whereas Stiglitz focused his attention on the material poverty and political unrest that resulted from this imposition of orthodox free-market principles on the Third World, other authors have concentrated on the destruction of local culture and the mass production of dislocation. Anthropologists and historians have described the appalling dislocation of approximately 1 billion human beings who have streamed from farms and villages to the slums, *favelas*, and garbage dumps of impoverished Third World cities, clinging desperately to fragments of their nuclear families and remnants of their ancestral identities.[75] Today's Third-World slums are full of moving stories of heroism and ingenuity, like Dickens' stories of the English slums of the 19th century. Yet the large-scale emergence of real psychosocial identity in these 20th-century slums is only a dream. Culture in Third-World slums, like housing, can only be built from remnants and desperation. Like the crumbling buildings, emerging local culture and community cannot survive the incessant influx of new, desperate people; or the destruction of national economies by economic shock therapy; or the continuing disasters of landslides, fires, and disease; or the intense individual competition expected by the new free-market economy; or the physical assaults by military and paramilitary enforcers of order and progress in the globalising economy.[76]

As a mainstream economist, Stiglitz thinks that the system can be fixed. He argues that the free-market principles that have been imposed by international financial aid agencies can be beneficial in the future, if administered by honest local governments. He suggests, always in a guarded way, that the failures of structural adjustments imposed by international financial aid agencies resulted not only from militant free-market orthodoxy, but also from the self-serving influence of private corporations.[77] He cites contemporary China as a positive example where the more careful imposition of free-market principles with outside 'help' has produced amazing increases in prosperity.[78]

Whereas more rational and honest imposition of free-market principles can reduce some adverse consequences, imposing free-market principles is bound to produce massive dislocation problems, even under more optimal conditions, such as those now prevailing in China. The evidence for this must await Chapter 6.

International humanitarian aid

Even purely humanitarian aid, given with the very best of intentions to improve health, increase crop production, raise educational standards, and establish basic human rights, sometimes has unintended, devastating effects on local cultures, spreading dislocation.[79] For example, child labour is a huge, heart-breaking problem throughout the Third World that is usually ignored in the rich countries or occasionally recognised in a spasmodic overreaction. In 1995, for example, the American television network CBS and *Life* magazine broke the story of child labour in the town of Sialkot, Pakistan, where most of the world's soccer balls were being manufactured. The details were horrendous. One well-known media figure wrote in *Life* magazine:

> As I travelled, I witnessed ... children as young as six bought from their parents for as little as $15, sold and resold like furniture, branded, beaten, blinded as punishment for wanting to go home, rendered speechless by the trauma of their enslavement.[80]

Naturally, readers were horrified. Many people and non-governmental organisations (NGOs) organised themselves to do something about it. Child labour was quickly banned in Sialkot, subsequent production monitored to ensure that children under 14 did not participate, and the problem was apparently solved.

Now, more than 10 years later, the details have been analysed and the effects of this instance of 'transnational activism' can be assessed more fully. It can now be shown that the sensationalised reports referred, at most, to a small number of isolated and correctable cases of heinous cruelty in the midst of a large cottage industry. The majority of sewing work was done in the homes of the poorest peasants where parents as well as children participated to supplement meagre family incomes. After years of investigation and monitoring, the NGO Save the Children described the general situation that had existed in 1995 quite differently from *Life* magazine:

> ... football stitching provided a regular supplementary income. All family members, even those with other jobs, would stitch footballs at home in their spare time to earn an extra 125 to 150 rupees daily. People described how they would stitch while they watched television in the evening.[81]

Subsequent to the banning of child labour in 1997, many peasant families suffered economic disaster. Average household incomes of people who were already living at or below subsistence levels fell by 25–30%. Work previously shared by children in a subsistence economy structured by family life is now done primarily by women outside their homes. Although the pay in the new labour market is somewhat higher than it was, it is difficult for the women to leave the children alone in order to go to the 'workshops' where the stitching is now done, and many women have been subjected to sexual harassment and a few raped on the way. Many who previously earned essential income as stitchers can no longer do so.

The irony of this is that the localised child abuse that did exist prior to 1995 might well have been corrected by the local community and government once it was publicised, or it might have been solved simply by raising the pay of the stitchers, so that the parents could have supported a family without being forced to depend on their children. This would have been relatively painless to the industry, since the stitchers' pay amounted to approximately 1% of the retail price of the finished soccer ball.[82] Instead, a precipitous international intervention, undertaken with the best of intentions, imposed a modern legal structure on a socially organised local economy. The new structure, imposed without consultation with the stitchers themselves, reduced many previously functional families to a state of dislocation and destitution.[83]

War

Free-market society is also being spread today by war, as it has been for centuries. Although this fact is fully documented,[84] there has been an almost complete blackout on it in the mainstream mass media. As examples, I have chosen two of the biggest wars that are underway as this book moves towards completion: the Iraq War and the War on Drugs as it is carried out in Colombia. *Both wars have the imposition of free-market economy among their primary goals.* Although the United States is the prime mover in both of these contemporary wars spreading free-market society, other great powers have carried out wars with similar goals since the beginning of free-market society.

The Iraq War

The Iraq War of George W. Bush has baffled almost everybody, because all of the highly publicised reasons for the invasion were false. There were no 'weapons of mass destruction' in the country; Iraq played no role in the attack on the American World Trade Centre in 2001; and the dictatorship of Saddam Hussein, although indeed vile, had been generously supported by the United States and its European allies in the years that it served their political purposes.[85] The creation of democracy in Iraq cannot be a pressing goal of the United States, which continues to support brutal dictatorships in the Middle East, Africa, South America, and Asia.[86] What then could have been the real purpose of the invasion?

No doubt, many advantages were considered by the planners, along with the risks and disadvantages. One major purpose was the opportunity to impose free-market economics on the people of the region.[87] The American government revealed its long-range plans to impose a free-market economy on the entire Middle East, including all the Arab countries along with Turkey, Iran, Pakistan, Afghanistan, and Israel, in a paper prepared for the G8 meeting in 2004. This paper sought to gain the cooperation of the world's richest industrial nations in this project.[88] The target area included Iraq, in which most of the major components of the economy, including the all-important oil business, were run by the state. The United States immediately imposed its plan once it had gained control of Iraq in 2003.

Within weeks of military victory in Iraq, the American occupation government had fired 500,000 workers at government agencies and state-owned factories; opened the border to completely unrestricted free trade without tariffs, duties, inspections, or taxes; tried to put all 200 of the major state-owned businesses, the heart of the Iraqi economy, up for sale; changed the law to allow foreign investors to buy 100% of Iraqi assets in any business outside the oil sector; and allowed foreign investors to take 100% of all profits made in Iraq out of the country without taxation and without any requirement for reinvestment in Iraq. American officials set out to establish institutional support for the expected flood of foreign investment, including a new stock exchange in Baghdad. Foreign businesses organised a flurry of 'Rebuilding Iraq' trade shows designed to attract capital to help them buy industries at bargain prices in the best imaginable economic environment. The occupation government imposed rules protecting patented and copyrighted 'intellectual property' that are among the strictest in the world. Paul Bremer, the leader of the United States occupation after 2 May 2003, declared that Iraq was 'open for business'. President George W. Bush proposed the establishment of a United States–Middle East free trade area within a decade.[89]

A major portion of this economic restructuring has been achieved, outside the battle zones.[90] Nonetheless, Iraqis fought back fiercely. So far, very little foreign investment has actually occurred, both because of continuing bloody chaos and because many of the economic changes imposed on Iraq are illegal under the terms of United Nations Security Council Resolution 1483, which sanctioned the occupation of Iraq by American and British forces. Foreign investors fear that investments authorised illegally could later be subject to legal forfeiture. However, as Naomi Klein predicted in 2004, even if the changes in Iraqi law imposed by the American occupation are all rescinded by a future Iraqi government, Iraq will remain a small country with an enormous public debt of US$120 billion. As the country will be able to avoid economic collapse only by further borrowing, it will come under the control of the IMF, which can be expected to provide loans only when it receives iron-clad promises of 'structural readjustments'—in other words, imposition of the most extreme form of free-market economy, with all the dislocation that this brings.[91] Klein's prediction was confirmed by the Iraqi government's latest report of its concessions to the IMF in 2007.[92]

Other probable purposes of the war in Iraq have come to light. One was to enrich American corporations close to the present American government.[93] Another was to further American ambitions for strategic control of the world's oil resources.[94] These possibilities, however, go beyond the scope of this book.

The War on Drugs

The governments of Colombia and the United States are carrying on a protracted war in Colombia ostensibly to protect American youth from the horrors of cocaine addiction. Again, the purpose of this war is not what it seems. During a decade of war,[95] cocaine consumption in the United States has not decreased and cocaine production in Columbia has actually increased.[96] However, the war is succeeding very well in securing existing oil pipelines and in clearing peasants from areas that are coveted for oil exploration. (Some multinational oil companies are proceeding less violently by acting legally through the Colombian courts to dislocate tribal people for purposes of oil exploration.[97])

Much of the fighting is carried out by mercenary armies of American corporations.[98] The motives of the war have been called into question on many sides.[99] The Colombian government is friendly with the United States and is willing to enact whatever free-market legislation the Americans want. However, it has been unable to enforce its economic legislation in remote areas where peasants and Indians do not want to open up their land to oil exploration or to be removed from places where the oil companies want to put pipelines. American military help has been needed to extend free-market society into the jungle and to subdue indigenous guerrilla armies under the convenient justification of a War on Drugs.

In sum, no corner of the earth is remote enough to escape from free markets and the mass dislocation that follows them in the era of globalisation. Today, 15 years after the private ownership of agricultural land was legalised in Cambodia, massive flows of capital and a rapidly increasing population are inexorably driving the peasants off their lands and into extreme poverty and dislocation.[100] Even remote Outer Mongolia is heavily marketised with mass dislocation of people from traditional lands and ancient cultures as a consequence.[101] This saga of contemporary dislocation repeats itself endlessly in today's Third World, almost entirely unreported by the mainstream media in free-market society and rarely connected, in the public mind, to the problem of addiction.

Dislocation of working people in today's developed world

A series of articles in the French journal *Le Monde diplomatique* has documented many causes of increasing dislocation among working people in France over the last few decades. For example, the replacement of family farms with industrial agriculture after World War II—accomplished through a combination of administrative pressure and irresistible glamourisation of the city lifestyle—has increased dislocation of small farmers. This process was accelerated by a new proposition accepted by the European Commission in 2003 that will reduce the amount of farming that occurs in France. However, the need for this reduction would have been avoided if the old, labour-intensive farming practices had been left in place.[102] A second example is the rapid growth in France since 1980 of the working poor (i.e. people who work for less than the monthly support provided for the unemployed). This group receives almost no attention in the French press. Perhaps because they are mostly women, it is easy for the larger public to assume, incorrectly, that most have freely chosen part-time or intermittent work in order to have more time for their families. On the contrary, most are forced by lack of other opportunities to take low-income jobs and many work on fragmented, irregular schedules that are likely to interfere with their family responsibilities.[103]

A detailed case study of the French company Moulinex, a manufacturer of kitchen gadgets and appliances, showed how French politicians eagerly opened the doors to global free markets and an international financial system without foreseeing the effect it would have on French industries and their workers. Administrators of Moulinex, working in the newly deregulated markets, were seduced by the success formulas of the 1980s—leveraged buyouts, restructuring, global acquisitions, etc. This had the effect of gradually demoralising the work force and bankrupting the company, multiplying the dislocation of workers and of the communities in which the company had functioned.[104]

A pan-European example is the campaign carried on since 1994 by the Organisation for Economic Cooperation and Development to dismantle various aspects of the European welfare state established after World War II. This campaign is explicitly justified on the ground that the European welfare state 'perturbs' the workings of the free market in labour. Detailed examination of the changes that are being made[105] reveals that they lead not only to material poverty for the unemployed, but also to loss of security and social identity in mainstream society—in other words, dislocation.

Dislocation of the poor in the developed world sometimes takes spectacular leaps during catastrophic events, such as Hurricane Katrina which inundated the American city of New Orleans in September 2005. Whereas the storm itself revealed that inadequate protection had been provided for the poorer districts of the city, the aftermath of the storm revealed city and state governments seizing the opportunity to redevelop the inundated quarters of the city in ways that destroyed the existing local culture of the urban poor—in this case, the world-famous home of New Orleans' heritage of jazz music. Tens of thousands of despairing, poor people will be displaced by federally funded redevelopment from property that has commercial potential to '... the periphery, at the edge of the bayous, in trailer parks and prisons'.[106] Naomi Klein has dubbed the opportunistic imposition of free-market society following catastrophes 'disaster capitalism'.[107]

Dislocation of the rich in today's developed world

The spread of dislocation is by no means confined to poor countries or to poor people. Throughout affluent free-market societies, dislocation plays havoc with delicate ties linking all classes of people to society, nature, and spiritual values. Although free-market societies produce both winners and losers as measured by economic success, they ultimately produce only losers when psychosocial integration is the measure. Polanyi perceived the growing dislocation among the rich as well as the poor from the earliest beginnings of the free-market system:

> ... the most obvious effect of the new institutional system was the destruction of the traditional character of settled populations and their transmutation into a new type of people, migratory, nomadic, lacking in self-respect and discipline—crude, callous beings *of whom both labourer and capitalist were an example.*[108]

Contemporary economists also see that dislocation is built into free-market society for the rich as well as the poor, although they never allow themselves to become overly concerned about it. Francis Fukuyama, famous for proclaiming 'the end of history', an expression of his conviction that no better social system than free-market capitalism and Western-style democracy could be imagined, nonetheless noted its 'emptiness at the core'.[109]

As the basic markets in goods, labour, and capital become securely established in more and more countries in the globalising world, new kinds of markets for services, intellectual property,[110] popular culture,[111] animal and plant varieties,[112] and intimate relations[113] have emerged with further devastating consequences for psychosocial integration at every social level.[114] In contemporary Canada, markets are encroaching everywhere: in the apparently ineluctable 'privatisation' of publicly funded medical care and education, which have been bedrocks of national identity and collective security for decades;[115] in the fiscal starvation of the Canadian Broadcasting Corporation, once a powerful voice of national identity now said to be competing unfairly with commercial broadcasters because it is publicly funded;[116] in the movement of high-paying jobs to low-cost workers in Ireland, China, and India; in the undermining of families by television advertisers who deliberately encourage 'rude, often aggressive behaviour and faux rebellion against the strictures of family discipline' in their child viewers in order to harass insecure parents into buying mass-produced junk food and toys;[117] and in the commoditisation of romantic love through Internet dating services,[118] romantic fiction,[119] Viagra,[120] Internet pornography,[121] and 'escort services'.[122]

As the market continues its encroachment into social life, rich and poor people are finding themselves capitalised as well as commoditised. Perhaps uncomfortable with being treated as 'labour', people find themselves upgraded to 'human resources' or 'human capital'. People's friends can be calculated along with other assets as 'social capital'.[123] Their emotional qualities can be calculated as 'emotional capital'.[124] Their writings become 'intellectual property', 'proprietary knowledge', and 'good will' that are parts of the capitalization of large corporations. Their songs, shorn of cultural meaning, become 'product' that is bought and sold in bulk lots. Even the ordinary words of their language, the ultimate commons, can be construed as private 'brands' and their use restricted by law for commercial purposes that profit their new owners. In Canada, which will host the Winter Olympics in 2010, the words 'medals' and 'winter' are now among those words that are legally protected as marketing tools.[125]

As markets extend their reach into society, governments extend their willingness to manipulate social life for the benefit of the economy, whatever the effects may be on psychosocial integration. The governments of rich countries employ carefully engineered management, advertising, taxation, and surveillance techniques to keep people buying, selling, working, borrowing, lending, consuming, moving, learning, immigrating, reproducing, and saving in ways that seem to benefit the economy and 'grow' the gross domestic product.[126] This economic engineering invisibly undermines both what remains of traditional culture and the new traditions that might otherwise spontaneously arise in the modern world.

At the international level, new 'free trade' agreements designed to accelerate international exchange and ramp up growth, open up a nation's businesses to takeovers by transnational corporations and 'buy-out funds' with no concern for local custom or utility, unless it makes a profit.[127] These agreements impose international regulatory panels with even less concern for traditional culture than domestic regulatory agencies.[128] The global market extends amoebic pseudopods, like eBay and Amazon, into everybody's home, providing instant access to all. Work is increasingly monitored by computers and 'micromanaged' to the specifications of unseen distant buyers, management gurus, investors, and corporate headquarters.[129] Thus, dislocation is on the march among the rich as well as the poor.

Free-market society not only manages people's personal and social lives in the interests of the economy, it also destabilises the economy itself. For rich and poor alike, in great cities and small towns,[130] people's jobs disappear at short notice;[131] life-long employees' pensions disappear;[132] families and communities live with financial uncertainty; people routinely change neighbourhoods, occupations, co-workers, technical skills, status, reference groups, languages, nationalities, priests, therapists, spiritual beliefs, and ideologies as their lives progress.[133] Deregulation of finance capital in the 1980s has enormously inflated the global free market in stocks, bonds, and debt obligations, bringing terrifying market volatility and long-term uncertainty into the domestic economy.[134] The corporate practice of 'transferring' workers and their families from place to place has produced an enormous amount of dislocation. In British Columbia, with a rich economy based on exporting natural resources extracted from forests and mines, entire towns appear and disappear when market prices fluctuate. Above all, workers are learning that their contribution is to be 'flexible'— that is to say, 'dislocated'.[135]

Although economic instability is partly an unplanned side effect of global free-market society,[136] it is also deliberately cultivated. Management literature encourages 'creative destruction' of 'subpar' workers and departments, and a reserve army of the unemployed is maintained to make the threat of being fired credible.[137] In Canada, the policy of artificially propping up the level of *unemployment*—for the purpose of controlling inflation by keeping down the price of labour—was federal government policy up until the late 1990s.[138] Thus, the economy, for which all social stability has been sacrificed, is itself unstable.[139]

Beyond economic instability, the integrity of the world's crucial ecological systems is seriously threatened. This goes far beyond the catastrophic consequences of global warming, to the destruction of adequate supplies of fresh air and clean water,[140] the extinction of irreplaceable forms of life, and much more. People are shorn of the security that once grew from a primordial identification with a wondrous and providential natural world, multiplying their dislocation in addition to threatening their survival.[141]

Contemporary forms of dislocation among the affluent have been brilliantly analysed by many contemporary authors. For example, the French philosopher Dany-Robert Dufour has shown how dislocation of prosperous citizens in wealthy countries has accelerated between World War II and the present because of the increasing dominance of free-market society.[142]

In Dufour's analysis, modernity gave way to post-modernity after World War II. The difference between the two is that, even though modernity destroyed tribal and medieval psychosocial integration, it maintained a symbolised environment, which at least offered people symbolic sources of belonging and identity. European people, for example, could identify themselves as members of the Church of Rome, or followers of a Protestant sect, or citizens of a powerful nation, or respected authorities in their field of knowledge, or part of the intellectual community, or strong fathers or nurturing mothers, or members of a proud race, or any combination of these. By contrast, post-modernity is a 'desymbolised' environment, in which the symbolic potency of religion, nationality, intellectual achievement, authority, gender, and race must be discredited in order to make people maximally responsive to a continually changing economy. People must be flexible workers and trendy consumers with all their options open.

Although desymbolisation may well mitigate some horrors of religious, nationalistic, and racial fanaticism, which reached a peak before and during World War II, fanaticism continues to spread in the desymbolising world of the 21st century, while the psychosocial integration afforded by a wholesome identification of people with deeply rooted symbols has been sacrificed to the needs of the market.[143]

Strange as it may seem, the need of the markets to desymbolise society was partly achieved through the hippie movements of the 1960s. This was:

> … a totally new form of domination which the 1960s (especially in California, Italy, England, and the French uprisings of May 1968) put into place. The new capitalism was in the process of discovering how to impose itself in a way that was less obviously authoritarian and onerous: No longer exercising the kind of domination that conquered people, but breaking down its established institutions and thus not obviously engaging in domination... in this manner producing a new kind of people who were flexible, uncertain, mobile, and thus open to all the fashions and changes of the market.[144]

Thus, post-modernism constitutes another great leap forward for free-market society and dislocation. Dufour and many others[145] believe that a new, post-modern, egocentric human species—with a short attention span and characteristic psychological afflictions—is coming into being:

> … I offer the hypothesis that an actual mutation of the human condition is happening right under our eyes, in our societies. This mutation is not a mere hypothetical construct; on the contrary, I think it is observable in a whole parade of changes, not all yet well understood, that are affecting the populations of the developed countries. These are familiar changes: preoccupation with merchandise, difficulties of self-concept and socialisation, drug addiction, hyperactivity and the appearance of what are called, rightly or wrongly, 'the new symptoms'.[146]

The next leap forward may result from a small step in biochemistry. Rapid-fire advances are already enabling wealthy people to hand-craft their own mood and personality, the genetic make-up of their children, and—with the help of a little surgical cutting and pasting—their own gender. The absence of any powerful restraints by religion or culture means that people can imagine that they are their own creators, once the biomedical techniques become available.[147] Whatever good may come from these innovations, they are surely bringing new levels of dislocation.

The dislocation engendered among the affluent citizens of wealthy countries, including Canada, is apparent in a recent interview and questionnaire study of 'cutting-edgers', the 15% of the population that is comprised of young adults working in information technology, aesthetics and design, food and drink, and personal care and health:

> ... cutting-edgers focus on bubbles of flexible groups composed of those with shared interests and friendships rather than on the conventional institutions and organisations of civil society.... They have no interest in ideals, ethics or societal issues or any belief that their participation in politics or civic life would make any difference.
>
> These are not the activist antiglobalisation disciples of Naomi Klein, but rather the apolitical crew of the Starship Enterprise. They are non-ideological and non-judgmental. They see nothing worth fighting for, no belief system, no country, no tribe. Life for them is an unending exploration of all the micropleasures the world has to offer them.[148]

Another index of dislocation among the rich is the spreading psychological and social problems of the United States middle class, arguably the pinnacle of success in the free-market world. The pressures of ever-increasing competitiveness, productivity, flexibility, overwork, downsizing, mobility, restructuring, surveillance, etc.[149] on the two working parents in American middle-class nuclear families are such that the children are deprived of essential time and support, even if a day-care centre keeps them occupied during the working day.[150] These children are further deprived because their upwardly mobile parents are often living far from their extended families. Richard DeGrandpre, commenting on the shocking number of American school children who are prescribed the stimulant methylphenidate (e.g. Ritalin®), has called this a 'culture of neglect' and a 'trickle-down theory of child rearing'.[151] These problems appear to be more severe in the wealthier suburbs than in the more average middle-class neighbourhoods.[152] Americans consistently receive the worst scores, relative to all other developed countries, on other indications of dislocation, including divorce, single parenthood, children in poverty, economic disparity, the prison population, and excessive television viewing.[153] Canada's middle-class plight is less extreme than that of the United States, but the trends are in the same direction.[154]

Dislocation of the rich is also evident in the growing discontent, stress, and workplace violence among corporate 'management'. An enormous 'management literature' abounds with discussions about how the army of stressed-out managers should themselves be managed, sometimes identifying dislocation as the root cause of the dysfunction.[155] The cause of this discontent is ingeniously lampooned in the American business cartoon, 'Dilbert'.[156] In the more dour terms of John Gray,[157] a former champion of the New Right, 'Businesses have shed many of the responsibilities that made the world of work humanly tolerable in the past.'

Of course, more esoteric explanations of the contemporary apathy that disregard the concept of dislocation abound. A psychologist recently claimed that a key cause of workplace bitterness is a traumatic event that occurred early in the bitter person's life. He proposed naming this problem, 'Post-Traumatic Embitterment Disorder'.[158] Canada's National Research Council, after a 4-year study of the discontents of people who work in 'open-concept' offices, concluded that morale and profits can be increased through application of a software program 'that will tell office designers whether their cubicles are too cramped, too dark, too noisy or too draughty. The program will also help employers avoid the all-too-common maze effect in many cubicle colonies'.[159] I think not.

Some economists admit to being shocked by the fact that the vast increases in wealth in the rich countries have not led to measurable increases in happiness.[160] However, they rarely recognise dislocation as a cause. More typically, they fall back on a supposed psychological principle to explain why depression is spreading where happiness should abound—people are naturally insatiable! No matter how abundantly the free market satisfies their deepest needs, people will not be happy, because they will always want more of what the free market can deliver.[161] However, innate human insatiability exists only in the imagination of economists. Historians, sociologists, and anthropologists report long periods of stability among various peoples outside free-market society, who seem to have achieved contentment without ever-expanding consumption. Psychologists have traditionally understood human motives as satiable.[162] As a single example, in Maslow's famous hierarchy of needs, the satisfaction of materialistic motives frees a person to move on towards other, more transcendent motives. Maslow thought that the materialistic motivations that economists say are insatiable would virtually disappear in affluent societies,[163] as they have for some people. Many people live modestly by choice and could never be considered insatiable in the sense that the economists propose, despite the fact that, like the rest of the population, they are subjected to ceaseless, sophisticated advertising throughout their lifetimes.[164] Only the most severely addicted people are truly insatiable, because their addictions never succeed in filling the void of dislocation. For this reason, the economists' prophecy of human insatiability may eventually become self-fulfilling, if an increasingly marketised world continues to raise the tide of dislocation.

There was a time when the spread of dislocation in Western society could be denied, but that time has passed for all but those who resolutely refuse to see it. Today, countless novels and short stories focused on the anguish of dislocation are popular in the richest countries.[165] The theme of dislocation is sometimes sensationalised and sometimes muted,[166] but clearly recognisable. Contemporary cinema abounds with powerful dramatisations of dislocation.[167] The second principle of the dislocation theory of addiction, like the first, is rapidly becoming commonplace. However, the third principle of the theory is not yet so widely accepted. It will require three chapters, rather than one, to lay out the evidence.

Endnotes

1   K. Polanyi (1944, p. 71).
2   Tawney (1926/1947), K. Polanyi (1944, pp. 3–4), Hobsbawm (1962, 1994), Berman (1982, p. 16), Klein (2007), Ramonet (2007), and many others cited in this book have outlined ways

in which free-market economics shapes all of the diverse aspects of modernity. Whereas it is generally recognized that free-market economics lies at the heart of globalisation, it can also be argued that globalisation (in the different sense of a single, seamless global market) has come to an end due to the rise of new forms of nationalism (Golub, 2005a; Saul, 2005). However, this does not detract from the fact that globalisation (in the sense of the domination of society everywhere by free-market economics) is stronger everywhere, including China, India, and Russia. K. Polanyi (1944), in his classic work, *The Great Transformation*, argued that the 19th-century globalised civilisation based on the gold standard, the ever-shifting balance of power between the European nations, the dominance of the liberal state model of government, and free-market economics had collapsed by the end of World War II. Whereas he may well be proved correct about the first three of these, it has become clear that the free market has risen from the ashes of this collapse and is rapidly expanding its dominance at the dawning of the 21st century. Bayly has pointed out, correctly, that there is more to globalisation than the expansion of free-market principles from west to east, but he acknowledges the centrality of free marketisation in today's globalisation nonetheless (Bayly, 2004, pp. 3–5, 290–292, 473–475).

3 An international example of the unpublicised advance of free-market society is the Multilateral Agreement on Investment (MAI), which was the topic of formal, but confidential, negotiations among the member nations of the Organisation for Economic Co-operation and Development (OECD) beginning in 1995. The MAI was designed to maximize profits for offshore investors, partly by giving them the legal right to sue governments if they felt their opportunity to make a profit had been compromised by government legislation or regulations. A draft copy of the agreement was leaked in 1997 and put on the Internet, bringing it to the attention of various NGOs and labour unions, which saw it as an abrogation of national sovereignty to foreign corporations. In the wake of widespread public protests, it was abandoned by the OECD in 1998. Since that time, several of its provisions have been added to other proposed trade agreements, notably by the World Trade Organisation (Barlow and Clarke, 2001, pp. 22–25).

A current Canadian instance of the lingering influence of the MAI is the Trade, Investment and Labour Mobility Agreement Between the Governments of British Columbia and Alberta (TILMA) in Canada, which was agreed upon between the two provincial governments without any real discussion in the mainstream media and came into effect on 1 April 2007 (Island Tides, 2007a). Its stated purpose is to substantially deregulate trade, investment, and labour movement between the two provinces (see Governments of British Columbia and Alberta, 2006, especially Articles 1, 3, and 5). Among its many provisions, the agreement creates a 'TILMA Panel' with the power to force local and provincial governments to overturn regulations that are seen to interfere unduly with the rights of property developers and other landowners to profit from the land they own. In the language of this book, this serves to remove many of the regulations that restrict the free market in land, although there are some explicit exceptions to the kinds of regulation that can be challenged. An agreement of this sort in the American state of Oregon enabled property developers to sue the state for billions of dollars over regulations on land use. In the end, the 'state's land use planning has become largely ineffective' (Patrick Brown, 2006, p. 2; see also E. Gould, 2006–2007; J. Hill, 2006).

4 Weber (1920/1958); Tawney (1926/1947); K. Polanyi (1944); M. Friedman and Friedman (1979); Fukuyama (1989, 1992); C. Taylor (1991); Ramonet (1994); Soros (1997); J. Jacobs (2000); J. Heath (2001); Dufour (2003a, 2005); Lordon (2003, 2004); Saul (2004); Beder (2006); Homer-Dixon (2006, pp. 203–204); Klein (2007).

5 Weber (1920/1958); Tawney (1926/1947, Chapters 1 and 5); K. Polanyi (1944); K. Polanyi *et al.* (1957); Heilbroner (1961); Wrightson (2000, p. 29); J. Heath (2001, pp. 117–122). Historians do not agree on why this novel form of society first appeared just when and where it did. K. Polanyi makes the case that free-market society was ultimately a consequence of the invention of expensive machinery, which produces an unacceptable risk to investors unless the supplies of raw material and labour are made as predictable as possible through the introduction of free markets (1944, pp. 40–42). Marx (1869/1978) attributed the dominance of free markets to the self-serving machinations of a bourgeois social class, an explanation that K. Polanyi refutes (1944, pp. 151–153). Contrary to the historians listed at the start of this endnote, J. Jacobs (2000) argues eloquently that free-market economy is the natural, ancient human form of social organisation. However, neither she nor others who have taken this position can support this empirically, because the bulk of existing historical and anthropological evidence indicates the contrary.

6 Retrieved 19 October 2007, from http://en.wikipedia.org/wiki/Reinheitsgebot.

7 Retrieved 30 December 2005, from http://www.american.edu/TED/germbeer.htm (see also http://en.wikipedia.org/wiki/Reinheitsgebot).

8 Wrightson (2000, Chapters 1–4) provides a number of examples of how these regulations and constraints operated in English markets around the year 1500. See also K. Polanyi (1944, 1957).

9 Tawney (1926/1947).

10 Tawney (1926/1947, p. 15); Bayly (2004, Chapters 1 and 2). The Dutch role was also extremely important at the outset, but is not discussed here.

11 Wrightson (2000, p. 72).

12 Philosophical foreshadowings of individualism and thus free-market economics can be found in Western classical philosophy, both pagan and Christian, and in the writings of the Italian Renaissance (Bayly, 2004, p. 286), but these theoretical adumbrations are beyond the scope of this book.

13 Enclosures of formerly agricultural land for sheep pasturage actually affected only a few small landholders before the late 1500s because most of the land enclosed before then had been abandoned in the aftermath of the huge population reduction caused by the Black Death after 1300 (Wrightson, 2000, pp. 98–104).

14 More (1516/1965, pp. 25–27).

15 K. Polanyi (1944, Chapter 3).

16 Tawney (1926/1947, Chapter 4).

17 Wrightson (2000, pp. 75–78, 108–112).

18 Similar shifts occurred in many societies besides the English.

19 Wrightson (2000, pp. 160–164).

20 For example, K. Polanyi (1944), C. Hill (1958, 1973), and Wrightson (2000, p. 213).

21 See K. Polanyi (1944), C. Hill (1958, Chapter 7), Neeson (1993), Wrightson (2000, pp. 320–330), and McQuaig (2001). Beyond England, a huge historical literature documents the fact that establishing a 'free'-market society regularly requires coercion on a massive scale, as most people resist dislocation fiercely (K. Polanyi, 1944; Agar, 1936/1999; C. Hill, 1958, Chapter 7; Prebble, 1963, 1971; McFeat, 1966; Tennant, 1990; Gray, 1998; McMurtry, 1998, pp. 259–296).

22 One such *parvenu* was Robert Owen who, as a hard-driving entrepreneur, exploited child labour in his factories and used the cheap cotton produced by black slaves long before he

became famous as a social reformer who deplored the ravages of the free-market system. His rise to wealth in the late 1700s is described by Donnachie (2000, Chapters 2 and 3).

23 Bayly (2004, pp. 59–64).

24 This has been described in meticulous detail by many historians of the left (e.g. Hobsbawm, 1962) and acknowledged without great elaboration by other historians (e.g. Bayly, 2004, p. 119).

25 See Heilbroner (1961) for a summary of the views of the classical economists on this topic. Robert Owen's growing opposition to the horrors of capitalism is summarised in Donnachie (2000, Chapters 7–13). Marx and Engels (1848/1948, p. 11) devoted some of the most powerful rhetoric in their *Manifesto of the Communist Party* to describing the dislocation that free markets produced in Europe. However, Marx also wrote with great conviction of the benefits that were created as the 19th century destroyed even the memory of past traditions. Although Marx was sympathetic about dislocation, he did not want to reverse the capitalist form of social organisation, only to put it under the control of the proletariat (Marx, 1869/1978, pp. 416–417, see also p. 503 including footnote).

26 For example, Klein (2000), M. Burke (2002), Cassen (2004a), Hourcade (2004), Jaffrelot (2004), Kristianasen (2004), and Bayly (2004, pp. 111–119, 300).

27 Wrightson (2000, pp. 238–239).

28 Prebble (1963).

29 Hughes (1987).

30 Doucet (2005); Ross and Deveau (1992).

31 Davis (2003).

32 Marx (1869/1978); K. Polanyi (1944, p. 180); Bayly (2004, p. 111).

33 Peter the Great acted on this insight even earlier in Russia, but less successfully (Toynbee, 1948, Chapter 9).

34 Bayley (2004, pp. 270–271).

35 Saul (2004).

36 Tawney (1926/1947, Chapter 5).

37 Polanyi (1944).

38 Soros (1997, p. 45). See also Fukuyama (1989, 1992).

39 Ashby (2004); Drohan (2004c); Nolen (2005).

40 Brook and Wakabayashi (2000); Yi-Mak and Harrison (2001). The latter authors argue that globalisation spreads addiction primarily by distributing addictive drugs at low prices. Whereas their investigation of the 'supply side' has added a dimension to the issue, Chapter 6 of this book will show that the effects of globalisation on the 'demand side' are more important.

41 The word 'clan' in Scottish history does not correspond to 'clan' in North American aboriginal history. A Scottish clan is equivalent to an aboriginal 'tribe' or 'tribal group'.

42 Prebble (1963, 1971); Herman (2001).

43 Wrightson (2000, p. 176).

44 Prebble (1971, Part 6).

45 Wrightson (2000, p. 71).

46 Prebble (1963, 1971, p. 299); Mathieson (2000).

47 Prebble (1963); Macinnes (1998, p. 170).

48 MacKenzie (1883); Mathieson (2000, pp. 114–116).

49 Mathieson (2000, pp. 9–12).

50 Prebble (1963).

51 Some of these first-hand observations were collected by MacKenzie (1883).

52 Prebble (1963).

53 Prebble (1963, p. 69).

54 Herman (2001).

55 See the autobiographical account of childhood in a Canadian–Scottish community by John Kenneth Galbraith (1985) and a magnificent Canadian novel, *No Great Mischief*, by Alistair MacLeod (1999).

56 Prebble (1963, pp. 114–115).

57 Prebble (1966, pp. 31–32; 1971, p. 24); Mathieson (2000, Chapter 7).

58 English historians sometimes described young Scots as if they were addicted to war, but this was universal among them and it was the honoured role that they were expected to play within clan society.

59 Prebble (1971, pp. 231–232).

60 Mathieson (2000, Chapter 7); Galbraith (1985).

61 Mathieson (2000).

62 As examples, see Klein (2000), M. Burke (2002), Cassen (2004a), Hourcade (2004), Jaffrelot (2004), and Kristianasen (2004).

63 Scholars who recognize the devastating effect of free-market society on traditional culture but nonetheless support it include von Hayek (1944), Beniger (1986, pp. 434–435), Fukuyama (1992, pp. xix, 77–79), Huntington (1996, pp. 76, 97–98), Giddens (1998, pp. 15, 63), T. Friedman (2000, pp. 11–12), and Herman (2001, pp. 85–88, 136). On the other hand, scholars who condemn free markets because of their devastating effects on traditional society include K. Polanyi (1944), Prebble (1963, 1971), Hobsbawm (1994, p. 16), Chossudovsky (1997), Bourdieu (1998), Gray (1998), Sassen (2000), McQuaig (2001), Edward Luttwak quoted in deGraaf *et al.* (2002, p. 50), Champagne (2003), Dufour (2003a, b), and Lordon (2003, 2004). Erikson (1959, pp. 158–159) recognized the effect of the 'technological and economic developments of our day' on 'all habitual group identities and solidarities', but seemed to view this cultural evolution without making any judgement of its value.

64 *Republic of East Vancouver* (2004).

65 Oborne (2002) and others have striven to soften Thatcher's meaning.

66 K. Polanyi (1944, p. 214).

67 Latte (2006); Monbiot (2006); Nolen (2006); Boal (in press).

68 Klein (2007, Chapter 19) has shown how aid money advanced to several South Asian countries after the tsunami of 2004 was used to force coastal villagers from their ancestral homes and to build five-star hotels where their villages had been. Vigna (2006) has shown that some 'ecotourism' is devastating native culture and the natural environment.

69 Donahue (2007).

70 Homer-Dixon (2006, pp. 148–151).

71 J. Perkins (2004); Klein (2007).

72 Chossudovsky (1997); Stiglitz (2002, pp. 15–17, 20); Bulard (2005); Caplan (2005); Klein (2007).

73 See Chossudovsky (1997).

74 Stiglitz (2002); Klein (2007).

75 Davis (2006a, b). The 1 billion number comes from Davis (2006b, p. 23) who cites the executive director of the United Nations Human Settlements Programme. Naturally, the urbanisation of the Third World cannot be blamed solely on structural adjustments imposed by international financial aid agencies, but many of the other causes, such as uncontrolled land speculation, also have their roots in free-market society.

76 Davis (2006a, b, especially Chapters 4 and 8).

77 Stiglitz (2002, pp. xiii–xiv, Chapter 1, pp. 206–213).

78 Stiglitz (2002, pp. 122–126 and Chapter 7).

79 Sogge (2004); Brauman (2005).

80 Schanberg (1996, p. 41).

81 Save the Children (2000, p. 19, as cited in Kahn, 2005, p. 10).

82 Kahn (2004, p. 140).

83 Kahn (2005).

84 See Chapter 3, endnote 38, point a.

85 Despratx and Lando (2004).

86 Achcar (2004); MacKinnon (2006).

87 P. Adams (2003); Achcar (2004); Klein (2004; 2007, Chapters 16–19); Warde (2004); Keyder (2005).

88 Achcar (2004).

89 All of the facts in this paragraph come from Klein (2004, 2007) except for the fact about intellectual property rights, which comes from Keyder (2005).

90 N. Reynolds (2007).

91 Klein (2004).

92 R. Weissman (2007).

93 Warde (2004); C. Simpson and Madhani (2005).

94 Chomsky (2003a, b); Dyer (2005); Roberts (2005).

95 'Plan Colombia', a Colombian–American war against cocaine production, was initiated in 1998. The military commitment of the United States has grown since that time, currently exceeding US$600 million per year.

96 Sanger and Forero (2004); Otis (2006); J. E. Gould (2007).

97 Chepesiuk (2001).

98 Ospina (2004).

99 Lemoine (2000, 2001); Ospina (2003, 2004); Leech (2004); J. E. Gould (2007).

100 de Dianous (2004).

101 Rufin (2004); G. York (2005d, e).

102 Champagne (2003).

103 Maruani (2003).

104 Lordon (2004).

105 Cordonnier (2006).

106 Davis (2005, p. 5); M. Siegel (2007).

107 Klein (2007).

108 K. Polanyi (1944, p. 128, italics added).

109 Fukuyama (1989). His full phrase was 'emptiness at the core of liberalism'. He used the word 'liberalism' in this context to encompass both free-market society and Western-style

democracy, which he perceived to be closely linked. J. Heath (2001, pp. 2, 39) also speaks of the emptiness of free-market society, which he advocates in a Canadian form that he calls the 'efficient society'.

110 Kapica (2003).

111 Fawcett (2004).

112 *Island Tides* (2007b).

113 Chang (2003); Mattelart (2003); Illouz (2007).

114 Dufour (2003a, b); Abley (2004); Fawcett (2004); Ticoll (2005).

115 The overwhelming majority of Canadian voters support the Canadian medical insurance system. While the federal and provincial governments have managed to create an illusion of concordant governmental support for it, the medical system is being dangerously starved of funds, requiring its gradual opening to private enterprise (Barry and Lombardi, 2004; Duhaime, 2004; Lee, 2004; Mahoney, 2004a; G. Smith, 2004a; Ibbitson, 2006; Mickleburgh, 2006a). However, this problem is not simply the government surreptitiously backing away from a service that the public considers essential. There are changes in the nature of medical needs, such as aging of the population and an explosion in the costs of new, sophisticated technology, that were not foreseen in the Canada Health Act. These may require some kind of fundamental change, no matter what economic ideology the government might support (Yalnizyan, 2005).

116 J. Simpson (2005).

117 deGraaf *et al.*(2002, Chapter 7, quote from p. 54). See also Brune (2004).

118 Andrews (2004); Traves (2006); Illouz (2007, Chapter 3).

119 Babineau (2004).

120 Viagra was introduced as a medicine for male 'erectile dysfunction', conceived as a medical problem. It is now widely used by young men and women as a 'lifestyle drug' that increases the quantity and quality of copulation on a mass scale (e.g. Mickleburgh and Giroday, 2004), thus changing the nature of sexuality itself for people who can afford the drug.

121 Valpy (2004a).

122 The 2006/2007 Vancouver telephone book lists over 35 enterprises under 'E' for 'Escort Services'.

123 Here is a standard definition of social capital:

> … a person's or group's concern, caring, regard, respect, or sense of obligation for the well-being of another person or group that may produce a potential benefit, advantage, and preferential treatment for another person or group beyond that which might be expected in an [economic] exchange relationship.

Veltmeyer (2005, p. 2).

124 Illouz (2007, pp. 62–67).

125 Industry Canada (2007a, b); Government of Canada (2007). The *Olympic and Paralympic Marks Act* makes several ordinary English words into protected trademarks that are owned by a corporation, the Canadian Olympic Committee, which is organising the Vancouver Winter Olympic Games in 2010. The use of numerous words and phrases, including 'Olympic Games', 'faster, higher, stronger', 'medals', and 'winter', is restricted to a greater or lesser degree under this law.

126 Beniger (1986); Bourdieu (1998); Dobbin (1998, Chapter 3); Beaud and Pialoux (2000); Ramonet (2000); G. MacDonald and Little (2001); R. Blackwell (2003a); Anderssen (2004b);

Immen (2004); Fritz (2005); Partridge (2005); Wegert (2005); *Globe and Mail* (2006a). This use of the word 'grow' has become common in financial writing in the last decade.

127 Reguly (2007).

128 Bourdieu (1998); Konrad (2003); Cassen (2004a); Erdman (2007).

129 Ansberry (2002); Linhart (2002); McWilliams (2002); H. Schachter (2003); J. Saunders (2003b); Immen (2005).

130 Dislocation might seem to be largely an urban phenomenon, but it is not. A good description of small-town dislocation is provided by Miles Orvell (as cited in Lackner, 2004; see also Mooers, 2004).

131 J. Saunders (2003b); Ramirez (2004); Pitts (2006).

132 *Globe and Mail* (2004b); McCarthy (2004a, 2005a, b); Atlas and Walsh (2005); Shalai-Esa (2006).

133 Bouffartigue (2002).

134 Lordon (2003, 2004); P. J. Davies *et al.* (2007).

135 Ramonet (2006a).

136 Schroeder (2003); Kolko (2006).

137 Bourdieu (1998); Dobbin (2003); Thomas (2003).

138 Dobbin (2003, pp. 56–61).

139 For example, Chang (2003).

140 Suzuki and McConnell (1997); S. Hume (2003a); Dolmetsch (2004); Homer-Dixon (2004; 2006, Chapter 6); M. Hume (2004b); Radford (2004); Sinaï (2004, 2006); M. Hume (2005c); A. Hurley and Nikiforuk (2005); D. Jones (2005); Freeman (2006).

141 Homer-Dixon (2006, p. 147).

142 Dufour (2003a, b) calls the dominance of free-market society 'le capitalisme total'.

143 One of the most contested topics of our times is the cause of the rise of fascism in 20th-century Germany. Two books written at the end of World War II, both still famous, advanced quite opposite interpretations of the rise of fascism and of economic history in general. K. Polanyi's (1944) position was that fascist leaders gained power by promising people grandiose symbols of national and racial magnificence to replace the symbols that had been shattered by World War I and by the invasion of free-market society (see also K. Polanyi, 1935). von Hayek (1944) argued that German fascism grew out of a fatal attraction to socialism. The historical evidence that supports K. Polanyi's position over von Hayek's lies beyond the scope of this book.

144 Dufour (2003b, pp. 234–235).

145 Pieiller (2007) reviews four recent books originally written in French, English, and Hebrew that share this point of view.

146 Dufour (2003b, p. 27).

147 Mahoney (2005c); McLaren (2006); Elie (2007).

148 M. Adams and de Panafieu (2003). I have relied on the newspaper report of this research because the original proprietary research is only available at a very high price.

149 Bulkeley (2004).

150 DeGrandpre (1999); Judith Warner (2005).

151 DeGrandpre (1999, p. 18).

152 Luthar (2003). Jong-Fast (2006) has written an autobiographical account of dislocation and addiction among the very rich.

153 Bronfenbrenner *et al.* (1996).

154 *Globe and Mail* (2002a); Mitchell (2004).

155 Of the following authors, I find Barbara Moses' three articles the most insightful: Church (1999); Gibb-Clark (1999); *Globe and Mail* (1999); Moses (1999, 2001, 2004); R. Schachter (1999); Sennett (1999); Huang (2001); Tapscott (2002); Harding (2003); S. R. Lewis (2003); Galt (2004a, b, c, d, 2005); Lowe (2004); Pinker (2005).

156 S. Adams (2002).

157 Gray (1998, p. 72).

158 S. Strauss (2003).

159 Galt (2004b, p. A1).

160 Anderssen (2004a); Homer-Dixon (2006, pp. 192–193).

161 J. Heath (2001, pp. 248–249, 305); A. J. Morris and Sayre (2004, p. 20).

162 See Cushman (1995, pp. 214–215). The traditional psychological model of motivation was 'homeostatic', meaning that people were only motivated when they were deprived and became content when their needs were met.

163 Maslow (1950/1973, p. 188).

164 Each year, twice as much is spent on advertising in the United States as is spent on all levels of education (Dawson, 2003, as cited in Eckersley, 2005, p. 161).

165 A list of Canadian novels that describe dislocation appears in endnote 46 of Chapter 4.

166 Berger (2003).

167 My three personal favourites: *Fight Club*; *The Big Lebowski*; *Goodbye Lenin*.

Chapter 6

Addiction is a Way of Adapting to Dislocation: Historical Evidence

The third principle of the dislocation theory of addiction is that addiction is a way of adapting to sustained dislocation. Modern history provides many examples of abrupt increases in dislocation in local societies being followed by dramatic increases in addiction, and at least one documented example of an abrupt decrease in dislocation followed by a decrease in addiction. Some of these instances are discussed in this chapter. The two chapters that follow this one draw additional evidence for the third principle of the dislocation theory from more conventional addiction research.

The historical correspondence between rises of mass dislocation and of mass addiction can be documented endlessly. For example, although daily alcohol consumption and drunkenness on festive occasions were common in Europe during the Middle Ages, and although unruly drunkenness sometimes caused problems, these were isolated occurrences. There was no 'alcohol problem' and no thought of a disease called 'alcoholism'. Free-market economics flourished in England before other European countries, and it was in England that alcohol addiction first emerged as a national problem.[1] It was not until the English 'gin craze' of the 1700s, however, that drinking became really devastating.[2] The gin craze followed a surge in religious support for enclosures and other free-market initiatives that began with the Restoration of Charles II in 1680.[3] Alcoholism reached epidemic proportions all over Europe after 1800[4] along with the mass dislocation that grew from the accelerating movement towards an encompassing free-market society.

Charles Dickens and many other social historians identified chronic drunkenness as a way of adapting to dislocation (along with material poverty).[5] Working as a freelance journalist in London in the 1830s under the pen name of 'Boz', Dickens acknowledged the tragedy of brilliantly illuminated, splendid 'gin palaces' in the most miserable slums of the city, and he described with horror the harm that the worst drunkards did to their own families. But he chastised the middle-class temperance societies, which were fulminating uselessly about the demonic properties of distilled liquor and the moral weakness of gin drinkers:

> Gin-drinking is a great vice in England, but wretchedness and dirt are a greater; and until you improve the homes of the poor, or persuade a half-famished wretch not to seek relief in the temporary oblivion of his own misery, with the pittance which, divided among his family, would furnish a morsel of bread for each, gin-shops will increase in number and splendour. If the Temperance Societies would suggest an antidote against hunger, filth, and foul air, or could establish dispensaries for the gratuitous distribution of bottles of Lethe-water,[6] gin-palaces would be numbered among the things that were.[7]

Contemporary historian Eric Hobsbawm expressed the same view of drinking among the 'labouring poor' in the early 1800s:

> ... faced with a social catastrophe they did not understand, impoverished, exploited, herded into slums that combined bleakness and squalor, or into the expanding complexes of small-scale industrial villages, [most of the labouring poor] sank into demoralisation. Deprived of the traditional institutions and guides to behaviour, how could many fail to sink into an abyss of hand-to-mouth expedients, where families pawned their blankets each week until pay-day and where alcohol was 'the quickest way out of Manchester' (or Lille or the Borinage). Mass alcoholism, an almost invariable companion of headlong and uncontrolled industrialisation and urbanisation, spread 'a pestilence of hard liquor' across Europe.[8]

European history was replayed in the United States. Abundant alcohol was consumed in American colonial society. In the 1600s, daily drinking was simply part of life in a religious and hierarchical colonial society. Individual episodes of drunk and disorderly behaviour were isolated occurrences that were tolerated or punished individually without arousing fears of any general problem of alcoholism. Taverns were centres of community life where good behaviour was the norm. Tavern keepers were expected to be reputable members of local society. As potent forms of liquor became more and more available, older norms of restraint broke down somewhat and drinking became more disorderly in the 1700s, but alcoholism did not emerge as a social problem for most of the century.

After the American Revolution freed the former colonies from the economic restraints and traditional values of a colonial system, however, life was transformed. Explosions of expansion, urbanisation, immigration, innovation, and wealth occurred within a scarcely regulated free-market economy. Along with its creative benefits, the new economic and social regime fractured the traditional society of former colonies. Michael Kenny describes the period between 1790 and 1820 as:

> ... a transitional phase between the corporatist ideas of classic republican thought that dominated the perceptions of the Revolutionary generation and the liberal ideology of nineteenth-century America with its exaltation of the individual in a free, competitive, aggressively entrepreneurial society.[9]

It was precisely in this period of American history that alcohol addiction came to be widely perceived as a grave menace to individuals and society. As the 1800s proceeded, the redoubtable American temperance movement rose to a position of such power that it was able to impose alcohol prohibition on the entire nation by 1919.[10]

A parallel shift occurred with opioid drugs in both Europe and the United States. Opium use, which had been widespread but unproblematic in Great Britain, became perceived as the root of a widespread addiction problem in the 1800s.[11] Similarly, by the end of the 1800s, opium and morphine use in the United States was no longer perceived as normal, but as the route to uncontrollable addiction. This new view of opioid use led to the first American outburst of repressive passion towards drugs around World War I.[12]

In China too, mass opium addiction arrived with free-market society, centuries after the Chinese began using opium regularly for medical and recreational purposes.

There were problems with opium addiction in the 1700s and early 1800s, but the overwhelming number of users partook in a way that was socially acceptable and healthful, and was an integral part of a well-established 'smoking culture'.[13] China's devastating epidemic of opium addiction followed the forced imposition of free trade after China's loss of wars to Great Britain in 1839 and 1858. Although these are known as the 'Opium Wars', their main effect was to force the opening of Chinese ports to the full range of commodities that the industrialised world wanted to sell. Opium addiction grew further, spreading to include morphine and heroin addiction, concomitantly with a series of bloody rebellions that were partly provoked by the further spread of capitalist and Protestant ideology.[14] Opioid addiction continued to flourish during the first half of the 20th century in an era of ruthless economic exploitation, including further expansion of forced free trade, by the Western powers and Japan.[15] This occurred both before and after the establishment of the Chinese Republic in 1911. According to Yi-Mak and Harrison:

> China had used opium since at least the Ming Dynasty (AD 1280–1326) without experiencing a drugs epidemic of the kind that overtook the nation towards the end of the nineteenth century … [16]

But was the spread of addiction in globalising Europe, America, and China a way of adapting to dislocation per se? Instead, could it have been a way of adapting to the starvation, material poverty, and disease that the switch to free-market economics brought? Or was it caused by the sudden availability of cheap distilled spirits and strong drugs? Or was it a consequence of panicky prohibitions of alcohol or drugs? Although these alternative hypotheses have been proposed by serious scholars, they do not find much support in historical fact. Working people were often poor and sick before free-market society began to emerge, but they were seldom dislocated or addicted.[17] Drunkenness began to emerge as a serious social problem in some places before cheap distilled spirits became available.[18] In other places, strong drugs arrived a very long time before addiction. Finally, where prohibition can be studied closely, as in the United States, it becomes evident that the prohibitionists acquired power long *after* severe addictive problems had become evident, even if heavy-handed prohibition remedies actually exacerbated the problems later on.

However, detailed studies of the historical record are needed to document the role of dislocation in the emergence of addiction as a massive social problem. The ideal historical case study would be one in which dislocation increased suddenly, but was unaccompanied by the other possible causes. The histories of Canadian Indians and of early European immigrants to Canada from the Orkney Islands of northern Scotland provide historical examples that approach this ideal type reasonably well. The mid-20th-century history of China provides a different sort of historical example that documents the effect of *decreasing* dislocation on addiction.

Canadian aboriginal peoples

The story of Canadian aboriginal people that follows is merely one of a series of stories about the fate of aboriginal people around the globe.[19] Prior to their devastation by Europeans, the diverse aboriginal cultures that were spread across Canada all provided a level of psychosocial integration that is unknown in modern society. Aboriginal people lived within stable tribal groups and distributed their resources within a matrix of responsibilities and privileges that grew from their family, clan, village, and religion as well as individual talents. There was considerable inter-tribal trade, as well as theft and warfare, but these too entailed well-established traditions and competition between groups, rather than between individual producers and consumers functioning in a free market.[20] After European contact, the various aboriginal people clung to their cultures with death-defying resolution. Although they valued European trading goods, they found European ways repellent.

Although I have searched the literature and questioned many anthropologists and Canadian native people, I have found no evidence of any behaviour that could reasonably be called addiction in pre-contact aboriginal cultures. This is despite the abundance of habits and pursuits that existed in those cultures prior to European contact that are addictive in free-market society, including gambling, sex, smoking tobacco, feasting, and status seeking.[21]

Canadian aboriginal people did not have access to alcohol before the Europeans brought it, but Indians in what are now Mexico and the American Southwest made their own alcoholic drinks without developing alcoholism problems.[22] Where alcohol became readily available to Canadian aboriginal people living in intact tribal groups, it was used peacefully and often ceremonially—but not addictively. For example, the Innu people of Northern Quebec and Labrador had centuries of access to whisky from traders who were eager to trade alcohol for furs and deliberately sought to develop dependence or addiction. Nonetheless, the great majority of Innu continued their traditional tribal existence as nomadic caribou hunters.[23] Colin Samson described this long period, which extended from the 1700s up to the 1960s, as follows:

> For most Innu currently living in Labrador, neither the fur trade nor white intrusion succeeded in changing their way of life. They were able to continue nomadic hunting and, as some ethnographers have pointed out, integrate alcohol into their religious lives. In the diaries of his 1927–8 ethnographic visit, American anthropologist, William Duncan Strong ... observed that the Mushuau Innu drank spruce beer and home brew to celebrate a big kill. He records no particular adverse effects other than mild chaos. Speck ... observed that after particular dreams, hunters would drink whisky to give their soul-spirits a libation to pay for the revelation of a caribou by a river and to induce its fulfilment. Similarly, Georg Henriksen ... argued that Innu used alcohol not only to celebrate but, along with drumming, singing and dancing, to communicate with the animal Gods.[24]

This is not to suggest that Canadian Indians were noble savages and cultivated social drinkers, or to argue that they were more moral than their conquerors. The history of Canadian Indians, like that of their European conquerors, abounds with brutal warfare, torture of prisoners, and slavery. Life spans were often short due to inter-tribal warfare and intermittent famine. Individual cases of murder, adultery, and insanity occurred.[25] Moreover, the Europeans claimed that Canadian Indians washed too seldom and smelled anything but noble. In short, the native people had most of the same problems that the Europeans had before the Europeans arrived, *but they did not have enough addiction that we can now document that it existed at all.*

The history of Canadian Indians differs from the more famous slaughter of aboriginal people in the United States and in some other parts of the world,[26] although it is ultimately a story of terrible dislocation nonetheless. Centuries before Vancouver was founded, both British and French trading companies in Canada established formal and mutually beneficial fur-trading relationships with many native tribes, primarily in eastern and central Canada. Because few European settlers then sought to settle in the inhospitable Canadian climate, there was no need to displace the natives. Later, the English colonial government formed indispensable military alliances with various aboriginal nations in several wars, primarily against the Americans.[27] After these crucial wars ended, it would have been unseemly for the Crown, as it began moving settlers into the vast native lands, to murder its former allies. Instead, British and later Canadian governments quietly pursued a policy, later called 'assimilation', intended to move aboriginal lands into the real estate market and aboriginal people into the labour market as peacefully as possible. This policy was explicitly intended to strip the natives of their culture as well as their land. One notorious instrument of this policy, among others,[28] was a network of 'residential schools' where children, often forcibly taken from their parents, were strictly trained to disdain their own language and customs, frequently alienating them from their own families in the process. An 1847 report of the colonial Canadian government explained:

> Their education must consist not merely of the training of the mind, but of a weaning from the habits and feelings of their ancestors, and the acquirements of the language, arts, and customs of civilised life.[29]

Although assimilation policy nearly succeeded in eliminating native languages and cultural practices, it failed to integrate most natives into free-market society, thus leaving them utterly dislocated.[30] As wards of the federal government, however, they were generally provided with food, housing, and social services.

In recent years, the policy of assimilation has lost its earlier legitimacy. The residential schools have all been closed as their intrinsic cruelty became more apparent. The government of Canada and the churches that ran the schools now face large numbers of lawsuits from individuals who claim that residential schools destroyed their culture and their individual mental health. Most of these claims are based on the physical and sexual abuse that occurred in many residential schools, but the case has been made, most eloquently, that the deliberate destruction of culture was the most harmful part of the residential school experience.[31]

Although Vancouver was settled much later than Eastern Canada, its native people experienced at least as much dislocation. The Vancouver area had a relatively minor history of fur trade and no history of military alliances between Indians and the Crown.[32] In the Canadian tradition, natives were dispossessed of their lands without military slaughter, although harsh examples were made by British warships, cannon, and hangmen when the natives became too unruly.[33]

Although there was no military slaughter of aboriginal people in the Vancouver area, deliberate destruction of aboriginal culture began immediately and was more stringent in many ways than it had been in the eastern provinces. The ability of Vancouver's Indians to defend their cultures was weakened by smallpox, an advance guard for European conquest that arrived well before the settlers themselves. Vancouver's Indians were given smaller allotments of reserve land than those given to Indians elsewhere in Canada, and most tribes and bands still have not been granted formal treaties that permanently establish their rights to the land that was left to them, leaving them in a state of perpetual uncertainty.[34]

The expropriation of native resources as needed by the free-market economy and the consequent dislocation of native people are proceeding as fast as ever in Canada today. Land essential to already-battered native cultures is being lost to hydroelectric flooding, urban sprawl, mineral exploration, toxic mining operations, clear-cut logging, military manoeuvres, industrial development, and waste disposal.[35] As a single example, in British Columbia today, wild salmon stocks, which have provided an essential economic and cultural basis for coastal and riverine cultures for countless centuries, are being destroyed by the wholesale introduction of salmon farms, which create breeding grounds for parasites that fatally infect nearby wild salmon migrations.

Salmon are not just food. They also figured prominently in aboriginal culture because it was necessary to develop elaborate technologies for capturing the fish, sophisticated conservation rules to preserve the stocks, and complex sharing arrangements between different aboriginal groups located at different points on the same river or stream.[36]

The disastrous effects of salmon farming on the migrating wild salmon have been amply demonstrated by careful research in Canada and Europe.[37] The dependence of native culture on the wild salmon stock remains undisputed. Many British Columbians refuse to eat farmed salmon. Yet the salmon farms apparently cannot be stopped. Governments deny, against the balance of independent science, that the farms will destroy the wild stock. They argue that the huge export income that comes from shipping farmed salmon to the world market is essential to the provincial economy. A large group of entrepreneurs, both in salmon farming and other enterprises, issue passionate statements in defence of a free-market approach to salmon farming, which the local media promulgate. Free-market ideology, which holds that markets must never be encumbered by mere tradition, biases public thinking in favour of the salmon farms and against the Indians who oppose them. Salmon farms provide only one example among many of the continuing dislocation of Canadian aboriginals by free-market society.

The progress of alcoholism and other addictions among Canadian Indians tracks the progress of their dislocation. Although some Canadian natives developed a taste for riotous drunkenness from the time that Europeans first introduced alcohol centuries ago, most individuals and tribes abstained, drank only moderately, or drank only as part of tribal rituals as long as they maintained an intact tribal culture.[38] It was only during periods of cultural disintegration that alcoholism emerged as a universal, crippling problem for native people, along with gambling and other forms of addiction, suicide, family violence, sexual abuse, and other ways of reacting to dislocation.[39] Samson observed of the Innu people discussed earlier in this chapter that:

> The adverse effects of drinking, including mass inebriation, social disorganisation, marital disharmony, child neglect and untimely deaths, coincide with drinking patterns since sedentarisation [i.e. removal from traditional hunting lands] in the 1960s and 1970s.

Sedentarisation put a final end to nomadic hunting as a way of life. It brought dependency on the Canadian government and other white intermediaries and occasioned a profound loss of meaning.[40]

Eventually, every tribal culture in Canada was broken down by the overpowering European culture, and every tribe succumbed to addiction and other ravages of dislocation.[41] Universal dislocation produced nearly universal addiction.[42] Addiction among Canadian natives has not been limited to alcoholism. It has kept pace with the times as addictions to the latest drugs, gambling, television, and video games have been added to the list. The causal relationship between dislocation and addiction has been apparent from the start.

Observing the alcoholism and violence that became, and remain today, rampant on native reserves, governments sometimes concluded that these problems were caused by poverty, and poured money onto the reserves.[43] Interventions of this sort sometimes worsen dislocation[44] and addiction problems. The Innu People of Davis Inlet in Labrador provide a highly publicised example. The Innu had been drawn into sedentary village life only in the 1960s as their land became desirable to Canada for hydroelectric, mining, and military purposes.[45] Once the Innu were settled in the village, their aboriginal culture quickly fell to ruin, making the 700 people of the village more and more dependent on government handouts. The federal government was spurred to action by a widely viewed videotape of six Innu children sniffing gas from plastic bags and screaming that they wanted to die. The government reacted to this international embarrassment by moving the entire village 15 kilometres away to a brand new village at Natuashish, built at a cost of C$150,000,000, a move that increased the people's material well-being, but seemed almost calculated to increase dislocation in people with strong ties to hunting on their own land. The move was completed in 2003. So much money was funnelled into the new village that some residents have four-wheel-drive pickup trucks and two-storey homes, and most have satellite television dishes in the yard. With the influx of money, the availability and the prices of drugs and alcohol rose sharply in the new village. The addiction problem did not diminish for either children or adults. Violence is as prevalent as before, and the local jail is full.[46]

Whereas interventions that do not recognise dislocation as a precursor for alcoholism in Indians have been minimally successful at best, initiatives undertaken by Indian bands that foster native cultural revival (often with a Christian component in addition to native spirituality) have been somewhat more successful.[47] Perhaps the most famous success story is that of the Indian band at Alkali Lake, British Columbia. This band went from virtually 100% alcoholism to 98% sobriety between 1972 and 1979. Under the leadership of a powerful chief and his wife, the people organised themselves to support one another's recovery efforts and to re-establish native spiritual practices while simultaneously relying on Alcoholics Anonymous, the Round Lake Treatment Centre, and the local police detachment to help enforce alcohol prohibition on the reserve.[48] An entire generation recovered from alcoholism at Alkali Lake. Most of these people remain sober today, although other serious problems associated with prolonged dislocation have become more visible, particularly the scars left by years of family violence and sexual abuse. Many of the community's youths are drinking heavily now, while their parents remain sober. It is perhaps too much to hope that the effects of cultural devastation can be overcome in a single generation, even with the best methods.[49]

Reflecting the partial success of the Alkali Lake band, the Round Lake Treatment Centre in British Columbia and other aboriginal institutions use the motto, 'Culture is treatment'.[50] Nonetheless, the problem of alcoholism and other forms of addiction among Canadian Indians remains massive, perhaps because even native-oriented treatment programmes treat alcoholism more as an individual disease than a social problem.[51]

Although dislocation is widely recognised as the root cause of addiction among Canadian aboriginal people, there is an even more common and convenient explanation. Aboriginal people are often said to have a racial and genetic inability to control alcohol. This convenient explanation is not tenable, as alcoholism was not a devastating problem among natives until destruction of their cultures subjected them to dislocation. Moreover, the addictions now experienced by natives extend far beyond alcoholism. Furthermore, if natives were handicapped by the 'gene for alcoholism', the same must be said of the Europeans who colonised them, since those subjected to conditions of extreme dislocation also fell into addiction, almost universally.

Canadian 'Orkneymen'

The history of the Hudson's Bay Company, the 'oldest continuous capitalist corporation still in existence'[52] provides an example where, at least for some employees, maximum dislocation was little confounded by poverty or violence. The Hudson's Bay Company was chartered by Charles II of England in 1670. Until 1987, a span of more than three centuries, it maintained forts and fur-trading outposts on the shores of Hudson Bay and throughout the Canadian north and west. Some of the company's traders were enlisted in London but more came from the Orkney Islands off the northern tip of Scotland, where the ships from London stopped en route to Hudson Bay to take on provisions and augment their crews.[53]

Preferred as employees because they were already accustomed to extreme northern latitudes and life at sea, and because of their characteristic sobriety and obedience, the Orkney recruits were mostly poor lads who volunteered for adventure and escape from the extreme poverty of traditional Orkney society. By 1779, 78% of the Hudson's Bay Company employees in Canada were Orkneymen. Whereas they did gain some of the high adventure they sought, they severed their ties to a close, traditional system based on both common land and cottar labour, which persisted in the Orkneys until the middle of the 19th century, long after the highlands had been flooded with sheep.[54]

As 'Bay men', the Orkneymen's only contact with home came once a year from a single ship that brought mail, supplies, and conversation, and then left in a few days with the pelts. When the annual ship disappeared, the men were alone again. Although fed and treated as well as circumstances permitted, their lives were prototypes of dislocation:

> With some exceptions, the Bay men became internal exiles in both their homelands, original and adopted. Never part of any society outside the fur trade, they gradually pruned

their ancestral roots, becoming bitterly aware of the true nature of any voluntary emigration: that one is exiled from and never to, and that disinheritance and marginality are all
too often the price of freedom. More than one loyal HBC trader faced the end of his days
with few close friends or blood relatives he wished to acknowledge and so bequeathed
whatever worldly goods he had gathered to the only family he had: the Company.[55]

One conspicuous aspect of the lives of the Bay men was intemperance. Alcoholism
was rampant:

> The Company quickly realised that liquor was a greater enemy than the climate to its
> trade on the bay, but no matter how many prohibitions it proclaimed and no matter how
> often it paid off informers to halt the smuggling of brandy cases on outgoing ships, the
> booze flowed steadily across the Atlantic. Exceptional was the Company [employee] who
> failed to organise surreptitious caches of several gallons or so of brandy for his private
> stock … [56]

The record of alcohol-related problems suggests almost universal alcoholism,
although the word, 'alcoholism' had not yet been invented.[57] The following was
written about an outpost on Hudson Bay named 'Moose Factory':

> Many of the work accidents at Moose were alcohol-related. One man consumed so much
> 'bumbo'—that fur-trade mixture of rum, water, sugar, and nutmeg—that he fell off the
> sloop and promptly drowned. With some regret and much haste, his mates lost no time in
> auctioning off the contents of his chest. The chief factors were always afraid that the men
> on watch, who were too often drunk, would spitefully or accidentally set fire to the build-
> ings. The courage to commit suicide could also be found in the bottle. 'Brandy-death' was
> common … [58]

But could the Bay men already have been alcoholic before they encountered the
supreme dislocation of Hudson Bay? Or could the extremes of northern life have
made them alcoholic? These explanations could work for the Londoners, but not
the Orkneymen. They were preferred employees of the Hudson's Bay Company
because of their sobriety in their homeland and because they were accustomed to life
at extreme northern latitudes.[59] Their alcoholism was a way of adapting to extreme
dislocation.[60]

However, the dislocation theory is not a theory of alcoholism alone, but a theory of
addiction in general. Alcoholism is an easy addiction to document, but there are signs
that the Orkneymen may well have been involved in others. They may have been so
dedicated to accumulating money, both for the company and for themselves, that they
qualified as addicted in this way too. The phrase 'sordidly avaricious' was applied to
them by one historian.[61] Certainly, local preachers in the Orkneys spoke of the returning Bay men in terms that suggest problems that went beyond simple alcoholism:

> … the Rev. Francis Liddell, minister of Orphir, launched into an impassioned diatribe
> against those who abandoned wives, children, and parents to enter the service of the
> Company, eventually returning home with enough money to out-bid honest farmers;
> they brought home none of the virtues of the savage, but all the vices—indolence, dissi-
> pation, and irreligion; 'My God!' he declaimed, 'shall man, formed in the image of his
> Creator, desert the human species and, for the paltry sum of six pounds a-year, assume
> the manners and habits of the brutes that perish?'[62]

China

The regime that ruled China from 1949 until Mao Zedong's death in 1976 has been discredited in the Western world in every conceivable way, except one. Even its worst enemies no longer deny that Mao's regime drastically reduced drug addiction in China in just a few years, after many decades of mass addictive misery. This is the only instance I have found of a modern nation bringing widespread addiction under control.

Analysing this unique historical event without inflaming political sensitivities requires dispelling two ideologically based myths and a major distraction at the outset. The first myth, which still has visceral appeal to the political right, is that Mao eliminated opium addiction through mass murder of drug users and dealers.[63] The second myth, once beloved of the political left, is that addiction cannot become a problem in a Marxist society. Both stories are false—the evidence is summarised below. The major distraction is the conflicting analyses of Mao's personal character, which has been alternately deified and demonized since the mid-20th century.[64] But Mao's personal qualities are not relevant here. The documented events of his regime are the topic of this account.

Despite their success in controlling addiction, the drug control methods of Mao's regime cannot be adopted in the 21st century. These methods were embedded in a unique era and a short-lived political system that began making disastrous economic mistakes within a decade of its establishment in 1949. Mao's regime failed politically as well, when the solidarity and optimism of the late 1940s and 1950s were overcome by economic setbacks, political division, corruption, and, after 1966, the bizarre mob politics of the Cultural Revolution.[65] Mao's regime did not lead the world to utopia, but it did demonstrate that, under certain circumstances, addiction problems can be solved on a vast scale, quickly and with relatively little violence.

Opium addiction had been spreading in China for a century prior to 1949, as discussed earlier in this chapter.[66] By the time that Mao's army gained control of the country, the Chinese masses were smoking great quantities of opium and consuming almost as much morphine and heroin—much of it by injection. Much of this drug use was seriously addictive, although some was recreational and medicinal.[67]

Despite continuing mass poverty, Mao's regime largely eliminated opium and morphine use between 1949 and 1953, a period of only 4 years, more than a decade before the protracted violence of the Cultural Revolution began. Moreover, the Maoist regime experienced no serious problem with alcoholism or other addictions. Drug addiction did not reappear as a serious problem in China until the 1980s under a very different regime.[68]

After taking control in 1949, Mao's new government immediately imposed its unique version of socialism throughout China. This approach to socialism had been described in Mao's earliest political writings.[69] It entailed gaining and maintaining power by working through existing forms of social organisation, as well as developing new social and political organisations particularly among poor peasants, industrial workers, and ethnic minorities, who together comprised the vast majority of China's population.[70] Regional social and political organisations were encouraged to make decisions democratically and some political influence was allowed to flow upwards to the government. Although the major decisions and mass propaganda were promulgated from the top down, and although the regime undoubtedly became a 'personality cult',[71] it was wildly successful for its first decade. The great mass of the population, which had endured decades of starvation, oppression, and war, found it natural to work together in support of a regime that gave them real collective power, led by an icon of iron courage who idolised common people and expressed his grand designs in simple poetry and parables. Starvation was largely overcome; education flourished; barefoot doctors brought medicine to the poor for the first time; prostitution and domestic violence were greatly reduced; people were proud to be Chinese again.[72] The gains were obvious and measurable. For example, the mortality rate fell from about 25 per 1000 of the population before 1949, to 17 per 1000 in 1951, and 10.8 per 1000 in 1957.[73]

In restructuring Chinese society, Mao's regime took great pains to preserve and strengthen the traditional village social structure of the peasants (minus the landlords, who were dispossessed and sometimes killed by peasants who redistributed their lands). Mao's regime also strove to support existing trade unions and the peasants' unions[74] and to organise and incorporate new associations both in rural and urban areas. The new associations included the Communist Youth League, peasant communes, women's associations, residents' associations, and associations of artists, intellectuals, and businessmen.[75] The principle of continuous discussion and mutual criticism, which had been successfully applied to the army and party members during the long revolution, was extended to the whole of Chinese society.

The pinnacle of this way of thinking was the official 'Great Leap Forward', which commenced in 1958. Rejecting USSR-style factory-based heavy industry, the great leap was to spring from rural communes that would simultaneously serve industrial, agricultural, trade, cultural, educational, and military functions. This was the era of smelting steel in thousands of 'backyard furnaces'. Although this Maoist rescripting of the industrial revolution became an economic disaster within a few years, and although many millions of people died in the ensuing famines, ordinary people working together locally comprised the very heart of the nation for a time, sharing the goals of social justice and prosperity. They succeeded or failed as a psychosocially integrated society.

Popular acceptance of Mao's regime grew from Mao's personal charisma as well as from the people's need for release from dire poverty and for renewed psychosocial integration in Chinese society. He used his enormous popularity to actualise his dream of a utopian society founded on collective ownership of all property by peasants and the urban poor (the overwhelming majority of the Chinese population at that time). Whatever Mao accomplished, he accomplished though social action. He emphatically denounced and discouraged individualism.

Mao himself was probably an egotist with a lust for power. It is also possible, as many people now believe, that he was also a cunning actor who fooled the people about his love for them. However, *their* love and admiration *for him* and their wholehearted enthusiasm for his dream of radical socialism leading to communism was absolutely real, contagious, and euphoric. Throughout the 1950s, the vast majority of the Chinese population joined his new organisations, worked long hours on his modernisation projects, sang songs, wrote poems, and lived in relative harmony with their neighbours. Huge improvements in nutrition, production, unemployment, health, and education materialised very fast in a country that had been devastated by exploitation, starvation, and war for as long as anyone could remember.

Many Chinese people were disillusioned by the failures of the Great Leap Forward and by the Cultural Revolution that began in 1966. Nonetheless, the regime held together. The basic social institutions introduced in 1949 and afterwards continued to function reasonably well into the 1970s, and there were even some modest gains.[76] Despite serious setbacks, substantial economic growth took place during this whole period and the condition of the poor was greatly ameliorated. For example, the World Bank reported that the net output of industry grew 10.2 % per year between 1957 and 1979, despite the Great Leap Forward.[77]

The psychosocial integration and solidarity that Mao's regime successfully fostered[78] throughout the 1950s and to a lesser degree in the 1960s and 1970s may have been the most important component of its successful control of opioid addiction.[79] The experience of living an encompassing social life left people with little need for addictive pursuits to fill a void of dislocation. Moreover, local society took a direct interest in preventing drug addiction. An American psychiatrist described Mao's social innovations in 1977 on the basis of an extensive literature review and a trip to China. Here is a portion of his description:

> The mechanism by which the reintegration of Chinese society was accomplished was the organisational leadership and ideology of the Communist Party. Small street committees offered political and cultural leadership and effective social pressure in many communities. The basic unit of government structure was based on a residential group of 100 to 200 people, which was part of larger community organisations. It was this basic residential unit that produced the 'mass line', a review, revision, and implementation of national health policies and other political decisions. Such a basic unit was effective in carrying out national decisions because members of every third or fourth family in such groups were neighbourhood activists. These local cadres were responsible for propaganda, agitation, and indoctrination in the anti-opium campaign and were also a source of information about and social censure of those who continued to use opium.[80]

Certainly, the effect of increased psychosocial integration on addiction was augmented with more direct deterrents: use of the social infrastructure as a bureaucratic channel for dispensing anti-drug propaganda (as well as other forms of propaganda), supportive treatment for addicts who were willing to give up their habits, surveillance for drug use, and, most famously, harsh punishment of major drug traffickers. Yet contrary to the myth of the political right, harsh punishment and the other direct methods cannot have been the whole story. Despite sensationalized reports of executions of Chinese traffickers during this period, capital punishment can be ruled out as an explanation of this unique success in eliminating opioid addiction. In fact, there were relatively few executions of addicts and traffickers in Mao's China. Of 10,000 addicts brought to public attention in China in the year preceding March 1951, 37 were executed. In Shanghai, the centre of the Chinese drug trade, only ten executions of major drug distributors took place between 1949 and 1951.[81]

The Maoist Chinese were probably no more punitive in their suppression of opioid addiction than several other Chinese regimes in the 19th and early 20th centuries. These regimes include the pre-1911 Qing Dynasty, the post-1911 Chinese Republic under Sun Yat-sen, the 1927–1949 Chinese Nationalist government under Chiang Kai-shek, the post-1949 nationalist government of Taiwan, and the British-controlled government of the Crown Colony of Hong Kong. Each of these Chinese regimes also made use of very harsh deterrents, including the death penalty[82] with no success.[83]

Mao's regime, although it visited murderous violence upon people who were perceived to be capitalistic, may actually have been no more violent in its drug enforcement than the American government in the corresponding post-World War II period. A War on Drugs was raging in the United States during these years, although the phrase was invented later. The United States, deep in a cultural revolution called 'McCarthyism', associated communism with 'narcotics', and cultivated fear of narcotics with a ferocious barrage of anti-drug propaganda. United States law allowed American juries to impose the death penalty for selling heroin to people under 18 years of age during this period.[84] Capital punishment was not the main deterrent in either China or the United States. Rather, both countries utilised long jail sentences, dramatic propaganda, brutal policing of recalcitrant addicts and traffickers, neighbourhood surveillance (primarily by neighbours in China and paid police agents in the United States),[85] and compulsory treatment. Whereas Maoist China essentially eliminated opioid addiction, the United States—too enmeshed in free-market economics to do anything that would increase psychosocial integration—failed completely, *using similar coercive techniques*.[86] Canada's approach to narcotics during this period, now mostly forgotten, was disturbingly similar to the punitive American one, although it did not include capital punishment. It too was completely unsuccessful.[87]

Contrary to the myth of the political left, Mao's success in controlling addiction cannot be attributed to Marxist society per se. In contrast to China, alcohol addiction was as widespread in the USSR in the years following World War II as it had been under the Tsars.[88] Although the regimes of the USSR and China can both be labelled Marxist in their attempts to eliminate private ownership and their ideological commitment to the proletariat, Mao's version of Marxism fostered psychosocial integration to a much greater degree than the Soviet version.

There is little in the basic literature of Marxism that commits a communist state to promote psychosocial integration. Although Marx and Engels devoted some of the most powerful rhetoric in the *Communist Manifesto* to the destructive effects of capitalism on traditional social structures, they expressed no expectation that a communist society would restore traditional social relationships. In fact, they distanced themselves from those socialists who believed that traditional social relationships could be restored, whom they disdainfully labelled 'utopian socialists'.[89] Marx and Engels famously stated that the 'real conditions of life' come to the fore when traditional social ties are broken.[90] In his writings on French history, Marx spoke eloquently of how it had been necessary for the bourgeois revolutions of the 19th century to destroy even the memory of past traditions and how the proletarian revolution that he believed would follow depended on this prior destruction.[91] Although Marx saw the misery of dislocation clearly, his concern was not to undo the capitalist form of social organisation that produced it, only to bring it under the control of the prole-tariat.[92] Engels, writing in 1891, argued that a just world would exist when workers, at last in control of the means of production, received the full value of their labour. He did not question the massive dislocation and environmental destruction that the capitalist economic system had produced and assumed that it would continue if the proletariat took charge.[93] Engels believed that compulsory collectivisation of peasants would proceed with a bare minimum of force, because the peasants' appreciation of the productivity of collective farming would overcome all contrary sentiments they might have.[94]

Although the overall intent of Marx and Engels can be interpreted differently on the basis of other writings that have a more humane tone,[95] Lenin was unambiguous.[96] He spoke of the development of monopolies, cartels, and colonial empires as the 'socialisation' of society under private ownership. All that remained to establish communism, he thought, was to transfer control of industry to the proletariat. He appeared unconcerned over either the dislocation that industrialisation caused in the developed countries or the dislocation that colonialism caused in the Third World.[97]

The Soviet Union took the hyperindustrialist strand of Marxist-Leninist doctrine to heart. The USSR's practice of destroying traditional society in the interest of tech-nological development is well known in the case of collective farms and has been doc-umented in many other instances.[98] Josef Stalin himself wrote a forceful argument for maintaining elements of the capitalist system and for seeking ever-increasing produc-tion in Soviet heavy industry.[99] Marxism in the USSR imposed the industrial revolu-tion under bureaucratic, rather than entrepreneurial, control.[100] The contemporary Russian philosopher Mejouev has said of the former USSR, 'Our socialism was actu-ally Russian-style capitalism in its technological structure and anticapitalist in its form.'[101] In addition, psychosocial integration in the USSR was undermined by the ubiquitous secret police, who made any relaxed association of people very dangerous.

If Soviet Marxism can be characterised as Russian-style capitalism, it still fell far short of the hypercapitalism imposed on Russian people by the government of Boris Yeltsin, beginning in 1992. This hypercapitalist 'shock therapy' impoverished the majority of the population leaving little discetionary money available for addictive habits. Nonetheless, alcohol consumption doubled between 1987 and 2003. Officially designated drug users increased 900% bewteen 1994 and 2004.[102]

Contrary to the USSR, China's approach to modernising the economy after 1949 valued many traditional forms of social organisation and introduced new ones. Opioid addiction and alcoholism remained a negligible problem in China from 1951 until 1980, when a new free-market economic system (ambiguously called 'market socialism') introduced under Mao's successor, Deng Xiaoping, began to take hold. The movement towards free-market society regulated by the Communist Party bureau-cracy became very rapid after 1990.

The economic system introduced by Deng has improved the economic status of China and raised the standard of living for the majority of Chinese people.[103] China has become a poster child for the success of free-market society in the Third World. However, Chinese free-market society produces dislocation just as relentlessly as any other. Psychosocial integration appears to be dying the death of a thousand cuts.

For example, China has now privatised or closed tens of thousands of state-owned enterprises that previously gave millions of industrial workers lifelong job security, secure housing, and medical care.[104] The damming and re-routing of Chinese rivers has flooded the homes and villages of many people. The Three Gorges Dam alone—just one of many massive projects—is expected to dispossess 1.2 million people.[105] A giant pincer movement of dislocation has been produced by inexorable population growth combined with increasing agricultural mechanisation. The result is that, since 1979, an estimated 200 million rural people have moved into cities, many of them new and unserviced,[106] and unemployment has become widespread, a new problem for modern China.[107] Millions of workers with no prospects for work must either settle down to a life of poverty and exclusion in their homelands or try to emigrate. Already, floods of clandestine immigrants, from China and other countries, are inundating the United States and Europe. Dislocation affects not only the migrating workers, but also the countries where they arrive as local society is destabilised.[108]

China has shown no signs of modifying its fundamental commitment to the new 'market socialism', even in the face of obvious environmental problems, economic disparities, and mass dislocation.[109] China's commitment to a market economy is carried out on a symbolic as well as a structural level. In September 2004, the Chinese Communist Youth League entered into a formal partnership with the Walt Disney Company 'to promote Mi Laoshu, or Mickey Mouse'.[110]

History thus provides a natural experiment. If the dislocation theory of addiction is correct, China will be unable to avoid massive increases in addiction of all sorts in the next few years. This prediction applies even if China continues to develop its free-market society pragmatically and successfully, avoiding the economically ruinous 'shock therapy' that devastated the economy of the USSR and other countries that let their globalisation be guided by Western economists.[111] For example, China is currently seeking a way to reduce the huge income disparities that have grown from market socialism.[112] Eliminating the extremes of poverty and wealth could increase social justice within the Chinese market system, but it would not eliminate the structural dislocation that is intrinsic to free-market society.

Signs of mass dislocation in China grew more and more evident in the 1980s among both rich and poor[113] and grew further following the entry of China into the World Trade Organization.[114] Current news reports indicate a shocking growth in alcoholism, gambling addiction, Internet addiction, heroin addiction, and obesity spanning China's emerging social class system.[115] The number of registered drug users in China increased from 70,000 in 1990 to 1.16 million in 2005, a 16-fold increase, which prompted China to establish a massive harm reduction programme.[116]

Today, three decades after Mao's death, the government of China applies the death penalty to at least four drug crimes: smuggling, selling, transporting, and manufacturing illegal drugs.[117] Although the current numbers of executions for drug crimes are secret, there are indications that they are large.[118] China is the biggest practitioner of capital punishment of any country on earth at this time. If addiction could be eliminated by mass execution, present-day China would probably have done it. However, the drug problem in China appears to be out of control.[119] It will take a few more years to establish whether or not China's addictive problems can be brought under control. I predict that they cannot, as long as China continues to expand its free-market society.[120] If this prediction is not borne out, the dislocation theory is wrong.

Endnotes

1 Jessica Warner (1994) provides a good survey of moral condemnations of drunkenness from English pulpits beginning in the 1600s.

2 Jessica Warner (2002).

3 Tawney (1926/1947, Chapter 4). Scholars have offered other explanations for the gin craze as well (e.g. Plant and Plant, 2006, pp. 6–11).

4 Austin contrasted drinking in medieval and 18th-century Europe as follows:

> Although chronic inebriety was a sin (in medieval Europe), occasional inebriety was accepted as a natural aspect of life. One of the few examples of legislation against drunkenness was a decree by Archbishop Theodore of Canterbury in the seventh century ordering that anyone who drank to excess must do penance for fifteen days. Because of the importance of beer and wine to the diet, drink controls largely focused on protecting the drinker from unscrupulous sellers, maintaining a good supply and a fair price, and reducing the adverse consequences (such as public disorders) of too much drinking. As in antiquity, inebriety was largely associated with occasional festivities and with a few specific populations (nobles, students, and clerics) who had the wealth, free time, or access to supplies that enabled more regular indulgence.... In the eighteenth century, concerns again rose as inebriety became more regular among more people, reaching unprecedented heights. The upper classes and the towns continued to lead the way, but chronic inebriety was no longer primarily the prerogative of the upper classes. The major development of the century was the expansion of drinking among the lower classes and into rural villages. It was most prevalent in England, but everywhere complaints about inebriety multiplied.

Austin (1985, pp. xviii, xx).

See also Jessica Warner (1992).

5 Charles Dickens (1833–35/1994); Hobsbawm (1962); Hughes (1987); Schivelbusch (1992); Mathieson (2000). Dickens described the terrible crimes that severe drunkards did to their own families with revulsion in his article *The Drunkard's Death* (pp. 463–472). However, he understood the cause as well, and described it in his article *Gin Shops* (quoted in the text above). British social reformer Robert Owen made the same observation about the cause of alcoholism slightly earlier than Dickens, but Owen was shouted down by his contemporaries (Donnachie, 2000, Chapter 7).

6 Waters from the mythological River Lethe were said to bring people forgetfulness of all that had happened in the past.

7 Dickens (1833–1835/1994, p. 185).

8 Hobsbawm (1962, p. 202).

9 Kenny (1994, p. 19).

10 Aaron and Musto (1981, pp. 131–139).

11 Sonnedecker (1962, 1963). Berridge and Edwards (1987) argue that rising concern with opium addiction was more a matter of class persecution and professional ambition of doctors eager to treat new types of patients than of a major increase in addiction. They also report, however, a substantial increase of opium use in 19th-century England and indications of increases in addiction as well.

12 Musto (1987); T. M. Hickman (2004).

13 Dikötter *et al.* (2004, Chapters 3 and 4).

14 Bayly (2004, pp. 148–155).

15 Gittings (1973, pp. 188–190).

16 Yi-Mak and Harrison (2001, p. 48). Dikötter *et al.* (2004) point out that many Chinese people used opium safely and beneficially for health and recreational purposes in the 19th century, that the Chinese government's horror of opium addiction in the late 19th and early 20th centuries served many political purposes, and that opium became a scapegoat for national decline. These qualifications are true, but they do not negate the devastation of opioid addiction in that period any more than similar exaggerations of temperance doctrine negate the devastation of severe alcoholism in the temperance era of the West.

17 K. Polanyi (1944, pp. 157–158); Wrightson (2000, p. 317). This conclusion remains debatable, however. See Bayly (2004, p. 119).

18 Jessica Warner (1992, pp. 422–423).

19 Bayly (2004, Chapter 12).

20 Among Canadian sources, I have drawn most heavily on sources that describe the social lives of southern British Columbia native people and the Innu people of northern Labrador and Quebec. See Jewitt (1824/1988), Sproat (1868/1987), McFeat (1966), Fisher (1992), K. T. Carlson (1997), and Samson (2003, 2004).

21 Sproat (1868/1987, esp. pp. 181–182). The only suggestion to the contrary that I have found concerns the avid competition for status among chiefs of western coastal tribes, which has been called 'megalomania'. Status arose primarily from ceremonial giving at potlatches. As Woodcock pointed out:

> At first glance it seems as though in every way the potlatches expressed and aggravated a desire for individual self-glorification rare among primitive peoples. Yet it should be cautiously remembered that the chief was only the temporary bearer of names and privileges belonging to the lineages, whose prestige was collectively enhanced by his actions—a fact recognized by his kinsmen who would eagerly share in his efforts to gather goods for the potlatch so that the honour of the house and the clan should be sustained.

Woodcock (1977, p. 18).

22 McAndrew and Edgerton (1969, p. 109); D. B. Heath (1987).

23 Fur traders were able to use alcohol and trading goods to lure a few Innu into becoming trappers in the 18th and 19th centuries, but most remained in their tribal groups, shunning both trapping and alcoholism (Samson, 2003, pp. 131–132). The Sekani people of northern British Columbia also used alcohol sensibly until the mid-20th century when they were driven from their traditional hunting lands. They are discussed in more detail in Chapter 15.

24 Samson (2004, pp. 150).

25 Jewitt (1824/1988); Sproat (1868/1987); Oberg (1934/1966, p. 193); McFeat (1966); McAndrew and Edgerton (1969, pp. 137–139); K. T. Carlson (1997).

26 Bayly (2004, Chapter 12); P. McKenna (2004).

27 P. C. Newman (1985); Allen (1992).

28 More examples are given in Chapter 1 under the heading *Probable Causes of Addiction in Vancouver*. Another instrument of this policy, which is now coming to light, is the systematic slaughter of sled dogs of Canadian Inuit people by Canadian police in the decades after World War II (Makin, 2005).

29 Quoted in Haig-Brown (1988, p. 25).

30 Haig-Brown (1988); Tennant (1990); Fisher (1992); Chrisjohn and Young (1997).

31 Chrisjohn and Young (1997).

32 K. T. Carlson (1997, Chapter 3). Although it is hard to be certain about tribal boundaries, as they were always contested, the Stó:lo people of whom K. T. Carlson and his colleagues wrote lived along the Fraser River, thereby probably occupying part, but not the whole, of the area of the present city of Vancouver.

33 Sproat (1868/1987, pp. 132–136); Arnett (1999); Warrior Publications (n.d.). It is impossible to know whether the native cultures lost their strength more from the devastation of their populations by smallpox, which eventually killed two-thirds of the aboriginal population, by the magical attraction of British trade goods, or by occasional demonstrations that resistance to traders and settlers would always encounter irresistible force.

34 Tennant (1990); Shields (2007).

35 Samson (2003); Pasco (2005); Reid *et al.* (2006); Séguin (2006); Mason (2007). A current example is the dumping of garbage from the Vancouver area onto native territory. This is explained eloquently and accurately in a pamphlet released at a public meeting in Vancouver on 16 March 2004 by native people who live close to the Thompson River, about 250 km upstream from Vancouver. Their position is documented by careful research on similar 'landfills' in British Columbia and elsewhere. The pamphlet begins as follows:

> Nlaka'pamux Fight Against the Ashcroft Garbage Dump. Would you like 80 million tonnes of garbage dumped in your backyard? Starting in 2007, the Greater Vancouver Regional District (GVRD) plans to dump 200,000 tonnes of garbage per year on the territory of the Nlaka'pamux Nation, directly beside the Ashcroft Indian Band community. The dump would operate for 100 years and threatens the life and health of the People, the Water, and the Land. The Nlaka'pamux Nation opposes the building of the garbage dump, and requests your assistance. The GVRD argues that the land is worthless, and does not see a problem with siting the dump on Nlaka'pamux territory because it is land covered with sagebrush, and in the drier part of the province. This is our homeland, and it is beautiful. The Ashcroft garbage dump has the potential to severely impact upon the Nlaka'pamux people, land, waters and resources. The garbage dump would alter the landscape and destroy sagebrush, bitterroot, deer and other wildlife habitat, as well as pollute the groundwater. The Nlaka'pamux Peoples do not consent to the building of the garbage dump on their Aboriginal Title territories.

36 Copes (2005). Salmon figured in the stories and myths of various tribes.

37 Union of BC Indian Chiefs (2002); Western Canada Wilderness Committee (2002); S. Hume (2003a); M. Hume (2005a); Morton and Routledge (2006).

38 McAndrew and Edgerton (1969, Chapter 6); Samson (2004, 150–151).

39 Sproat (1868/1987, Chapter 27); Kew (1990); Fisher (1992); Matas (2000). Sproat's account, originally written in 1868, indicates that dispossession from land was not necessary to produce a profound psychological demoralisation of native people once they witnessed the overwhelming power of nearby communities of English settlers and (he could have added) had witnessed the power of the Royal Navy to suppress any native uprising that might occur. He noted that alcohol became irresistible to Indians in this demoralized state (p. 191).

More quantitative evidence for this assertion comes from studies of the relationship between cultural integrity of native groups and both alcoholism and youthful suicide (D. B. Heath, 1987; M. J. Chandler and Lalonde, 1998). D. B. Heath also reviews 'a few interesting exceptions' in which the expected relationship between degree of dislocation and heavy drinking was not found (p. 39). Although some eastern tribes were ravaged by drunkenness and alcoholism centuries before assimilation was established as an official policy, the causal principle appears to be the same. For example, the Huron of eastern Canada, who were 'civilised' by the courageous devotion of French missionaries backed by the firepower of the French Army early in the 17th century, were famous for their drunken violence (McAndrew and Edgerton, 1969, pp. 124–126). 'Civilisation', as it came to these natives, was administered by militant Jesuits in a century of fanatical religious zeal. This meant destruction of the robust Huron religion and, hence, Huron culture itself, with dislocation as the consequence.

40 Samson (2004, pp. 150–151).

41 There are many other ways to react to dislocation besides alcoholism. For example, drug addiction of all sorts is rampant among aboriginal people. Recent data show that gambling addiction is about three times as prevalent among native people as other Canadians (G. Smith, 2003). Obesity is more common among aboriginal people living off reserves than any other ethnic group in Canada (Picard, 2005b). Aboriginal suicide rates have historically been much higher than the rates of other Canadians and are about six times higher today (M. J. Chandler *et al.*, 2003; Picard, 2005f).

42 Sproat (1868/1987, Chapter 27); May (1982); Tennant (1990, p. 72); Alfred (1999, pp. 34–35); Samson (2003, 2004); Menzies (2006). Charles Darwin himself apparently saw at least part of the connection, and used the natives of Vancouver Island in the 19th century as his chief example. The following is a quote from *The Descent of Man*, originally published in 1871:

> When civilised nations come into contact with barbarians the struggle is short, except where a deadly climate gives its aid to the native race. Of the causes which lead to the victory of civilised nations, some are plain and some very obscure. We can see that the cultivation of the land will be fatal in many ways to savages, for they cannot, or will not, change their habits. New diseases and vices are highly destructive; and it appears that in every nation a new disease causes much death, until those who are most susceptible to its destructive influence are gradually weeded out; and so it may be with the evil effects from spirituous liquors, as well as with the unconquerably strong taste for them shewn by so many savages. It further appears, mysterious as is the fact, that the first meeting of distinct and separated people generates disease. Mr. Sproat, who in Vancouver Island closely attended to the subject of extinction, believes that changed habits of life, which always follow from the advent of Europeans, induce much ill-health. He lays, also, great stress on so trifling a cause as that the natives become 'bewildered and dull by the new life around them; they lose the motives for exertion, and get no new ones in their place'.

Darwin (1871/1981, pp. 238–239).

43 *Globe and Mail* (2005f); J. Strauss (2005).

44 *Globe and Mail* (2005f); Picard (2005g).

45 Samson (2003, Prologue and Chapter 1).

46 D. Moore (2003); *Globe and Mail* (2005a).

47 Jilek (1981); Duran and Duran (1995, p. 105); McCormick (2000); Coyhis and White (2002).

48 Hodgson (1987). The community approached its problems on many levels. These included reintroducing traditional spiritual practices, such as 'sweat lodges'; showering social approval on people who gave up drinking; providing a house for band members who decided to continue their schooling; reintroducing the band's native language to the children through the schools; withholding the welfare cheques of alcoholics and instead issuing vouchers that could not be exchanged for alcohol; offering petty offenders a choice between accepting treatment for alcoholism and facing legal charges; laying charges against

people who sold alcohol in the community; creating employment by opening a local logging operation and a store on the reserve; organizing support groups for victims of physical and sexual abuse; caring for the families and fixing up the homes of people who left the reserve for treatment; and establishing Alcoholics Anonymous groups and social-skills training programmes on the reserve. All of these efforts were embedded in a matrix of native spiritualism and traditionalism. Professionals and law-enforcement officers were involved in this programme, but they operated under the control of the band, rather than representing autonomous, external institutions. Furness (2004) placed greater importance than did Hodgson on the simultaneously authoritarian and charismatic leadership of the Alkali Lake chief and his wife.

49 Four Worlds International Institute (n.d.).

50 Edgar (2003b).

51 Samson (2003, Chapter 8) has written a thoughtful critique along these lines of what is sometimes called 'pan-Indian healing'.

52 P. C. Newman (1985, p. 3).

53 P. C. Newman (1985).

54 Thompson (1987).

55 P. C. Newman (1985, p. 9).

56 P. C. Newman (1985, pp. 160–161).

57 There is some disagreement among historians on the issue of just how widespread alcoholism was among the Orkneymen. Although Burley (1997, p. 131) stated that 'alcoholism in the HBC was not widespread and drinking was rarely fatal', Burley's chapter on this topic is full of examples of drinking incidents recorded by company officials that sound exactly like alcoholism (see pp. 131–139). Some of these incidents involved men with characteristically Orkney names, like Flett. It is certainly not the case, however, that all Orcadians were debilitated by alcoholism. See also M. Payne (1989, p. 157).

58 Pannekoek (1979, p. 5).

59 Canadian winters were far colder though.

60 Although there is no doubt that the Hudson's Bay Company was quite convinced of Orcadians' sobriety (J. H. S. Brown, 1988), an Orkney historian has questioned whether Orkney sobriety was as consistent as they believed. Thompson (1993) concluded that Orcadians were generally sober by the end of the 18th century, but not at the beginning of that century, which was a period of heavy recruitment by the company in Orkney. Nonetheless, the Hudson's Bay officials were probably in a better position to make direct comparisons between the employees they found at Orkney and those available at English ports, and at the same time were highly motivated to obtain the best employees they could get.

61 J. H. S. Brown quoted a 1790 description of Orkney employees of the Hudson's Bay Company as follows:

> ... a close prudent quiet people, strictly faithful to their employers, and sordidly avaricious. When these people are scattered ... among the Indians ... their behaviour is conducted with so much propriety, as not only to make themselves esteemed by the natives, and to procure their protection, but they also employ their time in endeavouring to enrich themselves, and their principals, by their diligence and unwearied assiduity.

> J. H. S. Brown (1988, p. 5).

Phrases like 'sordidly avaricious' and 'unwearied assiduity' suggest that some Orkneymen were subject to work addiction rather than, or as well as, alcoholism. However, it may now be impossible to see clearly enough into the past to be certain about this.

62 Thompson (1987, p. 220). In a later article, Thompson (1993) pointed out that the same kind of transformation was observed by other ministers among their countrymen who went off for long periods with the fishing and whaling fleets that came to call at Orkney. However, he attributed part of the ministers' motivation to view the men thus was to discourage off-shore employment in the interests of local gentry who were then suffering from a shortage of local labour for their own projects.

63 Dalrymple (2006a, p. 38).

64 For example, Roux (2006).

65 Gittings (1973, pp. 196–212; 2005, Chapters 2, 3 and 5) pointed out that there were actually two Cultural Revolutions, but this book follows the conventional usage of referring to them in the singular.

66 Yi-Mak and Harrison (2001).

67 Dikötter et al. (2004, Chapters 8 and 9). These authors have argued that the cause of this addictive consumption was earlier attempts to impose prohibition by Chinese governments, but I do not accept this interpretation, for reasons stated earlier in this chapter.

68 S. G. Sullivan and Wu (2007).

69 Mao Tse Tung (1929/1966b, 1937/1966c, 1948/1966d). The first is a short article addressed to the military personnel and party cadres associated with the 4th Corps of the Red Army of China. It is explicit not only about Mao's belief in the absolute necessity of fostering and using local social organisations in the struggle against the Kuomintang, but also about con-tinuing group discussion and criticism to be carried out at all levels among the soldiers and political cadres themselves. This strategy seems to be a natural outcome of Mao's epistemol-ogy, described in the second article. His epistemology is a kind of Marxist social pragma-tism, in which valid knowledge only originated in, and was confirmed and refined in, multiple levels of social practice, including production, class struggle, and cultural activities (see Mao Tse Tung, 1937/1966c). The third article lays out the principles of government pol-icy always according with the evolving will of the masses (Mao Tse Tung, 1948/1966d).

70 Gittings (1973, pp. 107–172).

71 J. Wong (1996).

72 Gittings (1973, pp. 107–172, 206–207; 2005, Chapter 2).

73 Gittings (2005, p. 23).

74 See Mao Tse Tung (1927/1966a) for an account of the power of peasants' unions of the uprising of the 1920s and of his enthusiastic support for them.

75 Chen (1975, Chapter 3, esp. p. 59).

76 Gittings (2005, Chapter 5).

77 Gittings (2005, pp. 99–101).

78 See Bianco (1971, esp. Chapter 4) and Chen (1975, Chapter 3).

79 Jan Wong, a Canadian writer whom I greatly admire, may not agree completely with the interpretation of Chinese history that I have presented here. The difference between her and I may be because I am concentrating more than she does on the period before the Cultural Revolution.

80 Lowinger (1977, pp. 169–170).

81 Lowinger (1977).

82 Lowinger (1977); Brook and Wakabayashi (2000); Zhou (2000); Yi-Mak and Harrison (2001); Dikötter et al. (2004, pp. 115, 142–145).

83 A close comparison between the methods and efficacy of addiction treatment in Hong Kong and mainland China in the decades following World War II would be extremely valuable, although I do not have access to the information that is needed to make it. Hong Kong was a British Crown Colony, committed by British colonial policy to the purest form of free-market economics (M. Friedman and Friedman, 1979, Chapter 1), whereas the Chinese People's Republic prior to 1976 was committed to destroying free-market economics and re-establishing social solidarity. If the dislocation theory of addiction is correct, Hong Kong could not have succeeded in controlling addiction, no matter what methods it employed, whereas the Chinese People's Republic did succeed, and quickly.

84 Musto (1987, pp. 230–231); Alexander (1990, Chapters 1 and 2). I have found no record that anyone was actually executed in the United States under this law.

85 Alexander (1990, pp. 8–15).

86 Alexander (1990, Chapters 1 and 2).

87 Alexander (1990, Chapter 1).

88 Sysenko (1982, as cited in Orford, 2001a); Kort (1996, pp. 80, 285–286).

89 Marx and Engels (1848/1948, esp. pp. 39–42).

90 Marx and Engels (1848/1948, p. 12).

91 Marx (1869/1978, pp. 416–417, 503 including footnote).

92 O'Meara (2004, p. 6).

93 Engels (1891/1966).

94 Cited in Lenin (1918/1970, p. 40).

95 Thanks to Gabor Maté, whose knowledge of the Marxist literature is far more complete than mine, for this insight.

96 Lenin (1916/1966, pp. 154–155, 1918/1970, pp. 36–40). See also L. Harris (2003).

97 Lenin (1918/1970, pp. 36–40). In these pages, Lenin, outlining orthodox Marxism, explains how the industrialized family will thrive under the dictatorship of the proletariat.

98 See Gray (1998, Chapter 6); Ginisty (1999).

99 Stalin (1952/1974, esp. Chapters 5 and 7).

100 Lewin (2001).

101 Lewin (2001, p. 9). The English statement in the text is my translation of a French text that appears to be a translation of a Russian text.

102 Klein (2007, pp. 286–287, 596).

103 Ramonet (2004b).

104 Gittings (2005, pp. 256–257).

105 Gittings (2005, p. 286).

106 Davis (2006b, pp. 7, 11–12).

107 Gittings (2005, pp. 276–280). Between 1949 and 1990, there was relatively little unemployment in China. Even though many workers in state-owned industries and poor rural farms were badly paid, they were able to subsist and their lives were stable.

108 Ramonet (2006b).

109 Fu (2003); G. York (2003b); Célérier (2004).

110 Jiménez (2004).

111 Stiglitz (2002, Chapter 7).

112 Grimmer (2006); G. York (2006).

113 Weil (1996).

114 Cernetig (1999); Lew (2000); Mangin (2000); Rochon (2003); G. York (2004b); Attané (2006).

115 Weil (1996, pp. 69–70); Zhou (2000); McCoy *et al.* (2001); G. York (2003a); *Time* (2003); Xinhua News Agency (2003); Lim (2004); Gittings (2005, Chapter 13); G. York (2005a, b); Yamane (2007).

116 S. G. Sullivan and Wu (2007).

117 Undated Chinese government publication entitled 'White Paper on Narcotic Control'. Retrieved 8 April 2007, from http://english.people.com.cn/features/drugpaper/drugc.html.

118 Chu (2000).

119 S. G. Sullivan and Wu (2007).

120 A further prediction: the current attempt to adapt Maoist style methods of social control to a free-market society (G. York, 2005c) will also fail.

Chapter 7

Addiction is a Way of Adapting to Dislocation: Quantitative Research, Clinical Reports, and 'Spam'

The third principle of the dislocation theory is that people use addiction as a way of adapting to sustained dislocation. The previous chapter summarised some historical evidence supporting this hypothesis. The historical record shows that when dislocation increases sharply in a society, addiction also increases in that society, and vice versa.

The third principle, however, also leads to predictions about differences between individuals *within* a society. For example, it predicts that: (i) The individuals who are the most dislocated within any society, no matter what the cause, will be the most prone to addictions; (ii) Addicted individuals within any society will be using addiction as a functional way of adapting to their dislocation, either consciously or unconsciously; and (iii) Individuals should be able to overcome their addictions if their psychosocial integration is restored. These predictions from the dislocation theory can be evaluated with evidence from both quantitative social science research and clinical studies of individuals in treatment—the conventional sources of evidence in the addictions field. This evidence generally supports the three predictions above, and provides other kinds of support for the third principle of the dislocation theory as well.

This chapter is by no means limited to recent research. In many cases, the findings have been consistent over several decades, although they have usually been interpreted from the viewpoint of the conventional wisdom on addiction, rather than as support for the dislocation theory.[1]

Even though many predictions concerning individuals that are derived from the dislocation theory of addiction are testable in principle, evidence from social science and clinical research is far from conclusive by itself, for several reasons. First, since there has been no direct attempt to test dislocation theory, researchers have not developed quantitative measures of either an individual's dislocation or an individual's degree of addiction to the full range of possible habits and pursuits. The relevant research is generally based on assessment techniques designed for screening large numbers of people. These techniques are restricted to data that are easily attainable, such as information from official records or answers to simple questions in public surveys. Individual levels of dislocation and addiction are complex states that cannot be measured adequately in these simple ways. Although it is possible to assess dislocation and addiction in the clinical intimacy of psychotherapy and counselling sessions, clinical assessments are not hard data, even when dressed up in numbers. Furthermore, it is difficult for clinical researchers to prove *why* people become addicted or cling to their addictions. Human motives are always mixed and at least partly concealed, and, hence, endlessly arguable. Insightful clinicians may reach correct conclusions about people's motivations without being able to convince those who read their reports.

Another reason that social science and clinical research on this topic is inconclusive is that major portions of the variance in people's dislocation and addiction come from differences among societies, as the previous chapter has shown. This makes it difficult to test hypotheses about the residual variance between individuals within societies at a single point in history For example, it is difficult to determine the effect of dislocation produced by residential schooling of Canadian Indians by comparing those who went to residential schools with those who did not. Taking children from their families and educating them with alien ideas in a foreign language had the effect of fracturing families and entire communities, not only the particular children who were sent away to school.[2] For all these reasons, the social science and clinical research studies that support the dislocation theory of addiction are subject to conflicting interpretations and endless reanalysis. It is because of the inconclusiveness of this kind of research that this book is based primarily on historical evidence.

At its end, this chapter departs from the polite world of academic literature altogether, attempting to draw useful conclusions from farther afield, including the Internet and, at the very end, some of the 'spam' that greets me in such profusion whenever I turn on my computer. This sort of evidence is even more equivocal than quantitative social science and clinical research, but it is easier to collect.

Dislocated people are more likely to become addicted

If people become addicted as a way of adapting to dislocation, as the third principle of the dislocation theory maintains, then the most dislocated individuals in any society should be the most prone to addiction. People who have achieved and maintained psychosocial integration should not become addicted.[3]

Many studies demonstrate a correlation between dislocation and addiction.[4] The family backgrounds of people who have become addicted to alcohol or drugs are frequently marked by child abuse, incest, exclusion from mainstream society, debilitating poverty, parental delinquency, family breakdown, too much or too little parental control, failure of secure attachment in childhood, and overdependence of parents on offspring.[5] People who have drug problems, including addiction, are less likely to be part of an organised religion than those who do not.[6] For a single example among countless others, one American study found that 34% of alcoholic women had been victims of childhood incest, whereas 16% of non-alcoholic women reported having been victims of childhood incest.[7] The difference between the two samples is in the expected direction, since those who have become alcoholic are more likely to have been dislocated by their personal history of incest during childhood.

Obviously, this illustrative study is not encompassing enough to confirm the general prediction that people who are dislocated, no matter what the cause, are the most likely to become addicted, over the whole range of addiction$_3$. However, hundreds of studies with results of this sort do provide support for the prediction.[8]

Whereas no one indication of dislocation is by itself a powerful predictor of later addiction, people who have been exposed to several of them are much more likely to become addicted subsequently than those who have been exposed to none or only a few.[9] For example, in a recent retrospective study, 8,667 medical patients were asked to describe their childhoods on an 'adverse childhood experiences' scale of ten items. The items included emotional abuse, physical abuse, sexual abuse, mental illness in the family, loss of a parent, etc. Each of the ten items could reasonably be taken as an impediment to the psychosocial integration of the patients who had experienced them during their childhood. The patients were also asked to state whether they had ever been addicted to a street drug. Less than 1% of those who reported no adverse childhood experiences reported ever having been addicted. The more of these ten adverse childhood experiences the patients reported, the higher the percentage of reports of street-drug addiction. More than 9% of those who reported five or more of the adverse childhood experiences had been addicted.[10] This same research group found a similar relationship between these same risk factors (as they are often called) and self-reported adult alcoholism, smoking, injection drug use, and obesity.[11]

In addition to indications of dislocation in the life circumstances of people who later become addicted, there are frequently visible indications of dislocation in their individual temperaments. Visible temperamental problems that are likely to precede addiction include depression, hyperactivity, chronic pain that interferes with normal life activities, a reduced attention span, heightened emotionality, alienation, personal insecurity, anxiety, conflict with parents, a sense of meaninglessness, and a perceived loss of control.[12] A different line of research reveals that a variety of minor biological abnormalities and certain 'endophenotypes' are correlated with the occurrence of alcoholism. These include low platelet monoamine oxidase levels, hormonal abnormalities, tremor, and electrophysiological 'disinhibition'.[13] Even left-handedness and a family history of left-handedness appear to correlate with the severity of alcoholism.[14] The fact that such an extraordinary diversity of minor problems correlates with later addiction fits the dislocation theory, if it is assumed that almost any deficit, even one as minor as left-handedness, decreases the prospects of complete psychosocial integration.

Studies of Latin American immigrants to the United States shed a different kind of light on the relationship between dislocation and addiction. If it can be presumed that Latin Americans who migrate to California are generally moving from Third-World regions of relatively high psychosocial integration into the very heartland of affluent dislocation in the modern world, the third principle of the dislocation theory would predict that individuals who make this move would be more likely to become addicted than individuals who do not. This is generally true, although a great variety of diverse explanations have been advanced to explain why.[15]

A 1998 study of Mexican immigrants to California compared the prevalence of a series of mental disorders in large populations arranged along a scale according to their degree of absorption into the United States way of life. The study compared the following five populations: Mexican people currently living in Mexico city; Mexican immigrants to the United States who had lived in Fresno County, California, for less than 13 years; Mexican immigrants who had lived in Fresno County for more than 13 years; Mexican-Americans born in the United States who lived in Fresno County; and the general population of the United States.

Generally speaking, the further along this scale towards absorption into the United States mainstream, the higher the average educational attainments and incomes *and* the higher the frequency of substance abuse, substance dependence, alcohol abuse, and alcohol dependence.[16] Mexican immigrants who had lived in Fresno County, California, for less than 13 years had relatively low mean prevalences of these four addiction-related types of problematic drug use, similar to the prevalences found in Mexicans in Mexico City. Mexican immigrants who had lived in Fresno County for more than 13 years had levels of problematic drug use that were intermediate between the first group and Mexican-Americans born in the United States. Mexican-Americans born in the United States had rates of problematic drug use similar to those of the general American population. These rates were nearly three times as high as the rates of the Mexican-American immigrants in the first group.[17]

This and other studies of immigrants to California support the conclusion that dislocation, more than poverty, is the precursor of addiction. On the other hand, the results can be interpreted in other ways. For example, it could be supposed that simply increasing people's wealth increases the likelihood that they will be able to afford drug addiction, although this seems unlikely, since rich people are generally less likely to be addicted to drugs than poor people. Moreover, along with higher levels of drug problems, Mexicans who were absorbed into American society also had a higher prevalence of mental disorders that are independent of personal wealth (e.g. depression, anxiety disorders, and antisocial personalities).[18] Another alternative explanation attributes the problematic drug use of Latinos born in the United States simply to the disruption of families that move from any culture to any other. This explanation would imply that the children of families moving to *more* psychosocially integrated cultures would become more vulnerable to addiction as their parents became more absorbed into the local culture. The dislocation theory would predict the opposite.

Relapses to addiction following treatment frequently occur in situations that suggest a breakdown of psychosocial integration. Interviews with patients who relapsed following treatment for alcoholism, smoking, heroin addiction, compulsive gambling, or overeating revealed that the majority of relapses occurred during 'negative emotional states'. Relatively few relapses of drug users could be associated with simple withdrawal symptoms or spontaneous craving for drugs.[19]

A comprehensive book by Jim Orford[20] has reviewed a large number of studies, many of which showed that people who become addicted are likely to have been dislocated beforehand. The more recent studies that Orford reviewed were not limited to alcohol and drug users. Problematic users of food and gambling (many of whom are likely to be addicted₃) are consistently more likely to report events in their lives that would naturally generate dislocation than are non-problematic users. Such experiences include childhood sexual and physical abuse, depression, low self-esteem, and serious problems in their family of origin. Childhood abuse is consistently reported as one of the strongest predictors of adult addiction.

One clearly measurable aspect of dislocation is unemployment. It is certainly the case that some people who lose their jobs sink into alcoholism and other kinds of addiction. For example, case studies of workers conducted 3 years after a 'plant closing' in a rural area of the United States provide clear evidence that unemployment can increase heavy smoking and alcoholism, as well as a variety of other personal problems. Because the abrupt closing of the factory resulted in all of the workers being out of work, it is clear in this instance that unemployment led to addiction, rather than the other way around. As this research was a collection of case studies, it provided no count of the total number of workers who responded to their abrupt dismissal in an addictive manner.[21]

Unfortunately, most studies of the relationship between unemployment and addiction are not completely clear. In most situations, unemployment may be a result of alcoholism and other forms of addiction as well as a cause. Often, the loss of an onerous job, while producing financial crisis, leads to an *increase* in psychosocial integration, as people become active in other types of social groups; for example, cooperative or political protest groups. The dislocation theory would predict that dislocation produced by unemployment might instigate any kind of addiction whatsoever. However, most of the research studies focus their attention on alcoholism or just on the amount of alcohol consumed, whether the consumption actually constitutes an addiction or not. Although quantitative studies in this area tend to show an association between sustained unemployment and heavy drinking, the effects are often small, and there are studies that do not find the expected relationship at all. Orford's thoughtful analysis of studies relating unemployment and heavy drinking[22] points out the many complicating factors in such research and suggests that no clear conclusion can be reached because of the inconsistent findings of the existing research.

At a more cognitive level of investigation, self-reports of a state of mind that would seem to reflect dislocation correlate with the occurrence of addiction. A 'Purpose in Life Scale'[23] has been developed to measure the extent to which people experience their life as meaningful. If it can be assumed that dislocation is the antithesis to purpose or meaning in life, then scores on this scale should correlate negatively with addiction. A dozen quantitative comparisons have shown that addicted people score lower on the Purpose in Life Scale than non-addicted people.[24]

Jan Blomqvist has pointed out that, despite the correlation between dislocation in early family life and later addiction in his Swedish longitudinal data, there were also many addicts whose early lives appear to have been normal and happy.[25] This finding is concordant with the dislocation theory, which does not assume that dislocation necessarily begins either early in life or within the addict's family of origin. Often, for example, rejection by peers and teachers in adolescence can be as powerfully dislocating as childhood events that occurred within a nuclear family.

Finally, the view that dislocation is a pre-condition of addiction and of other personal tragedies is stated explicitly in the modern public health and 'primary prevention' literature. Cassell has stated this view succinctly:

> A remarkably similar set of social circumstances characterises people who develop tuberculosis and schizophrenia, become alcoholic, are victims of multiple accidents, or commit suicide. They are individuals who for a variety of reasons ... have been deprived of meaningful social contact.[26]

It is important to remember at this point that the third principle of the dislocation theory does not predict a connection between dislocation and drug use, but between dislocation and addiction₃. Some support for this prediction can be drawn from the 2007 report of the UK Drug Policy Commission, which reached the conclusion that adults who suffer from 'social exclusion' are no more likely to use drugs than other people, but are more likely to be drug dependent.[27]

People use their addictions to adapt to dislocation

Many clinical-interview studies confirm that addicted individuals within any society use addiction as a functional way of adapting to their dislocation. For example, Chein and colleagues, in a classic psychological study of adolescent heroin addicts in New York City, reported:

> The adolescent addict has a weakened sense of, and a deep-lying disturbance inhibiting the acquisition of, personal identity. Perhaps this is why the almost exclusive identification—'I am a junkie'—is so supportive. It is often observed that an exclusive, affect-laden, predominant group identity can conceal or substitute for a weak sense of personal identity ... [28]

The fact that Chein et al.[29] also described other adaptive functions of heroin addiction that are not so easily connected to dislocation does not constitute evidence against the dislocation theory of addiction. The dislocation theory does not maintain that addiction *only* serves as an adaptation to dislocation. Indeed, it would be an extraordinary lifestyle that served only one function. The dislocation theory maintains that adaptation to dislocation is the *raison d'être* for addiction, not that addiction cannot serve other adaptive functions as well.

Other reports describe many additional ways in which addiction can help people cope with dislocation. Addiction can function to provide an 'illusion of potency and social recognition',[30] to produce a feeling of 'community and acceptance... when with other users',[31] to solve many of the 'dilemma's of modernity',[32] to 'handle existential agony',[33] to control aggressive impulses,[34] to provide a substitute 'career' where legitimate opportunities are few,[35] to gain power over others,[36] to buffer dislocation from local culture and from nature that has been caused by exploding technology,[37] to prevent neurotic disintegration of the ego,[38] to divert attention from interpersonal problems that threaten to split up a precarious family,[39] to cope with loneliness,[40] to alleviate crippling personal insecurity,[41] to energise people who are chronically depressed,[42] to control intolerable self-hate, shame, and guilt,[43] to fill a perceived spiritual vacuum,[44] to masquerade 'as a zest for living',[45] to regain an intensity of feeling that has been repressed as a consequence of childhood abuse or humiliation,[46] to gain a purpose in life,[47] to provide 'a passage into a respected identity',[48] or to reduce the pain that results from the instinctual repressions necessitated by modern civilisation.[49] Although most of the adaptive functions of addiction cited above are drawn from studies of drug addicts, a few are from studies of addictions that do not involve drugs.[50]

In my role as a psychologist,[51] I have listened to people explain the adaptive functions of their own addictions on countless occasions. They have explained how addictions help them cope with the lack of a sense of belonging or meaning in life and the pain of repeatedly hurting those whom they love. Their stories have taught me much about the inadequacy of addictive lifestyles to fill the void of dislocation, even in cases where their addiction was approved by their society; for example, in instances of addiction to overwork, scholastic achievement, or personal beauty.

On a few occasions, addicted individuals have sought out my help as a researcher. These people were not seeking to improve their lives so much as to unravel the impenetrable mystery of why they had chosen to live in an addictive and self-destructive way when other alternatives were possible. The most recent person was an injecting drug addict in Vancouver's Hastings Corridor with a terminal case of AIDS. A man of about 50, he was from an upper middle-class family and had not been abused in any way prior to becoming a life-long drug addict in his late teenage years. As his AIDS symptoms worsened and the end of his life approached, he desperately wanted to understand why he had thrown his opportunity for happiness and privilege away, and why he was living as a junkie to the very end, when he could easily return to his family's home at any time.

At the end of a series of about ten meetings, interspersed with periods of reflection and recollection on his part, he and I were both satisfied that he had found the explanation that he was seeking. He had come to understand his drug addiction on two levels: first, as an adaptation to the social fragmentation caused by continual travel during his childhood as his father acquired prestige and wealth as a well-known European clergyman and philanthropist; secondly, as an adaptation to the impossibly high set of family expectations that made it impossible for him to achieve a life that he could himself respect. He did not feel that his intelligence fell short of what was expected, but that his moral character did. Junkie life was his refuge from the suffering that he believed, rightly or wrongly, he would have to inflict on his 'saintly father' (this is his phrase) because of the moral shortcomings that he would have inevitably displayed to the world in the life he was expected to live.

It seemed both to him and to me at the end of our discussions that, although the mystery was solved, we had not found a cure for his addiction or even a reason for him to change his life. AIDS will kill him. All indications are that his will be an addict's death, for all his bridges to the kind of life that both he and his family wished for him have long since been burned. He could only be an object of pity and shame if he returned to his parents' home now. He has, however, found a place in the junkie community, where he is respected both as a clever thief and a good companion. Thanks to a local housing society, he has a stable place to live. His resolution of the mystery of his life gives him a visible sense of relief. He understands his own previously inexplicable decisions. He agreed that a summary of our discussions could be published.

Addiction is sometimes seen as a means of controlling any type of emotional and physical pain whatsoever, whether or not the pain originates in dislocation.[52] For example, it has been observed that cancer patients and others with uncontrollable pain often become obsessed with prescription narcotic drugs and appear addicted to others,[53] although there is no indication that they are severely dislocated. This observation is often taken to show that addiction is a form of self-medication, and this is sometimes formalised as a self-medication or a coping theory of addiction. Where the self-medication theory provides a good explanation for the drug consumption of medical patients, it does not explain the overwhelming involvement of addiction$_3$. People who are self-medicating insist on using certain drugs, even when there are obvious adverse side effects and when sometimes they are illegal. However, they quickly stop using them if the pain or other symptoms that they are medicating go into remission. They do not take up other addictions in their place. This crucial distinction was discussed at length in Chapter 2 under the heading *The Importance of Distinguishing Addiction$_2$ from Addiction$_3$*.

Psychosocial integration makes recovery from addiction possible

If addiction is a way of adapting to dislocation, individuals should be able to overcome their addictions if their psychosocial integration is restored. Although this prediction contradicts the still widely held views that addiction is an incurable disease or a disease that is curable only by expert treatment, it finds abundant support in social science and clinical research.

Full recovery from mild and severe addictions quite often occurs without any professional treatment whatsoever. This phenomenon is variously called 'natural recovery', 'spontaneous recovery', 'spontaneous remission', 'maturing out', and so forth. Natural recovery from addictions to food, love, gambling, compulsive shopping, and so forth hardly require formal documentation, since they are part of many people's experience. However, people believed for many decades that drug and alcohol addictions were somehow a different species, and natural recovery was impossible. Steadily accumulating documentation that natural recovery from drug addictions frequently occurs and that it follows the same course as recovery from non-drug addictions has finally overcome this erroneous belief.[54]

Natural recovery frequently entails either the adoption of a new way of living or a period of reorientation to a familiar, non-addictive lifestyle. This reorientation is usually aided by the addicted person's family or close friends and by the supportive institutions of their culture with little or no involvement of addiction professionals.[55] The essential role of family, friends, and society is evident even for people who attribute their recovery to a miraculous personal epiphany or to divine intervention.[56] People who recover from addiction find what Cloud and Granfield have called 'a renewed stake in conventional life and in their social relationships'[57] and a new identity to go with it.[58] Often, the identity shift is so dramatic that it can be likened to a religious conversion experience.[59]

Sometimes, natural recovery is instigated by 'hitting rock bottom', but it is more likely to be instigated by *positive* social events that open the door to renewed psychosocial integration.[60] Of course, some people have more access than others to the social, cultural, and personal supports that enable a non-addictive way of life to be built or rebuilt, and these people are more likely to recover from their addictions.

Within the broad category of natural recovery, there are, of course, a huge variety of individual recovery stories.[61] A study by Paris and Bradley[62] illustrates some diverse paths to natural recovery with the lives of three American women who, after their graduation from Mills College in the United States, had descended into alcoholism. The descriptions were based on interviews conducted approximately once each decade between the ages of 21 and 60 by a variety of interviewers. Paris and Bradley analysed these three histories of addiction within Erik Erikson's theoretical framework. Each woman's alcoholism was understood as a consequence of a failure of psychosocial integration that had its beginnings in a disturbed relationship with her parents. In each case, the woman described herself as using alcoholism to fill a void in social relationships and self-confidence. In each case, the woman's recovery entailed a re-establishment of psychosocial integration and a revitalised identity. For one woman, the new psychosocial integration and identity centred around the woman's 'family' in Alcoholics Anonymous (AA) and her profession; for the second, it centred around her work, her friends, and an appreciation of the arts; and for the third, it centred around her husband, her work, and her step-children.

Further support for the prediction that psychosocial integration makes recovery from addiction possible comes from research on the 'moral communities theory', which shows that post-treatment reductions in consumption of crack cocaine and alcohol are correlated with increased church attendance and increased participation in 12-step groups, but not with religious belief alone.[63] The relatively new 'Community Reinforcement Approach' to treatment for alcoholism and drug addiction is explicitly designed to help the client to establish new drug- and alcohol-free social contacts and to strengthen and improve the relationships between clients and their families and friends.[64] Therapists enlist the help of members of the clients' communities to help with the recovery project wherever possible. The Community Reinforcement Approach consistently outperforms most conventional types of treatment that are not directed at re-establishing psychosocial integration.[65]

If people completely recover from addiction without establishing or re-establishing psychosocial integration, the dislocation theory is wrong. In evaluating this possibility, it is important to remember that people often stop overtly engaging in an addictive habit, but remain fully addicted. Many members of AA and other 12-step groups recognise that they have not overcome their addictions, even though they have completely stopped using alcohol, drugs, or whatever. This is why many members of AA who have been 'in recovery' for long periods remain totally abstinent and eternally vigilant, and regularly use the famous AA introduction: 'My name is … and I am an alcoholic,' although they never drink. There is great wisdom in such a phrase for people who are still dislocated. However, there is no reason for people who have actually overcome addiction by re-establishing psychosocial integration to use this phrase, or to be total abstainers.

Addicted people are not 'out of control'

The third principle of the dislocation theory depicts addicted people as responding adaptively to their state of dislocation. If addicted people are behaving adaptively, they are not 'out of control', even though it is sometimes natural for others, and even for themselves, to perceive that they are. The conventional claim that addicts are out of control must, therefore, be examined critically.

Serious logical problems with the claim that addicted people are out of control were discussed in Chapter 3 under the heading *False dichotomy 2: 'Out of control' or 'acting of their own free will'*? In addition, several experimental studies have thrown serious doubt on this claim. When severe, chronic alcoholics were given unlimited access to alcohol in an experimental setting, they typically did not drink 'to oblivion'. One experimental study showed that alcoholics given free access to 32 ounces of liquor per day for 9 to 12 days maintained remarkably stable blood-alcohol levels. They accomplished this by varying their consumption of both alcohol and food and generally not consuming all of the alcohol available to them.[66] Other experimental studies have shown that alcoholics are able to moderate their drinking for many reasons; for example, to reduce the discomfort of anticipated withdrawal symptoms or to obtain small monetary rewards offered by experimenters.[67] Alcoholics in treatment who were allowed to drink for 2 days in the middle of their treatment regimen were able to stop drinking again when the period of allowable drinking ended, even though they were free to leave treatment and continue the binge.[68] If the language of 'control' is useful at all, the alcohol intake of alcoholics appears to be under the same kind of partial control as other types of human adaptive behaviour.

Adaptation is a 'lesser evil'

How can a lifestyle that, in extreme forms, is so obviously harmful to an addicted person and his or her society ever be called 'adaptive'? The answer to this perplexing question rests on a full understanding of the nature of adaptation. By the time people reach a state of severe dislocation, they have usually tried all the harmless roads to psychosocial integration they could find and have found them blocked, leaving only harmful substitutes to chose from. Under these circumstances, the only adaptive response is to choose the lesser evil—the least harmful lifestyle. This use of the term 'adaptive' is commonplace in modern behavioural theory outside the field of addiction. For example, George Vaillant, in his book *Adaptation to Life*, pointed out that a self-deceptive ego defence mechanism like 'denial' may help a person adapt to especially difficult circumstances by censoring thoughts that are too threatening, even though denying reality entails a harmful inflexibility.[69] In addition to their beneficial functions, other commonly used coping mechanisms have obviously detrimental side effects. These mechanisms include overeating, undereating, and Type A behaviour.[70] The dislocation theory adds addiction to this list of harmful ways of living that become adaptive when less-harmful solutions prove unworkable.

This view of adaptiveness is also compatible with evolutionary theory. A fox caught in a leg-hold trap might behave adaptively by gnawing off its own foot rather than dying of starvation in the trap. This behaviour would only appear maladaptive to an observer who does not discern the trap beneath the snow. Even addicted persons may not clearly see the hidden trap of dislocation that incapacitates them, and may only perceive a fatal attraction to a harmful lifestyle that is inexplicable even to them.

Even the fact that addiction sometimes has fatal consequences does not necessarily mean that it is maladaptive in general. A similar danger inheres in other adaptive responses to emergency situations. For example, the 'general adaptation syndrome'[71] is a complex of physiological responses that is adaptive because it protects the body from a variety of stressors. In cases where the stress persists for too long, however, the flow of hormones produced by the adaptive syndrome sometimes causes so-called 'diseases of adaptation' that can be fatal.[72]

This is not to imply that all self-destructive behaviour is adaptive. Evolutionary biologists might think of a self-destructive behaviour as 'maladaptive' if it were caused by a deleterious mutation or if it had evolved in a species under one set of conditions and then become dysfunctional when the species' environment changed. But such maladaptive traits would tend to be eliminated rapidly through natural selection in the new environment. Therefore, behavioural capacities that have been relatively common throughout long historical periods, such as addiction in human beings, would normally be considered adaptive by evolutionary biologists unless some reason to think differently was apparent.[73]

Hibernation is a familiar instance of a costly adaptive process. Hibernation protects animals from the harshness of winter or other environmental stringencies through a pre-programmed reduction in food intake and diminution of metabolic activities. This protective retardation of function comes at the cost of weakening the hibernating creatures, taxing their physiological systems to the limit, and making them vulnerable to predators. Yet hibernation and other lengthy types of 'animal anorexia' are recognised as adaptive in large numbers of vertebrate species.[74] According to the third principle of the dislocation theory, addiction, like hibernation, occurs when an individual cannot meet the demands of the environment and survives by adopting a diminished mode of functioning until the opportunity for more complete activity reappears.

Addictions are interchangeable

Another implication of the third principle of the dislocation theory is that the successful prohibition of one addiction is likely to result in a person switching to another addiction, unless the dislocation that was the precursor of the original addiction has been relieved. It is addiction itself that substitutes for psychosocial integration in addicted people, not any particular drug or other habit. My own experience with heroin addicts in Vancouver over the decades is that they respond to periodic short supplies of heroin in part by augmenting their drug consumption with alcohol, cocaine, or a variety of other drugs that are available to them. Research in the United States has shown that former patients whose methadone programme had been shut down for administrative reasons consumed much more alcohol and heroin than patients who continued to have access to legal methadone.[75] Naturally, addictions are not totally interchangeable, as each addicted person finds some addictive pursuits repellent or impossible.

A related implication of the third principle is that a person might respond to dislocation with several habits, forming them into a single addictive complex that provides a substitute for psychosocial integration, rather than a singular addiction. This scenario fits with the well-known fact that street addicts are more likely to use a large number of drugs with quite different effects, rather than to restrict their habit to a single drug, like heroin or cocaine.[76] Addictions among university students, which are quite often not addictions to drugs, tend to cluster in particular individuals. Generally, students who report addiction to one habit also report addictions to two or more others.[77] The concept of the 'addictive complex' was introduced in Chapter 2 and will be illustrated with a biographical study in Chapter 9.

Social worlds of addiction: real and imaginary

The third principle of the dislocation theory holds that addictions are adaptive specifically because they provide a partial substitute for the psychosocial integration that the addicted person lacks. Many, perhaps most, types of addiction actually provide a kind of community or subculture that entails some real psychosocial gratifications. Psychosocial benefits are readily visible in people who are addicted to drinking together at parties and clubs or people who gamble together. This section describes hidden psychosocial benefits of some addictions that might otherwise appear to be quite solitary.

Communities of drug addicts

The hackneyed image of junkies as loners who live only for their drugs is false. During decades of contact with injecting heroin addicts in Vancouver, I gradually came to perceive the importance of addiction-centred communities with norms, rituals, values, stable social relationships, and certain areas of mutual trust. These junkie groups afford addicted people some sense of belonging, for they are truly members of a society of outcasts from mainstream culture. Historian Catherine Carstairs[78] has described the devotion of an earlier generation of Vancouver heroin addicts to their junkie subculture in the years 1945–1961. In addition to actual community membership, there is a junkie mystique that provides junkies with a kind of imaginary membership in a company of fearless rebels. The function of the junkie mystique as an identity will be described at some length in Chapter 8. It is not only addicts to heroin who form communities. Philippe Bourgois[79] provided a detailed look at a close-knit, though sometimes violent, society of crack cocaine users and dealers in New York City.

The psychosocial function of heroin addiction helps to explain a fact that defies explanation within the conventional wisdom. When heroin is in short supply, dealers 'cut' their product with inert white powders, sometimes to the extent that the pharmacological potency of the 'heroin' sold on the street becomes negligible for extended periods of time. The adulterated drugs are not strong enough either to produce significant euphoria or withdrawal symptoms. When this happens, many heroin addicts continue to buy almost as much 'heroin' as before, although they are well aware that it has little or no effect. They usually supplement it by heavy drinking or using other street drugs.[80] This suggests that the primary motivation for heroin addiction—like other kinds of addiction—is psychosocial, whether or not the addicts are conscious of this fact. The drug loses its pharmacological effects at low doses, and laboratory animals that are being reinforced with heroin quickly cease pressing the levers in their Skinner boxes when the doses are cut. However, for many human heroin addicts, the primary function of 'pressing the lever' is undiminished, because using heroin is the badge of membership in the junkie subculture. Likewise, the junkie mystique continues to serve its adaptive function whether or not there is any heroin in the white powder that is injected.

There is another fact that is hard to explain if it is believed that drug addicts live only for their drugs. A 1959 study[81] showed that only half of prison volunteers who were considered 'incurable heroin addicts' wanted to repeat injections of heroin given to them in the prison hospital under double-blind conditions. The drug was unappealing to them outside of the junkie culture.

The appeal of junkie subculture seems further confirmed by the way heroin addicts speak. It is quite common for street addicts in Vancouver and other places to describe themselves with what ought to be embarrassing epithets like 'junkie', 'hype', and even the otherwise archaic phrase 'dope fiend'.[82] They apply these labels to themselves without visible shame or regret but, rather, like personal logos that signify their toughness and tragic depth of character. They heap disdain upon heroin users who think they are junkies but are really not, who they call 'joy poppers', 'skin poppers', 'chippers', or 'pseudo junkies'.[83]

Society can deliberately undermine the appeal of the junkie subculture. When it does, there are fewer heroin addicts. In 1991, the city of Zurich, Switzerland, adopted a policy of freely providing methadone and buprenorphine[84] under deliberately sterile and institutional conditions to anyone who was a regular heroin user.[85] Heroin too was sometimes dispensed, but also under conditions that were equally sterile and institutional.[86] In effect, 'this medicalisation of opiate dependence changed the image of heroin use as a rebellious act to an illness that needs therapy. Finally, heroin appears to have become a "loser drug" with its attractiveness fading for young people.'[87] Crime and overdose deaths linked with heroin use have fallen in Zurich, and the number of heroin users has declined sharply and steadily since 1991.[88]

Many non-addicted users of heroin who have not fallen into addiction even after many years of regular or even daily use avoid communities of addicts. These non-addicted heroin users are mindful that excessive heroin use would cause serious problems to other aspects of their lives. Authors of a recent study of non-addicted heroin users observed that 'rejection of the "junkie" identity played an important role, albeit subconsciously in many cases, in maintaining their control over heroin use'.[89] They avoided becoming addicted to heroin by rejecting the junkie identity and subculture rather than by rejecting heroin use!

There are also drug-centred communities that are not communities of addicts. Recent quantitative studies have provided counts of the number and types of drug-using societies in different cities.[90] I have personally observed two quite independent subcultures of marijuana users in Vancouver that include only a few people who can reasonably be considered addicted to marijuana and a large number of other marijuana users who are definitely not addicted. There is also a worldwide 'rave' culture, with a distinctive set of rituals and a special language, some members of which are addicted to crystal methamphetamine or to polydrug use, although many others are not.[91] In these cases, membership in the community is not necessarily defined by addiction but by the use of a particular exotic drug.

Co-dependence

The family therapy literature affords evidence of a different kind of social system that can serve heroin addicts as a substitute for genuine psychosocial integration. A surprisingly large number of heroin addicts, possibly a majority, play the role of an errant child in their family of origin for many years, long after their non-addicted brothers and sisters have become independent adults. These enduring, if dysfunctional, social relationships are in part based on addiction, with the addict adopting the role of the endangered child and the parents playing the heroic role of the rescuing, all-giving protectors.[92] In such cases, both the heroin users and their parents receive the social benefit of membership in an intense, if dysfunctional, family relationship.

There is an extensive literature on the phenomenon of 'co-dependency', or the supportive relationship between addicts of all sorts and other family members. Such relationships are usually analysed with the aim of discouraging non-addicted family members from 'enabling' the continuing addiction, and there are co-dependency support groups, which function with the aim of keeping co-dependent family members from falling back into enabling. In the context of this chapter, however, the difficulty of weaning both addicts and non-addicted family members from such relationships is more important as evidence that social relationships are a major part of the pay-off of addiction.

Imaginary or virtual communities

Substitute communities provided by addiction need not be composed of real people. In fact, substitute communities often seem at least partly imaginary or 'virtual'. For example, participation in religious cults, which grows to addictive proportions in some participants, often involves interacting with 'spirits' who do not actually exist for any but the members of the cult. Of course, cults generally involve face-to-face interactions between people as well, so the substitute community in the case of addictive religiosity is only partly imaginary. More extreme cases in which the community that substitutes for psychosocial integration is *predominately* imaginary include addiction to video games, pornography, and, possibly, anorexia.

The alarming spread of addiction to video games was discussed in Chapter 3. The video and Internet role-playing games that I have observed in action, under the expert guidance of my youngest son—who plays but is not addicted to them—engage their players in a primordial world of unrestrained individual competition usually set either in the future or in the middle ages. The competition frequently entails fighting to the death, but also involves buying and selling weapons and other paraphernalia in the many markets of these fantasy worlds between mortal combats. Although this virtual world simulates the dog-eat-dog individualism of free-market society, the games are constructed so that players cannot feel dislocated. For example, impossibly voluptuous maidens and their allies frequently pop out of nowhere requesting help and suggesting missions. Richly ornamented symbols of magic and virtue imbue the endless combat with a powerful, but completely abstract, sense of meaning. In the virtual world of these role-playing games, players can put all of their energies into individual competition and expect that psychosocial integration will follow, gratuitously.

The producers of such games for teenagers and adults are offering dislocated people an opportunity for overwhelming involvement with a computer-enhanced fantasy life that is more appealing than real life. In virtual life, gamers are never isolated. They interact with other characters (or 'avatars') generated by a computer program and with characters that are controlled by other gamers who are participating at the same time. Interactions may be combative, commercial, friendly, or even vaguely sexual. Hundreds of thousands of players 'are not just consumers of game content; they are developers, community members, entrepreneurs'.[93] However, the dangers that accompany human interaction in the real world are largely eliminated by the avatars taking all of the risks. Real names are proscribed. As killing is a primary pastime,[94] there is a constant risk of death, but death in these fantasy worlds is only a brief time-out. Within seconds, the avatar is reincarnated and life resumes as before. Characters may be seriously embarrassed at times in the eyes of other human players, but it is simple for the humiliated player to completely abandon his temporary avatar identity and assume a different one at any point.

Video simulation games do not end. They do not offer the gamer a delimited contest, but an alternative to life. This appears to make these games ideally suited for the addiction of children and adults. It is impossible to make an accurate guess about the prevalence of serious addiction to video games, but there are innumerable anecdotal reports and first-hand accounts. Self-help websites dedicated to gaming addiction, like Gamers Anonymous, and others dedicated to addictions to a particular game, like EverQuest Widows, claim thousands of subscribers.[95] The word 'addicting' frequently appears in advertising for video games, not as a warning but as an attraction. My expert guide informs me that the biggest and best source of free video games for teenagers is a website called www.addictinggames.com.

Yet even games centred on virtual reality can offer some real social interaction. Flesh-and-blood friends discuss each other's achievements in virtual worlds, and can plan encounters of their avatars there, acting as allies. Players can visit innumerable chat rooms where they can discuss their games with people who, although invisible, are still acting as human beings rather than avatars. The discussions of these chat rooms seem vacuous to me, but no more vacuous than discussions between strangers about imaginary things would normally be.

A challenge to the idea that addiction provides a social benefit arises in connection with addiction to pornography and masturbation, which would at first appear to be entirely solitary.[96] Although I have not researched this form of addiction in the academic literature, the merchants of Internet pornography have thoughtfully deluged my e-mail inbox with relevant data in the form of pornographic 'spam' for several years. (Recently, the daily serving of spam has shifted its contents more towards obscene wealth to be obtained from underrated stocks and from several Nigerian benefactors who are dying to send me their millions for safe keeping.[97])

In the pornography spam, I found at least two kinds of invitation to *psychosocial* intercourse that arrived with the visual representations of sexual intercourse. In the first kind, the advertising text appeared to be written by a very young girl who revealed her coy hopes that the pictures or videos that she had crafted with her equally coy and gymnastic girlfriend would please me and make me excited. The page that followed asked for my credit card number, and if that detail was taken care of, I was assured that things were going to get better and better between us in ways that I could not imagine.

The second kind of psychosocial invitation arrived in the voice of a lascivious pornography merchant rather than that of a coy maiden. The merchant frequently encouraged a comradely disdain for the 'tramps' or 'sluts' that were to be viewed once the credit card number was entered. He expressed a keen enthusiasm for viewing and masturbating that he leeringly shared with me. Advanced practitioners of these arts make their own pornography and exchange it with each other over the Internet.

Thus, addictive Internet pornography viewing and masturbation can evoke at least two alternative imaginary communities. One community comprises the viewer and imaginary girls who love to be viewed as they disport themselves, and will probably come coyly knocking on his door, once the credit card detail is out of the way. The second imaginary community comprises the viewer and fellow voyeurs who foster their macho camaraderie by mocking the imaginary unquenchable lust of women for penetration by everybody in every conceivable position.

The Internet has an enormous capacity to enhance the illusion of interactivity at low cost to the merchant, and thus can provide highly profitable mass substitutes for psychosocial integration. Therefore, it can serve an addictive function very well. Perhaps this is the reason that Internet pornography has been so much more addictive than books or magazines of the sort that little boys guiltily passed from hand to hand in earlier generations.

In the case of anorexia, there are at least 20 so-called 'pro-ana' websites that offer an online sense of community to young women who are anorexic and intend to remain so. These websites are not designed to overcome anorexia, but to encourage young women to maintain their self-imposed semi-starvation. They offer 'thinspiration' through a sense of membership in a sort of spiritual sorority and painful pictures of emaciated role models.[98] This is not to say that anorexia, which is often understood as a form of addiction to starvation, is entirely motivated by the virtual communities provided on the web, but only that a virtual community can be part of the substitute gratification that addiction provides.

In general, free-market society seems to be generating ever-more-effective substitutes for psychosocial integration to fill the needs of the people that it dislocates. These newer substitutes may soon replace drugs as the most important objects of addiction.

Conclusion

This chapter and the previous one summarised evidence from historical, social science, and clinical research supporting the principle that addiction is a way of adapting to sustained dislocation that provides a substitute sense of community. One more line of evidence must be considered to complete the argument for this principle. This final line of evidence has a more ghostly quality than the first two.

Endnotes

1 See Granfield and Cloud (1999, Chapter 1); Felitti (2003).

2 This methodological problem has been discussed in the particular case of residential schools by Chrisjohn and Young (1997) and in more general terms by Gmel et al. (2004).

3 If, as the dislocation theory claims, addiction only occurs as an adaptation to severe dislocation (see Chapter 3), there should be not one single addicted individual who was not severely dislocated beforehand. This stronger prediction cannot be tested with the kind of evidence that is presently available.

4 Most of these studies are more concerned with addiction$_2$ or simply drug and alcohol use, rather than addiction$_3$. I have chosen studies and reviews for discussion here in which the dependent measure is defined in such a way that high scores are likely to include a reasonable number of addicted$_3$ people, but this is speculation.

5 Chein et al. (1964); Braucht et al.(1973); Alexander and Dibb (1975); Helzer et al. (1976); Wurmser (1978); Yeary (1982); Browne and Finkelhor (1986); Cook (1991); D. L. Hurley (1991); Siegrist (2000); and Bradley (2001); S.R. Friedman (2002); von Sydow et al. (2002); Blomqvist (2004); Reuter and Stevens (2007, p. 33).

6 This literature is reviewed by W. R. Miller (1998, pp. 981–983).

7 Covington (1982).

8 See the collection of studies reviewed by Orford (2001a).

9 Bry et al. (1982); Timmer et al. (1985); Tucker (1985); Newcomb et al. (1986); Dube et al.(2002, 2003); Felitti (2003).

10 Dube et al. (2003).

11 Dube et al. (2002); Felitti (2003).

12 Peele and Brodsky (1975); Kielholz and Ladewig (1977); Tarter et al. (1985); Newcomb and Harlow (1986); Deyken et al. (1987); Peele (1987); Tarter and Edwards (1987); D. Hurley (1991), Rosenblum et al. (2003).

13 Tarter and Edwards (1987); Nernberger and Bierut (2007).

14 London (1986).

15 Vega et al. (1998, 2003).

16 These researchers used the definitions in the DSM-III-R, which do not differ from those in the DSM-IV in any way that is important here. The DSM-IV is discussed in Chapter 2 of this book under the heading Addiction$_2$.

17 Vega et al. (1998).

18 Vega et al. (1998, Table 4).

19 Marlatt (1985b, c).

20 Orford (2001a).

21 Strange (1977).

22 Orford (2001a, pp. 191–192).

23 Crumbaugh and Maholick (1964, as cited in W. R. Miller, 1998).

24 Black (1991, as cited in W. R. Miller, 1998).

25 Blomqvist (2004).

26 Quoted in Albee (1986, p. 893).

27 Reuter and Stevens (2007, p. 33).

28 Chein *et al.* (1964, p. 216).

29 Chein *et al.* (1964, especially Chapter 9).

30 Quote from Dewey (1922, p. 148). See also Davidson (1964) and Blomqvist (2004, pp. 147–148).

31 Granfield and Cloud (1999, p. 46).

32 Svensson (1996).

33 Giddens (1994). See also Dalrymple (2006a, pp. 104–106).

34 Khantzian (1974).

35 Coombs (1981).

36 Adler (1934/1954).

37 Glendinning (1994, Chapter 7).

38 Wurmser (1978).

39 Alexander and Dibb (1975).

40 Working in a pastoral rather than a clinical context, Jean Vanier (1998), the founder of l'Arche, a Christian organisation that provides long-term care for intellectually disabled people, reached the conclusion that 'loneliness', which he understands in much the same sense as the term 'dislocation' is used in this book, is a root cause of addiction. Vanier (1998, p. 8) wrote: '[Loneliness] can be a source of apathy and depression, and even of a desire to die. It can push us into escapes and addictions in the need to forget our inner pain and emptiness.'

41 Peele and Brodsky (1975).

42 Khantzian and Khantzian (1984); Zinberg (1984, p. 76).

43 McFadden (1987); Cook (1991).

44 Woodman (1982).

45 Chein *et al.* (1964, pp. 245–246).

46 A. Miller (1981).

47 Dalrymple (2006a, p. 108).

48 Granfield and Cloud (1999, p. 46).

49 Freud (1929).

50 Peele and Brodsky (1975); Glendinning (1994).

51 I am not currently a practising clinician or counsellor. However, people often approach me as a psychologist wanting to talk about addictive problems. I do not try to change or cure them, but listen to their stories at length, often over several meetings. Although I think of this as research rather than treatment, people sometimes find it helpful.

52 Khantzian and Khantzian (1984); Hadaway *et al.* (1986).

53 Tuttle (1985, p. 122).

54 Winick (1962); Robins and Murphy (1967); Pattison *et al.* (1977, Chapter 6); Zinberg *et al.* (1978); J. S. Blackwell (1982); S. Schachter (1982); Vaillant (1983); Alexander and Schweighofer (1988); Biernacki (1986); Granfield and Cloud (1999); Klingemann *et al.* (2001); Blomqvist (2004); Cloud and Granfield (2004); Öjesjö (2004); Warburton *et al.* (2005); Dalrymple (2006a, pp. 38–39).

55 Cameron *et al.* (2002); Blomqvist (2004, pp. 151–153); Cloud and Granfield (2004).

56 Granfield and Cloud (1999, Chapter 5, esp. p. 149).

57 Quote from Cloud and Granfield (2004, p. 200); see also W. R. Miller (2004).

58 Biernacki (1986); Koski-Jännes (1998); Granfield and Cloud (1999, pp. 63–68, 73); Cameron (2004); Hänninen and Koski-Jännes (2004); Hecksher (2004); Warburton *et al.* (2005).

59 Granfield and Cloud (1999, pp. 63–68, 73).

60 Granfield and Cloud (1999); Blomqvist (2004, pp. 151–152); Öjesjö (2004).

61 Recovery stories have been classified into types by Blomqvist (2004, pp. 153–155). All of these types seem to me concordant with the dislocation theory of addiction.

62 Paris and Bradley (2001).

63 Richard, Bell, and Carlson (2000).

64 The theoretical basis for the Community Reinforcement Approach is entirely different from the dislocation theory of addiction, however. It derives from Skinnerian behaviourism and Cognitive Behaviour Therapy.

65 W. R. Miller and Meyers (1999); J. E. Smith *et al.* (2001).

66 Mello and Mendelson (1971).

67 Mello and Mendelson (1972); Fingarette (1988).

68 Pattison *et al.*(1977, Chapter 5).

69 Vaillant (1977).

70 Roskies and Lazarus (1980).

71 Selye (1946).

72 The demonstration that the general adaptation syndrome itself can cause severe disease if it continues long enough was part of the theory of stress propounded by Hans Selye (1946). Since that time, the ideas of 'stress' and 'diseases of adaptation' have become enmeshed in a confused philosophical debate in which Hans Selye himself was an active participant (G. Weissmann, 2007). These terms have no generally accepted meaning today.

73 Darwin (1871/1981, p. 381); Symons (1979, p. 46); W. J. Bock (1980); Mayr (1982, p. 132).

74 Mrosovsky and Sherry (1980).

75 McGlothlin and Anglin (1981).

76 Tarter and Edwards (1987, p. 75).

77 Cook (1987); Alexander and Schweighofer (1988).

78 Carstairs (2006, pp. 75–76, 90).

79 Bourgois (1997).

80 Lindesmith (1968, pp. 38–39); Primm and Bath (1973); DeGrandpre (2006, Chapters 4 and 7). I have observed this myself in Vancouver.

81 Beecher (1959, pp. 330–341).

82 Lindesmith (1968, p. 63).

83 I learned the first three of these terms from discussions with junkies. The fourth comes from an academic study entitled *The Pseudo Junkie: Evolution of the Heroin Lifestyle in the Non-Addicted Individual* (Gay *et al.*, 1974). Hammersley and Reid (2002, p. 23) mentioned the scornful label 'giro junkie', which appears to have the same meaning in the UK junkie world.

84 Methadone and buprenorphine have very similar effects to heroin, as will be explained in Chapter 8.

85 Nordt and Stohler (2006).

86 M. Hickman *et al.* (2006); Laurance (2006).

87 Nordt and Stohler (2006, p. 1834).

88 Nordt and Stohler (2006).

89 Warburton *et al.* (2005, p. 29).

90 Orford (2001a, pp. 188–190).

91 Placonouris (1998). See also Shewan *et al.* (2000) who did not analyse their ecstasy-using population specifically as a subculture, although their transcribed interviews suggested the existence of one.

92 Alexander and Dibb (1975); M. D. Stanton *et al.* (1982).

93 Tapscott and Williams (2006, p. B2).

94 In some games, the player never sheathes his or her sword, although the game may go on indefinitely. There is always someone new to fight to the death.

95 See endnotes 71 and 79 in Chapter 2.

96 Valpy (2004a). Another kind of addiction that seems to be solitary is online gambling. Some indication that it is not as solitary as it seems comes from Robbeson (2004).

97 My spammers also seem to be concentrating more on vending prescription medication.

98 Norris *et al.* (2006); Shimo (2006).

Chapter 8

Addiction is a Way of Adapting to Dislocation: The Myth of the Demon Drugs

Although most medieval superstitions have died out, the myth of demon possession was revitalised in the 19th century in a new, pharmacological form.[1] As that century progressed, more and more people came to believe that anyone who drank distilled liquor fell permanently under its control, a helpless slave to drink, possessed by 'demon rum'. Unless drunkards were saved by Christian conversion, they remained under the control of booze forever after, until the story ended with their ghastly deaths.

If this myth were true, the third principle of the dislocation theory of addiction would be false because alcoholism would inexorably afflict all people who had exposed themselves to alcohol, including the most psychosocially integrated. Addiction would be a reflexive reaction to an addictive drug, rather than a way of adapting to dislocation. However, the belief that mere exposure to alcohol causes alcoholism was a wholly unsubstantiated myth.

The myth was preached from pulpits and printed in tracts in its full-strength, hellfire-and-damnation form. A representative snippet of this long-winded rhetoric from an 1847 temperance tract reads:

> A father took a little child by his legs and dashed his head against the house, and then, with a bootjack, beat out his brains. Once that man was a respectable merchant, in good standing, but he drank alcohol.[2]

Outside of religious contexts, the myth was often stated more cautiously or vaguely, or merely implied. However, a number of scientific authorities and journals of the day offered supposedly objective proofs that it was true.[3] Here is one scientific version of the myth from an 1890 American book:

> The liquor has the power of stimulating the nervous system, and by means of this excitement it causes a degree of pleasure. This pleasurable excitement is soon followed by a corresponding degree of languor and depression, to obtain relief from which, resort is again had to the intoxicating draught. This results not only in restoration, but in exhilaration of spirits; which is again followed by depression and distress. And thus, resort is had, time after time, to the strong drink until an appetite is formed, so strong as to subdue, lead, capture, and brutalise the subject of it.[4]

The myth of demon rum, adorned with religious and scientific endorsements, was proclaimed endlessly with the intention of scaring the populace so badly that they would never touch a drop. The myth gradually came to be believed, or at least half-believed, by millions of otherwise sober citizens. With the myth of demon possession came other lurid tales about the horrendous effects of liquor on the body and mind that fleshed out temperance doctrine.[5] Although this doctrine was most floridly expressed in the rhetoric of the American temperance movement, it appeared in many other countries as well.

From the late 19th century into the 21st, the myth of possession by a demonic substance was applied, essentially unchanged, to a parade of new drugs that aroused public concern. This parade included, but was not limited to, morphine, heroin, cocaine, marijuana, meprobamate, barbiturates, 'speed' (i.e. amphetamines, including methamphetamine), benzodiazepines, crack (i.e. cocaine again), ecstasy, and 'crystal meth' (i.e. methamphetamine again).[6] At one time or another, each of these has been said to take control of the people who use it, just as medieval demons were said to possess their victims. Here is an early example of this rhetoric as applied to morphine, from the *Journal of the American Medical Association* of 1894:

> The subtly ensnaring power of morphia is simply incredible to one who has not had personal observation or experience … I make bold to say that the man does not live who … can bear up against it … Let him not be blinded by an underestimate of the poppy's power to ensnare. Let him not be deluded by an over-confidence in his own strength to resist, for along this line history has repeated itself with sorrowful frequency and, as my experience will well attest, on these two treacherous rocks hundreds of promising lives have gone awreck.[7]

The myth of demon drugs survived modern scepticism because it was—and still is—spread by governments as official warnings, by media as news reports, by churches as gospel truth, and by medical authorities as scientific fact.[8] The myth is easier to believe when applied to illegal drugs than to alcohol because many people have personally experienced harmless alcohol consumption, but have never seen drugs like heroin, cocaine, and methamphetamine, much less experienced their effects. Moreover, the myth is highly serviceable. For example, if the myth is believed, addicted criminals can credibly claim to be 'out of control' and therefore deserving of sympathy, rather than punishment, for their misdeeds.[9]

If the myth were true, enforced prohibition of alcohol and drugs would be necessary and right, because substances with demonic powers can never be tolerated. More importantly for this book, if this myth were true, even for a single drug, the dislocation theory of addiction would be false.

Some advocates of the demon-drug myth still apply it to some illegal drugs in florid and simplistic language scarcely different from that of the original anti-drug militants.[10] However, most current statements of the myth, particularly by scientists, are stated more calmly, more vaguely, or in a watered-down form.[11] Here is a full-strength version of the myth stated in calm medical language that appeared in *Science* in 1997:

> That addiction is tied to changes in brain structure and function is what makes it, fundamentally, a brain disease. A metaphorical switch in the brain seems to be thrown as a result of prolonged drug use. Initially, drug use is a voluntary behavior, but when that

switch is thrown, the individual moves into the state of addiction, characterized by compulsive drug seeking and use.[12]

A more watered-down statement of the myth appeared in another *Science* article. Whereas this article asserted that 'cocaine causes a neurophysiological addiction', it also acknowledged that not all those who experiment with cocaine become addicted. The article explained the unreliability of this phenomenon by suggesting the possibilities that those who do not become addicted do not have the normal euphoric reaction to cocaine, cannot find or afford additional supplies of cocaine, or recognise that they are becoming addicted early in the process and 'are able to cease use'.[13] Although this article takes into account the fact that many people who use cocaine do not become addicted, it still harbours the essential kernel of the demon-drug myth. A physiologically normal person, dislocated or not, will be transformed into an addict if he or she uses it more than a few times, unless he or she either lacks the financial means to afford an addiction or stops using before crossing the invisible threshold.

An even more watered-down, and vaguer, form of the myth, still retaining its essential kernel, appeared in an authoritative article in the *Journal of the American Medical Association* in 2000. According to the authors of this article, 'Few people who try drugs or regularly use drugs become dependent.'[14] However, the authors also point out that '… repeated doses of alcohol and other drugs produce paradoxically increasing tolerance to the effects of those drugs concurrent with decreasing volitional ability to forgo the drug.'[15] In other words, if a person becomes addicted to alcohol or drugs, it is the drug that has been the active agent by increasing the person's tolerance and decreasing their 'volitional ability'. Even in this minimalist form of the myth, the cause of addiction lies in the power of the drug to control a person's brain, and, thus, their mind. When addiction occurs, the drug is the active agent, rather than the person. Drugs and alcohol are 'no ordinary commodity'.[16]

The myth of demon drugs survives and prospers in the 21st century in forms that range from full strength to highly dilute. For many concerned citizens, some form of this myth has acquired the status of an established truth that requires no critical examination. For others, it is accepted as a truth of convenience—dubious if one thinks too hard about it, but reckless to ignore, like religious stories of heaven and hell.

No drug has ever been convincingly shown to have the demonic power portrayed even by the calm and watered-down form of the demon-drug myth.[17] This chapter will use heroin as an example to demonstrate the falsity of the myth. This is anything but a new discovery. On the contrary, there never was any really solid evidence for the myth,[18] and counter-evidence has steadily accumulated for nearly a century, during which it has been officially ignored, denied, explained away, and occasionally suppressed by government intervention.[19] Despite its insubstantiality, the myth lingers on, like a ghost, materialising in the middle of rational discussions, distracting people from more careful analysis of the growing threat of addiction in a globalising world.

Although there is only room in this book to assess the validity of the demon-drug myth in relation to a single drug, heroin, a thorough consideration of heroin requires discussing several other opioid drugs that have very similar effects. There is no space, however, to survey the mountain of evidence on cocaine, 'crack', benzodiazepines, 'speed', methamphetamine, and all of the other drugs that have been demonised in the same way as heroin at one time or another. I have learned, as a university professor, that a comprehensive tour of the demonised drugs is extremely helpful for students, but a semester-length walkabout would require an entire book, whereas this one has a different road to travel. There is now enough high-quality, published evidence to convince even the most sceptical reader of the falsity of the myth with respect to all of the drugs to which it has been applied. This voluminous evidence has been published by medical practitioners (including psychiatrists),[20] psychologists and social scientists,[21] medical historians,[22] political scientists,[23] investigative journalists,[24] psychopharmacologists,[25] and expert panels.[26] Most readers of this book will probably not know of this voluminous literature. This is because, unlike the myth that it debunks, the actual evidence is rarely publicised in the mainstream media, taught in schools, proclaimed by politicians, or solemnized in church services. The ending of this chapter discusses one of the reasons that the mainstream institutions of modern society would like this evidence to just go away.

Whereas this chapter is meant to lay a ghostly myth to rest, it is not intended to launch a counter-myth. The mood-altering drugs that have been demonised are not wonder drugs, keys to enlightenment, sacred herbs, or symbols of human liberty, although they are sometimes portrayed as such by their champions. They are just drugs. Their effects are occasionally deadly, occasionally wondrous, but usually quite mundane. They produce much the same range of costs and benefits as other consumer goods, although they have much more symbolic impact. As with many other consumer goods, a small percentage of their users do become tragically addicted or otherwise harmed. They have appropriate and inappropriate uses and reasonable people often differ on which is which. The terrifying demon-drug myth did not arise from any intrinsic demonic property of any drug, but from the capacity of human society to express its deepest fears symbolically and to use drugs to symbolise one of the gravest of all modern tragedies, spreading impoverishment of the spirit.

Two more disclaimers are needed on this sensitive topic. First, heroin truly is a 'drug of addiction'. All over the world, people who are drifting towards serious addiction are drawn to it, despite its high cost. In some degree, this is because heroin has properties that suit it well for addictive use, but, to a much greater degree, it is because heroin has become a universal symbol following a century of unrelenting, worldwide publicity about the incredible euphoria it allegedly produces and the mystique of the junkie. During the same century and for similar reasons, thirsty people all over the world have learned to reach for a Coca-Cola when they are thirsty. It is as wrong to attribute heroin's spread as a drug of addiction to a unique pharmacological property of the drug as it would be to attribute Coca-Cola's spread as a popular drink to a unique thirst-quenching quality of that particular flavour of carbonated sugar water.

The second disclaimer is that this chapter is not anti-scientific. Of course drugs have physiological as well as psychological effects and of course the response to drugs is influenced by a person's genes. Of course addictions of all sorts can be explained scientifically as well as historically, psychologically, and socially. On the other hand, some excellent biomedical research has been appropriated to provide untenable scientific justifications for the myth that certain drugs, particularly heroin, cocaine, and amphetamine, have irresistible powers to induce addiction in people.[27] Highly qualified scholars have pointed out serious problems with these appropriations of biomedical research,[28] but this does not mean that they have turned against science.

Science is likely to serve the field of addictions well in the future. The adaptive mechanism that regularly gives rise to addiction under conditions of sustained dislocation can almost certainly be explained in terms of evolutionary, genetic, and physiological science. Individual differences in susceptibility to addiction and to various specific addictions can be investigated genetically, physiologically, and psychologically.[29] The appropriation of biomedical research as a justification for the demon-drug myth reveals more about how science can be seconded to the service of mythology than about the scientific respectability of those who seek a more useful analysis.

The opioid family

Heroin cannot be fully understood in isolation, because it is a member of a large family of drugs called the 'opioids' or 'opiates'. The members of this family of drugs all have similar effects on human beings.[30] Several are essentially indistinguishable from heroin in their psychological effects, although they differ from it chemically. Even though heroin and a few other individual members of this family have acquired demonic reputations, their reputations have more to do with historical circumstances than with any unique pharmacological quality.

The opioid family tree has distinct branches all stemming, in one way or another, from opium itself. The pain-relieving and soothing qualities of the dried sap of the opium poppy have been known throughout history, as has the fact that some users become addicted to it. Opium's primary psychoactive component is morphine, which constitutes 10–15% of its weight. One branch of the opioid family tree that is highly relevant to this book includes drugs that are extracted from opium with little or no modification,[31] starting with morphine, which was first extracted in 1806. These drugs also include codeine, buprenorphine, heroin, and oxycodone. A second branch includes molecules with very similar pharmacological effects to the first branch. Although they generally have a chemical resemblance to morphine,[32] they are ultimately synthesised from chemical precursors that are not found in opium. This second branch includes methadone, fentanyl, meperidine, pentazocine, and dozens of others. A third branch includes various polypeptide compounds collectively known as endorphins,[33] which are naturally synthesised within the body of vertebrates, including human beings. These have no chemical resemblance to any constituent of opium, although they are almost indistinguishable[34] from opium-derived drugs in their psychoactive effects. Endorphins serve as natural painkillers and play a complex role in the emotional life of human beings and other animals; for example, in forming the attachment relationship between mothers and infants.[35] A fourth branch is the opiate antagonists, which are essentially antidotes to the rest of the opioids.

All of the opioids mentioned above, except the antagonists, have similar pain-killing and soothing effects, and similarly unpleasant side effects. Large overdoses of any of them can be fatal. However, all of the opioid agonists (i.e. opioids that are not antagonists), including heroin, are used safely by the great majority of consumers in both medical and recreational contexts. Where they are hard to obtain legally, most of them, except the endorphins, are bought and sold illegally for the full spectrum of recreational, self-medicating, or addictive purposes. Some of the opioid agonists are indistinguishable from heroin, others are readily distinguished from it, but medical, recreational, and addicted users are not terribly fussy in this regard. Even though many of them express a preference for heroin or for one of the others, they are generally willing to use any of them.[36]

Throughout the 20th century, pharmaceutical companies organised extensive research projects to discover an opioid painkiller that was as effective as morphine or heroin but did not attract recreational and addictive users. Concurrently, recreational and addictive users undertook their own kinds of research and found virtually all of the new opioids worthy additions to the family.[37] Members of the opioid family are strictly regulated everywhere, although many of them, sometimes including heroin, are available by prescription.[38]

Opioids are carried in the bloodstream throughout the body. How they enter the bloodstream does not matter much—they can be injected, smoked, swallowed, snorted, absorbed rectally from a suppository, or synthesised in the body itself. Their pathway into the bloodstream does not influence their effects, although it does influence their strength and speed of action.[39] For example, the effects of most opioids are weaker and slower if the drug is swallowed rather than injected because some of a swallowed dose breaks down in the digestive system before finally being absorbed into the bloodstream.

Opioid agonists are powerful painkillers and tranquillisers because they inhibit neurons involved with pain and emotion. The major sites of opioid binding are the so-called mu, kappa, and delta receptors[40] in the brain. These receptors are mostly located in the paleospinothalamic pain pathway, which mediates chronic pain, and in portions of the limbic system, which mediates emotion. These opioid-binding areas are also considered the 'reward centres' of the brain. This means that laboratory animals will press levers at high rates to produce an electrical stimulation in the same areas. Opioids also bind in some spinal-cord regions that are implicated in transmitting pain signals to the brain. Like all drugs, opioids travel through the entire bloodstream and bind in numerous places other than just those concerned with pain and emotion. They also bind, for example, on the large intestine and, in males, on the vas deferens.

Like most drugs, the opioid agonists have some harmful side effects. These effects can include vomiting, depressed breathing, 'pinpoint pupils', constipation, depressed activity levels, excessive sweating, decreased sexual libido, cessation of menstruation, withdrawal symptoms, increasing tolerance to the effects of the drug, and overdose.[41] These side effects are a source of considerable discomfort to regular opioid users, but despite the 'fried-egg' claims of drug-war propaganda, result in no known permanent damage[42] except in the case of fatal overdose. However, some people become addicted to each of the opioid agonists, sometimes for a lifetime.

The black sheep

Several members of the opioid family have embarked on glorious careers, only to later fall into scandal and disrepute. Morphine was the first to fall into disrepute in modern times. Widely regarded as a wonder drug because of its miraculous ability to control pain, coughing, and diarrhoea, morphine quickly replaced opium in many forms of medical treatment and as an everyday tonic. It was freely available throughout much of the 19th-century world at very low prices.[43] However, by the end of the 19th century, some patients had become seriously addicted to it and suffered from excruciating withdrawal symptoms when they quit. Addiction spread rapidly. At its peak, it is estimated that nearly 0.5% of the American population were either addicted$_2$ or addicted$_3$ to morphine.[44] As a consequence, the former wonder drug was demonised in the United States, and the strictest controls were applied, to the point that medical patients sometimes died in agony because of groundless fears that administering enough morphine to control the pain would make them addicted.[45]

The curse struck again when heroin was substituted for morphine near the beginning of the 20th century. This substitution was vigorously promoted by heroin's manufacturer, the Bayer Company, and by some physicians, partly on the grounds that heroin did not have the habit-forming properties that had been associated with morphine.[46] So high were the expectations for the new wonder drug that its proprietary name was adapted from the German word *heroisch*, meaning heroic. Within a decade, however, the glory days were over. As many patients were becoming addicted to heroin as had previously become addicted to morphine, and heroin was becoming fashionable as a recreational drug in the criminal underworld in the United States.[47]

There were major economic reasons to lash out against opioids at that time in history. These included a desire to restrict the growing immigrant Chinese population, which constituted an economic threat to white workers and merchants in the United States and Canada,[48] and a great enthusiasm in the United States to establish trading relations with China, which was seeking international support in its struggle against opium addiction in the aftermath of the Opium Wars with Britain.[49] It is sometimes argued that economic reasons were the primary motivation behind the American and Canadian attack on heroin, but, even if this is so, the concern about addiction and other health issues was genuine. Anti-drug propaganda featured health concerns and many people cared about them wholeheartedly.

Although the number of medical patients who became addicted to heroin was a very small fraction of the number who benefited from its medical properties, governments, particularly in the United States and Canada, enacted a series of ever-stronger laws restricting its use. The public hysteria that had been directed at morphine was largely redirected towards heroin, with a vengeance.

The United States soon began a century-long campaign[50] to persuade and pressure other countries to ban all use of heroin. This international campaign was founded upon a false, but endlessly repeated claim that all users eventually became addicts of the worst sort—depraved criminals directly or indirectly serving an international conspiracy of evil. It was further claimed (also falsely) that heroin caused irreversible damage to the brain and virtually every other organ of the body. In the language of the day, anyone who used heroin was likely to become a 'drug fiend' under control of 'the ring' that monopolised distribution of the drug that enslaved their soul and destroyed their body.[51] These florid descriptions were ultimately recycled from the temperance literature where the same sort of language had been used to describe the inevitable fate of people who experimented with 'demon rum'.[52] Thus, heroin went from being celebrated as a new panacea to being demonised as a mass murderer. In reality, it is neither.

Although there were genuine instances of ruinous addiction among those who used heroin prior to its prohibition early in the 20th century, they were few relative to the total number of people who used the drug either medically or recreationally. The great majority of medical patients used the drug only to relieve coughing, diarrhoea, or pain. Most of those who began using it non-medically continued to live normal lives. Their drug use was either unnoticed by their friends and family or subject to the same kind of everyday disapproval as any other dubious habit.[53] This could reasonably be called addiction$_2$, but not addiction$_3$. Of those few who became addicted$_3$, the larger number experienced addictions that were short-lived, harming only themselves and their immediate family by cutting off the opportunity for a fuller, more productive, and happier life. Of those who became more seriously addicted, some actually did became violent, depraved drug fiends, but this was rare until heroin had been demonised and prohibited. Thereafter, users were subject to harsh judicial punishments as well as brutal treatment by police officers determined to protect the public at any cost. At this point, larger numbers of addicted heroin users became desperate criminals, fulfilling the prophecy of the demon-drug mythology.[54]

The pyramid of drug use, with a large base of users benefiting from the valuable effects of a drug and a few desperate addicts at the apex, is typical of all opioid drugs and of many other kinds of drugs as well.[55] Currently, the percentage of heroin users who become seriously addicted is larger than the percentage of users of the other opioids who do, but this is not because of any uniquely addictive pharmacological quality. All opioid drugs agonists can make suffering people feel better for a time, all can cause withdrawal symptoms, all can produce overdose, and all can be drugs of addiction.

People's way of responding to opioids, exactly like their way of responding to other drugs and ordinary consumer goods, is powerfully conditioned by their expectations. In 1898, when heroin was introduced as a cough suppressant and painkiller by the same trusted company that distributed Aspirin®, most users were seeking a remedy for their coughs and pain. A few became addicted to it, just as a few of the millions of users of other opioid drugs and of other painkillers become addicted to them now.[56] A couple of decades later, when heroin was sensationalised as a demon drug in the international press and was said to cause the most spectacular kind of addiction, many seriously dislocated people turned to it as part of their transition to a lifestyle of reckless addiction, although others continued to use it solely for medical or recreational purposes.[57] All drugs are subject to placebo effects—not just sugar pills. People who experiment with heroin today are much more likely to become addicted to it because every respected source of knowledge is telling them that they will experience irresistible bliss and unbearable withdrawal effects. Richard DeGrandpre has labelled this powerful social influence on the effects of heroin a 'placebo text'.[58]

The myth exposed

The myth of demon drugs can be broken down into five component ideas, each of which contributes some demonic images to the overall picture. To the degree that they are testable, all five ideas have proven false for heroin and the other opioids. The evidence refuting them was published in a large number of research articles and scholarly books throughout the last half of the 20th century and is summarised below.

'It's so good, don't even try it once.'

This compelling phrase, which served as the title of an American book on heroin written in the early 1970s,[59] states the first component of the myth of demon drugs. The phrase implies that any use of heroin will induce an irresistible euphoria, leaving users with uncontrollable cravings to repeat the experience. Lurid descriptions of the mysterious euphoria are frequently associated with heroin even now, with the word 'orgasmic' often included once or more for emphasis.[60] Heroin's actual hedonic effects are not nearly as gratifying as the myth would have it.

It is true that some junkies are rapturous about the euphoria produced by their first exposure to heroin, and that the opioid experience is often described in very positive ways by patients suffering from post-surgical pain. I have experienced the post-surgical euphoria myself. However, the effects of heroin and other opioid drugs are quite different under the more ordinary circumstances in which most people might have occasion to 'try it once'. When people experiment with opioids, either out of their own curiosity or the curiosity of researchers who provide the drug in laboratory settings, the overwhelming majority do not experience any extraordinary kind or degree of euphoria. Although this fact may surprise many people, it has been known for a very long time. Medical researcher Lawrence Kolb summarised it succinctly in 1925: 'Only in rare instances, if at all, does anyone except the emotionally unstable, the psychopath, or the neurotic [experience euphoria from morphine].'[61]

The best laboratory experiments on this topic were conducted in the 1950s and 1960s at the Harvard Medical School. They could not be done now because of today's stringent ethical restrictions on human experiments. Yet these experiments of half a century ago proved safe and informative. They were carried out with scrupulous attention to detail, because of the controversial nature of the topic. They used double-blind procedures in which neither the experimental subject nor the medical technician knew what was being injected. They used placebo controls to factor out the power of suggestion.

The results were consistent. The great majority of ordinary volunteers (i.e. normally healthy people or chronically ill people without a past history of drug addiction) did not experience any mysterious euphoria *or even ordinary pleasure* from heroin or morphine, and expressed no desire to repeat the experience.[62] The few who did report pleasure did not describe it as an unusual euphoria, but in ordinary terms. The most consistently reported reactions to heroin were mental cloudiness, lethargy, and somatic discomfort (e.g. itchiness, nausea, and dizziness). The volunteers' performance in tests of attention and arithmetic calculation decreased somewhat, about 7% on average for heroin.[63] In one experiment, amphetamine was also used as an experimental drug, and the volunteers consistently reported a pleasurable response to it, showing that the experience of pleasure is possible, even in the sterile atmosphere of a medical school research laboratory. (It does not follow from this that the demon-drug mythology is true of amphetamine, however.)

These classic experiments have been confirmed outside the laboratory as well. An American scholar who spent many years in Laos investigating opium use and addiction in treatment facilities described the results of his investigation of experimental use of opioids, conducted far from a medical school laboratory. He visited local opium dens with his friends on a few occasions and described the results as follows:

> Of my eight Caucasian fellow visitors, six did try smoking opium. None had ever used opium before, and to the best of my knowledge none has ever used it again. They inhaled relatively small doses, apparently more from curiosity and to say 'I smoked opium' than from any fervent wish to make this ritual part of their regular lives. All were married, in their thirties, employed, getting along well in their lives, and mostly in professional fields; and they did not live where they had ready access to opium or opium dens.... Among my adventuresome friends and acquaintances, a few non-smokers could not inhale the smoke deeply into their lungs and keep it there. A few others felt nothing after one or two inhalations. And a few more experienced some nausea and lethargy after finishing a pipe or two. None of them reported anything resembling pleasure or euphoria. One man having a bout of diarrhea at the time found that two pipefuls greatly relieved this condition (much as one would expect from the old nostrum, tincture of opium). I have followed the lives of these eight people (seven men and one woman) over a six-to-ten year period since their smoking opium in one or another Laotian den. None has become an opium addict, or, for that matter, an abuser of any other substance.[64]

It might be objected that it takes more than one or two exposures for the euphoric effects of opioids to be appreciated, or that repeated injections are required to produce the irresistible euphoria, but this possibility has been investigated as well. A careful study of experimental injection of heroin in two volunteers over a period of several days that was reported in the *British Medical Journal* in 1969 included the following first-hand report:

> We've been on heroin a week now, Stuart and I. Seven days of voluntary illness. And how ill we feel ... My personal view at present is just one made grey and utterly grim by heroin.
>
> The extraordinary thing is that it brings no joy, no pleasure. Weariness, above all. At most, some hours of disinterest—the world passing by while you feel untouched.
>
> Even after the injection there is no sort of a thrill, no mind-expansion nonsense, or orgasmic heights, no Kubla Khan. A feeling of oppressed breathing, a slight flush, a sense of strange unease, almost fear unknown ... how can people want to take the stuff? To escape to all this—life must be hell if they can want to escape to all this ...
>
> It's a month now since we've stopped the stuff, though some measurements continue. It's been wonderful to feel fit and to relish life again. To be once again in the regular sequence of clinics, wards, and teaching makes one realise the satisfaction within the routines of work. I'd taken some comfort during that week by quietly pottering in the garden, but how much richer is enjoyment now. The late October roses have liked this dry,

still week, and the autumn foliage beside the river as I sit and look at it this Sunday afternoon brings a greater peace than known to any poor devils who take heroin. We condemn them and despise them, but we forget to appreciate how fortunate we are to find our joy in life and not be driven to escape it.[65]

I have personally had the opportunity to 'try it once' myself. In fact, suitable opportunities have presented themselves more than once in my life. The first took me by surprise after oral surgery to remove an impacted tooth. After the procedure was finished, the dental surgeon's assistant gave me an injection and I felt a warm glow and sense of well-being along with the welcome pain relief. Although my mind had been wholly on my tooth problem, my inner researcher sprang to life. When I asked the dental assistant what the injection was, she responded that she wasn't supposed to tell. She eventually revealed that it was meperidine, an opioid usually known under the name Demerol® that is so attractive to heroin addicts that it has been included in the demands by desperate prisoners in some hostage-taking incidents in Canadian prisons. My experience of well-being mixed with pain relief is common among patients who receive opioid drugs for post-surgical pain, and helps to explain the important place that opioid drugs, including heroin, still play in medicine around the world. It is now well established that there is only a miniscule danger of medical patients who enjoy opioids under these conditions becoming drug addicts afterwards, and I am happy to confirm this personally.

The other three experiences were quite different from the first. As they were similar, I will describe only one of them, the most recent. Several years ago, I was contacted by an ex-student, a man of 25 years who suffered chronic back and neck pain from a car accident. He controlled the pain with a variety of painkillers that he received by prescription, including OxyContin®, a time-release form of oxycodone, which had recently received some notoriety when the well-known American television personality and political commentator Rush Limbaugh became addicted to it. My friend noted that the various opioid drugs relieved the pain effectively but also provided a feeling of well-being that he valued highly. He thought he would probably continue taking the drugs even if the pain were to subside (which was not likely). He invited me to take one of these drugs with him for an evening because he thought, correctly as it turned out, that I would enjoy the experience.

I was delighted at the opportunity to use opioids in a friendly setting with a regular user who was experiencing pleasure from his own use. I asked that we use OxyContin®, which was at that time first coming to public notice as 'hillbilly heroin'. Not only are the effects essentially identical to those of heroin when it is administered in equivalent doses,[66] but it is frequently sold to junkies on the street.[67]

I took a few tablets during the course of a pleasant evening with my young friend. I enjoyed the wide-ranging discussion that ensued at least as much as discussions that I had had with him in my office when he was a student. He was definitely an interesting man, and he had already endured a number of serious disappointments in his young life, deeper than the shock and pain of the car accident, that drew me to him. I know that I took enough of the opioid drug to be affected physiologically, because I had the best known of all the opioid side effects. I vomited—just once, and without residual nausea. This unpleasantness did not seriously detract from my enjoyment of the experience.

I definitely felt the effect of the opioid drug, but I did not experience anything that I would call euphoria, beyond the pleasure of sharing the evening with an interesting person participating in a ritual that was important to him. The nature of the opioid experience became clearest to me after the social evening was over and I had gone home to bed. I slept reasonably well and dreamed, as I often do. The dreams, however, had an eerie quality to them that might be called 'euphoria', although that is not the word I would choose. My dreams normally have a surface action and an emotional underlay. The underlay is quite often anxiety. On this night, I encountered the usual kind of dream, but without the anxiety underlay. This experience was so unusual that I awoke two or three times, surprised by the absence of anxiety. All things considered, I prefer my normal style of dreaming, which somehow seems richer, despite, or perhaps because of, its emotional complexity. I have not tried opioids since that experience several years ago, although I probably will if there is a good opportunity to try a new one in a suitable environment. My young friend still suffers chronic pain and still relies on legally obtained drugs to control it, but his professional and family life is busy and full and he has not become a drug addict.

In contrast to all of the reports cited above, glowing memories of extraordinary euphoria produced by their first opioid experience have been recalled by many (but not all) opioid addicts.[68] A study of the first experiences of polydrug addicts with heroin also found a much higher frequency of euphoria than had been found with the volunteers in the studies above.[69] Thus, while the large majority of people do not experience powerful euphoria when they 'try it once', some definitely do, and some of these become addicted. It can be argued from this that there are *some* people who will, in fact, be transformed into addicts by the euphoria of one or a few exposures to heroin. It can further be argued that, since it is impossible to predict who they are, the myth of demon drugs is essentially true for heroin, although it does not apply to everybody.

However, the logic of this version of the myth is as watered-down as the claim that it makes. Pleasure, even very great pleasure, is not normally addicting. If it were, almost everybody on earth would become addicted, because most people occasionally experience joy and ecstasy; for example, in their music, religion, sexuality, celebrations with families and friends, and moments of personal triumph. Even the most exquisite pleasures do not draw the majority of people into addiction. Rather, they enrich mundane life with colour, vitality, and the hope that more special moments may come. If some people experience great pleasure from heroin, this only shows that heroin is no more (or less) addictive than a thousand other activities that occasionally cause great pleasure and to which a few people become addicted.

That some people do experience euphoria from heroin whereas most do not is an important fact that requires explanation. Although the demon-drug myth does not explain it, the dislocation theory of addiction does. Heroin, like the other opioid agonists, is extraordinarily effective in relieving both physical pain and emotional anguish. The relief it provides is experienced as intensely pleasurable. Anguish is the dominating emotion in people suffering from dislocation, as shown in Chapter 3. The most likely conclusion is that people who experience intense pleasure from heroin are severely dislocated. The argument that applies to emotional anguish also applies to severe boredom, although it is not as fully documented. Heroin effectively relieves boredom,[70] and boredom is common in people who are vulnerable to addiction.[71]

Heroin withdrawal is unbearable

Another component of the myth of demon drugs holds that ceasing to take heroin or another opioid after a period of regular use causes excruciatingly painful withdrawal symptoms that force users to recommence their habit at any cost. This part of the myth, which was the dominant one for decades, has been quietly abandoned in recent years by researchers in the field and is no longer published in textbooks on addiction. However, it is still portrayed floridly in popular media and still widely believed.[72] It is impossible for me to take it seriously because I have observed heroin addicts in withdrawal many times.

The word that Vancouver addicts most often use to explain the nature of withdrawal symptoms is 'flu'. Sometimes they compare withdrawal to mild influenza and sometimes to severe influenza. Their choice of the word 'flu' fits well with my own observations of them. For example, a heroin addict who appeared as the guest speaker in a university class that I was teaching some years ago was asked, among many other questions, if it was true that withdrawal symptoms were not as serious as their depiction in the media would indicate. He answered by asking if anyone had been aware that he was undergoing withdrawal himself as he had been addressing the class. No one had guessed it, including me, although he was persistently sniffling as he spoke and looked very tired.

Three decades ago, Canada's Commission of Inquiry into the Non-medical Use of Drugs reported, ever so cautiously, that:

> The classical, severe opiate narcotic withdrawal syndrome … seems to be the exception rather than the rule; much milder, flu-like symptoms are typically described by clinicians and the drug users themselves. This may be due to the relatively low purity of street heroin in some areas, and the light and intermittent use patterns which have developed, but more likely reflects an overemphasis of extreme cases in the earlier literature.[73]

The dislocation theory of addiction implies that withdrawal symptoms are in no way necessary to the existence of any addiction, since the primary motivation for addiction is maintenance of a lifestyle and an identity that provides a dislocated person with a substitute for psychosocial integration. Direct evidence that withdrawal symptoms are not necessary to addiction comes from the fact that, in past decades, American and Canadian addicts often passed through periods of days or weeks when the heroin sold on the street was so weak that it could not have caused withdrawal symptoms. Nonetheless, these addicts continued to live the junkie lifestyle and to buy and use drugs that were essentially placebos.[74] Alfred Lindesmith described an example of this during a period of greatly reduced heroin importation into the United States shortly after World War II as follows:

> … addicts who believed themselves to be addicted were in fact using such a heavily diluted product that they were not getting enough to maintain physical dependence. Some of these users were themselves surprised and humiliated when, after claiming to have big habits, they experienced little distress upon withdrawal.[75]

It remains possible that even mild withdrawal symptoms could cause people to continue taking a drug, despite all the harm that it causes them. However, common sense points in the other direction. Outside the credulous climate that surrounds the myth of demon drugs, the belief that people would endure a life of misery because they could not endure a few days of predictable sickness from withdrawal symptoms is simply unbelievable. Countless people willingly submit themselves to sickness that is worse than withdrawal symptoms in order to achieve important goals. For example, the sickness caused by chemotherapy used in the treatment of cancer involves nausea, hair loss, and prolonged and extreme discomfort. People voluntarily accept chemotherapy repeatedly and endure the consequences bravely, in order to live. Heroin addicts would do the same thing if heroin addiction were merely a disease that could be overcome by enduring its normally mild withdrawal symptoms.

Beyond common sense, much hard evidence shows unequivocally that addiction is not maintained by withdrawal symptoms. Countless involuntary withdrawals were forced on drug-addicted prisoners in the 20th century, in the belief that overcoming withdrawal symptoms would cure addiction. Almost invariably, these addicts returned to their drug use after their withdrawal symptoms had passed.[76] A wide variety of drugs to which people do not ordinarily become addicted do produce severe withdrawal symptoms,[77] including one of the most widely prescribed anti-depressants.[78] People do become severely addicted to cocaine, although it 'does not cause gross physiological withdrawal symptoms'.[79] Withdrawal symptoms produced by prolonged exposure to heroin and other opioid drugs in medical settings are easily managed with sedative drugs or with the power of suggestion or hypnosis.[80] They rarely, if ever, cause iatrogenic addiction.[81] Relapses of opioid addicts do not usually occur when people are suffering from withdrawal symptoms, but rather when they are suffering from anxiety and stress of other sorts.[82] So-called 'controlled dependent users' of heroin experience withdrawal symptoms when they stop using, but are not addicted$_3$, although they can reasonably be called addicted$_2$.[83] Although they must suffer from withdrawal symptoms in the process, many regular heroin users change their pattern of use and become intermittent recreational users.[84] The great majority of heroin-addicted American soldiers returning from the war in Vietnam gave up their addictions when they reached home, even though heroin was often easily available to them.[85]

None of this is meant to deny that withdrawal symptoms can be extremely uncomfortable if the person has been taking high doses of heroin for a long time, or to deny that withdrawal symptoms are mentioned by many heroin addicts as the reason for continuing their addictions. However, it has become absolutely clear that withdrawal symptoms are neither necessary to cause opioid addiction nor sufficient to maintain it once a person has become addicted. The cause of opioid addiction lies elsewhere.

Heroin causes addiction, even in the absence of euphoria and withdrawal symptoms

The third component of the myth of devil drugs draws its credibility from behavioural theory. Addiction researchers point out that the 'reinforcers' that presumably cause addictive behaviours are not necessarily experienced as pleasurable and do not necessarily produce withdrawal symptoms.[86] If all or most people who experiment with opioid drugs become addicted, it would be reasonable to conclude that the drug is extraordinarily reinforcing, whether euphoria and withdrawal symptoms play a role in this process or not. However, notwithstanding the scientific language that is used to explain why opioids are extraordinarily potent reinforcers, the vast majority of people who take opioid drugs, including heroin, have no later problems with drug addiction.[87] The small number who do become addicted generally show signs of having problems related to dislocation beforehand.[88]

The use of heroin, morphine, and opium in the United States, Canada, and Great Britain during the 19th century was far greater than it is now. These drugs were available in the form of inexpensive pills and patent medicines that were available at most pharmacies, grocery stores, and general stores,[89] and as physician-prescribed injections. Many of the commercially available preparations were used for non-medical purposes. Although some users did become dependent or addicted to these preparations, the combined incidence of addiction$_2$ and addiction$_3$ to opioid drugs probably never rose above 0.5% of the total population in the United States where the most complete statistics were compiled.[90] The incidence of addiction was declining there by the end of the century as the risks of addiction became publicised, well before the harsh anti-drug laws were passed. Similarly, widespread use of opium in China since the Ming dynasty did not lead to addiction in the vast majority of the population,[91] although opioid addiction did become a serious problem late in the 19th century after China was forced into free trade with the West, as discussed in Chapter 6. It has long been known that members of opium-producing societies in India, Turkey, and Southeast Asia use opium as part of the normal routines of village life, from childhood to old age, with only a very small incidence of addiction.[92]

In the UK, heroin continued to be used widely as a medication for cough, diarrhoea, chronic pain, and other conditions throughout the 20th century, in spite of the hysteria about its irresistible addictiveness that had spread around the world. In 1972, for example, British physicians prescribed 29 kg of heroin to medical patients, enough to provide over 7 million 4 mg injections. After a careful examination of the British statistics on iatrogenic addiction, Arnold Trebach concluded, 'there is a virtual absence of addicts created by this singular medical practice'.[93] Heroin has remained a staple drug in British medical practice along with morphine and other opioids. It is currently used primarily to relieve pain associated with cancer, childbirth, physical trauma, and heart attack. It is given to children as well as adults.[94] Fears of heroin-induced addiction continue to be minimal among British physicians, although this may change amidst the current explosive increase in heroin addiction.[95]

About 25 years ago, an American research team began experimenting with a Canadian invention, a bedside self-medication machine programmed to deliver about 1 mg of morphine intravenously to patients who pressed a hand button. The machine limited infusions to one every 6 minutes. In one early study, 50 patients were kept on the regimen for between 1 and 6 days. The self-administered doses were considerably less than the maximum the machine would allow. Rather than increasing as patients continued the regimen, the doses progressively declined.[96]

In the last 10 years, this machine, now widely known as the patient-controlled analgesia (PCA) machine, has come into general use in hospitals. In spite of the misgivings of hospital workers who believed that exposure to opioid drugs would cause addiction in many patients, the development of addiction has been rare, even among those patients who were allowed larger doses over longer time periods.[97] The only patients deemed unsuitable for PCA are those with concurrent medical conditions that could be exacerbated by analgesics and, in some institutions, patients with a history of addiction to drugs or alcohol.

A number of careful field studies have described people who have become casual or regular users of heroin and other opioids and have remained unaddicted for the length of the study, in spite of their frequent exposure to opioids.[98] For example, Norman Zinberg studied both addicted and non-addicted users of heroin, whom he labelled 'controlled users'. These non-addicted users were not 'overwhelmingly involved' with their drug. It did not consume their lives, they did not steal to obtain it, and they were not criminalised.

The non-addicted users described by Zinberg were no more likely to escalate to addictive use than to reduce their use or become abstinent. Zinberg followed up a group of non-addicted users of opioids 12–24 months after an initial interview. He was able to re-interview 60% of the original group. Of these, 49% were using drugs in the same way as at the first interview, 27% 'had reduced use to levels below those required for them to be considered controlled users', and 13% had increased their opiod use above the controlled level. The remaining 11% were still controlled opiod users, but had begun to consume another drug too heavily to be considered a controlled drug user.[99]

Even today, when every schoolchild is conditioned to associate heroin use with inevitable addiction, it seems that most regular users of heroin do not become addicted or socially degenerate. In a 2005 study, Shewan and Dalgarno located 126 people in Glasgow, Scotland, who had used heroin and other opioid drugs for an average of 6.8 years and who had neither been incarcerated nor in treatment for drug misuse. As many as possible of these people were interviewed two times, with an average of 15 months between the two interviews. The purpose of the study was to document the addiction and other problems that arose within this group both before the first interview and between the two interviews. Of the original 126 users, 85 were located again for the second interview.[100]

These heroin users were unexceptional in employment, occupational status, housing status, and living arrangements compared with UK and Scottish norms. For example, at the first interview, 74% had jobs at all levels of occupational status except the very lowest, 11% were occupied as full-time students, and 15% were unemployed. At the first interview, 64% had some post-secondary education; 89% were settled in their own living accommodations, which they either rented or owned; 11% lived with family or friends; 57% were 'in a relationship'; and 33% had children. This picture was essentially the same at the second interview, except that average incomes and occupational status had risen somewhat.

Among the participants, heroin consumption ranged widely from 35 people who had consumed heroin on an average of 13 days in the past 2 years to 29 people who had consumed heroin on an average of 536 days in the past 2 years. In addition to heroin, the participants had used several other opioid drugs, generally in lesser quantities. Virtually all of them had at some time used marijuana, ecstasy, amphetamine, LSD, or cocaine either in the form of powder or 'crack'. In response to a Severity of Dependence Scale[101] administered at the first interview, the participants reported a mean self-rating of dependence on heroin of 4.7 (out of a possible 15). They gave higher mean self-ratings of dependence to tobacco (8.3), cannabis (5.6), and alcohol (5.6). The normal cut-off for recognising a person as dependent is 5.0.

Between the two interviews, six participants had entered treatment because of increasing heroin use and deteriorating health. All of these had become daily or nearly daily injectors of heroin by the time they entered treatment. Of these six, five were receiving methadone. None of the remaining 79 follow-up participants perceived a need for treatment.

Most participants reported a similar level of heroin consumption at the two interviews. There was no statistically significant increase in the frequency or amount of heroin use from the first to the second interview. Six were regular injectors at the first interview and four at the follow-up (not counting those who had presented themselves for treatment). Of the 85 follow-up participants, 17 did not use heroin at all between the two interviews, although only two said they would definitely not use it again in the future.

These results showed conclusively that it is possible for many people to use heroin regularly, even to inject it, without needing treatment for addiction and without experiencing serious health problems. Regular use of heroin is not a sufficient cause of addiction.

The main findings of the Glasgow study have now been confirmed in England by a study sponsored by the Joseph Rountree Foundation.[102] The English study solicited volunteers who had used heroin at least once in the previous 6 months but were experiencing no legal or medical problems connected with heroin use. The 123 volunteers in the Internet sample responded to a questionnaire on the World Wide Web. The 51 volunteers in the face-to-face interview sample were all from the UK, and 32 were re-interviewed 24 months later. Whereas the English study pursued some ideas that were different from the Glasgow study, it replicated the finding that regular use of heroin is not a sufficient cause of addiction.

Of course, a few of the heroin users in these two studies did move from incipient addiction to full-blown, catastrophic addiction. The authors of these studies did not deny the dangers of heroin addiction, but they did reject the myth that all or most regular users of heroin become out-of-control junkies. The percentage of heroin users who remain occasional users or controlled dependent users, rather than junkies, may be unknowable, since people's use of heroin is normally shrouded with secrecy. However, these authors pointed out that existing quantitative studies suggest that 'non-dependent or controlled users outnumber those whose use is uncontrolled and problematic'.[103]

Junkies know best

The fourth component of the demon-drug mythology as applied to heroin does not rely on austere scientific language, but on a shocking story. Throughout the 20th century, countless heroin addicts have recounted this familiar story, with a thousand variations. They were living normal, heroin-free lives when, for some reason—a pusher, a false friend, a painful illness, a foolish impulse—they tried heroin and were caught in its grip, forever 'hooked' with a 'monkey on their back'. Sometimes the story was told in the uneducated language of the street and sometimes in the eloquent prose of the highborn and well-educated, most famously William S. Burroughs, an American writer of the 20th century.[104] Taken together, these wrenching tales constitute powerful testimonials for the myth of demon drugs. They have been treated as serious evidence by leading authors in the addictions field.[105]

It may seem arrogant in the extreme to dispute the testimony of sincere and knowing voices. However, this story must be disputed, because there are at least as many testimonials by junkies against the myth of demon drugs as there are for it, although this counter-evidence has not been given the same play in the popular media. In decades of close contact with junkies, I have heard many retellings of the myth of demon drugs, but I have heard more stories that contradict it. Some heroin addicts have tried very hard to make me understand why they chose to maintain the life of a junkie and others have confessed that they were confused about their own reasons. Occasionally, one has invited me to explore his or her subconscious motivations for his or her addiction, which I have tried to do. Just as there are countless variations of the myth of demon drugs, there are countless stories told by drug-addicted people who do not believe that they have been possessed by drugs.[106]

Some people's adoption of a junkie lifestyle is easier to understand than others'. People whose self-respect has been shattered by childhood abuse and destitution have little to lose by joining a junkie subculture and much to gain from the camaraderie and social support of their fellow junkies, as well as the broad-spectrum anaesthesia that the drug provides. However, many junkies come from prosperous, apparently harmonious families.[107] Why would they become junkies? I have had the opportunity to work with several junkies with upper middle-class backgrounds and with their parents during my years as a psychologist. Among such junkies, dislocation sometimes grows from devastating inabilities to meet highly internalised standards of achievement, rendering them unacceptable failures in their own estimation. In addition, some prosperous but frigid families maintain an impenetrable veneer of warmth that camouflages subtle cruelty or dysfunction.[108] Alternatively, dislocation in junkies-to-be may come from painful rejection by their peers.[109] In free-market society, dislocation among the offspring of rich families is often as bad as that of poorer families.[110] For such people, becoming a junkie may be the most workable alternative to deep depression or suicide.

Besides the adaptive benefits that every other addiction could provide children of prosperous families, being a junkie offers a unique, if perverse, boost to self-esteem, which was labelled 'junkie mystique' in Chapter 7. Embracing the most feared and despised of all drugs is a bold counterattack upon the emptiness and boredom that often fills an affluent life. To be a junkie is to kick sand in the face of 'respectability' with its myriad hypocrisies. It is to work a terrible revenge on resented parents. To be a junkie is to be feared as well as pitied, to provoke awe as well as to endure humiliation. It is a starkly honest position. Whereas many affluent people struggle to deny and conceal their addictions, junkies flaunt theirs. Junkies can share a sense of camaraderie with other adventurers of the counterculture. Former heroin addict William Pryor[111] coined the insightful phrase 'devoted scapegoat' to describe some of the perverse pay-offs that rebellious children and junkies from prosperous families may receive along with their suffering.

Of course, it is better to be famous than to be infamous, but it is preferable to be infamous than to be utterly inconsequential or 'a contradictory bundle of identity fragments', as Erikson put it.[112] The psychosocial benefits of being a junkie, including a compelling sense of purpose, a well-recognised identity, the relief of boredom, and the power to shock and horrify 'straight' people, have been extensively documented by therapists and social scientists[113] and by junkie authors.[114] Being a junkie is painful, and may eventually be fatal, but it provides a blockbuster substitute for psychosocial integration for people who cannot escape chronic dislocation.[115]

It remains logically possible that there are two fundamentally different kinds of junkie: those who have been possessed by a demon drug and those who use their addiction as a form of adaptation. The former kind would account for the seemingly incontestable testimonials of drug possession that impassioned junkie authors have written. But impassioned testimonials do not provide convincing evidence for the myth, *even in the junkie authors' own lives*. This does not mean that the authors are lying. Since Sigmund Freud first revealed the power of unconscious motives, it has been necessary to view even the most sincere claims of being controlled by an alien force with scepticism. From a sceptical perspective, there are plausible explanations for a junkie having the powerful experience of being possessed by a drug, as well as for a society accepting these testimonials credulously.

Psychologist John Davies and others[116] have shown that the attribution of irresistible addictive power to drugs by addicts can best be explained by a set of psychological principles known as 'attribution theory'. Most people, consciously or unconsciously, attribute qualities to people and things more to maximise their personal gains than to describe reality objectively. Thus, what addicts say and experience about themselves could serve more to excuse their deviant behaviour than to actually describe the cause of their addiction. To claim that one has been transformed into an addict by a drug has all the advantages of pleading guilty to a lesser offence. Rather than accepting responsibility for actions that offend society, addicts need only admit to the unwise experimentation that got them hooked, after which the responsibility was no longer theirs, but must be attributed to the 'monkey on their back'. Davies reviewed research showing that addicts more often describe themselves as being under the control of the drug when they are being interviewed by an authority figure than when they are speaking to another drug user.[117]

In many instances, the self-perception of being under a drug's control may not result from shame about the behaviour that has occurred, but from shame about the motivation behind it. People often experience dislocation as a social rejection caused by their personal unworthiness. Such thoughts can cause unbearable shame.[118] If a person becomes addicted, it is less painful to attribute their life of addiction to possession by a demon drug than to face the shame of enduring, irremediable dislocation. Drugs that society defines as 'addictive' may be particularly appealing to dislocated people for this reason.

The addicted person's parents and other family members also must deal with the shame. Parents are inevitably prone to blame themselves for their child's addiction. What greater shame and horror could there be for them than to perceive that the family environment that they have provided is so repellent that their child prefers the squalid life of a junkie? It is more merciful to believe that drugs have demonic powers and that their wayward offspring is out of control. Believing junkies' stories about being controlled by drugs has a certain benefit for overworked and frustrated treatment professionals as well, because it frees them of the anguish of repeated therapeutic failures and allows them to place their faith in simpler, more program-matic solutions.[119] For the same reason that parents and therapists must sometimes repress too-painful reality, the larger society must repress the idea that it is unfit for habitation by many members of the new generation. Thus, addicts, their parents, treatment professionals, and the larger society can all agree with the myth of the demon drug for a similar reason. All four collude to conceal the real or imagined aspect of addiction that is the most shameful to them.

'Once a junkie, always a junkie'

The phrase 'once a junkie, always a junkie' was part of the folklore about heroin for many decades and was endorsed by some of the most respected scholars on the topic.[120] The phrase adds a particular dramatic bite to the myth of heroin as a demon drug, because it means that the mysterious transformation caused by using heroin is not only profound but permanent. A precious human soul has been lost, and the loss is irrecoverable, unless a miracle occurs.

This claim is demonstrably false. The evidence is now overwhelming that many people who have been severely addicted to heroin cease to use heroin entirely and cease to have any residual cravings for it. Evidence of recovery from heroin and other kinds of addiction was reviewed in Chapter 7 under the heading *Psychosocial Integration Makes Recovery from Addiction Possible*. In addition to junkies who become abstainers, many become intermittent users or 'regular controlled users' who are not addicted$_3$.[121]

Ghostly evidence

So far, this chapter has concentrated on the evidence that disproves component ideas of the demon-drug myth, as applied to heroin. It now turns to two widely accepted aspects of the conventional wisdom on addiction that provide popular support for the myth. These aspects of conventional wisdom have stood, rarely contested, for decades. I believe that, in the future, both of these aspects will be recognised as cultural relics, like medieval lore on demon possession and witchcraft.

The American Civil War

For many decades, the most powerful proof for the demon-drug myth as applied to opioid drugs was an imagined epidemic of addiction to morphine during the American Civil War of 1861–1865. Battlefield doctors, in their zeal to spare the wounded from suffering, supposedly pumped so much morphine through their newly invented hypodermic syringes that they created a generation of morphine-addicted war veterans. This story was told and retold throughout the 20th century, steadily growing in scope and certainty.[122] In the United States, opioid addiction was sometimes referred to as 'soldiers' disease'.

However, this urban myth, as it could now be called, was without substance, as American medical historian David Musto showed years ago by compiling a few historical facts.[123] Whereas it is true that there was an increase in morphine addiction in the late 19th-century United States and that many battlefield doctors used morphine to treat the wounded, the use of morphine in battlefield medical practice did not cause the increase of addiction.

Consumption of morphine and opium climbed steadily between 1840 and 1896 in the United States, but there was no sign of a spike during the Civil War. In fact, the great surge in consumption occurred in the 1870s, well after the war had ended. There were no quantitative studies supporting the claim of a cohort of addicted veterans. In fact, American historians writing shortly after the Civil War about increasing morphine consumption made little or no mention of wartime battlefield injection as a cause, although later historians made much of it. Before moral panic ruled out rational debate, a number of influential American doctors and writers argued that the rise of addiction to opioids in the late 19th century could best be understood as a natural response to the strains of modern life and the fragmentation of identity that accompanied it.[124] Moreover, the myth of demon morphine:

> … does not explain the relatively few addicts proportionally or absolutely in such nations as France, Germany, Great Britain, Russia, and Italy, which also fought wars during the latter half of the nineteenth century and also used morphine as an analgesic.[125]

Addicted rodents

The demon-drug myth is frequently justified by reference to research on the self-administration of drugs by experimental animals. When carefully scrutinised, however, this evidence also proves vaporous.

In the early 1960s, researchers at the University of Michigan perfected devices that allowed laboratory animals to inject themselves with drugs simply by pressing a lever in what was called a 'Skinner box'. By the end of the 1970s, hundreds of experiments with this apparatus had shown that rats, and occasionally mice and monkeys, would self-inject large doses of heroin, cocaine, amphetamines, and a number of other drugs.[126]

Many people concluded that these data constituted proof for the demon-drug myth. If most animals inject an opioid drug avidly and to the detriment of their health, as they did under some of the experimental conditions, does it not follow that these drugs instil a need for addictive consumption that transcends species and culture, and is simply a tragic fact of mammalian destiny? Eminent American scientist Avram Goldstein put it this way in 1979:

> If a monkey is provided with a lever, which he can press to self-inject heroin, he establishes a regular pattern of heroin use—a true addiction—that takes priority over the normal activities of his life…. Since this behaviour is seen in several other animal species

(primarily rats), I have to infer that if heroin were easily available to everyone, and if there were no social pressure of any kind to discourage heroin use, a very large number of people would become heroin addicts.[127]

Although many scholars still accept this conclusion, it does not fit with human history, which shows that when heroin and morphine are freely available, only a very small percentage of people became addicted. It does not fit with reports of moderate, non-addictive use of heroin over long periods. It contrasts with observations of people who are given relatively free access to opioid drugs either by physicians or through PCA machines.

Could it be that heroin is more addictive to laboratory animals than to people? If so, what possible point could there be in reaching conclusions about human addiction from the behaviour of rats? It now appears, however, that the research was misinterpreted and that the demon drugs are unable to possess even the most compliant of all mammalian species, the laboratory rat.

Critical scholars have asked how it can be known that a rat has become addicted. This is more than an academic quibble. It requires personal knowledge and sensitivity to distinguish a person who gambles regularly from a gambling addict or a person who loves intensely from a love addict. Some doctors argue that the distinction between medical patients who are desperate for opioid medication to relieve pain and those who are seeking narcotics to sustain their addictions is so difficult that an entire medical team, rather than a single doctor or nurse, is required to make it accurately.[128] How many doctors and nurses might it require to distinguish between addicted and non-addicted rats in a Skinner box? In fact, a Skinner box would be the last place to try to make this subtle distinction, because it is designed specifically so that it is not necessary for the experimenter to actually look at the experimental animal. The only output from a Skinner box that researchers normally see is a piece of paper with cumulative lever-press data. Could anybody tell from such data if a rat had become so overwhelmingly involved that its life centred on drug use? Can such terms even be applied to laboratory rats? Addiction can only be studied in a Skinner box if it is defined in a simple, operational way that would be useless for human beings.[129] By the Skinner box definition, every diabetic is addicted to insulin, every assembly line worker is addicted to work, and every 'dry' Alcoholics Anonymous member who introduces himself or herself as an alcoholic is lying.

Other critical scholars suggested that opioid ingestion by laboratory animals could be understood as a way that the animals coped with social and sensory isolation that was imposed by the Skinner box itself. Laboratory rats are gregarious, curious, active creatures. Their ancestors, wild Norway rats, are intensely social and, despite generations of laboratory breeding, their albino descendants retain many of their social instincts. Therefore, it is conceivable that rats may self-administer powerful drugs simply as a response to stress when they are housed in isolated metal cages, subjected to surgical implantations, and tethered to a self-injection apparatus by a cannula implanted in their jugular veins. The results of self-injection experiments may show nothing more than that severely distressed animals, like severely distressed people,[130] will seek pharmacological relief if they can find it.

To determine whether the self-injection of opioids in these experiments could be something other than a sign of addiction, my colleagues Barry Beyerstein, Robert Coambs, and Patricia Hadaway and I carried out a series of experiments beginning in the late 1970s. Albino rats served as subjects and morphine—which is interchangeable with heroin for most human addicts—as the experimental drug. We put one group of rats in the most natural environment for rats that we could contrive in the laboratory. 'Rat Park', as it came to be called, was airy and spacious, with about 200 times the square footage of a standard laboratory cage. It was also scenic, with a peaceful, British Columbia forest painted on the plywood walls, and rat-friendly with empty tins, wood scraps, and other desiderata strewn about the floor. Finally, relative to the standard laboratory housing of its day, it was a psychosocial paradise, with 16–20 rats of both sexes in residence at once.

We compared the morphine consumption of Rat Park rats with that of rats housed in individual cages. For the individually caged rats, we fastened two drinking bottles, one containing a morphine solution and one containing water, on each cage and weighed them daily. In Rat Park, we built a short tunnel leading out of the residential area that was just large enough to accommodate one rat at a time. At the far end of the tunnel, the rats could release a fluid from either of two drop dispensers. One dispenser contained a morphine solution and the other an inert solution. The dispenser recorded how much each rat drank of each fluid.

A number of experiments were performed in this way,[131] most of which indicated that rats living in Rat Park had little appetite for morphine compared with the rats housed in isolation. In some experiments, we forced the rats in both groups to consume morphine for weeks before allowing them to choose so that there could be no doubt that they would develop withdrawal symptoms. In other experiments, we made the morphine solution so sweet that no rat could resist it, but we still found much less appetite for the morphine solution in the animals housed in Rat Park. Under some conditions, the rats in the cages consumed nearly 20 times as much morphine as those in Rat Park. Nothing that we tried instilled a strong appetite for morphine or produced anything that looked to us like addiction in the rats that were housed in our approximation of a normal environment.

These results have subsequently been replicated, extended, and analysed by other psychologists.[132] Therefore, the intense appetite of isolated experimental animals for opioid drugs in self-injection experiments does not prove that opioid drugs have an irresistibly addictive quality, even for rats. As shown earlier in this chapter, psychosocially integrated people ignore opioids, even when they are abundant in their environment. Even people who use opioids medically or recreationally rarely become addicted. The inhabitants of Rat Park appeared to be no less discriminating.

A myth cycle

One final important question remains concerning the myth of heroin as a demon drug. If heroin is not the irresistibly addictive drug that the myth portrays, why do millions of intelligent people, including recognised authorities and political leaders, believe that it is? Why do some of these people go to heroic lengths to convince others of their unfounded belief? Why do governments and media appear to ignore or even hide facts that contradict the myth? Scholars have suggested several historical factors that may well contribute to this phenomenon,[133] but this chapter focuses only on the one that is most directly relevant to free-market society. The stranger-than-fiction history of what is here labelled a 'myth cycle' shows how most people can be deceived about 'addictive' drugs most of the time, and why honest, intelligent people unwittingly take part in the deception. It may be difficult for people who have not studied the history of drugs over the last two centuries to believe this story. However, the facts are a matter of public record. They were first outlined in a classic work by Thomas Szasz in 1975[134] and updated in a 2006 book by Richard DeGrandpre.[135]

In the 19th and 20th centuries, several psychoactive drugs came to be seen, at various times, as magical happiness potions that could make people feel much better than they ordinarily do. This mythical view of certain drugs as pharmacological panaceas existed independently of the genuine utility of the same drugs in medical practice. Because each panacea seemed at first to relieve modern society's deepening poverty of the spirit, these marvels were eagerly embraced by unfulfilled people, welcomed by the governments of their day, and energetically merchandised by the drug companies. At various times, these highly publicised panaceas have included opium, morphine, heroin, cocaine, amphetamine, various synthetic opioids, the barbiturates, the 'tranquillisers', and a series of anti-depressants. For example, Sigmund Freud was one of several well-known public figures who took it as their duty to spread the good news about cocaine to the world, beginning in the 1880s. Upon first discovering cocaine's effects on himself and a few patients, Freud wrote to his future wife, 'I am just now busy collecting the literature for a song of praise to this magical substance.'[136] As Freud was a doctor, his 'song of praise' appeared in the form of an uncharacteristically lyrical article in a German medical journal.[137]

Each of the panaceas that seemed to relieve the malaise of life in free-market society eventually fell into disrepute. (This process may be just getting underway with the selective serotonin reuptake inhibitors or SSRI anti-depressants.[138]) The downfall of each pharmacological panacea came about because of an increasing awareness of the side effects that had been largely forgotten in the initial enthusiasm and because, apparently, there is no pharmacological antidote to poverty of the spirit.

When society eventually turns against its overrated panaceas, sometimes decades later, the rejection is often violent, like the casting-off of a false lover. Formerly overrated drugs come to be perceived as causes of addiction, brain damage, fetal damage, and criminality. Panaceas are transformed into scapegoats. Exaggerated scare stories about the new scapegoats serve to counteract the allure that they retain from the past. The myth of demon-drug possession re-energises with a vengeance at these times! A century after Sigmund Freud's song of praise for cocaine, cocaine was a drug that stood for everything bad, and above all, a cause of addiction. In the 1980s, governments, the pharmaceutical companies, doctors, and scientists were frantic in their condemnation of the former panacea, especially in its smokable form of 'crack', which was said to produce 'instant addiction'.[139]

The full myth cycle, however, goes one step beyond this. Governments, the pharmaceutical companies, and the general populace change their collective minds *three times.*[140] The first change establishes the myth that a particular drug is a panacea. The second change establishes the myth that the exact same drug is demonic and must be prohibited. The third change establishes that, despite their previous disappointments, a newly discovered happiness drug is a *true* panacea. The demonisation of cocaine in the 1990s was accompanied by the spectacular rise to prominence of a new class of panaceas that would make the population of free-market society feel 'better than normal'—the SSRI anti-depressants. When the myth cycle moves to the third stage, traffickers and users of discarded panaceas are punished and forced into treatment because by selling or using the demonic drug, they are proving themselves to be evil or sick, or both.

In each iteration of this cycle, the media and public-spirited citizens help first to spread the good news, then the bad news, then the new good news. People become genuinely excited by the promise of a new drug that can help them to feel better than normal, or whatever the slogan of the day may be. Their excitement is greatest when social conditions are most dismal, putting realistic ways of attaining happiness out of reach. When people turn against the former panaceas, they are genuinely terrified by the newly discovered side effects, which generally include addiction. They exaggerate the dangers of the former wonder drug in good faith, because they now fear it, not only for themselves, but for their children. The use of terrifying myths to alert children to danger is a widespread human practice, and not a bad one—if the danger is real.

In reality, however, the stories of demon drugs are just as mythical as the stories of drug panaceas. In every case, the drugs are being used to advantage by some people and ineffectually or harmfully by others, regardless of whether they were being glorified or demonised at the time. But mere facts have little influence when people's fondest hopes and darkest fears are manipulated by governments and drug companies hungry for power and profit. The pharmaceutical industry does not mind demonising some of their old products when they fall into disrepute, especially if they are no longer patentable, because they are able to sell very similar drugs with different names and fresh patents afterwards. They especially do not mind if people go to jail for selling their old drugs outside the legal market.

This cycle has repeated itself several times in the 19th and 20th centuries.[141] The most recent episode of the myth cycle, as this book nears completion, is the downfall of the drug OxyContin®. OxyContin® is a commercial preparation of the opioid oxycodone, discussed earlier in this chapter. OxyContin® is prepared with a time-release coating designed to slow its action, making it unsuitable for use by opioid addicts. However, 'experienced drug abusers and novices, including teenagers, soon discovered that chewing an OxyContin® tablet or crushing one and then snorting the powder, or injecting it with a needle produced a high as powerful as heroin.'[142]

Following society's violent rejection of a series of opioids (morphine, heroin, dolophine, and several synthetic opioids) that were first heralded and then fell into disrepute, Purdue Pharma, an American pharmaceutical company, introduced OxyContin® in 1996. The company contended that 'because of its time-release formulation, [OxyContin®] posed a lower threat of abuse and addiction to patients than do traditional faster-acting painkillers.'[143] This claim became 'the linchpin of the most aggressive marketing campaign ever undertaken by a pharmaceutical company for a narcotic painkiller. Just a few years after the drug's introduction in 1996, annual sales reached $1 billion.'[144] The company 'heavily promoted OxyContin® to doctors like general practitioners, who often had little training in treating serious pain or in recognizing signs of drug abuse'.[145] The next stage in this myth cycle was a growing number of complaints and lawsuits launched against Purdue Pharma in the United States. Eventually, 'skyrocketing rates of addiction and crime related to use of the drug'[146] were reported. In 2007, Purdue Pharma pleaded guilty in a United States court to the crime of 'misbranding' and the corporation was fined US$600 million. Three executives of the company were also fined for a total of US$34.5 million.[147] Will there be a new pharmaceutical wonder to replace OxyContin®? There are many indications that the dream of a pharmacological panacea is as strong today as ever,[148] and that the cycle will repeat yet again.

Conclusion

The myth of the pharmacological panacea and its counterpart, the myth of demon drugs, are still believed or half-believed by many serious people around the world, including some highly qualified researchers. Those who know better generally see no way to show their more credulous neighbours what is wrong with this thinking. However, good-natured indulgence of this myth cycle has serious costs.

Just as the myth of the pharmacological panacea distracts people from efforts that will truly increase their own happiness and the well-being of society at large, the myth of demon drugs exacerbates the addiction problem. By its power to dominate and confuse rational debate, it blocks the path towards more useful and badly needed knowledge. The myth of demon drugs, in both its strong forms and its watered-down forms, and the uncritical science that has grown up around it, constitute a great amorphous blob of pseudoknowledge that shields free-market society from the kind of scrutiny that could reveal its crucial role in the causation of dislocation and addiction.

The influence of deeply entrenched mythology cannot be ended easily by scholarship or research. It is possible to hope that it will one day be ended by a gifted comedian, who will find a way to show on global, prime-time television that the drug myths are not only disastrous, but also painfully, tragically, insanely funny.

Endnotes

1 There are also ancient superstitions about plants with magical powers to control people (DeGrandpre, 2006, Chapter 4) so the myth of demon drugs may have historically complex origins.

2 J. Edwards (1847, p. 37, as cited in Aaron and Musto, 1981, p. 144).

3 Kobler (1973, pp. 125, 127, 170–171); Aaron and Musto (1981).

4 Chenery (1890, pp. 167–168).

5 Aaron and Musto (1981, p. 147).

6 This literature has been reviewed by Lindesmith (1968, esp. pp. 109–112), Musto (1987, Chapter 2, especially p. 147), Schaler (2000), Hammersley and Reid (2002), and DeGrandpre (2006, Chapters 5 and 6). Psychiatrist Mark Gold (1984) promoted the modern form of this demon possession myth with particular fervour and authority for cocaine in the 1980s.

7 Mattison (1894, as cited in Lindesmith, 1968, p. 110). Lindesmith (1968) gives several other examples from this era on pp. 107–112.

8 E. Murphy (1922/1973); A. Goldstein (1979, p. 342); Washton (1989); Gawin (1991, pp. 1580–1581); Henningfield *et al.* (1991); Inciardi (1992, pp. 62, 246); Leshner (1997). Musto (1987, Chapter 11) has suggested that the authorities who circulate these stories do not necessarily believe them, but are acting out of a variety of motives, including a desire to control dangerous drug use, even if it must be at the expense of the truth.

9 J. B. Davies (1992, 1997), Hammersley and Reid (2002), and Dalrymple (2006a) have elaborated on this and other social functions that this myth serves. Some of the others will be discussed later in the chapter.

10 Gold (1984); Booth (1996, pp. 83, 85, 91, as cited in Sullum, 2003, p. 223); Leshner (1997); Drug Free America Foundation (2007). Sullum (2003, Chapter 1) also cited contemporary anti-drug crusaders who regard all drugs, including the opioids, alcohol, and marijuana as causing addiction. The most recent statements of the strong form of the demon-drug mythology are usually directed towards methamphetamine.

11 Lindesmith (1968, p. 3); Washton (1989, p. 57); Addiction Science Network (2000); McLellan *et al.* (2000); Courtwright (2002, p. 6); C. Chandler (2006). Babor *et al.* (2003, pp. 24–26) apply the watered-down form of the myth to alcohol.

12 Leshner (1997, p. 46).

13 Gawin (1991, pp. 1580–1581). Gawin's watered-down version of the demon-drug myth as applied to cocaine is essentially the same as Lindesmith's version of it as applied to heroin (Lindesmith, 1968, Chapters 4 and 5).

14 McLellan *et al.* (2000, p. 1693).

15 McLellan *et al.* (2000, p. 1691).

16 This phrase is taken from the title of a book by Babor *et al.* (2003).

17 It is true that there are some people who will predictably become addicted to drugs and should stay away from them (Maté, 2008, Chapter 12), but these unfortunate people are so dislocated that they are vulnerable to addiction to many non-drug pursuits as well. The fact that they are vulnerable to drug addiction does not result from any uniquely addictive powers of drugs.

18 The most solid argument for it in the case of heroin was perhaps given by Lindesmith (1968) and was based primarily on individual cases as interpreted by the junkies themselves and by their doctors. I will show later in this chapter why this evidence can now be disregarded.

19 The example of government suppression of which I have first-hand knowledge was the suppression by the United States Government of the World Health Organisation's international study of cocaine use that was completed in 1995 (S. T. Martin, 2001; DeGrandpre, 2006, Chapter 1). I was the principle investigator for the World Health Organisation in the Vancouver portion of the international study. Other examples directly involving heroin are discussed by Musto (1987, pp. 132–134).

20 Szasz (1975); Zinberg (1984); Khantzian (1985); Dalrymple (2006a, pp. 16–20).

21 Chein *et al.* (1964); Erickson and Alexander (1989); Peele (1989); Alexander (1990, 1994); P. Cohen and Sas (1993); Hammersley and Ditton (1994); Erickson *et al.* (1994); Mugford (1995); J. B. Davies (1997); Hando and Hall (1997); Klee (1997); Reinarman and Levine (1997); Granfield and Cloud (1999); Schaler (2000); Klingemann *et al.* (2001); Blomqvist (2004); Coomber and South (2004); Granfield (2004); Dalgarno and Shewan (2005); Shewan and Dalgarno (2005); Warburton *et al.* (2005); DeGrandpre (2006); Fish (2006).

22 Musto (1987). Although Musto wrote as if he assumed that heroin and cocaine cause addiction, he debunked some of the most powerful evidence against this claim, such as evidence against the claim that prescription of morphine during the American Civil War caused an outbreak of addiction (Chapter 1).

23 Trebach (1982, 1987).

24 Brecher (1972); Treaster (1992); Sullum (2003); Osborne (2005); Tierney (2005). Brecher (1972) thought that the demon-drug myth was true as applied to heroin, but untrue with respect to a number of other drugs that he investigated.

25 J. P. Morgan and Zimmer (1997a, 1997b); S. Siegel (n.d.).

26 These go back to the 19th century, notably the British Royal Commission on Opium of 1894–1895 and the *Indian Hemp Drugs Commission Report* of 1894. The newest at the time of writing was the *Report of the British Royal Society for the Encouragement of Arts, Manufactures and Commerce Commission on Illegal Drugs* (Press Association, 2007; Royal Society for the Encouragement of Arts, Manufactures and Commerce, 2007, see Summary, item #6, p. 2). See also Reuter and Stevens (2007).

27 For example, studies of self-administration of heroin by rats in Skinner boxes have been used to argue that heroin and cocaine are irresistible to rats, and, therefore, to all mammals (A. Goldstein, 1979, p. 342). The ability of cocaine and heroin to enhance the action of dopamine in the brain has been used to argue that exposure to these two drugs causes addiction (Leshner, 1997; Addiction Science Network, 1998, 2000).

28 Orford (2001a, pp. 208–214, 234–244); DeGrandpre (2006, Chapter 7).

29 Maté (2008, Chapter 21).

30 For simplicity, the antagonist branch of the family is left out of this account.

31 For most of these, morphine is the precursor molecule, but some are modifications of codeine or thebaine, also found in raw opium.

32 The similarities are not always obvious when structural formulas are examined visually, but chemists can see them (Perrine, 1996, p. 58).

33 I use this word in its collective sense to include the enkephalins and dynorphin.

34 Perrine (1996, p. 54).

35 Maté (2008, Chapter 14).

36 Shewan *et al.* (1998, esp. pp. 220, 222); Shewan and Dalgarno (2005, esp. p. 38); Fischer *et al.* (2006b).

37 Perrine (1996, Chapter 1); Meier (2007).

38 Heroin is available by prescription in many countries, including Canada and the UK. It is totally prohibited in the United States.

39 I am bypassing the famous 'rush' of injected or smoked drugs because it has little effect on addiction per se (Alexander, 1990).

40 In addition, there is a sigma receptor to which some opioids bind. However, when opioids bind only to the sigma receptor, none of the psychological responses normally associated with opioid drugs are induced (Perrine, 1996, pp. 56–57).

41 Lindesmith (1968, pp. 39–40); Ledain (1973, p. 308).

42 Ledain (1973, p. 309).

43 Brecher (1972, Chapter 1).

44 T. M. Hickman (2004).

45 Alsop (1974); Health and Welfare Canada (1984); Musto (1987, Chapter 1); D. E. Weissman and Haddox (1989); Porter-Williamson *et al.* (2003).

46 DeGrandpre (2006, Chapter 4); Musto (2002, p. xv);.

47 Courtwright (2002); Musto (2002).

48 N. Boyd (1984); Carstairs (2006, Chapter 1). In Canada, these ulterior motives also included efforts by the medical profession to suppress the patent medicine industry, as many of the popular patent medicines contained heroin (Murray, 1988).

49 Musto (1987).

50 Musto (1987, Chapter 2).

51 Silver and Aldrich (1979) have provided a useful compendium of newspaper accounts of this florid propaganda in the United States. Similar images were popularised in Canada in a series of articles and a book by Emily Murphy (1922/1973).

52 The similarity of language used to describe drunkards and drug fiends is easily seen by comparing Charles Dickens' (1833–1835/1994, pp. 463–47) *The Drunkard's Death* to Emily Murphy's (1922/1973) *The Black Candle*.

53 Brecher (1972, Chapters 2, 3).

54 Brecher (1972); Musto (1987, pp. 69–77); Alexander (1990, Chapter 1); DeGrandpre (2006).

55 DeGrandpre (2006, Chapter 5)

56 Alexander (1990, Chapter 6) summarised the literature on acetylsalicylic acid addiction.

57 During the decades of the mid-20th century when heroin was exclusively understood as a drug of addiction in the United States and Canada, it was used safely and beneficially as a prescription medicine in the UK (Trebach, 1982).

58 DeGrandpre (2006, Chapter 4) argued convincingly that heroin was actually made more addicting for medical users by the 'placebo text' that was being circulated in the mass media, which convinced people that they could not overcome withdrawal symptoms once they were established.

59 D.E. Smith and Gay (1972).

60 This is easily confirmed by search on Google™ for the words 'heroin' and 'orgasmic' together.

61 Cited in Beecher (1959, p. 334).

62 Beecher (1959, Chapters 10 and 14); G. M. Smith and Beecher (1959, 1962a).

63 G. M. Smith and Beecher (1962b).

64 Westermeyer (1982, pp. 165–166).

65 Oswald (1969, p. 438).

66 Zhukovsky *et al.* (2000); Meier (2007); T. McLaughlin (2007).

67 Fischer *et al.* (2006b).

68 Chein *et al.* (1964, pp. 157–158); Ledain (1973, p. 307).

69 McAuliffe (1975).

70 G. M. Smith and Beecher (1962a).

71 Alexander and Dibb (1977); Gosline (2007).

72 Dalrymple (2006a, pp. 122–139).

73 Ledain (1973, p. 318).

74 Lindesmith (1968, pp. 38–39); Primm and Bath (1973); DeGrandpre (2006, Chapters 4 and 7). See also Gay *et al.* (1974) who describe 'pseudo-addicts' who live the junkie lifestyle but do not choose to use enough heroin to produce withdrawal symptoms.

75 Lindesmith (1968, pp. 38–39).

76 Musto (1987).

77 Jaffe (1985, p. 534); Henningfield *et al.* (1991, p. 567).

78 DeGrandpre (2006, Chapter 2).
79 Gawin (1991, p. 1580).
80 DeGrandpre (2006, Chapter 4).
81 Schug *et al.* (1991).
82 Marlatt (1985b, c).
83 Warburton *et al.* (2005).
84 Warburton *et al.* (2005).
85 Robins *et al.* (1975).
86 T. E. Robinson and Berridge (2001, pp. 108–109).
87 Lindesmith (1968, p. 3); Hunt and Chambers (1976); Anthony *et al.* (1994); McLellan *et al.* (2000, p. 1693).
88 This is documented at some length in Chapter 7 under the heading *Dislocated people are more likely to become addicted.*
89 Brecher (1972, Chapter 1).
90 The exact percentage cannot be known, and the 0.5% figure, although widely cited, is an educated guess based on a hodgepodge of scattered records summarized in historical sources such as Brecher (1972), Ledain (1973), and Courtwright (1982). See T. M. Hickman (2004) for a more recent, authoritative discussion of this issue.
91 Yi-Mak and Harrison (2001, p. 48); Dikötter *et al.* (2004, Chapter 4).
92 Westermeyer (1982); Ganguly (2004).
93 Trebach (1982, p. 83).
94 Gossop and Keaney (2004).
95 White *et al.* (1991).
96 Bennett *et al.* (1982).
97 Schug *et al.* (1991).
98 J. S. Blackwell (1982); Zinberg (1984); Treaster (1992); Shewan and Dalgarno (2005).
99 Zinberg (1984, p. 71).
100 The authors attributed this low re-interview rate to the confidentiality requirements of the study. They kept no records of their participants' whereabouts but relied on 18 participants in the experiment as contacts. Two of these participant contacts left the country in the interval between the first and second interviews: one took a job abroad; the other, a soldier, moved abroad with the armed forces. In addition, some of the other participant contacts lost track of their contacts (Shewan and Dalgarno, 2005, p. 36).
101 See Gossop *et al.* (1995). This five-item scale could be construed either as an index of 'dependence' or as an index of addiction₃ as these terms are defined in Chapter 2.
102 Warburton *et al.* (2005); McSweeney and Turnbull (2007).
103 Warburton *et al.* (2005, p. 4). For more detailed analyses, see Lindesmith (1968); Hunt and Chambers (1976); Anthony *et al.* (1994); Makkai and McAllister (1998, p. 45); McLellan *et al.* (2000, p. 1693).
104 Burroughs (1967, as cited in Lindesmith, 1968, p. 171). For other testimonials to the myth of demon drugs, see Brecher (1972) and Courtwright *et al.* (1989, Chapter 3).
105 E. Murphy (1922/1973); Lindesmith (1968); Brecher (1972, Chapter 10).
106 Published accounts of clinical investigations that contradict this component of the myth of demon drugs are discussed in Chapter 7 under the heading *People use their addictions to adapt to dislocation.* In addition, Shewan and Dalgarno (2005, p. 44) provide evidence

against this component in data that was gathered for a different purpose on the attributions of causes of heroin use given by light heroin users and heavy heroin users.

107 Pryor (2003); Blomqvist (2004).

108 Pryor (2003) points out that wealthy families may take it as their social obligation to create an illusion of harmony that conceals deep dysfunction. See also Alexander and Dibb (1975).

109 Simmons (2002); Pryor (2003).

110 Luthar (2003).

111 Pryor (2003).

112 Erikson (1968, p. 88).

113 The appeal of this mystique to junkies quickly becomes evident in face-to-face contact with them. It has been described by Chein *et al.* (1964, p. 216), Lindesmith (1968, pp. 100–103), Gay *et al.* (1974), and Dalrymple (2006a, Chapter 2), and mentioned in passing by Hammersley and Reid (2002, pp. 23–24). It is shown in a negative way by Warburton *et al.*(2005, p. 29) who point out that heroin users who do not become addicted even after many years of daily, or near daily, use reject the junkie identity. See Chapter 7 under the heading *People use their addictions to adapt to dislocation.*

114 Pryor (2003).

115 See also Laurance (2006).

116 J. B. Davies (1992, 1997); Hammersley and Reid (2002); Dalrymple (2006a).

117 J. B. Davies (1992).

118 This way of looking at the psychology of shame was elaborated by Cook (1991) and others.

119 Hammersley and Reid (2002).

120 For example, Lindesmith (1968) uses this phrase with approval.

121 Winick (1962); Robins and Murphy (1967); Pattison *et al.* (1977, Chapter 6); Zinberg *et al.* (1978); J. S. Blackwell (1982); S. Schachter (1982); Vaillant (1983); Biernacki (1986); Alexander and Schweighofer (1988); Granfield and Cloud (1999); Klingemann *et al.* (2001); Cloud and Granfield (2004); Blomqvist (2004); Öjesjö (2004); Warburton *et al.* (2005).

122 Musto (1987, p. 279 endnote 2).

123 Musto (1987, pp. 1–2, p. 279 endnote 2).

124 T. M. Hickman (2004).

125 Musto (1987, pp. 1–2).

126 J. H. Woods (1978).

127 A. Goldstein (1979, p. 342).

128 Kowal (1999).

129 The invalidity of this operational definition has now been acknowledged by some psychopharmacology researchers (T. E. Robinson, 2004).

130 D. E. Weissman and Haddox (1989); Porter-Williamson *et al.* (2003).

131 For a more detailed summary of the experiments and their results, see Alexander *et al.* (1985). For an example of an individual study, see Alexander *et al.* (1981).

132 Not all of the following replications were successful, but the majority were: Petrie (1985); Schenk *et al.* (1987); Bozarth *et al.* (1989); Shaham *et al.* (1992). See also L. Slater (2004, Chapter 7).

133 As examples, see Gusfield (1963), Bulych and Beyerstein (1989), Beyerstein and Hadaway (1990), and Chomsky (1998).

134 Szasz (1975).

135 DeGrandpre (2006).

136 As quoted in Brecher (1972, p. 273).

137 Freud (1884, as translated in Byck, 1974).

138 DeGrandpre (2006).

139 Gold (1984); Alexander (1992); Reinarman and Levine (1997).

140 There is a huge literature on the unscrupulous means used by pharmaceutical companies to control governments, science, and public opinion for their own enrichment. See for example Szasz (1975), Healy (2003), Motluk (2004), Lippman (2005), and DeGrandpre (2006, Chapter 1).

141 Szasz (1975); DeGrandpre (2006).

142 Meier (2007, p. 2). See also T. McLaughlin (2007).

143 Meier (2007, p. 1).

144 Meier (2007, pp. 1–2).

145 Meier (2007, p. 2).

146 Meier (2007, p. 2).

147 Meier (2007).

148 For an expression of this dream in a recent popular science magazine, see Elie (2007).

Part 2

The Interaction of Addiction and Society

Part I of this book showed that the current globalisation of addiction is largely the result of people adapting to the globalisation of free-market society. However, addiction is surely a *cause* as well as an effect of today's social reality. How could a multitude of addicted people fail to shape and colour their world? How could mass addiction fail to exacerbate society's other problems? How could addicted individuals fail to create more dislocation and, thus, a vicious cycle? Part II considers, most basically, whether the current spread of addiction can be tolerated as a manageable side effect of civilised progress or whether—as I have come to believe—it is the manifestation of a crippling and unendurable poverty of the spirit.

Part II takes the dislocation theory of addiction as given, and uses it as a tool to analyse the complex interrelationship between addiction and society. As well as today's society, two earlier periods of widespread dislocation in Western civilisation will be included in the analysis: the period just before the collapse of the Athenian Empire around 400 BC and the period just before the collapse of the Western Roman Empire around 400 AD. The interaction of addiction and society in every era of extreme dislocation involves not only people whose addictions are easily identified (Chapter 9), but also those whose addictive dynamics are masked by other conspicuous features (Chapter 10), and even those who have mastered dislocation well enough to become models of success and happiness (Chapter 11). The phrase 'addictive dynamics' is used throughout Part II to refer to people's ways of finding addictive substitutes for psychosocial integration, whether or not their dislocation is publicly visible, and whether or not their addiction is severe enough to be recognised as such. It is possible that large numbers of slightly addicted people could have a greater destructive impact on society than smaller numbers of severely addicted people.

Addiction shapes not only social life, but spiritual and secular philosophy as well. The attempts of the Roman world to comprehend addiction through Christian and other forms of spirituality have become embedded in today's conventional wisdom on addiction (Chapters 9 and 12) with some beneficial consequences and some detrimental ones. On the other hand, Socrates' comprehensive analysis of the reciprocal relationship between addiction, society, and human nature, written 24 centuries ago (Chapter 13), is currently being ignored. Part II will show why Socratic wisdom on this topic is important now.

For the last two centuries, conventional wisdom has limited public understanding of addiction to an individual problem of alcohol and drug use. This misrepresentation has kept today's scholars futilely searching for a technological fix somewhere in the individual brain or genome, today's spiritual leaders focused on individual spiritual interventions that have been demonstrating their worth—but also their limitations—for millennia, and today's politicians vainly trying to solve the problem by purging the world of drugs. It has kept people who experience addictive problems from understanding the broader context of their personal suffering. A full comprehension of addiction as a problem of modernity can point society towards fresh approaches. The last two chapters, Chapters 14 and 15, sketch some of these out.

Chapter 9

Addiction and Society

This chapter explores the complex interrelationship of addiction and dislocated societies using five addicted people in three different societies as examples. Two of these addicted people are historical figures. I know the other three personally. All five have used their addictions to adapt to their own dislocation. The two historical figures have had universally recognised impacts on society that were unmistakably shaped by their addictions. The impacts of the three living addicted people cannot yet be known, but their lives illustrate some diverse ways in which addiction may shape and colour society in an era of mass dislocation.

The first addicted person in this chapter is St Augustine of Hippo, a renowned father of the Roman Catholic Church, as well as history's first documented love and sex addict. The second is Sir James M. Barrie, whose account of his own addiction to children and childish fantasy, personified in Peter Pan, has charmed audiences for over a century. Of the remaining three, one is a former crystal methamphetamine addict who is putting his life back together, one is a recently graduated honours student who feels addicted 'to herself', and one is an engineer and single father who spent most of his career in the military before taking up civilian employment and grappling with a terrifying addictive complex.

St Augustine: addiction in the last days of the Roman Empire

Aurelius Augustinus, a Roman born in 354 AD, is known to history as St Augustine of Hippo. Beyond his leadership as a bishop and his brilliant theological writings, St Augustine is famous for his amazingly frank descriptions of his own early life. His best-known book, *Confessions*,[1] describes his utterly dislocated childhood in a disintegrating empire, his agonising inner struggles with severe addictions both to love and to worldly success, and his recovery through conversion to Catholic Christianity.

St Augustine described his own addictions on two levels: first, as understandable human responses to a world of dislocation, and, secondly, as abominable sins against God. In the process of analysing his struggles, St Augustine created major foundation stones of Christian thinking, and, thereby, of all Western thought. St Augustine's ideas remain a powerful influence within today's conventional wisdom on addiction and within global philosophy in general.

A dislocated world

Centuries before St Augustine was born, the Roman Republic had been an efficient and prosperous society, bound together by a rational legal system and a rigid code of military honour. Under the emperors, however, Imperial Rome gradually lost these stern virtues. The late Roman Empire of St Augustine's day was hell on earth. On the eve of its final collapse, Roman society was fractured by incessant civil wars, barbarian invasions, gruesome mass executions, brutal slavery, ubiquitous secret police, institutionalised torture, religious intolerance, brutalising entertainment (the gladiatorial games), and base corruption at the highest levels of authority.[2] Although collapse was imminent, there were no alternative political models to provide hope or inspiration, for the civilised world was entirely Romanized. Beyond the Imperial borders lay only empty sea, endless dessert, black forest, and the dreaded barbarians.

Roman Christians sensed the danger and predicted the end of the world in the mystical language of their religion. In an important sense, they were right. After St Augustine's death, the Western Roman Empire was trampled and pulverised by the Four Horsemen of the Apocalypse. The world they had known had, indeed, ended.

Although the collapsing Roman Empire was in no sense a free-market society, its prolonged descent into chaos created profound mass dislocation. St Augustine described the Romans of his day as follows:

> … always rolling, with dark fear and cruel lust, in warlike slaughters and in blood, which, whether shed in civil or foreign war, is still human blood; so that their joy may be compared to glass in its fragile splendour, of which one is horribly afraid lest it should be suddenly broken in pieces.[3]

His descriptions of extreme dislocation were by no means limited to those directly exposed to military violence, slavery, or poverty, but encompassed the free, well-to-do citizens as well. He described the breakdown of intimate social life as follows:

> On all hands we experience these slights, suspicions, quarrels, war, all of which are undoubted evils; while, on the other hand, peace is a doubtful good, because we do not know the heart of our friend, and though we did know it to-day, we should be as ignorant of what it might be to-morrow. Who ought to be, or who are more friendly than those who live in the same family? And yet who can rely even upon this friendship, seeing that secret treachery has often broken it up, and produced enmity as bitter as amity was sweet, or seemed sweet by the most perfect dissimulation? … If, then, home, the natural refuge from the ills of life, is itself not safe, what shall we say of the city, which, as it is larger, is so much the more filled with lawsuits civil and criminal, and is never free from the fear, if sometimes from the actual outbreak, of disturbing and bloody insurrections and civil wars?[4]

It was not only Christians who sensed that their souls were under siege in the chaos of the late Roman Empire. Secular philosophers like Stoics and Neo-Platonists also lamented the anguish of the Roman soul and proposed remedies in their own, non-Christian terms.[5]

Beyond his observations of collapsing Roman society, St Augustine recounted his personal dislocation and misery.[6] He grew up in a North African colony, whose rulers were puppets of a distant Roman state. In an age where people fought to the death over matters of theology, his mother and father were so fundamentally at odds in religious belief that he had to take sides, repudiating his father.[7] He was cruelly beaten by his masters at school for his intellectual independence. He left the security of his provincial homeland early to pursue a prestigious career as a rhetorician in the cosmopolitan cities of Rome and Milan. He soon became aware that rhetoric was itself corrupt, because rhetoricians, including himself, achieved the greatest rewards by lavishing praise on degenerate emperors. Before becoming a staunch Roman Catholic, St Augustine was a Christian Manichaean and he also explored other sects and philosophies, each of which viewed the others as heretical.[8] Both his father and his best friend died when he was in his twenties. After being domestically settled for 15 years with his common-law wife, whom he dearly loved, he felt so pressured by his mother and by his own ambitions for wealth and status that he sent his beloved away in order to undertake a more religiously and socially appropriate marriage. Rather than converting and marrying immediately, however, he exploded into furious promiscuity. Shortly after he finally converted and achieved celibacy, both his mother and his son by his common-law wife died. He did not complete the marriage that his mother had arranged, but retreated from the world in celibacy and seclusion with a few Christian philosophers. He then returned to his home city in North Africa where he was called to serve the Church as a priest and bishop at Hippo, a nearby port city. At the time of his death, Hippo was besieged by Barbarians, who would soon lay waste to the city—a routine tragedy in the collapsing Roman world. To say the least, St Augustine was exposed to more than his share of 'risk factors' for addiction.

Beyond circumstantial evidence of his dislocation, St Augustine's writing exposes his impoverished inner life through the incessant, tearful self-abasement that fills his written prayers. In one prayer, for example, he describes himself to God thus:

> … when my groaning bears evidence that I am displeased with myself, you [God] shine out on me and are pleasing and loved and longed for, so that I am ashamed of myself and renounce myself and chose you and, except in you, can please neither you nor myself.[9]

In modern times, universal dislocation is accompanied by near-universal addiction. St Augustine's writings indicate that this was equally true in his times. He vividly described addictions to love, worldly success, wine, gladiatorial games, food, friendship, music, pseudoscientific intellectuality, and other pursuits among the inhabitants of his dislocated world. He gave colour to his descriptions by enlisting himself and his friends as prime examples, often presenting himself as a pathetic, tearful sinner, begging God for help in overcoming his addictive sins. He observed that all earthly pleasures can become uncontrollable distractions from religious life, and preached that all must therefore be renounced in order to achieve a redeeming and fulfilling personal relationship with God.

Confessions of a sex and love addict

St Augustine centred his book, *Confessions*,[10] on his personal addictive cravings for sex and love, which he saw as the final obstacles (along with worldly ambition) to his conversion.[11] He movingly described the inner void that his early sexual enthusiasms filled and the short-term joy that they gave him. However, he also described the jealous anguish of his dysfunctional attachments, the inconsistent feeling of being out of control at some times but not at others, and the misery that irrepressible craving caused him long after he became celibate. He found it necessary to turn from excessive indulgence to complete abstinence. In short, his descriptions are strikingly similar to the reports of contemporary sex and love addicts.[12]

He described the inner void that his sex addiction filled for him as a young man as follows:

> I was starved inside me for inner food…. And for this reason my soul was in poor health; it burst out into feverish spots which brought the wretched longing to be scratched by contact with objects of sense…. It was a sweet thing to me both to love and to be loved, and more sweet still when I was able to enjoy the body of my lover.[13]

St Augustine explicitly described the dysfunctional suffering of his overheated love life, again in a way that is reminiscent of contemporary sex and love addicts. In fact, he thanked God for imposing so much suffering on his love life, for otherwise he might not have been able to achieve celibacy, an indispensable step in his religious conversion:[14]

> Desiring to be captivated in this way, I fell headlong into love. My God and my mercy, how good you were to me in sprinkling so much bitterness over that sweetness! For I was loved myself, and I reached the point where we met together to enjoy our love, and there I was fettered happily in bonds of misery so that I might be beaten with rods of red-hot iron—the rods of jealousy and suspicions, and fears and angers and quarrels.[15]

Using only the austere language of a churchman, St Augustine managed to reveal his extreme involvement with sexual excess. He discreetly describes an incident from a period of wild promiscuity as follows, leaving the reader to imagine the details:

> Once when your solemnities were being celebrated within the walls of your Church, I actually dared to desire and then to bring to a conclusion a business which deserved death for its reward. For this you lashed me with punishments that were heavy, but nothing in comparison with my fault … [16]

In a calmer moment, on the eve of his conversion, St Augustine found that his needs for sex and love were concentrated on his common-law wife, to whom he was bound in faithful, mutual devotion:

> But I was still closely bound by my need of woman …. I lacked the strength and … because of this one thing everything else with me was in confusion; I was tired out and wasted away with gnawing anxieties, because I was compelled to put up with all sorts of things which I did not want simply because they were inseparable from that state of living with a wife to which I was utterly and entirely bound.[17]

As he struggled to put aside his wife, he found himself in long inner dialogues with his sexual fantasies, which he described with both retroactive horror and pious euphemism:

> Toys and trifles, utter vanities had been my mistresses, and now they were holding me back, pulling me by the garment of my flesh and softly murmuring in my ear: 'Are you getting rid of us?' and … 'From this moment will you never for all eternity be allowed to do this or to do that?' My God, what was it, what was it that they suggested in those words 'this' or 'that' which I have just written? I pray you in your mercy to keep such things from the soul of your servant.[18]

After St Augustine converted and became chaste, he discovered the torture of craving, which extended into his dreams throughout the remainder of his long life, and he found it natural to medicalise this craving as one of the 'sicknesses of my soul':

> Almighty God, surely your hand is powerful enough to cure all the sicknesses of my soul and, with a more abundant measure of thy grace, to quench even the lustful impulses of my sleep. Lord, you will increase your gifts in me more and more, so that my soul … may follow me to you; so that it may not revolt against itself and may not, even in dreams, succumb to … those degrading corruptions which by means of sensual images actually disturb and pollute the flesh.[19]

Like many contemporary addicts, St Augustine was torn on the topic of whether or not his sexual addiction was 'out of control'. As a Christian, he had to believe that all evil was caused by free will. If heredity or environment had a causal role, the evil of addiction would have a natural cause. But if the proximal cause was nature, the ultimate cause must be the Divine Creator of nature—a blasphemous thought. Therefore, St Augustine had to experience his addictive sexuality as under the control of his own free will. However, he often experienced himself either as out of control completely or as under the control of a dark force, which he sometimes called 'the enemy'. His writing on this topic is intellectually brilliant, but uncharacteristically tortuous and confusing.[20] For example:

> … I was held back [from conversion to Christianity] not by fetters put on me by someone else, but by the iron bondage of my own will. The enemy held my will and made a chain out of it and bound me with it. From a perverse will came lust, and slavery to lust became a habit, and the habit being constantly yielded to, became a necessity. These were like links, hanging each to each … and they held me fast in a hard slavery. And the new will which I was beginning to have and which urged me to worship you in freedom and to enjoy you, God, the only certain joy, was not yet strong enough to overpower the old will which by its oldness had grown hard in me. So my two wills, one old, one new, one carnal, one spiritual, were in conflict, and they wasted my soul by their discord.[21]

St Augustine never succeeded in explaining the cause of his own addictions in a lucid way. His more theological analyses of the question of free will in general[22] were as murky as his self-analysis.[23] Often, as in the preceding quotation, he described himself as having two wills, or a conflicting will and habit.[24] Thus, today's inconsistency about whether or not addiction is 'out of control' has ancient, Christian roots that are tangled in theological issues. Moreover, millennia of abstract philosophical debate concerning free will and determinism have roots in arguments that St Augustine laid out as a way of analysing his experience as an addict.

Confessions of addiction to worldly success

After sex and love, St Augustine's most significant addiction was his feverish pursuit of worldly success as a rhetorician. His confession of this addiction parallels self-reports of contemporary work addicts.[25] Although he did achieve wealth and fame as a teacher of rhetoric and a public intellectual, he recognised the addictive quality of this career and dramatised it by comparing himself, unfavourably, to a drunken beggar:

> It was on a day when I was preparing a speech to be delivered in praise of the emperor; there would be a lot of lies in the speech, and they would be applauded by those who knew that they were lies. My heart was all wrought up with the worry of it all and was boiling in a kind of fever of melting thoughts. I was going along one of the streets of Milan when I noticed a poor beggar; he was fairly drunk, I suppose, and was laughing and enjoying himself. It was a sight which depressed me, and I spoke to the friends who were with me about all the sorrows which come to us because of our own madness. I thought of how I was toiling away, spurred on by my desires and dragging after me the load of my unhappiness and making it all the heavier by dragging it, and it seemed to me that the goal of this and all such endeavours was simply to reach a state of happiness that was free from care; the beggar had reached this state before us, and we, perhaps, might never reach it at all. With the few pennies that he had managed to beg he had actually obtained what I, by so many painful turns and such devious ways, was struggling to reach—namely, the joy of a temporary happiness.
>
> No doubt the beggar's joy was not true joy; but it was a great deal truer than the joy which I, with my ambition, was seeking. And undoubtedly he was happy while I was worried; he was carefree while I was full of fears. And if I were asked which I would prefer, to be merry or to be frightened, I should reply 'to be merry.' But if I were asked next whether I would prefer to be a man like the beggar or a man like I then was myself, I should choose to be myself, worn out as I was with my cares and my fears. Was not this absurd? Was there any good reason for making such a choice? For I had no right to put myself in front of the beggar on the grounds that I was more learned than he, since I got no joy out of my learning....
>
> So I will not allow my soul to listen to those who say to her: 'The difference is in the source of a man's happiness. That beggar found his joy in being drunk, you were looking for your joy in winning glory.' What glory, Lord? A glory that was not in you. For just as the beggar's joy was not true joy, so my glory was not true glory. Moreover it had a worse effect on my mind. The beggar would sleep off his drunkenness that very night; but I had gone to bed with mine and woken up with it day after day after day and I should go on doing so. Certainly it makes a difference what is the source of a man's happiness. I know it does. And the joy of a faithful hope is incomparably beyond all such vanity. Yes, and so was the beggar then beyond me; without any doubt he was the happier, not only because he was drenched in merriment while I eaten up with anxieties, but also because he by wishing people good luck had got some wine for himself while I by lying was seeking for an empty bubble of praise.[26]

Although St Augustine was not tempted by alcohol addiction, there were many other addictive pleasures that he felt he could only resist because of God's grace. These included the attractions of passionate (but non-sexual) friendships with men and of food.[27] Another almost-irresistible pleasure for him was Ptolemaic astronomy, a useful and highly sophisticated science in his day, although it was eventually superseded by modern astronomy.[28] St Augustine was a man of extraordinary intelligence who, in his state of dislocation, might easily have become overwhelmingly involved with the grand intellectual designs of science, as many contemporary scientists have.[29] He expressed his horror at this danger rhetorically, referring to science as 'the lust of the eyes',[30] and elaborating on his fear that love of science could draw him from God.

He laid the foundation for an opposition between Church and science that has coloured much of Western history.

Addiction as sin

St Augustine believed that all possible objects of worldly pleasure led to unhappiness, because they led to addictive craving but were apt to disappear when they were most needed. Therefore, in a strictly pragmatic, secular sense, he thought addiction to any worldly pleasure was ruinous to happiness on earth.[31] This was an accurate reflection on an historical period of universal dislocation in which unrelenting crime, state persecutions, disease, civil war, invasion, and so on made any source of addictive solace utterly unreliable.

However, addiction was much more than just a mistaken lifestyle choice for St Augustine. He expressed the deeper tragedy in theological language. Addiction was a fatal distraction from lifelong communion with God in favour of pleasures of the flesh. Addiction, for St Augustine, was equivalent to voluntarily forsaking God, a revolting sin and abomination. A similar moralism can be discerned in the supercharged rhetoric of the 19th-century Christian-dominated temperance movement and some anti-drug movements of today.[32] The phrase 'besetting sin' is still used interchangeably with 'addiction' by some contemporary Christians.[33] A besetting sin is a powerful compulsion[34] that besets a particular person. Other people may find no attraction to it, although they may be beset by sins of their own.

Of course, modern moralistic intolerance of drug addiction cannot be attributed directly to the influence of St Augustine's words, written 16 centuries ago. Yet it would seem that St Augustine and other early Christians broke a theological trail by classifying addiction as an object of righteous condemnation as well as compassionate pity, and that this trail has felt natural for some later Christians to follow at times, like ours, when addiction has reappeared as a menacing problem. St Augustine is part of the reason that today's conventional wisdom on addiction is as much about moralism as scientific medicine. Anti-alcohol and anti-drug moralism are often called 'Puritanism' today, but their Christian origins are far older than the actual Puritan movement that sprang from the Protestant Reformation.

I believe that there is deep wisdom within St Augustine's understanding of addiction, in addition to its dangerous moralism. St Augustine explicitly documented his personal dislocation as well as the universal dislocation of the collapsing Roman Empire in which he lived and showed how addiction functioned to fill the void. He acknowledged the fleeting pleasure that he had found in his addictive pursuits in his early life, and dwelt at great length on the misery that resulted from these earthly pleasures in the long run—as it must, if addictions are only overworked substitutes for psychosocial integration. St Augustine insisted that alcohol and drug use were no more addicting than other pleasurable pursuits. He insisted, on principle, that he was never out of control in his periods of severe addiction, although he also revealed that he felt out of control at times. Like many addicted people, St Augustine testified that he was able to find lasting earthly happiness only in a life of complete abstinence. Even when abstinent, he was still subject to strong cravings, and he recognised that he was still addicted.

Despite the dangerous moralism that it can incite, I believe there is important wisdom St Augustine's theological revulsion towards addiction. Whereas history has proven that moralistic cruelty and self-righteousness do more harm than good as a solution to addiction, *understating* the tragedy of addiction is not productive either. For St Augustine, addiction could never be simply a disease that the doctor could cure or a suboptimal lifestyle choice to be avoided wherever possible. Rather, addiction involved forsaking that which is most worthwhile in life in the futile pursuit of trivial pleasures. For St Augustine, this meant forsaking communion with God. For the dislocation theory of addiction, addiction entails forsaking psychosocial integration. Although they are worlds apart metaphysically, these two ways of looking at addiction are fundamentally similar, because the meanings of 'communion with God' and 'psychosocial integration' overlap substantially in this context. St Augustine's conversion was a spiritual transformation, but it did not isolate him in an exclusive tête-à-tête with God. Rather, it immersed him in the affairs of a thriving Christian community. Within 5 years of his conversion, he had become a popular priest and bishop, integrated in the social world of his city. Correspondingly, according to the dislocation theory, psychosocial integration stands for much more than outward social interaction because the members of functioning societies reinforce a shared sense of inner purpose, identity, belonging, and meaning in each other.

Although many aspects of St Augustine's thought fit well with the analysis of addiction in this book, his theology contradicts it at points. St Augustine did not believe that human beings could ever enjoy any earthly pleasures in a wholesome, non-addictive way, not even the pleasures of faithful mutual love! He did not regard widespread addictive sin as the product of particularly dislocated earthly societies like his and ours, but as the invariant human weakness since the expulsion of Adam—and thus of all mankind—from the Garden of Eden.[35] St Augustine's theology also contradicts the dislocation theory because, whereas the dislocation theory readily envisions an addictive form of Christian faith, St Augustine could never envision *too much* devotion to God. These aspects of his thinking continue to perplex the issue of addiction in modern times.

However, St Augustine's account of addictive sinfulness has rung true to countless people across the centuries, and many aspects of it fit comfortably within the dislocation theory of addiction. The religious conversion that ultimately subdued his addictions provided the model of recovery from addiction that is still used by many Christians, and his thinking led to major principles of addiction treatment that remain influential in secular treatment.[36] Chapter 12 of this book will show that, whereas St Augustine's descriptions of addiction have not lost their timeless resonance, his solutions have, unfortunately, proved insufficient for the addictive problems of this era.

James M. Barrie

James M. Barrie was a Scottish author of popular articles, novels, and plays in the late 19th and early 20th centuries. His masterpiece, *Peter Pan*, was introduced on the London stage in 1904 to immediate acclaim, and soon became a classic. Although both

Peter Pan and Barrie's own life story are often served up as sugary confections in today's global popular culture, Barrie was a serious writer with a mission. Beneath the sweet fluff, even *Peter Pan* is full of protein.[37] Much as St Augustine translated his personal addictive story into serious theology, Barrie translated his addictive story into meaningful art, including an enduring myth that shapes the minds of children throughout the world today.[38]

The parallels between the addictive dynamics of the fictional Peter Pan and the real-life James M. Barrie are striking. Peter Pan could not bear to face the responsibilities and conflicts of adult life, so he remained overwhelmingly involved with Never Land forever. Although Barrie, as a popular author, was careful not to let tragic overtones spoil the magic of his story, he explicitly identified Peter as a lost soul who was incapable of understanding his own tragedy.[39] Reworkings of the story in today's popular culture tend to bury Peter's addictive tragedy more deeply than Barrie himself did, or leave it out entirely.

Like the fictional Peter Pan, the real James M. Barrie was terrified of adulthood and did not grow up in some important ways. At least three powerful addictions provided him with substitutes for mature psychosocial integration. The best known was his overwhelming involvement with children and childish fantasy. Of the other two addictions that will be discussed in this chapter, one made him rich and the other may have killed him. He documented his addictions in exquisite detail in his personal notebooks, his autobiographical fiction, and in the story of Peter Pan. As with Peter Pan, the tragic, addictive component of Barrie's life can be either emphasised, as it is in this chapter, or sugar-coated, as it often is in popular culture.

Barrie's biographers have shown that it is a mistake to pathologise Barrie as a paedophile, as some popular writers have. It would be no less mistaken to pathologise him as an addict. However, addiction is not a pathology, but rather a widespread way of adapting to dislocated societies like our own and like Barrie's turn-of-the-century London, dead centre of global free-market society until World War I. Although Barrie did not suffer from a disease of addiction, he experienced the anguish of dislocation more acutely than most people and he brilliantly described his natural inclination to seek out substitutes for psychosocial integration in childish fantasy and other addictions.

The dislocation theory of addiction provides a useful tool for analysing Barrie's life (although his life has also been perceptively analysed from other angles by his many biographers). Barrie's life was one of extraordinary dislocation. He explained in detail how at least three of his addictions provided substitutes for the psychosocial integration that he lacked. He wove his addictions together into a unique addictive complex.

Dislocation

Barrie was born to a prosperous linen weaver's family in the lowland Scottish village of Kerriemuir, where his parents and grandparents had also been born. His cultural identity was not drawn from Scottish clan society, which had been expunged from the lowlands for centuries, but from Scottish Calvinistic Protestantism, which was at once ascetic, devout, and oriented towards individual achievement in a rapidly industrialising society.[40] Although the members of Barrie's family were ambitious and upwardly mobile, both his family and village society remained largely intact during his lifetime, their social life centred by the Kirk.[41]

The best-known source of dislocation in Barrie's life was a series of unique events that began when he was six. His next older and highly gifted brother, David, his mother's favourite, died in a skating accident at the age of 13. Barrie's mother was laid low with grief and hardly even recognised the young James Barrie for months afterward. She mourned David for the rest of her long life, her chief comforts being an increasingly intimate, special relationship with Barrie and the belief that, as David had died a child, he would remain happy in childhood forever. In Barrie's words:

> She lived twenty-nine years after his death … But I had not made her forget the bit of her that was dead; in those nine-and-twenty years he was not removed one day farther from her. Many a time she fell asleep speaking to him, and even while she slept her lips moved and she smiled as if he had come back to her, and when she woke he might vanish so suddenly that she started up bewildered and looked about her, and then said slowly, 'My David's dead!' or perhaps he remained long enough to whisper why he must leave her now, and then she lay silent with filmy eyes. When I became a man … he was still a boy of thirteen.[42]

As a child, Barrie strove feverishly to resuscitate his relationship with his mother by wearing David's clothes, imitating his posture and whistle, and trying to remind her of him. He also questioned her extensively about her own youth and avidly read fantasy and adventure books with her. Her intense involvement with this sad relationship, together with her preaching of the sanctity of motherhood and the repulsiveness of adult sexuality[43] led one biographer to characterise her as 'an emotional boa constrictor'.[44] Barrie's passionate devotion to his mother and to motherhood in general became lifelong trademarks.[45]

Barrie developed a terror of growing up, apparently as a consequence of this experience with his bereaved mother.[46] He described his aversion to normal adult functioning in painful detail in his personal notebooks and autobiographical novels—particularly with respect to sexuality, to establishing a mature identity, and to opening a bank account.[47] He recognised that his overwhelming involvement with childish play overruled his craving for normal adulthood,[48] although he did not claim to understand why.

Little is known of Barrie's relationship with his father. Although Barrie's voluminous writing maps out every square inch of his emotional life, it reveals virtually nothing of his feelings for his father.[49] Whereas he romanticises motherhood incessantly in his stories, his fictional fathers, including Mr Darling in Peter Pan,[50] are generally treated with distaste or ridicule. It is quite possible that Barrie's father's rise from a poor cottage weaver to an employer of other weavers and onward into the middle classes[51] required such prodigious efforts that he had little contact with his youngest son, but this is speculation.

If maternal constriction and paternal distance were the most important causes of Barrie's failures to achieve mature psychosocial integration, there were other causes as well, including the dour life of work and asceticism that was envisioned by his Calvinistic faith and his unusual physical stature. Although the young Barry was healthy and athletic, his body joined in the conspiracy against his growing up. At 17, barely 5 feet tall, he had not begun to shave, but had finished growing. He saw himself as diminutive, unhandsome, and utterly without sexual magnetism. Using a fictional name, 'Anon', he wrote of himself as a young man:

> Did Anon ever hear ladies discussing him for the briefest moment in a train or anywhere else? Alas, his trouble was that ladies did not discuss him … I remember (I should think I do) that it was his habit to get into corners. In time the jades put this down to a shrinking modesty, but that was a mistake; it was all owing to a profound dejection about his want of allure. They were right those ladies in the train; 'quite harmless' summed him up, however he may have writhed (or be writhing still) … If they would dislike him or fear him it would be something, but it is crushing to be just harmless.[52]

Addiction to work

Barrie eventually became famous for his overwhelming involvement with children and childish fantasy, but his most obvious addiction as a young man was to work. Barrie's history demonstrates how harmful work addiction can be, even though it made him rich and famous. Barrie graduated from university in 1882 as an M.A. By 1887, he had rejected his family's deeply felt ambitions for him to enter a profession, abandoned his rural Scottish culture, and somehow climbed the top of the journalistic ladder in London, contributing articles to virtually every prestigious periodical in England. He accomplished this by sending off a barrage of articles to the best journals, enduring rejections, personally charming hesitant editors, and prodigiously rewriting material even after it was accepted for publication. By 1890, only 8 years after completing university, he had published six books, almost completed another, and produced a mountain of published and unpublished journalistic writing. During part of this same period, he had produced two newspaper articles a day and four columns a week. His work was not limited to writing. He was also active in civic societies and in charity, and was a diligent social climber who, despite his humble origins, consorted with the great figures of his day. He attended church twice or more on Sunday when he was visiting his family, although not in London.[53]

Why did he work so hard? Andrew Birkin writes: 'Hard work took Barrie's mind off his increasing bouts of depression, when he would "lie awake busy with the problems of my personality".'[54] Barrie was depressive and morose from an early age, suffering chronic headaches, deep depressions, and recurrent nightmares throughout his life.[55]

Barrie's autobiographical writing makes it clear that his overwhelming involvement with work served in part as a substitute for adult sexuality. In the following passage, he says this explicitly, referring to himself in the third person:

> If you could only dig deep enough into him you could find first his Rothchildean ambition, which is to earn a pound a day; beneath that is a desire to reach some little niche in literature; but in the marrow you find him vainly weltering to be a favourite of the ladies. All the other cravings he would toss aside for that; he is only striving for numbers one and two because he knows with an everlasting sinking that number three can never be for him.[56]

In a public speech, Barrie took the next obvious step and feminised work:

> The most precious possession I ever had [was] my joy in hard work. I do not know when it came to me—not very early, because I was an idler at school, and read all the wrong books at college. But I fell in love with hard work one fine May morning.... Hard work more than any woman in the world, is the one who stands up best for her man.[57]

He also feminised work in one of his novels:

> Ah work, work, there's nothing like it! The sparkling face of her when she opens your eyes of a morning and cries 'Up, up, we have a glorious day of toil before us.' I have run back to her from dinners and marriages and funerals. How often she and I have sat up through the night on tiptoe, so as not to wake the dawn![58]

In fact, Barrie did run back to his work after his marriage, and to childish fantasy as well. In 1894, at the age of 34, he married a beautiful actress, Mary Ansell, then starring in one of his plays. Although the new couple succeeded brilliantly in the London social world, the marriage was childless and passionless, according to the guarded account in Barrie's notebooks and autobiographical novels.[59] Barrie gave more and more of his attention to his work and social life, and less and less to his wife. His tormented ambivalence is detailed in his autobiographical novels. Shortly after his marriage, he published *Sentimental Tommy* about a man who couldn't bear to marry. Four years later, he wrote *Tommy and Grizel*, a novel about a man who could not experience sexual passion for his wife, but only for his work. Barrie's biographers regard these two novels as shockingly autobiographical,[60] and Barrie himself said as much.[61]

The protagonist in the latter novel, Tommy Sandys, a famous writer of love stories, says of his wife, Grizel:

> Oh, so exquisite a flower! he cried, for he knew his Grizel. But he could not love her. He gave her all his affection, but his passion, like an outlaw, had ever to hunt alone.[62]

Barrie makes it clear in this novel that, although he feared mature love and sex, he also desperately wanted to experience it:

> He would have done it if he could. If we could love by trying, no one would ever have been more loved than Grizel.[63]

In the same novel, Grizel sees clearly that she will never be loved by her husband:

> He did not love her. 'Not as I love him,' she said to herself,—'not as married people ought to love ...'
> 'He would love me if he could.' She was certain of that. She decided that love does not come to all people, as is the common notion; that there are some who cannot fall in love, and that he was one of them. He was complete in himself, she decided.[64]

But Tommy *was* capable of love, in the manner that work-addicted people are. He realises it when the irreplaceable lost manuscript of his next book momentarily seems to reappear:

> It was alive—his manuscript was alive, and every moment brought him nearer to it. He was a miser and soon his hands would be deep among the gold. He was a mother

whose son, mourned for dead, is knocking at the door. He was a swain, and his beloved's arms were outstretched to him. Who said that Tommy could not love?[65]

In *Tommy and Grizel*, Grizel is forced to accept that her husband's work is his true love,[66] but she loyally resolves to be content with the childish adoration that Tommy lavishes on her in lieu of mature love, passion, and babies. Her admirable resolve is not tested for too long because, after learning that his missing manuscript has been burned, Tommy dies in a freakish accident (or suicide)—the fictional marriage did not have to endure the withering death that passionlessness might bring over time.

Barrie's own marriage was not saved in this convenient way. Barrie's wife, Mary, a loyal and devoted companion despite her growing frustration with the marriage, eventually ceased to love him[67] and took up a passionate affair with a younger man. She refused Barrie's offer of forgiveness, insisting instead on a scandalous divorce in 1910 in which she confessed her infidelity openly. She also testified that her 15-year marriage to Barrie had never been consummated,[68] a fact long known to her close friends.[69]

Addiction to children and childish fantasy

Publicly humiliated and wracked with despair, Barrie continued his formidable output of work and intensified his involvements with children. He was already famous for his ability to charm children in endless games and fantasies and to lose himself with them. Some of the most powerful passages in his writing eloquently describe his passionate infatuations with little boys. There are no indications that his relationships with children were ever overtly sexual, but there are many indications of overwhelming emotional involvement.[70] A well-known hostess noted in her diary in 1908:

> Mr. Barrie arrived in the evening. He was quite talkative at dinner … We talked a great deal of Sylvia's boys & it is extraordinary to see how they fill his life and supply all his human interest.[71]

Barrie's many descriptions of his own involvement with 'Sylvia's boys' were no less equivocal than that of his hostess of that evening. Shortly before the end of his marriage he wrote:

> How I wish I were going down to see Michael and Nicolas … I feel they are growing up without me looking on, while I grudge any blank day without them. I can't picture a summer day that does not have Michael skipping in front. That is summer to me. And all the five know me as nobody else does.[72]

'The five' were the five sons of Arthur and Sylvia Llewelyn Davies. Barrie and his then-wife Mary befriended the Llewelyn Davies family in 1898, 6 years before the first performance of *Peter Pan* and 12 years before his divorce. Barrie, Sylvia, and the children soon became inseparable, with Mary on the sidelines.

The Llewelyn Davies family was marked for catastrophe. Arthur, the father, died a lingering death from cancer in 1907 with Barrie in constant, devoted attendance as a family friend. Upon Arthur's death, Barrie essentially took over much responsibility for raising the boys as well as increasing his filial devotion to their mother. Sylvia, however, also contracted cancer and died 3 years later, shortly after Barrie's divorce.

Barrie became the boys' guardian through an act of forgery. Sylvia had written a will, but it was not legally witnessed. Barrie found it months after her death and produced a hand-written copy for the family. It was a true copy except that the name 'Jenny', one of Sylvia's two preferred caretakers for the boys, was changed to 'Jimmy', the family's familiar name for Barrie. Jenny was the sister of the boys' nanny. Sylvia had envisioned the two sisters as paid caretakers for her orphaned sons under the supervision of her large extended family, with Barrie included only as one of many overseers.[73]

Under Barrie's guardianship, the five Llewelyn Davies boys became the second great love story of Barrie's life, after his relationship with his mother. He freely devoted his fortune to providing for the boys' needs and his time to helping them recover from the loss of their parents in a world of games, holidays, and fantasy. He depended on their love and attention to sustain his own equilibrium. For example, he wrote a letter to the second youngest of the boys, Michael, every day, without fail, while Michael was attending Oxford, and expected one in return. Although this unusual relationship between Barrie and the five brothers was one of touching, mutual devotion, it had a darker side that grew from Barrie's possessiveness, emotional dependence, and ultimately oppressive attempts to prolong the boys' childish fantasy lives beyond all reasonable limits.[74]

Barrie had attended Sylvia daily during her last few months of life and stated afterwards that she had promised to marry him if she survived. Much of Barrie's personality and the dark side of his expanding relationship with the boys come through in the later thoughts of one of the brothers, Peter, on the possibility of this marriage:

> Others may well say, and doubtless did, that it would have been the most natural thing in the world: that she was already more intimate with him than with any other living being, that he had adored her for years and loved her children, that she was taking so much from him that she could scarcely refuse if that was what he wished, and in fact it was much the best solution. All this is true enough. But I think that to Jack [another brother]... the thought was intolerable and even monstrous; so much so that he could not refrain from expressing himself in the most forcible manner to that effect when [Barrie] in an unguarded moment spoke to him of it. To me too, I confess, the idea of such a marriage is repugnant. Up to a point, perhaps, this is mere sentimentality ... But it does seem to me that a marriage between Sylvia, the widow, still so beautiful in her forty-fourth year, of the splendid Arthur, and the strange little creature who adored her and dreamed, as he surely must have dreamed, of stepping into Arthur's shoes, would have been an affront, really, to any reasonable person's sense of the fitness of things. And I do not believe that Sylvia seriously contemplated it ... Let me not be thought unmindful, in writing what I have written, of the innumerable benefits and kindnesses I have received, at one time and another, from the aforesaid strange little creature, to whom, in the end, his connection with our family brought so much more sorrow than happiness.[75]

Another view of the excessive and addictive nature of the attachment between Barrie and the boys is provided by a close friend of Michael, the second youngest of the five brothers, during his years at Oxford:

> Michael took me back to Barrie's flat a number of times, but I always felt uncomfortable there. There was a morbid atmosphere about it. I remember going there one day and it

almost overwhelmed me, and I was glad to get away. We were going back to Oxford in Michael's car, and I said, 'It's a relief to get away from that flat', and he said, 'Yes it is'. But the next day he'd be writing to Barrie as usual … It was an extraordinary relationship between them—an unhealthy relationship. I don't mean homosexual, I mean in a mental sense. It was morbid, and it went beyond the bounds of ordinary affection. Barrie was always charming to me, but I thought there was something twisted about him. Michael was very prone to melancholy, and when Barrie was in a dark mood, he tended to pull Michael down with him … I remember once coming back to the flat with Michael and going into the study, which was empty. We stood around talking for about five minutes, and then I heard someone cough: I turned round and saw Barrie sitting in the ingle-nook, almost out of sight. He'd been there all the time, just watching us … He was an unhealthy little man, Barrie: and when all is said and done, I think Michael and his brothers would have been better off living in poverty than with that odd, morbid little genius. Yet there's no doubt that Michael loved him; he was grateful to him, but he also had an affinity with him that ran very deep.[76]

The eldest and most accomplished of the Llewelyn Davies boys, George, died in World War I. Barrie was laid low with grief, but the worst was still ahead. Barrie's favourite, Michael,[77] drowned at Oxford in 1921. Those most acquainted with the circumstances of Michael's death recorded suspicions that it was a suicide, partly on the grounds that Michael suffered from chronic depression.[78] Barrie never fully recovered from Michael's death.[79] Meanwhile, the three remaining boys had continued to grow up. Two of them maintained close relationships to Barrie, but not close enough to fulfil his extravagant emotional needs. He spoke—generally in whimsical ways—of their deserting him in favour of maturity and their own marriages.[80] Barrie sank into deep despair, although he pursued various other consuming involvements, including infatuations with new children, until his own death in 1937. Peter, the brother who was so repulsed by the possibility that Barrie could have married his mother, eventually committed suicide in 1960.

Barrie essentially divided his fortune in cash and literary rights between Cynthia Asquith, who had become his personal secretary and emotional crutch in his old age, and the Great Ormund Street Hospital for Sick Children. There were only nominal bequests for the surviving Llewelyn Davies brothers.[81] The five boys who had served to 'fill his life and supply all his human interest'[82] for more than two decades had been replaced. It might be said that Barrie's addictive relationship with them had more to do with involvement than attachment.

Addiction to tobacco

Barrie was also addicted to tobacco. One of his early books, *My Lady Nicotine*,[83] is a droll description of overwhelming involvement with tobacco shared by a small group of young, middle-class men that included Barrie. The men earned livings as writers and other types of white-collar workers and sometimes had girlfriends, but they shirked the real complexities of life in favour of sitting, alone or together, to smoke the wonderful 'Arcadia' tobacco mixture in their pipes and cigarettes and to enjoy their cigars. Barrie reported that severe chest pains, which he attributed to smoking, made him fear for his life at times,[84] and that sometimes he and his smoking companions paid a high price for neglecting serious problems, but they always returned to their smoking and did not seem to mind bearing the consequences too much. Thus, tobacco addiction$_3$ is presented in an insouciant and humorous light that would be shocking today, although it is comparable to the humorous way people sometimes now speak, for example, of overwhelming involvements with 'blogging' or video games. *My Lady Nicotine* exposes the dangers of addiction, but, as usual in Barrie's writing, the grim warning is muffled by sugary confection.[85]

The title, *My Lady Nicotine*, feminises tobacco, as Barrie's other writing in that period feminised work. Throughout the text, he favourably compares the merits of tobacco-addicted male society to those of marriage and a sober acceptance of adult responsibility, despite the fact that he was terrified by his lack of sex appeal and marriageability at the time he was writing the book. In short, the book is a romanticised description of addiction$_3$ to tobacco.[86]

It became less and less possible to romanticise Barrie's tobacco addiction as he aged. He remained an incessant smoker and a devotee of smoking society throughout his life, in spite of repeated medical warnings, a chronic, racking cough, and serious bouts of bronchitis and pneumonia. He tried unsuccessfully to give up smoking many times,[87] but it probably killed him in the end.[88] Barrie's friend and biographer, Denis Mackail, described a typical evening visit with Barrie, then in his seventies, as follows:

> It seems that he has finished his after-dinner cigar, and has gone straight, and inevitably, to the tin of tobacco—John Cotton, it has been now, for many years—and one of his enormous bull-dog pipes. Many years ago, also, he gave me one of these ... But though I smoke pipes—and although Heaven knows I wanted to smoke that one—its capacity, its calibre, and above all the leverage which it exerted on the jaw, proved only too well what I should certainly have already known. That it was the gift of no ordinary smoker.
>
> And of a smoker to-night with, alas, no ordinary cough. It comes on him again now as he stands there clasping the great bowl, racking him and choking him. Filling us also with sympathy and alarm ... It is painful and pitiful, but we know, somehow, that it is better to let our eyes wander round the room again than attempt to go to his aid. For though the cough is an old enemy, it is also, in another sense, a very old friend ...
>
> The paroxysm is over. Our host, looking faintly surprised and, as almost always nowadays, sad and weary beyond belief, hasn't only filled the pipe but is recklessly lighting it.[89]

Late in his life, intermittently afflicted with physical disease, insomnia, and depression, Barrie was prescribed heroin several times, a routine and safe practice of British physicians of that day, as discussed in Chapter 8 of this book. However, Barrie was the exception to the rule:

> Instead of tranquilising him, the drug had the opposite effect. Repeatedly he failed to sleep, became intensely agitated, and then euphoric. The next morning he would suffer terribly the after-effects of such a 'high'. Miserable, irascible, clamorous, he was frequently confined to bed. Regularly demanding more heroin, no matter how Cynthia reasoned with him, Barrie obstinately forgot its lethal after-effects in favour of the temporary release it gave from his mental and physical anguish. He had to be monitored with care.[90]

Barrie's addictive complex

Barrie's plurality of overwhelming involvements suggests that the word 'addiction' is too singular to describe his lifestyle. All of his addictive pursuits seemed necessary for his addictive complex to compensate adequately for his unbearable lack of psychosocial integration. If he were alive today, Barrie might well be diagnosed as a 'tobacco addict', but that would be simplistic. Had Barrie been able to quit smoking, he would no longer be diagnosable as a 'tobacco addict', but his addictive complex would have continued to dominate his life as it did when Michael Davies died at a time when he was the main focus of Barrie's addictive energy. Barrie was devastated by Michael's death, but not cured of his addictive complex. Many absorbing alternative involvements were available, including, perhaps, his own histrionic grief itself. Other opportunities for involvement included writing, public-speaking projects, intense personal relationships with children or beautiful actresses, and heroin, all of which could be expanded to addictive proportions.

An addictive complex such as Barrie's could never be considered fortunate—Barrie was miserably lonely and unhappy, despite his fabulous literary and social attainments.[91] Throughout his life, he was subject to deep depression, chronic headaches, insomnia, and nightmares. He had some long-term adult friends, but he was often an object of pity to them, and sometimes of distaste, because of his possessiveness, domination, and moodiness.[92] He was loved by a much larger social circle, but, it seems, mostly for his theatrical charm, his fame, and his great financial generosity.

Addiction and society

Much of Barrie's hugely successful writing—certainly including *Peter Pan*—consisted of veiled or romanticised accounts of his own addictions. The success of *Peter Pan* shows that stories of addiction can have a powerful, lasting appeal in a dislocated society, as long as they are sufficiently sugar-coated that they amuse more than threaten. Barrie's artful personification of addiction in a boy who refused to grow up provides a metaphor that extends the understanding of addiction beyond the limits of more prosaic language.[93]

Barrie's life shows that addiction is a tragic waste of human potential, even among those who reap the highest rewards of their society. Society may applaud severely addicted people like Barrie, but those who know them well know the depth of their misery.

Barrie's ingenious images—Peter Pan, Tinker Bell, Captain Hook, the crocodile that swallowed the clock—have been so completely adopted by the globalised world that they are everybody's property now, copyright laws notwithstanding. The future impact of these images cannot be foretold. They can be used to romanticise escape from reality through childish fantasy, a form of escape that constitutes a growing addictive danger in a society that is saturated with mass-produced entertainments and diversions. Alternatively, the images can be used in more constructive ways.[94]

The main source of Barrie's dislocation appears to be different than that of most other addicted people discussed in this book. His dislocation may simply have been the product of a fiercely possessive mother who single-handedly crippled his potential for growing up.[95] Therefore, his addiction can be understood as having little to do with the fact that he lived in the centre of an empire at the pinnacle of a global free-market system. On the other hand, Barrie's dislocation can be seen as having many causes including the irresistible lure of wealth and fame in the free-market society of his day. Moreover, his mother's possessiveness could be traced back to anxieties rooted in the continuing marketisation and industrialisation of Scottish society of which she was a part. There is not enough information to decide this issue either way here, nor does it need to be decided. Neither way of resolving the issue would contradict the dislocation theory of addiction, which recognises that there are many potential sources of dislocation.

A former crystal methamphetamine addict

I wrote this account about a former crystal methamphetamine addict in the form of an interview for an East Vancouver newspaper, the *Republic*, a couple of years ago. It was not submitted for publication at that time because Raphael was afraid of the consequences of his history as a drug addict becoming widely known at a sensitive point in his career. He has agreed to publishing it now, but several facts have been changed to protect his identity. This story of a former crystal methamphetamine addict is particularly relevant now because the growing public hysteria in Canada over methamphetamine is rejuvenating the demon-drug myth with an apparently new demon. But, as Raphael pointed out during my interview with him, methamphetamine has been a popular drug since the 1930s, and it does not become demonic when used in the smokable form called 'crystal'. Crystal methamphetamine acts very quickly, but no more quickly than injected methamphetamine, dexamphetamine, or amphetamine, all of which have been in use for decades. Methamphetamine addiction is best understood, like other addictions, as a way that severely dislocated people struggle to adapt. Like heroin and cocaine, methamphetamine is demonised for reasons that have little to do with its pharmacological properties. Raphael's interview also reveals some unintended effects of demonising a drug.

The interview that is recorded here was done in two sessions of about 2 hours each. However, I had spoken with Raphael many times before, over a 10 year period. During most of that time, he was a heavy amphetamine user and sometimes a student at my university.

Raphael's earlier life had been a study in dislocation. He was born in England, spent part of his childhood in Africa, and then moved to Canada at the age of nine where his parents lived in several different places. His parents spoke different languages when they met each other in language school in England. He ran away from home at 15, and although he is now reconciled with his parents, he was still estranged from his brother at the time of the first interview. His parents separated for a year when he was an adult, but are now together again. He travelled by himself to India and Korea, where he taught for a time, but always returned to Vancouver where he found a place with his girlfriend in a group of 'ravers' whose drugs of choice were crystal methamphetamine and ecstasy, although they used many other drugs as well.

First interview: December 2005

Republic: As a crystal methamphetamine user, you must find all the sensational stories about methamphetamine and methamphetamine users these days a bit daunting.

Raphael: Actually, they make angry. But I am not a crystal user any more. I haven't used any since November 23, 2004, a little over a year ago.

Republic: Did you have some form of treatment?

Raphael: No.

Republic: Am I wrong to think that you were using crystal methamphetamine all the times that I spoke to you since you were an undergraduate student at the university?

Raphael: I snorted and swallowed meth from 1996 to 2000. I didn't start heavily smoking it until 2000 and continued for 4 years until I quit in 2004. In India, I drank liquid speed on several occasions. Between the years 1997 and 2005 I was using legally prescribed dexedrine (amphetamine pills) when I wasn't smoking. I was also using ecstasy, LSD, and marijuana regularly and other drugs as well during that 10 year period. I experimented with heroin for a few months. I injected it twice. There were short intervals when my only source of income was dealing drugs. But I quit all this, except marijuana, when I began to see that this life was going to do me serious harm.

Republic: Could we come back to quitting later and first talk about the years when you were using methamphetamine? Did you ever overdose?

Raphael: No, the reality with meth is that one cannot overdose.

Republic: But what happens if you take too much by mistake?

Raphael: You would have serious hallucinations. Some people might panic, but you definitely wouldn't pass out. Methamphetamine has been used to revive people who have overdosed on heroin. By the way, most of this information is published in a book by Lester Grinspoon called *The Speed Culture*.[96]

Republic: Would you say that you were addicted?

Raphael: I guess that depends on how you define the word.

Republic: To me the word 'addicted' means that your life is taken up with doing something even though it harms you and those around you.

Raphael: I was definitely addicted by that definition. I used very large amounts, primarily by smoking. I was often awake for 2–3 days at a time from its effects and I frequently danced all night at raves and then went on to so-called 'aftershows'. I spent most of my time with other meth users, including my girlfriend. During the period between my first use of methamphetamine in 1993 and when I quit in 2004, I gradually became more and more addicted, using your definition, to the point that I began to fear for my health. My teeth were damaged so badly from the smoke that I had to have four of them extracted and now I wear a denture all the time. I was homeless off and on for a period of 2 years and was on welfare whenever the government would support me. On the other hand, I remained reasonably healthy and I found time to complete my undergraduate degree in English with honours and to finish a graduate degree. Towards the end of this period, I wrote a short book on methamphetamine users.

Republic: You gave me a copy in 2000, and I still think it is a fine little book. It gives me a bit of insight into a subculture that I have not seen first-hand. The people are all young and their lives seem to centre around dance parties and raves. I like the way you write at some points in the book in the intoxicated voice of an all-out raver and in others with the reflective voice of a concerned scholar. It was after re-reading it recently that I decided to call you about an interview, thinking that you were still using crystal methamphetamine. But how could you write a book when you were that addicted?

Raphael: Well, I'm sure you know that Jack Kerouac, Hunter S. Thompson, Jimi Hendrix, Lou Reed, and many other successful authors were all heavy users of amphetamine—of course I'm not that talented.

Republic: If our readers want to buy a copy, what should they do?

Raphael: It's out of print. I am in a state of transition and it is very difficult to re-enter the straight world and get a real job after being a methamphetamine addict. I do not want you to print my name[97]—even to sell books—because it might jeopardise my ability to get a job. Even other drug users tend to look down on meth users. I am not sure why. It makes me sad.

Republic: Is there no good reason for other drug users to look down on meth users?

Raphael: Not that I can understand. It is true that some meth addicts are in really bad shape, and the most extreme could be considered dangerous. But that is also true of the most extreme drinkers, smokers, fundamentalists, politicians, and probably university professors…

Republic: Sure, but …

Raphael: On the other hand, most methamphetamine users simply use the drug for fun from time to time, like most users of other pleasurable commodities. Then there is a grey area of users who have a little problem of control or of insomnia, but no big deal. Then there are serious addicts—like myself—who have definitely hurt themselves and alienated their families. But I never stole anything or committed any violent crimes. I was never arrested and I never received any treatment for drug addiction, even when I decided to quit permanently. Some addicts do wind up in prison or in mental health treatment though, including the brother of a good friend of mine who was eventually diagnosed as paranoid schizophrenic.

Republic: Do you think that methamphetamine or any of the other drugs could have made him schizophrenic?

Raphael: It is possible, of course, but I don't think so. He had psychotic episodes before he began using methamphetamine and during fairly long periods when he was not using as well. But the meth may have precipitated some psychotic outbreaks.

Republic: Is it easy to quit methamphetamine?

Raphael: Not for me. I am now totally abstinent because I fear that if I even smoked once I would go back. That happened on previous occasions when I quit. I miss the exciting life of the rave scene and the pleasure of the drug itself. It is hard for me to get interested in much of anything right now, and I have to worry about getting a teaching job. I have been teaching as a sessional instructor in night school, but I am not satisfied with that. I want to be a full-time high-school teacher and a literary scholar, but at night I still dream about meth. In my dreams, people are trying to smoke but something is wrong. The pipe is clogged up or broken or something.

Republic: What keeps you from going back?

Raphael: Fear! I remember the loss of my teeth, and how they were all brittle and cracked up when they were finally extracted. I remember the way my friend's brother suffered from his psychosis. And I could see that I was sinking deeper and deeper into a dark way of living. On the positive side, I was able to successfully quit because I had wonderful support from a couple of true friends when I was first coming off the drug. That really made a difference. And I am reconnecting with my parents in a good way and they are really supportive now. They helped me pay my denturist. I am capable of having a full life, but I am not there yet. I need to find a good job and establish a long-term relationship. I have student loans to repay. I am feeling a bit shaky. I take an anti-depressant every day.

Republic: Is crystal meth worse than other drugs?

Raphael: I would say it is as bad a drug as heroin and cocaine. But heroin and cocaine are no worse than alcohol or any number of other strong psychoactive drugs and powerful forms of seduction. Most users of every drug, including crystal meth are safe, recreational users, and a few users of each of them are seriously self-destructive. It is not the drugs that make them self-destructive, it is their heavy personal problems. This is true of me too. We gravitate to whatever strong drug works for us because nothing else does. We understand that we have to pay the price, although they may deny how serious it is for a while. Methamphetamine is probably better than some drugs because it doesn't seem to do much physical damage—except to your teeth if you smoke it—and people are not likely to stay addicted to it as long as some of the other drugs. And it does not cause overdose. If the public is in a panic about crystal meth in particular, they are making a mistake. It's just another strong drug.

Republic: Are you addicted to anything at all now?

Raphael: Not in the sense that you defined addiction before. But I do take my anti-depressants every day... I'm afraid I will have to end the interview pretty soon. I have to catch a plane to join my parents in Atlantic Canada for the holidays.

Republic: Merry Christmas!

Second interview: August 2006

Republic: It's good to see you. How is everything?

Raphael: Pretty good, but I may be leaving town. I am applying to do a Ph.D. in English literature at a university in Atlantic Canada.

Republic: Is that because you want to be near your parents?

Raphael: No. They will still be 80 km away. I am getting along much better with them, but the real reason that I am applying is that it is a good university for 20th-century Canadian poetry. I love reading poetry and writing and I want, more than anything, to be a university professor. Right now, I teach mostly ESL classes and that is partly because I only have a Master's degree. As you may imagine, there is not much academic depth in the conversations that take place in an ESL class, although I teach them quite well and get excellent ratings from my students.

Republic: Are you getting along better with your brother too, or are you still at odds?

Raphael: We get along well now. We e-mail each other and send birthday greetings.

Republic: Is that a real reconciliation? Could it be just politeness?

Raphael: You need to understand that we are very different people. He was always the political conservative and athlete, whereas I was the student radical and poet. I won prizes for writing poetry in high school, when he was on the football team. And there are old scars that have not completely healed. I wasn't invited to his wedding. But I will see him and his wife at Christmas time, and we may bury some of the past then.

Republic: Is your amphetamine use still under control?

Raphael: Yes, but I am not abstaining any more. I used on about six weekends since the last time we spoke. However, I have not become re-addicted. Each time, I used a moderate amount and stayed away from the kind of people who go crazy when they are using. Each time, I went back to work the following week. The 'coming off' was very unpleasant, however.

Republic: I guess I am a little shocked. Does it show?

Raphael: A little. Some former addicts can use recreationally, and some cannot. It's beginning to look like I can. Actually, I would rather not use at all, but all my friends do.

I have not succeeded in making many friends among people who do not use amphetamine, although this is my goal. It is depressing that I have not succeeded very well at this yet.

Republic: Are you sure people can use amphetamine recreationally, without getting addicted?

Raphael: Oh, there is no question of that. I personally know people who have done it for years. One man who I know well, for example, uses amounts that would be insignificant for an addict and does not take part in the rave scene or any other activities of heavy users. He just uses the drug, as other people might use anti-depressants or whatever. There is no doubt that many people can use methamphetamine without becoming addicted, the question is whether or not *I* can.

Republic: Can you?

Raphael: I think so. Time will tell. I do know that if a crisis comes up, I must not use at all, because that is when I have re-addicted myself in the past. But of course, that is when it is most difficult not to use.

The illegality of amphetamine may help me to quit completely. Because the drug is so illegal, it is impossible for me to know what I have bought. Sometimes it has the desired effect, but sometimes it does not. Besides, the police could come crashing through my door, which would end my dreams of getting a Ph.D. and establishing myself in an academic setting.

Republic: Do you know of some research studies that would confirm that people can use crystal meth without falling into addiction? I know there are some, but at the moment I can't remember where. Could you send me some specific references after the interview so that I can document this?

Raphael: Yes, I will send you some of the references.

[He brought them over to my house in October 2006. They document his point fully. The most directly pertinent are now cited in the reference section of this book.[98]]

Republic: Why is it so difficult to make the kind of social connections that would lead you away from methamphetamine, rather than towards using it, even recreationally? There must be whole groups of people who are fascinated by Canadian poetry and literature in general.

Raphael: I don't know the answer. Partly it is because I carry the stigma of having been addicted to amphetamine, and many people who knew me then do not seem to want to take a chance on me now. I think it will take time. I am still separated from my girlfriend from the years when I was taking methamphetamine, and I miss her badly. I think she has been having a tough time but we are not in touch.

I have been writing quite a bit, maybe you would be interested in seeing some of what I have done.

Republic: It would be a pleasure. Do you write poetry, or only prose?

Raphael: Both.

Republic: Is all your writing about drugs?

Raphael: Oh no. I have a fascination for the drug use of famous authors and artists, because I think that many of them provide proof that it is possible to use drugs in considerable quantities without becoming addicted, and some of the addicted ones prove that it is possible to become addicted without ruining your life or becoming a vicious criminal. But I have many other interests. I am interested in the various theories surrounding post-colonialism and the novel in the 20th century—the study of Conrad, Rushdie *et al.* This will be the topic of my Ph.D. dissertation, I hope. I like the theoretical analysis of this issue that was laid out by Edward Said and Homi K. Bhabha. I think you would find their work interesting too.

Raphael illustrates and documents the falsity of the myth of demon drugs in its latest, methamphetamine, reincarnation. All addicts are understandable human beings, rather than drug zombies. In addition, this brief introduction to Raphael further illustrates the intricate interplay of addiction and society. If Raphael becomes a high school or university teacher or a poet, his work will bear the imprint of his history of dislocation and addiction as much as St Augustine's and James M. Barrie's works do, although not necessarily in as transparent a manner. If Raphael falls back into a severe addiction, it will be in some part because of the way people in society have learned to react to those who have been addicted to a demonised drug.

A university student

An honours student who attended my university and now attends graduate school in California wrote the following. She is a beautiful and talented woman from a prosperous family. Both of her parents were born in Eastern Europe and she, like many others of her generation, may be caught between two powerful cultures with conflicting values, both of which have strong claims on her identity. A couple of years ago, after studying Freud in a history of psychology course, she asked if I would read a paper that she intended to write on the unconscious life of addicts, using herself as subject. This unconventional method seemed reasonable enough because introspection was one of the methods that Freud himself used. However, I was shocked that she labelled herself as an 'addict'. I challenged her self-diagnosis. She responded to my challenge in her paper, and ended it with a challenge of her own. Part of her paper is printed here—shortened, but otherwise just as she wrote it.[99] I have spoken with her at length, and reflected on her paper often. I have come to think that she has shown brilliantly how one of the defining qualities of the current era, flamboyant narcissism,[100] can be understood. Here is a portion of her paper:

> Addiction was an alien term to a sheltered and scrubbed suburbanite like me. Sure, I knew the images. I'd driven through Vancouver's Downtown Eastside. But addiction didn't touch people like me.
>
> My recollections of early childhood and adolescence chronicle a series of conflicts over the construction of a coherent identity and the search for that elusive sense of place. I didn't want to be who my parents wanted me to be. They wanted me to be the best. So I was stuck, ill fitting and awkward, somewhere in the middle.
>
> I was a bright child, definitely. I just never felt excellent, the way that maybe I could have been, if only I had done everything right. I was so stubborn—blindly stubborn—to protect my autonomy, my sense of self, even when I knew I was wrong.
>
> I drew hundreds of pictures of perfect WASP-type North American families. Hundreds of portraits of moms, dads, and their perfect, beautiful, glistening children. I was captivated by this image of the perfect family, and perplexed with why mine never resembled what I'd continuously produce on paper.
>
> And then, tragedy struck my imperfect family. Death and illness plagued us for years, and I went through the stages of child to teenager to adult, quickly, clumsily, and feeling entirely isolated. I grew up in a context of grief, the burden of responsibility, and the great art of pretending we're all OK. I plunged in and seemingly never out of long bouts of sub-clinical depression. I was numb when I started high school that summer (an event

traumatic in and of itself). I did my work and slipped into routine again, but there never was comfort. Whatever 'normal' was, I never felt it again.

I watched too much TV, bought too many useless handbags, and I spent hour upon miserable hour locked to the computer playing Tetris, Solitaire, Minesweeper, and FreeCell. I couldn't play just one game. I had to play and play until I felt that my victories outweighed my failures. 'You are a winner: faster, stronger, and smarter', the computer would tell me. A sense of urgency crept up in me when my mind wasn't distracted by tedious and senseless work, so I'd go on clicking the 'yes' button to the computer's requests to disengage me from real life, to take me into another game.

But these were minor habits.

I am, essentially, addicted to myself.

It sounds ridiculous. You probably think it is.

I'm not 'addicted' in the sense that the public is generally familiar with. People don't drive by me and think 'poor girl, if only she came from a good family.' No one feels sorry for me, and they shouldn't. I'd say they should worry about themselves. My addiction feels unfamiliar only in its familiarity. My addiction is to my Self, an embedded Self in our modern society.

My overwhelming involvement is with the creation and manipulation of a coherent fantasy self. I want to be *somebody*: an individual, a team player, a positive attitude. A quirky, eclectic, passionately devoted citizen. A happy and successful and complete person. A person who genuinely *is* what I've only played at. Someone who doesn't act, doesn't pretend, and doesn't make excuses. Someone without darkness. But I am not.

My preoccupation with myself performs several functions. The preoccupation in general, anaesthetises my awareness of experiences in the world, allowing me to live in my own skin/masks without bearing full responsibility to myself and my relationships as a daughter, sister, friend, partner, worker, or whomever. My reification of a certain self allows me the satisfaction of owning and controlling a self that's wholly mine. I am my most important project, one that I work on constantly, with every conscious action, and through every lived experience. I'm imagining the people of the world in a race to win, not by swiftly crossing any finish line, but by collecting the right tokens in a maze full of useless treasures. I believe that any freeze-frame moment, he/she with the best overall collection of experiences (e.g. network of personal relationships, the path chosen and travelled, and the attitude adopted to play the game) is the fittest to survive. I strive to be the strongest person that I can be in the areas deemed important to my identity and development. I need to build accolades and live a respectable life so that, on paper (e.g. résumés, transcripts), I have lived a life other people thought was worth living. My life and will are contained within those boundaries of adding wins, subtracting losses, and the numbing of consciousness.

My endless self-analyzing tires me, annoys me, curses me. I'm compelled always to know, to control, and to understand. The riddle is thus: how can I stop myself from thinking inside this elaborate world of mental structures that I've built up? Cogito ergo sum; I think, therefore I am. My existence rests upon these elaborate structures, such that my psychological being is orphaned without its shelter. I fear the thought of being stupid and being out of control of my actions. But what I fear the most, is that I'll be found out. People can trace my intentions, my motivations, my mechanisms for making the decisions that I've made in my life and know exactly why I've done the things I've done and forfeit my rights to participate in their game.

I say all this with love and disgust, but ultimately self-love wins in the end. I've contrived my own religion, where I worship myself (a false god). But I'm proud of my faith.

Everywhere, people tell me I should love myself, and I should stand strong no matter what, and I've created this identity in the image of good, and shunned away evil. But when I can't fall asleep at night because I'm tearing apart my closet in my head, trying to put together the perfect 'costume' for tomorrow's day, or I spend three hours after phone calls in a catatonic state because I want to know what the caller really thinks of me, I know I have to stop. That's it. It's that simple. Just stop.

It's not that simple. I obviously can't rid myself of myself. I can't stop myself from being a thinking person. It's a futile fight.

I recognise addiction as some overpowering force that manifests in the surrendering to total need. It drives, compels, and exerts its power over a person, sneaking behind them and stringing them along from the inside. With this surrender come complex relations with comfort, a sense of place, power, and control. Lived experience becomes organised along one central theme, where mortality swings like a pendulum from those highs and those lows. Life becomes predictable in this frenzy. Control becomes possible.

Above all, my addiction confronts darkness. Addiction is a way of denying or flinching at human darkness in all its significance, darkness in its twisted monstrous form, and darkness as close as our own shadow.

Carl Jung writes 'How can I be substantial if I fail to cast a Shadow? I must have a dark side also if I am to be whole'. The Shadow is emphasised as an essential component of the Self. The wisdom of darkness rests firstly on the recognition of its fundamental existence as a constituent of a whole identity.

The addiction question really lies in how we choose our poisons. Compulsion and the need for oblivion can easily be included in the tale of modern life. The constraints of modern living have resulted in bounded individuals with dim memories of More. I'm afraid to get dirty only because I'd forgotten that we were never born clean. I want our denied freedom, our repressed desires crave fulfilment, and forays into Darkness allow us to accept the unacceptable and meet the lost arts of the Self, our estranged Shadows.

Don't tell me how or what I am, because you're wrong. I can see just fine; I know what I'm not seeing. This road I've taken isn't a shortcut, isn't a hide-away, isn't an excuse. It does not lead to some pleasure-dome, twisted hell, or satisfaction guaranteed. I am not your Shadow-Beast.

This extraordinary student's document raises the possibility that the often-lamented narcissism of our age can best be understood as addiction to a culturally sanctioned kind of self-improvement. When dislocation puts a more balanced identity out of reach, self-absorption can partially fill the void and keep the fear at bay and can itself provide a kind of identity. This possibility fits Dufour's even more radical characterisation of this era as one of desperate self-creation.[101] It also fits with autobiographical accounts of oppressive self-absorption by more conventionally addicted people. For example, the eloquent Patrick Lane used the phrase 'my endless preoccupation with myself' in describing his lifetime of severe alcohol and drug addiction.[102]

The social and personal costs of this student's addictive self-absorption may be large. She described herself as giving all of her energy and talent to projecting a variety of personally gratifying public images. Because she is a talented person, she will probably succeed both in her career and in her social life in a way that maximises her self-gratification, whether or not it does anybody else much good. Her potential to contribute to the greater good, which is unusually large, may be seriously compromised.

On a personal level, it is hard to see how she can know contentment unless she overcomes her overwhelming self-absorption.

Because this student is on the way to becoming a professional psychologist, her account raises questions about the influence of dislocation and addiction on the discipline of psychology. The following speculation has nothing directly to do with the student herself because I have no way of predicting her future.

A new form of 'scientific psychology' became popular the late 19th century, with the United States as its primary homeland. This new psychology deviated radically from many centuries of philosophical inquiry about human nature that preceded it. The new psychology did not envision human beings as purposeful, rational, or moral beings, as had most previous philosophical inquiry, but as collections of psychological elements (e.g. sensations, perceptions, stimuli, and responses) that interacted with each other according to simple mechanical laws (e.g. the laws of association or of conditioning). The leaders of this new psychology strove to demonstrate that aggregations of elements following mechanical laws could behave in a way that fooled centuries of philosophers of human nature into regarding people as unitary beings.

Books on the new elementalist psychology by John B. Watson, B. F. Skinner, and others captured the imagination of millions of people and were acclaimed for a time as a revolutionary achievement in psychological understanding, usually called 'behaviourism' or 'behaviouralism'.[103] The social implications were huge. For example, it followed from the principals of behaviourism that the behaviours of people—conceptualised as nothing more than collections of impersonal psychological elements—could be radically shaped in whatever way was good for the robust free-market economy of the early 20th century.

Fortunately, the most extreme forms of behaviourism lost their popular appeal after World War II when it became evident that people were far less responsive to conditioning techniques than the theory predicted.[104] Nonetheless, a generalised version of this elementalist psychology remains an important influence among many professional psychologists and their followers today. Today's psychological elements are not mechanical stimuli and responses, but neurotransmitters, receptor sites, traits, attitudes, disorders, and quotients (e.g. intelligence quotient, emotional quotient, assertiveness quotient). Yet, the elementalist message remains. Many psychologists still do not strive to comprehend people as unitary wholes, but confine their attention to measuring, understanding, and modifying one or more of the supposed elements.

How can psychologists with a strong sense of personal identity be entranced by an elementalist psychology that either ignores concepts like purpose, self (i.e. soul), reason, morality, and meaning or treats them as unscientific illusions? Perhaps the highly successful hypercapitalism of the United States in the late 19th and early 20th centuries weakened the psychosocial foundations of identity—both in psychological researchers and in their followers—to the point that the idea of unitary, purposeful, rational, moral human beings could be plausibly dismissed as a mere philosophical speculation.

Perhaps the rest of the world, now in a state of dislocation similar to that of the United States in the late 19th and early 20th centuries, is producing young psychologists whose identities are similarly weakened. Perhaps many of this cohort of psychologists will be drawn to psychological elementalism because accepting an elementalist, selfless theory can conceptually protect them from the addictive self-absorption that has made at least one young psychologist feel addicted to herself.

A technical communicator and single father

The following autobiographical essay was written by a professional technical communicator who worked in Vancouver until 2 years ago. Lanny had completed 13 years in the Canadian Forces and retired as an engineering officer at the age of 30. He cannot find fulfilment in his apparently successful achievements as a single parent, a homeowner, and a technical writer. His story is not a colourful one, but it is a frightening one in its implications.

Lanny finds relief from his fears through addictive involvements both with seeking approval from the people around him and with television and other diversions. He thought these problems might wane when he moved from Vancouver to an eastern Canadian city, but they have not. More and more, dread permeates his relatively successful addiction strategy. Death has started to appear inviting to him, and suicide has appeared among the alternatives he contemplates:

Fear is at the root of my addiction. I fear rejection and failure, and so find reasons not to risk experiencing either one. As well, I fear not being able to know who I am—but I also fear finding out, because it could lead to self-condemnation. Hamstrung by incapacitating fears, I attempt to attract and retain validation from others. I work for approval. Then, since I am also terrified of success, I sabotage my chances of really succeeding, and engineer a set of excuses to escape the fearful prospect of personal responsibility for failure.

I want to see life as a drive along a good road in a perfect vehicle with great weather, while I fear the fact that it is more akin to a controlled skid down a snow-covered hill in whatever vehicle is available. Because I crave a controlled Sunday Driving experience, I avoid life's extremes. I seek to fit in and avoid both hope and hopelessness—but it's really quite futile because my nature is such that I cannot fit in with the mainstream for long. It's like putting a poor quality bandwidth modulator on the human experience: I try to cut off the highs and lows, but end up just burning out the limiting device. The highs and lows remain unrestrained, while I sniff about trying to figure out where the familiar smell of burning electronics is coming from. I'm trying not to face the hopes, dreams, challenges, and setbacks that are my own.

What do you do when you are imprisoned in a trap of your own making? If I can't fill the void by getting approval from others, then I look for excuses through which I can escape my abysmal self-esteem and my failures in the eyes of others. And if excuses do not bring escape, then there are other more primitive ways of escaping. *And the escape itself brings pleasure, whatever method I use.* This then is my addictive cocktail: approval and escape.

And addiction it is. There's a reason why I can't have cable TV hookup or a satellite dish at my home. I've used alcohol and marijuana, yet TV watching is what I find most difficult to control. The key is escape—time wasting—and DVDs, books, TV, computer games, cooking, running. Actually, anything will suffice. But TV is the worst—even with just four television channels, courtesy of rabbit ears carefully arranged on my son's piano organ near the window. When I'm really down, I can spend countless hours numbing my mind in a concerted effort to avoid thinking; and that's when I find TV most pleasurable. I become involved with the characters, and the stories seem like real life to me. When I feel more healthy, I lose interest in shows that I absolutely had to follow only a few weeks before.

I delay starting projects or getting back to them because I'm terrified of failure, which my live-in little demon quietly makes sure is forefront in my mind. To me, real work means facing the wall of self-doubt—that's why I procrastinate by watching television, and a thousand other ways.

There are significant consequences to this addictive procrastination, not the least of which is that when the really important tasks pile up, I have to rise to the occasion and do an inordinate amount of work in a short period of time ... thus looking pretty good for a while. It's a boom and bust life, though, and it makes me feel unstable. Drug addicts do the same kind of thing for as long as they can. Which leads me to the Magic Cloak of the Secretly Self-Loathing.

If you are going to engage in this game, then the central survival trick is surrounding yourself with a richly embroidered Magic Cloak that fools all those targets from whom you want money (employers) or approval (friends, family, institutions). You need to build up credentials, reputation, defined skill sets, and a nice aggregate of achievements and illusions to give you the safety buffer you need. Do enough—do very, very well when it is critical to do so, but relax and swirl the cloak whenever you can get away with it.

If I were truly stupid I'd feel like I was getting away with something, but alas I'm denied that simple joy. There is no satisfaction—just a constant, slow drip as the level of frustrations and self-loathing goes up, ever so slowly. Addicts try to protect certain aspects of their lives from these effects more than others, until at last the addiction pervades their entire lives. With me, my most protected area is my role as a father. I try as hard as I can to prevent this role being damaged.

It's not as if I can't handle challenges. Physical, psychological, emotional—I've been tested by life in many, many ways and have found it within me to meet the challenge. In the military, in hiking/camping, in single parenting, in flying, in academics ... from the career-changing to the heart-breaking, and all the way to having my life and someone else's in real, immediate danger.

Nevertheless, avoiding self-worth has made it impossible for me to develop enduring self-confidence in day-to-day humdrum normality. Even if I've overcome a challenge or even just done a fairly mundane job a thousand times before, I always approach it as if I will fail. My creativity and skills are hamstrung every time by having to fight the fear of complete inadequacy. It can become so much easier, then, to avoid the fear—to be distracted, interested, or enthralled by something else, especially television.... I've practiced this kind of avoidance so intensely at times that I get very little sleep while accomplishing not too much at all. This makes me even more afraid of responsibility, of facing the fear. I feel myself shrinking. My options are diminishing, my ability to wrap my mind around difficult concepts is eroding, and my ability to multitask is reducing. And what do I do when I am wasting time, personal resources, and potential? I make *more* excuses, and the wheel turns again. Day to day events lead me through serpentine contortions as I avoid having to define myself in my own terms, manage to twist myself into whatever shape I perceive is expected or desired by the people who care about me and create an image that I hope people believe. Sometimes the result is an overwhelming feeling of panic, mixed with hopeless anger.

I used to seek imposing goals which glittered with false hope from my Magic Cloak—academics, qualifications, licenses, wealth, etc. These do not motivate me much any longer, because if I put my mind to it, I can get anything I really want out of an institution—and at this point, what will it really give me? If you don't believe in your own worth, and if the attraction of doing something for approval has waned, then what keeps you in the game? I could go back to school and get a doctorate, but unless something in me changes, half way through the process I'd lose all momentum in face of the utter emptiness of the endeavour. I'd finish it, to be sure, but it would become a hollow, bitter, and extremely arduous test of endurance.

Yet without these goals, I am doomed to a life without challenge. My ego won't let me believe it: a life without challenge? Now that would be cowardly, wouldn't it?

Indeed.

I know with certainty that not much seems new to me anymore, and that new beginnings are not going to help—not if they start and end in the same places, for the same reasons, over and over again. I am conscious that I want to change because I want to be happier with myself. A more powerful motivation is the terror I feel when I ask myself what kind of example I am setting for my sons.

It's a battle for something more than just survival.

There have been times when I can see my own doom but feel powerless to do anything about it—and what's more, feel that it's useless to try. At these times it's like a dream, and I can't get my dream-self to listen or wake up. It's like I'm spending so much time and effort looking after the small things, the ultimately meaningless details, that I'm distracted from the horrible truth that the whole shebang is about to go revolving down the toilet.

There is a familiar poem about taking the road less travelled. I like to think that the fork in the road actually has three prongs, instead of two: on the left, a safe one; in the middle, a less travelled one to goodness knows what; and on the right, another less-travelled one that leads to one of Hollywood's high cliffs with jagged rocks at the bottom.

So it appears that the decision is between three alternatives: stumble blindly towards meaningless survival; change the cycle of these dynamics and find some sense of self-worth, and possibly purpose; or take the really big escape.

Lanny could be called merely a television addict, but this would force an overly simplistic label onto a complex and potentially fatal problem. Nobody labels Lanny as an addict except himself. He is far too normal to be tarred with such a fearsome brush. His friends value him and do not think of him in the ways he fears they might. Yet he is certain that he is addicted, and he explains the reasons for his periodic overwhelming involvement with television and other procrastinations with the matter-of-fact precision of an engineer. Although his addiction is invisible to others, he is not really engaged with the world, but is instead fixated on, horrified by what he perceives to be his and his children's descent. What if he is only one of millions or billions of people who live at this level of quiet addictive desperation? Who then will be the thoughtful concerned citizens who rise to rescue our endangered civilisation in the age of unprecedented challenges?

This final life story serves as a transition to the next chapter, which is not so much about addicted individuals, as about a civilisation in which ubiquitous addictive psychodynamics contribute substantially to the dangers that threaten its continued existence.

Endnotes

1 My analysis is based on the *Confessions* (St Augustine, 397 AD/1963) and *The City of God* (St Augustine, 426 AD/2000).

2 St Augustine and later historians concur in describing the rampant violence and corruption of the late Roman Empire in abundant detail (St Augustine, 426 AD/2000, Book 1 Chapters 5 and 6, Book 19 Chapter 6; Gibbon, 1776/1974; Kiefer, 1934; Peter Brown, 1967, esp. p. 25).

3 St Augustine (426 AD/2000, p. 111).

4 St Augustine (426 AD/2000, pp. 680–681, see also pp. 676–677).

5 See Marcus Aurelius' *Meditations* (Aurelius, 170 AD/1964) for a presentation of this aspect of late Roman Stoicism. The views of the Neo-Platonists were extremely important to St Augustine. They are described in Peter Brown (1967, pp. 244–245, Chapter 9)

6 I have drawn this partial list from his *Confessions* (St Augustine, 397 AD/1963) and from an authoritative modern biography (Peter Brown, 1967).

7 St Augustine (397 AD/1963, p. 29).

8 St Augustine (397 AD/1963), Peter Brown (1967, Chapters 4–8).

9 From *Confessions of St. Augustine* by St. Augustine, translated by Rex Warner, copyright © 1963 by Rex Warner, renewed © 1991 by F. C. Warner. Used with permission of Dutton Signet, a division of Penguin Group (USA) Inc. (St Augustine, 397 AD/1963, p. 210.)

10 The word 'confession' does double duty in the title of St Augustine's book. The book is a 'confession' in the sense of a statement of a particular form of Christian faith as well as a 'confession' of personal sins.

11 St Augustine (397 AD/1963, p. 161).

12 Peele and Brodsky (1975), Anon. (1986).

13 From *Confessions of St. Augustine* by St. Augustine, translated by Rex Warner, copyright © 1963 by Rex Warner, renewed © 1991 by F. C. Warner. Used with permission of Dutton Signet, a division of Penguin Group (USA) Inc. (St Augustine, 397 AD/1963, p. 52.) For simplicity, I have omitted sections of this paragraph in which he interprets the starvation of his soul as an as yet unrecognized craving for God. His discovery that devotion to God could cure his earthly addictions will be considered in Chapter 12 of this book.

14 See also St Augustine (397 AD/1963, Book 2, Chapter 2).

15–19 From *Confessions of St. Augustine* by St. Augustine, translated by Rex Warner, copyright © 1963 by Rex Warner, renewed © 1991 by F. C. Warner. Used with permission of Dutton Signet, a division of Penguin Group (USA) Inc. (St Augustine, 397 AD/1963, pp. 52–53, 55, 161, 180, 237–238.)

20 St Augustine (397 AD/1963, pp. 138–139; 426 AD/2000, p. 463).

21 From *Confessions of St. Augustine* by St. Augustine, translated by Rex Warner, copyright © 1963 by Rex Warner, renewed © 1991 by F. C. Warner. Used with permission of Dutton Signet, a division of Penguin Group (USA) Inc. (St Augustine, 397 AD/1963, p. 168.) This quote is taken from Book 8 of *Confessions of St. Augustine*, a chapter-long description of St Augustine's conversion experience, which is surely one of the most powerful ever written.

22 His lengthy theological analysis of this issue centred on the proposition that, although all evil must be caused by free will, contemporary man's evil impulses were caused by Adam's free will, which led him to sin in Paradise. Adam and Eve were created naked, but without sexual lust, although they were capable of reproduction in service of God's desire to populate the earth with people. When Adam sinned by eating the forbidden apple, at Eve's prompting, both were punished. Part of the punishment was that they were afflicted with sexual lust, which neither they nor their descendants could overcome, even though they tried, first by covering their sexual organs with fig leaves, and later by stronger measures. All living men and women are afflicted with sexual lust as a continuing consequence of this original sin. In heaven, however, where the souls of the righteous live eternally, their bodies are restored without the burden of sexual lust or other excessive appetites. Righteousness, the key to admission to heaven, cannot be achieved unless sexual lust and other immoderate

appetites are suppressed on earth, requiring continuous vigilance and fortitude (St Augustine, 426 AD/2000, Book 13).

The remarkably severe but apparently unjust punishment of Adam and Eve naturally raises other theological questions since, in Christianity, God is merciful and just. St Augustine tried to answer these questions but, in my reading, eventually gave up. On the issue of why lustful sexuality was sinful in the first place, St Augustine explains that, more than any other earthly pleasure, sexual intercourse draws the mind from contemplation of God to which it should be devoted without interruption (St Augustine, 426 AD/2000, Book 14, Chapters 9 and 16).

23 Part of the reason for this confusion is that the debate between free will and determinism played an important role in fierce doctrinal rivalries in which St Augustine played a leading role. In his attacks on the Pelagian schism (which was later declared heresy), St Augustine took a complex position that leaned heavily towards determinism, while still maintaining a theoretical allegiance to the inviolable principle that God could not create evil (Peter Brown, 1967, Chapters 29–31).

24 St Augustine (397 AD/1963, Book 8).

25 Killinger (1991).

26 From *Confessions of St. Augustine* by St. Augustine, translated by Rex Warner, copyright © 1963 by Rex Warner, renewed © 1991 by F. C. Warner. Used with permission of Dutton Signet, a division of Penguin Group (USA) Inc. (St Augustine, 397 AD/1963, pp. 119–120.)

27 St Augustine (397 AD/1963, Book 4, Chapters 4 *et seq.*).

28 The astronomy of St Augustine's time was a well-developed science that the Romans had inherited from the Egyptians and the Greeks. It was based on the assumption that the planets and the sun rotated around the earth, but nonetheless proved useful for navigation and accurate in predicting eclipses (Kuhn, 1970).

29 See Land (1971) for a case study.

30 St Augustine (397 AD/1963, pp. 92–93, 245–246).

31 He showed this individually for several addictions, but he also stated it in general terms: 'For you [God] have commanded it to be so, and so it is, that every inordinate affection should be its own punishment.' (St Augustine, 397 AD/1963, p. 30)

32 American psychologist W. R. Miller (1998, p. 981) has described this modern Christian view precisely, although he does not express it in a moralistic manner.

33 F. E. Payne (1993).

34 Peter Brown (1967, p. 173).

35 The Biblical account of the Garden of Eden is an epic story of collective dislocation, although St Augustine would not have seen it that way.

36 Orford (2001a, pp. 17, 332–340).

37 Chaney (2005, pp. 1–3).

38 See Alexander (1982, 1990, pp. 244–252 for earlier discussions of this topic).

39 This is clearly seen in the stage directions of the published version of the play *Peter Pan* (Barrie, 1928, e.g. pp. 154–155). See Chaney (2005, pp. 229, 238, 353) for a description of Barrie's allusions to Peter's tragedy in versions of the story that were published before the play itself.

40 Chaney (2005, pp. 12–13); Weber (1920/1958).

41 Chaney (2005, Chapter 1). The social structure was gradually breaking down as the cottage weaving industry was industrialised. Barrie's father was not a victim of this industrialisation, but rather earned a modest profit by hiring other weavers, and later joined the white-collar workers as a bookkeeper.

42 Cited in Birkin (1979, p. 5).

43 Chaney (2005, Chapters 1 and 2).

44 Dunbar (1970).

45 Mackail (1941).

46 Chaney (2005, p. 21) offers a convincing argument that Barrie was rejected by his mother long before the death of David, rather than only after his death. This seems plausible to me as well, but, for present purposes, the cause of the intense maternal rejection that he experienced does not matter.

47 His resistance to growing up sexually is documented later in this section. For his inability to develop a mature identity, see Chaney (2005, pp. 47, 57, 60, 71, 136, 247, 329). For the bank-account story, see Chaney (2005, pp. 61–62).

48 Chaney (2005, pp. 40, 70–71, 121).

49 A. Wright (1976, p. 69).

50 Barrie (1928).

51 Chaney (2005, Chapters 1 and 2).

52 Barrie (1937, pp. 132–134).

53 Mackail (1941); A. Wright (1976); Chaney (2005, Chapter 3, p. 79).

54 Birkin (1979, p. 16).

55 Chaney (2005, p. 39).

56 Barrie (1937, p. 134).

57 Cited in Birkin (1979, p. 16).

58 Cited in A. Wright (1976, p. 23).

59 Dunbar (1970).

60 Chaney (2005, p. 129).

61 Chaney (2005, p. 137).

62 Barrie (1900/1929, pp. 511–512).

63 Barrie (1900, p. 168, as cited in Chaney, 2005, p. 163).

64 Barrie (1900/1929, p. 493).

65 Barrie (1900/1929, p. 515).

66 Birkin (1979, p. 65).

67 Chaney (2005, pp. 242–244).

68 Chaney (2005, Chapter 19).

69 Dunbar (1970, p 230–231).

70 Mackail (1941); Birkin (1979, pp. 73–76); Chaney (2005, pp. 209–216).

71 From Dolly Ponsonby's *Diaries*, as quoted in Chaney (2005, p. 267).

72 Birkin (1979, p. 174).

73 Chaney (2005, pp. 284–285).

74 Chaney (2005, Chapter 18, see also p. 286); Dunbar (1970, pp. 317–318).

75 Cited in Birkin (1979, p. 192).

76 Cited in Birkin (1979, pp. 282–283).

77 Chaney (2005, pp. 298–299, 342); Birkin (1979, pp. 195, 285).

78 Birkin (1979, p. 293).

79 Birkin (1979, pp. 291–300).

80 Chaney (2005, pp. 205–206, 294).

81 Dunbar (1970, pp. 391–395); Chaney (2005, pp. 369–371).

82 See endnote 71 of this chapter.

83 Barrie (1892). Actually, most of the chapters of *My Lady Nicotine* were written earlier than 1890 when they were regularly published as newspaper and magazine articles that Barrie later collected for his book.

84 Barrie (1892, Chapter 1).

85 To add to the ambiguity, Barrie later claimed that he was not a smoker when he wrote *My Lady Nicotine*, although a friend of Barrie's from those years said that 'he hardly ever went without, and he smoked all day' (Hammerton, 1929, p. 154).

86 Jack (2006).

87 Barrie (1892); Mackail (1941, pp. 2–4, 537).

88 Mackail (1941).

89 Mackail (1941, pp. 2–3).

90 Chaney (2005, p. 365); see also Dunbar (1970).

91 Chaney (2005, pp. 329, 354).

92 Chaney (2005, pp. 254–255, 354).

93 Many people now include this metaphor in their understanding of addiction (Peele *et al.*, 1991, p. 166).

94 In my opinion, the American film *Hook* is an example of a more constructive use of these images.

95 As stated earlier in this chapter, little is known of Barrie's relationship to his father, but there are indications that it too may have been problematic. See Chaney (2005, Chapters 1 and 2).

96 The book is Grinspoon and Hedblom (1975).

97 As stated in the *Author's Notes*, all names used in biographical accounts are pseudonyms.

98 The references he provided document his claim with journalistic observations (Osborne, 2005), qualitative research (Klee, 1997; Hando and Hall, 1997), and quantitative research (reviewed by Sullum, 2003, pp. 235–238). He supplemented this published evidence with descriptions of several long-term recreational users of crystal methamphetamine among his friends.

99 I made a few suggestions after reading her first version, to which she responded. These changes are included here.

100 Lasch (1991).

101 Dufour's (2003a, b, 2005) work is discussed in Chapter 5 under the heading *Dislocation of the rich in today's developed world* and in Chapter 11 under the heading *The 'tragically cool'*.

102 Lane (2001, p. 14; see also 2004). Many other addicts display this self-preoccupation in their eloquent but narcissistic accounts (see Crozier and Lane, 2001). Canadian author Jacques Ferron (1968/1993, pp. 56–59) crystallised this addictive narcissism in a short story.

103 Leahey (2001).

104 Leahey (2001, Chapter 9).

The Role of Addiction in the Civilised Madness of the 21st Century

During the 1930s, a cultured, scientifically advanced European nation flew into a mad frenzy, led by a racist egomaniac named Hitler who was taken to be an infallible genius. This outbreak of civilised madness was eventually curtailed, but only at an obscene cost in terms of human suffering and material destruction. At the end of World War II, many people turned to psychiatrists and psychologists for an explanation of Nazism, because it seemed that what had occurred could not be understood logically, but only psychologically.[1] Within a few decades, Germany had recovered its sanity and rejoined the leading nations of the world. Civilised madness can be bizarre and deadly, but it is not necessarily permanent.

Although Nazi Germany provided the textbook case of civilised madness for the 20th century, there were many other outbreaks. Moreover, many people, including me, believe that globalising world civilisation has entered the 21st century in a state of advanced lunacy.[2] Environmental destruction provides the most obvious example of today's civilised madness. What rational explanation could our descendants possibly find for their ancestors who knowingly depleted and fouled their planetary home?[3] Surely, they will turn to psychiatrists and psychologists for an explanation of us.

Civilised madness has many causes that lie outside the bounds of this book. For example, the madness of Nazi Germany can be partially attributed to innate human proclivities for racism, to a diabolical propaganda machine, to unscrupulous politicians, to the disasters of the Weimar Republic, and so forth. However, Nazi Germany could not have conquered western Europe if a substantial number of ordinary people had not become so overwhelmingly involved with its mad dogmas that they enthusiastically laboured, organised, killed, tortured, and, when necessary, sacrificed their own lives for the cause. Moreover, the people who manifested this overwhelming involvement were not simple thugs, because much of the work they did required great intelligence. How can highly intelligent and cultured individuals become overwhelmingly involved with simplistic, hateful dogmas? This question must be answered if civilised madness is to be fully comprehended.

This chapter shows that fanatical devotion to socially destructive ideas can be a desperate attempt to adapt to severe dislocation—the same dynamics that underlie addiction. Because this is so, the spread of addictive dynamics in a dislocated society is a far more deadly issue than society recognises, even during a War on Drugs. Addiction is more than a medical problem that afflicts unfortunate individuals and leaves the rest in peace, and more than an inescapable glitch in human nature that must be endured with grudging good humour. Addiction exacerbates the madness of the modern world, at times producing misery, death, environmental destruction, financial instability, and further dislocation. Because it exacerbates dislocation, addiction is self-perpetuating. Thus, addiction contributes handsomely to the lunacy that is currently drawing an already weakened civilisation towards self-destruction.

This chapter describes the role of addictive dynamics in several kinds of civilised madness, starting with a well-known Nazi bureaucrat, Adolf Eichmann. Other examples will include environmental madness and the fanaticism on both sides of the 'War on Terror'.

Bureaucratic madness in Nazi Germany

Everybody encounters 'heartless bureaucrats' who seem oblivious to the dire effects of the assignments that they carry out with unswerving devotion. Some of the harm they do is trivial and even funny; some is tragic on a massive scale. In some cases, overwhelming involvement with bureaucratic heartlessness is a way that a person adapts to sustained dislocation. This and the next section offer two examples; one well known, one previously unpublished.

The most notorious 'heartless bureaucrat' of the 20th century may have been Adolf Eichmann. With the aid of his subordinates, Eichmann organised the roundup and transportation of about a million Jewish men, women, and children to the extermination camps of the Third Reich. Virtually all of them were killed there, as Eichmann fully understood they would be. Many Jewish people who were beyond Eichmann's reach lost their families, their local culture, their nationalities, and their trust in mankind. Thus, he may have caused as much dislocation as death.

It was not just the importance of Eichmann's role in this 'bureaucratic massacre'[4] that made his trial and execution in Jerusalem in 1961–1962 a memorable event in that era, but also the wealth of detail that was unearthed and read into the record about his early life, his motives, and his later reflections on what he had done. This story appeared in a famous 1965 book, *Eichmann in Jerusalem: a Report on the Banality of Evil* by the German–American philosopher Hannah Arendt.

Arendt attended the entire trial and read the voluminous documentation in German and Hebrew. She wanted to discover how a human being could have done what Eichmann did. She succeeded, at least in a negative sense, by ruling out all the obvious possibilities. She found that Eichmann was not insane, sadistic, psychopathic, ideological, or even anti-Semitic, although some of his Nazi colleagues obviously were. Arendt's final conclusion about Eichmann's psychology is astounding:

> ... when I speak of the banality of evil, I do so only on the strictly factual level, pointing to a phenomenon which stared one in the face at the trial ... Except for an extraordinary diligence in looking out for his personal advancement, he had no motives at all ... He *merely*, to put the matter colloquially, *never realised what he was doing* ... It was sheer thoughtlessness—something by no means identical with stupidity—that predisposed him to become one of the greatest criminals of that period.[5]

'No motives at all'? 'Sheer thoughtlessness'? Can a person collaborate in the execution of nearly a million innocent people without thinking about it? Although Arendt did not explicitly state how such an extraordinary state of 'thoughtlessness' could come about, the elements of an explanation are present in the multitude of documented facts that she archived in her book.

It is necessary first to look at what Arendt discovered that Eichmann was *not*.

Not insane

The Israeli court employed six psychiatrists to look into Eichmann's sanity. He spoke to them freely, apparently welcoming the opportunity to unburden himself before his inevitable execution. Their unanimous verdict was that he was normal and agreeable. One complimented him on his positive attitudes towards his family.[6] Hannah Arendt herself agreed that he was in no way insane, although she pointed out that he was extraordinarily shallow and spoke in clichés.

Not sadistic

Although Eichmann organised transportation of huge numbers of people to brutal death camps, he did not personally torture or murder any of them, nor give orders for anybody to be tortured or murdered. He refused to witness actual exterminations, because they horrified him. Nothing in Eichmann's actions revealed any desire to torment the people he was conducting to their deaths. He disdained notorious Nazi sadists. The Israeli prosecution, eager to convict Eichmann of something more dramatic than being a heartless bureaucrat, struggled hard to prove that he had murdered a single Romanian boy with his own hands, but the evidence was indirect and unconvincing. Hannah Arendt, fully in accord with Eichmann's ultimate execution on the main charges, believed him innocent of this one.

Not psychopathic

Eichmann acknowledged the criminality of exterminating Europe's Jewish population.[7] He expressed guilt over what he had done, although he refused to publicly grovel.[8] He was loyal to Hitler to the end, and expressed disdain for other German bureaucrats who betrayed their *Führer* when the war was lost. He admired 'idealism', and regarded himself as an 'idealist' who only destroyed Jewish people in the service of a higher cause. Although his conscience primarily functioned in service of Hitler, it led him on a few occasions to make feeble efforts to save Jewish lives that he believed did not need to be taken.[9] He was loyal to his extended family in Germany, especially his own wife and children. He fled to Argentina at the end of the war, but found a way for his wife and children to join him there, where the couple had a fourth child. At the trial, he made the same plea to every charge, 'Not guilty in the sense of the indictment.' His German attorney explained: 'Eichmann feels guilty before God, not before the law.'[10]

Not ideological

When Eichmann was considering joining the German SS in 1932, he faced a difficult choice. He also wanted to join a light-hearted, fraternal lodge in his home city.

The lodge, however, was a branch of the Freemasons, which the SS despised. The lodge inadvertently resolved the dilemma by expelling him for a petty breach of etiquette, so he joined the SS.[11] Although Eichmann developed an overwhelming personal loyalty to Hitler, as did millions of other German people, he was never an enthusiastic Nazi. His 'idealism' was mostly limited to the cause of expanding the *Lebensraum* of the German people, in the service of his *Führer*.

Not anti-Semitic

Eichmann was not drawn to the Holocaust out of anti-Semitism. He was simply bored as a soldier in the SS and found an opportunity to become a bureaucrat because of an opening in the department of Jewish affairs. He had no personal interest in harming Jews. When he joined the department in 1934, it was not yet practising mass murder as the solution to the 'Jewish problem'. He worked for several years deporting Jewish people to Palestine and other possible havens, and, according to Arendt, was shocked when the orders for the genocidal Final Solution were announced in 1941.[12] (Mass executions had taken place earlier, but not within his jurisdiction.) Several members of Eichmann's extended family were Jewish, and they had helped him to find employment earlier in his life, for which he was genuinely grateful. Eichmann's personal interactions with Jewish people were never abusive; in fact, they were as cordial as the grotesque circumstances permitted.

Bureaucracy as a substitute for psychosocial integration

Many people attending Eichmann's trial in Jerusalem found it difficult to believe the ordinariness of Eichmann's character as it unfolded in the testimony.[13] Arendt described the three trial judges who:

> ... were too good, or perhaps too conscious of the very foundations of their profession, to admit that an average, 'normal' person, neither feeble-minded nor indoctrinated nor cynical, could be perfectly incapable of telling right from wrong. They preferred to conclude from occasional lies that he was a liar—and missed the greatest moral and even legal challenge of the whole case.[14]

Arendt became convinced that Eichmann, neither insane, sadistic, psychopathic, ideological, nor anti-Semitic, was simply not thinking about the mountain of corpses he was producing. The explanation for this monumental act of inattention appears to be that in Eichmann's desperate state of personal dislocation, banal personal matters assumed a far greater importance than the suffering of a multitude of innocent victims.

Adolph Eichmann entered his adulthood in an era of chaos for Germany following the loss of World War I, the imposition by the great powers of a vindictive peace, and the miserable failure of the Weimar Republic. Battered by every possible form of instability, including revolution, attempted coups, a general strike, hyperinflation, depression, and unemployment, Germany became a heartland of dislocation.[15]

Eichmann's personal characteristics compounded the collective dislocation of his circumstances. He was born in 1906, the eldest son of a solid, middle-class family with great expectations that Eichmann himself shared. However, he discovered little that

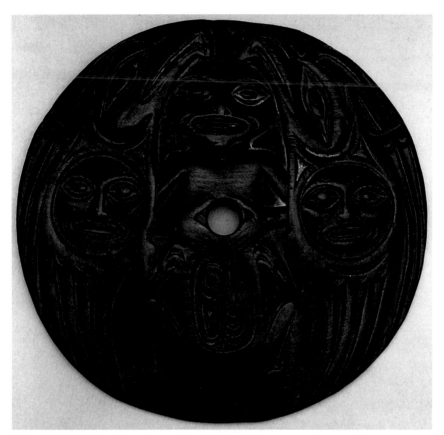

Plate 1 Spindle whorl, Northwest Coast Salish culture, wood, diameter 22 cm, early 19th century. (Private collection, courtesy of The Menil Collection, Houston, TX, USA. Photographer: Hickey-Robertson.) (See page 16.)

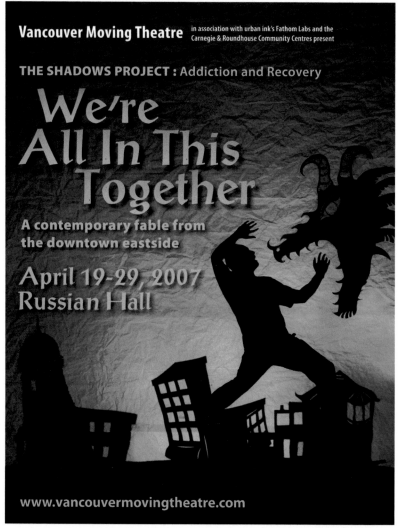

Plate 2 Programme cover for *We're All in This Together*. (Courtesy of Vancouver Moving Theatre. Image conception: John Endo Greenaway and Terry Hunter. Graphic design and photography: John Endo Greenaway. Shadow images: Tamara Unroe. Actor: Michael McNeeley.) (See pages 372–375.)

interested him in school, did not apply himself, did not graduate, was financially supported by his parents during his early adulthood, boasted to strangers and friends about non-existent achievements, could not get a good job, could not keep the low-status work that his family found for him occasionally, joined social clubs willy-nilly, and was always uncomfortable with others of his social class whose intelligence and learning seemed deeper than his own. He did manage to hold a job as a salesman for 5 years before losing interest in 1932 and being fired. Later in 1932, he joined the SS and there found meaning, order, and status—in short, a substitute for a deeper sort of psychosocial integration that was beyond his reach under the circumstances of his life. He pursued respectability in his corrupt world with 'extraordinary diligence', skilfully climbing a career ladder that eventually terminated on his scaffold.

In a passage that resonates with the dislocation theory of addiction, Arendt summed up Eichmann's work as a bureaucrat in the SS as follows:

> ... he had been an ambitious young man who was fed up with his job as a travelling salesman even before the Vacuum Oil Company was fed up with him. From a humdrum life without significance and consequence the wind had blown him into History, as he understood it, namely into a Movement that always kept moving and in which somebody like him—already a failure in the eyes of his social class, of his family, and hence in his own eyes as well—could start from scratch and still make a career. And if he did not always like what he had to do ... if he guessed, rather early, that the whole business would come to a bad end, with Germany losing the war, if all his most cherished plans came to nothing ... and if, to his greatest 'grief and sorrow', he never advanced beyond the grade of *S.S. Obersturmbannführer* ... in short if ... his life was beset with frustrations, he never forgot what the alternative would have been. Not only in Argentina [where he fled after the war], leading the unhappy existence of a refugee, but also in the courtroom in Jerusalem, with his life as good as forfeited, he might still have preferred—if anybody had asked him—to be hanged as *Obersturmbannführer* ... rather than living out his life quietly and normally as a travelling salesman for the Vacuum Oil Company.[16]

Eichmann's own words, describing the significance of Germany's military defeat in 1945 confirm Arendt's analysis of him:

> I sensed that I would have to live a leaderless and difficult individual life, I would receive no directives from anybody, no orders and commands would any longer be issued to me, no pertinent ordinances would be there to consult... [17]

Eichmann admired 'idealists' intensely, and identified himself as one. German literature is full of heroic idealism. Part of Hitler's political genius may have been to provide ersatz idealism that would prove irresistible to dislocated people like Eichmann. Arendt's account of Eichmann's version of idealism comes very close to a description of addiction₃.

> An 'idealist', according to Eichmann's notions, was not merely a man who believed in an 'idea' or someone who did not steal or accept bribes, though these qualifications were indispensable. An 'idealist' was a man who *lived* for his idea—hence he could not be a businessman—and who was prepared to sacrifice for his idea everything and, especially, everybody. When he said in the police examination that he would have sent his own father to his death if that had been required, he did not mean merely to stress the extent

to which he was under orders, and ready to obey them; he also meant to show what an 'idealist' he had always been. The perfect 'idealist', like everybody else, had of course his personal feelings and emotions, but he would never permit them to interfere with his actions if they come into conflict with his 'idea'... [18]

It is important not to push this analysis too far. I have no desire to insist that Eichmann should be labelled 'addicted' by future historians, although he clearly fits the definition of addiction$_3$. Why add to the litter of labels that lie at his feet, having failed to stick? Addiction is not a diagnostic label, but a human quality that comes to the fore in periods of extreme dislocation. He needs no label beyond that of human being.

Arendt's haunting phrase 'the banality of evil' has become familiar in the English language. Arendt documented the many ways in which Eichmann qualified as 'banal'. He was not an adventurous thinker in any way, nor an interesting person. One of my first great surprises in working with hard-core heroin and cocaine addicts over the decades was learning that these people, who have been portrayed as vicious evil-doers in the media, are similar to Eichmann in this way too. For the most part, they are neither vicious nor evil, but simply human beings struggling desperately to survive and maintain some sort of identity, blanking out awareness of the harm that they do as much as possible. The word 'banal' is perhaps too unkind, but it comes close to the mark.

Whereas it is quite probable that other people committed Nazi crimes for reasons that had little or nothing to do with addictive dynamics,[19] there are many reasons to conclude that Eichmann's motives were not totally idiosyncratic either. Eichmann belonged to a generation of Germans fated for the most extreme dislocation, many of whom found meaning and identity—ersatz psychosocial integration—in service to the Nazi movement. If doomed from the outset, the Nazi movement still provided a believable caricature of German strength, intelligence, and *gemütlichkeit* for those in whom more genuine national identity had been crushed by global geopolitics. Because this movement provided their only reliable source of identity and belonging in the world, they performed their bureaucratic functions with diligence and zeal. The horrible consequences drifted to the periphery of their consciousness, as they do in addictive denial.

Perhaps Eichmann did not differ much from many other middle-class bureaucrats of his unfortunate generation, and perhaps he differs less than one might expect from those of our own. Whether in Nazi Germany or in the contemporary world, a person who relies on a corrupt system as a substitute for psychosocial integration becomes a menace because corrupt systems grant acceptance and status only to those who serve their corrupt purposes.[20] It may be that Eichmann's personal dislocation was greater than the norm, leading him to greater crimes than most of his contemporaries, or perhaps it was just his bad luck to wind up in a highly visible role that would leave him condemned for all time.

An academic bureaucrat

The following is a stitched-together account, originally received in French as a series of letters and later e-mails from a friend of over 40 years. He and I have always written in French in our largely futile attempt to improve our writing skills in that language since graduate school. I have translated and consolidated some of his writing for this book and invited him to edit it, which he did. The author is currently a Professor of Experimental Psychology at a very large American university. He is devoted to the final years of his academic career to the degree that he and his academic colleagues often describe him as a 'workaholic'. He had not read any account of Adolf Eichmann's life when the material below was written.

I went to the University of Wisconsin, as my father had. There I found myself friendless, unable to gain acceptance in the cool, complacent American campus life of the 1950s. I was the opposite of 'cool'—aflame with acne, glistening with nervous sweat, habitually flexing my intellectual musculature, such as it was. I now think of my insecurities as the residuum of an unhappy childhood in a dysfunctional family in the transient world of American Army camps during and after World War II, although their source was a mystery to me then. One year after I entered university, I became a psychology major, hoping to find out what was wrong with me, and I have. I continued to study psychology through the BA, MS, and PhD at the same university and have never changed my career.

In both of my professional roles, as a teacher of university students and as a researcher in scientific psychology, I have acted in a corrupt way, although I have stayed within the guidelines and expectations of my profession. Even as a student it was completely obvious to me that alphabetical university grades—A, B, C, D, and F—did more harm than good to the students. I was a straight-A student in physics and psychology until my final under-graduate year, when I experimented by striving to learn what the professors were suggest-ing in their lectures was important, instead of studying what was going to be on the exam. I learned much more, but my grades fell sharply. I replicated this experiment during my first year in graduate school and came within a hair of flunking out. Chastened by this, I have been the equivalent of a straight-A student in my career ever since, although I hope to find some time when I retire to dig into some matters that seem more important to me.

When I became a university instructor in 1969, I had to teach four separate courses, finish my PhD dissertation, and help to care for my two young daughters. This was the normal load for new professors, but, like my colleagues, I found it impossible until I learned to cut corners.

I learned to reduce sleep to an absolute, unhealthy minimum. I learned to repeat the lectures that I actually had time to prepare to several classes. Even where they were irrelevant, I transparently insisted to the students that the lectures were, somehow, vitally important in their class. I learned to kill class time with pointless technicalities and pronouncements that I intended to sound intellectually impenetrable rather than simply meaningless. I learned to give trivial exams that could be marked quickly and that argu-mentative students could be forced to regard as 'objective' and therefore unchallengeable by the empirical conventions of the day. I learned not to be critical of faculty members who cut corners other than the ones I was cutting. To my secret astonishment, I was paid without question for doing all this; I finished my dissertation and was promoted to Assistant Professor.

I was no more corrupt than was necessary to keep up appearances and retain my job. I was too embarrassed to show the perfectly stupid classroom movies that were made available to us or to do what the students call 'reading right out of the textbook' from the lectern. One day, a student told me that if I didn't change his mark from 'F' to 'C', he would be drafted and sent to Vietnam as a soldier where he might well die. This could have been true in those days, or he could have been lying. I explained to him how the university would lose its reputation if we did not keep up our grading standards, how other students would soon learn that I had done this special favour and flood me with requests, and blah-blah-blah. He was not impressed, but I did not change his 'F'. After I had reflected for a few days on the look on the student's face while I recited the catechism to him, I realized that my corruption had some limits. My justifications were nonsense and he knew it. Although I thought the course I was teaching had some real value, and although he had wounded my vanity by not studying for it, I realized that capital punishment was too cruel and unusual a penalty for this offense. A few more Vietnam-fearing students came to me over the years and each time I secretly changed their grades. I felt good about that. Other cannon fodder was found, the Vietnam War ground on, and I got a substantial pay raise and a job at a better university.

To this day, I continue to grade students, knowing that the grades have less meaning than the same letters, A, B, C, when they are assigned to corporate bonds or supermarket beef. I also know that the course of the students' lives will be affected in significant ways by my alphabetic choice. Once I had a small seminar class that was so genuinely inspired and hard-working that I turned in a grade of 'A' for all 20 students. My department chairman let me know very nicely that this was unacceptable. 'Your job is to discriminate,' he said. A long pointless discussion followed, in which I politely forced him to admit that he could not tell me what it was that I was supposedly discriminating or why it was impossible that 20 people with an 'A' level of whatever-it-was could turn up in the same seminar. He was being polite too, since professors do not like to speak openly about the meaninglessness of the grades they give. He was letting me save face at his expense. He also pointedly let me know there would be consequences if I did not comply. I complied. I didn't feel good about it. I got a nice raise that year too.

I try to compensate for my corrupt teaching practices by giving the students information and ideas that are interesting and that they are not likely to hear elsewhere. All the same, the way that I grade my university classes does the students more harm than good, because it forces most of them to learn facts that are of no significance to them to pass my exams. Most students do not get the 'A' that they so desperately want, and suffer the consequences in self-esteem and professional advancement. Ivan Illich pointed out that the principle product of the educational system is failure, and I help to manufacture it.

Although my grading practices do more harm than good, this might be counterbalanced by the content of my teaching. However, my discipline, psychology, also does more harm than good no matter how it is taught. [There is enough material in this psychologist's letters to argue this point on a serious level, but that would lead to controversies that fall beyond the scope of this book. It is enough for this book that he believes for coherent reasons that both his socially acceptable careers, as a teacher and as a researcher on the visual systems of rhesus monkeys, are equally corrupt.]

Now, after a professional lifetime of this, I continue as professor and psychological researcher. I know that the futility of protest cannot be the entire explanation for my consistency. Surely futility in a good cause feels better than standing idly by. Why then do I remain in my profession? I have ascended the entire academic ladder from first-year undergraduate to full professor. I am at the top of the salary scale. I do not respect university administrators, and therefore, logically speaking, my self-esteem cannot be seriously wounded if I speak out and lose my job. My parents are dead, so I cannot break their hearts anymore. My wife would understand completely if I retired and would tolerate me, even as an outcast from my profession. We can afford retirement. My friends and family would probably enjoy having me around a bit more. I am dying to build the sailboat that I have designed, but my eyesight is beginning to fade. That project can't wait too much longer.

Then why don't I at least quit? Because, at the deepest level I still feel the same fear as the isolated, anxious 18-year-old who changed his major to psychology four decades ago. For whatever reason, I still need the acceptance of mainstream legitimate society to bolster my confidence. I need to become a Professor Emeritus, although I know the title to be ridiculous under the circumstances. I need the security that work brings, although the pension that I have already earned would be perfectly adequate. There is a terrible fragility that stands between me and a less corrupt existence. I feel bad about this, but I do not think it will change now.

I went into psychology to find out what was wrong with me, and psychology has given me the answer.

Obviously, the self-labelled corruption of this workaholic professor is less lethal than Eichmann's, although one young man could have died on a remote battlefield as a direct result. Moreover, the addictive dynamics of the corruption seems about the same. Who is to say that the madness of the 21st century owes more to a small number of high-level bureaucrats like Adolph Eichmann than to a large number of mid-level contributors like the professor in question?[21]

None of this is meant to imply that everybody who violates his or her own conscience at times is addicted. People have to earn a living and they sometimes compromise their values in order to support their families. However, family responsibilities do not require people to become driven participants or workaholics to rise to the top of a corrupt system by extraordinary devotion and zeal, or to enthusiastically carry out the shameful assignments that others find a way to avoid. Only the driven devotion and zealous enthusiasm of large numbers of people could have enabled Nazi Germany to transform itself from the demoralised loser of World War I to a brutally efficient military machine that almost conquered the whole of Europe. The same driven quality seems apparent in the more ordinary case of the professor examined here and others like him.

Environmental madness

Irreversible harm has been done to vital ecosystems everywhere: the atmosphere, the oceans, the rivers, the forests, the grasslands, the polar regions, and even the miraculous hidden life of the desert. Moreover, the rate of damage is increasing steadily, and some of the most circumspect scientists believe that the consequences soon will be catastrophic.[22] Yet the earth's political leaders and popular media have had little to say about it, except during occasional waves of public panic. For decades, political leaders and media have reported the evidence, if at all, in a scattered way, as if they want it never to reach a critical mass that would set off public alarm. The public has tolerated this, at least until very recently. Who really wants to know too much about that tiresome topic? Who wants to be labelled a 'tree hugger' or to become depressed and gloomy?

But what greater madness is there than to ignore cascading, irreversible damage to our planetary home?

How is environmental madness possible?

When our descendants look back from the despoiled planet that they will inherit, they will want to discover how human beings could possibly have done what we did. In their search for an explanation, they are likely to make the mistake of thinking of today's people as so consumed by greed as to be completely evil or stupid. But that conclusion would not be right, because we are also generous, good, and wise, much of the time.[23] We who have been party to the current madness may be able to discover the answer to their question by reflecting on the motives that underlie our individual ecological crimes and misdemeanours. The answer to the question of how we could have done it may be surprisingly simple.

Free-market society requires the sacrifice of psychosocial integration for the benefits of wealth. The resulting poverty of the spirit leaves each person, to a greater or lesser degree, desperate for something that will provide a sense of meaning and belonging. At the same time that the free market dislocates people, it proffers pseudosolutions for the misery of dislocation. As corporations know that affluent people's real material needs are already satisfied, they peddle a multitude of consumer products that are designed to fill the void of dislocation: enormous houses, modish clothing, personal beauty products, lottery tickets, electronic games and gadgets, gas-guzzling cars, sexual enhancements, exotic foods, weight-loss schemes, and on and on. Because these products can only partly or temporarily fill the psychosocial void, they are difficult to consume in moderation.[24] When they are consumed in excess, their ever-increasing environmental and social costs must be pushed to the periphery of consciousness, as in addictive denial.

Some of the excess consumption that is leading towards environmental catastrophe has an obviously addictive nature and carries labels like 'shopaholism', 'compulsive shopping', 'credit card addiction', and in the criminal form, 'compulsive shoplifting'. These obviously addictive forms of acquisition fit the dislocation theory of addiction well, since the people who engage in them are often clearly dislocated and their acquisitions give them a sense of importance, identity, and belonging that they cannot otherwise obtain, even if they lead to bankruptcy or prison. This sort of obviously addictive consumption is the topic of an enormous literature and the focus of thousands of 12-step groups.[25]

The larger portion of the world's excessive shopping is not carried out by 'shopaholics', however, but by people who buy only what they can afford and who would never dream of shoplifting. I believe that the great majority of them display the same addictive dynamics that are evident in severe 'shopaholics', although to a lesser degree. I base this conclusion on decades spent in affluent, North American suburbs, although I no longer live there. It also seems probable that the harm done to the environment by multitudes of minor addicts of this sort is likely to be far greater than the damage done by a relatively small number of severely addicted shopaholics.

If we take the time to really get to know the overweight couple taking the four-wheel-drive car to the superstore to stock up on superfluous merchandise in apparent ignorance of the environmental costs, we will see that their motivations originate in the same addictive dynamics as clinically diagnosed 'shopaholics'. This couple[26] truly *needs* to consume excessively. No matter how much they buy, they never get the feeling of personal satisfaction and social importance that they are seeking. They *need* to own that lavish home-entertainment centre, because if they could not dull their wits with incessant television and other entertainments, they might become horrified by the state of the world and the role of their own country in it. Their fragile, but essential, sense of the rightness of things as they are could be shattered. Besides, keeping up with the media really helps them to participate in conversations with their media-savvy friends. They *need* the big car to feel safe as they drive, because people drive these days as if nobody cares whether they live or die. In addition, having those other vehicles in the garage for when they might be needed gives them a sense of freedom, and without freedom what would they have, really? They *need* to buy materials to expand their already excessive house, because it will then express the unique sense of taste that they have so much trouble getting people to notice in other ways. They *need* more high-protein food and medical care for the two dogs than is available to most families in the Third World. Frankly, those precious little yappers have a bigger place in their lives than most of the people they know in the First World, never mind the Third.

They consume energy with the same avidity that they consume material goods. After all, people who have worked hard to put their money in the bank need some kind of recognition and reward. If it seems they have every electrical appliance and electronic gadget imaginable in their house, all flashing, whirring, heating, and cooling at once, it is only their due. Besides, hydroelectricity is still cheap.

They have their separate needs too. He *needs* to have all sorts of esoteric tools that he doesn't use now, because it will enable him to serve a real function in the community when he can eventually afford to retire from his job, finish fixing up the house, get away from the TV, and then turn to what has most fascinated him, in the background, all his life. She knows he will not have time to master any significant portion of that complicated stuff, but she senses his yearning for a sense of worth, knows his sensitivity to criticism on this topic, and values the stability of their marriage. Besides, if she is considerate about his stuff, he won't be mean about her little indulgences.

She needs to keep the fridge packed with meat and vegetables to feel like a good wife and mother, although most of it gets thrown out after a while. It's just that it's impossible to say when family or friends might show up unexpectedly for dinner or when she might get back to regular cooking. Besides, vegetables these days go all spotty; it seems like the restaurants buy all the good stuff. Plus, the clerks at the supermarket are so nice and chatty they almost seem like friends. And isn't there just a good feeling in knowing you're all stocked up? Taken together, all their scarcely used merchandise constitutes the material scaffolding for the construction of a fulfilling life that they genuinely need—but that, somehow, never gets built.

Of course, they do not consume every product in grossly wasteful or addictive ways. And—you must understand—they already know about the environment and they care.[27] They recycle. They only consume the products that satisfy real needs, and view the inexplicable, overconsumption of others with bitter disdain. They would not buy things that are environmentally destructive unless they were really necessary, as a buffer against depression and the other ravages of dislocation. They are not greedy, evil, or stupid. Rather, they are desperate to be recognised, to belong, to have a purpose.

They have been told throughout their lives that they can achieve these goals if they just purchase the right merchandise. They are as much victims of dislocation as the junkies who sleep in abandoned buildings. I would imagine that they are also just as loved by the Christian God for they, too, are poor in spirit[28]—even if their oversized house is stuffed with enough merchandise to enable some homeless, starving people to survive, and even if their addictions are, collectively, more environmentally and socially destructive than those of the much smaller number of heroin junkies. They suffer by comparison with drug-addicted people in another way, too: their plight seems more hopeless. Although there is no way that they will be able to buy a cure for their dislocation, they are doomed to keep trying because so many voices are encouraging them to make another trip to the mall.

Many affluent people have a smaller number of grossly wasteful habits than the composite couple described here, but they are part of environmental madness too. It matters little whether this style of life is formally labelled 'addiction' or not. The essential facts are that the fundamental motivation to relieve dislocation is the same as the motivation for addiction to drugs or anything else, and this couple's destructive way of life is as intractable as any other kind of addiction, even now, as the polar ice caps melt.

Wasteful consumption is essential for the survival of a bloated economy. There must be affluent people to consume the products of the factories as wastefully as possible so that more can be manufactured, because corporations that do not grow must die. The eternal expansion of the free-market society requires that people learn new needs and try the new products that are continually being invented for their consumption. The composite couple described here must be able to believe the barrage of propaganda that incessantly asserts that the way they consume is not madness, but is ultimately for the best, in some deeper sense. Multiplied by millions, they form a perfect vicious cycle. They work compulsively; they consume compulsively; the gross domestic product rises; the environment deteriorates; the poor get poorer; everyone feels more dislocated; they work *more* compulsively; they consume *more* compulsively, the gross domestic product rises *further*…

It is not innate wickedness or stupidity that is destroying our planetary ecosystem, so much as it is the increasingly desperate response of countless people to the dislocation of their lives.

Religious zealotry

In the midst of a War on Terror, Western mass media have tried to portray religious fanaticism as the natural product of bellicose Muslim religious texts or of the innate viciousness of Muslim people, but this is nothing more than propaganda. Most Muslims, like most Christians and Jews, are humane and non-violent people, notwithstanding certain ultra-violent passages that appear in the holy writings of all three of their religions. Even fundamentalist believers in each of these three religions are generally humane and non-violent.[29] However, fanatical religious zealots, usually drawn from fringe fundamentalist groups of all three religions, have shown themselves capable of utter disregard for human life. Religious fanatics of this sort are changing the world in major ways at the start of the 21st century. It is not inconceivable that they will precipitate World War III. This section is limited to Muslim and Christian fanaticism.[30]

Muslim religious fanaticism and suicide bombing

Muslim fanaticism is now a matter of intense study. It has come to be understood, both on the political left and right, as a way that severely alienated Muslim youth adapts to the dislocation that follows the collapse of their traditional societies and to the expanding free-market society that marginalises them. This dislocation is experienced both among the youth in Muslim countries and among the Muslim youth who have emigrated abroad.[31]

The conceptual bases of the most violent forms of Islamic fanaticism—sometimes called neo-fundamentalism—have been described thus:

> Different types of religion can serve the needs of the new population of Muslims dispersed around the world, but Muslim fundamentalism is perfectly suited for this, because it can transform the experience of dislocation into a step towards the refoundation of universal Islam, stripped of its exotic clothing and traditions, and therefore acceptable in every society. Islamic neofundamentalism sees earth as a potential Muslim world, waiting to be brought into being by the effort of all Muslim people. Neofundamentalism doesn't address itself to existing Muslim sects, but to isolated individuals who, through it, rejoin their faith and their identity. The Islamic neofundamentalists have found a way to 'Islamise' globalisation by finding within it the bases for the reconstitution of a universal Muslim community, requiring, of course, dethroning the dominant world culture of American-style Westernism.[32]

A study of Muslim suicide bombers[33] provides a more detailed description. Potential suicide bombers are not necessarily poor, young, or male, but they are people who experience hopelessness as their families, their cultures, their religion, their identities, and their futures are destroyed by foreign encroachments. Often they are people, like young Palestinians, who have been subjected to complete foreign domination for more than a generation, and who have, therefore, never known real hope of living in a viable culture.

If only the single act of suicide bombing is considered, a suicide bomber could hardly be compared with an addict because overwhelming involvement can only be demonstrated over time. However, the social life of the suicide bomber is rich with substitutes for psychosocial integration, which may last for a considerable period before suicide actually occurs. In the suicide bomber's religious vision, this rich social life may last for all eternity. Thus, the mere fact that they are destined to die does not prevent suicide bombers from being analysed in terms of addictive dynamics. Assigning life a lower priority than the substitute lifestyle is typical of many forms of addiction, such as addiction to illegal drugs, tobacco smoking, thrill-seeking, overeating, and so forth. Some kinds of addiction entail a high risk of sudden death, whereas others can be described as a slow suicide.

There are both real and imaginary psychosocial benefits in adopting the role of a suicide bomber. Future suicide bombers form close relationships with fellow fanatics in resistance groups that often last for many years. They may also find prophetic leaders who praise their courage and promise them psychosocial integration, either in paradise or in the theocratic world that is to come. Their fantasies are rich with the glory that they will receive from their families and friends after they have made their single supreme sacrifice because Muslim societies have developed a deep admiration of martyrs during long periods of oppression. In addition, suicide bombers feel a sense of identity with a powerful ethnonationalist collectivity for which they are proud to give their lives.

The popular misapprehension that Muslim suicide attacks can be explained adequately as a consequence of sinister messages in the Koran, innate viciousness of Muslim people, or diabolical leaders that hypnotise unwary people into carrying out their evil designs[34] bespeaks an unwillingness to acknowledge the basic psychology of people subjected to extreme and sustained dislocation. If society is willing to understand suicide bombers as real human beings, then it will acknowledge that they will not volunteer to kill and be killed except in a state of desperation.

Christian fanaticism

Most Christians, like most Muslims, are repelled by violence. Nonetheless, Christian fanaticism has broken out at many points in the long history of Christianity and it too can be understood as a way of adapting to dislocation that has at times exerted a profound influence on world events. For example, Christian martyrs in the Roman Empire were often brought before courts charged with heresy to the Roman gods. In this situation, many of them refused to make even minor, symbolic concessions to Roman magistrates who held the power of life and death in their hands. The martyr's willingness to accept the torture and public execution that resulted from defying all-powerful magistrates created a sense of awe among the non-Christian Romans that contributed to the successful overthrow of the Roman state religion well before the end of the Roman Empire.[35] Once Catholicism became the state religion of Rome, some Catholic Christians devoted themselves to murderous repression of competing religions, including other followers of Jesus.[36] St Augustine himself was a leader in the violent suppression of the Christian Donatists after he became Bishop of Hippo, although he resisted the most fatal measures.[37] Christian zealotry waxed and waned for 17 centuries through the various crusades, inquisitions, witch hunts, and religious wars of western Europe and its colonies.[38] Many Christians who did not participate in physical destruction of heretical groups nonetheless condoned these fanatical practices.

The dislocation theory of addiction implies that the inexorable dislocation produced by contemporary free-market society would engender Christian fanaticism for exactly the same reasons that it engenders Muslim fanaticism.[39] In fact, fanatical commitment to apocalyptic Christianity is widespread in the most highly marketised segment of the contemporary world, the United States. It has been particularly well documented among the American developers of atomic weapons and 'star-wars' technology, some of whom understand their technological achievements as leading the world through nuclear Armageddon to divine resurrection.[40] Christian literature of the American right provides another kind of example. The *Left Behind* series of novels envisions the world in a state of imminent apocalypse (the 'Rapture') that requires violent political action against the 'enemies of God' from true believers now.

The immense popularity of these novels indicates that ecstatic Christian zealots may exist by the millions in the United States.[41] The more sober political planning of extreme groups like Christian Exodus suggests the existence of a more earth-bound brand of Christian zealotry as well.[42] Recent American polls suggest that a combination of religious fanaticism and uncritical American patriotism may have become a majority position in the general population, although many American Christians have nothing to do with either.[43]

Contemporary Christian fanaticism is not limited to the United States. A fanatical religious order, *Opus Dei*, was influential in the Papacy of John Paul II.[44] *Opus Dei* and other secret orders are today exerting a powerful influence on the structure of the European Union as it grows and expands.[45] However, this fanaticism has not reached the extremes of mass violence of the better-known forms of Muslim and Christian fanaticism in this era. In the extremes, international aid agencies have reported that fanatical Christian groups currently seek to lift the 'curse' from the devastated city of Kinshasa by torturing and murdering children who they believe to be witches,[46] recapitulating the witch-hunting era of early modern Europe.

Political and economic fanaticism

Millions of staunch capitalists and communists rest their world views on faith rather than empirical evidence. Although faith is a part of human experience and has no necessary connection to addiction, some people's faith in their political and economic ideologies becomes so overwhelming that it is properly understood as addiction (or fanaticism, which means approximately the same thing in this context). Political and economic fanaticism play an important, sometimes decisive, role in the political madness of the modern era.

The Communist 'vanguard'

The fanatical devotion of some Communists, both leaders and ordinary party members, played decisive roles in the political struggles of the 19th and 20th centuries. The fanaticism of the Leninist Vanguard was vital to the establishment of a Communist regime in Russia. The willingness of devoted European and North American 'Reds' to suffer privation, beatings, and the risk of execution; to maintain unswerving loyalty to the perpetually swerving party line; to sacrifice their families' basic needs to the cause; and to overlook the mounting evidence of murderous repression in Stalin's Soviet Union illustrates a kind of political fanaticism that has the essential characteristics of religious zealotry, lacking only a deity. The heroic devotion of these committed Communists was perceived as fanaticism by outsiders at the time, and, in the aftermath, was described by some of the disillusioned participants in a similar way. A well-known collection of autobiographical accounts by former Western Communist activists is entitled, *The God that Failed*. It explicitly identifies the Communist zealotry of the mid-20th century both as a religion and as a severe form of addiction.[47]

Faith in the 'Market God'

Whereas true believers in free-market society correctly recognise the religious and addictive qualities of fanatical Communists, they generally perceive themselves quite differently—as rational proponents of objective economic science. However, many of them display unmistakable signs of faith and addictive devotion. This has been noted by scholars for at least a century, as has the flimsiness of the scientific evidence for the simplistic economic models of hypercapitalism.[48] This section first describes free-market doctrine as a faith, and then shows that extreme forms of this faith fully qualify as addiction.

Harvey Cox, a distinguished American Christian scholar, provided a theological analysis of free-market doctrine in his famous article, 'The Market as God'. He recounted how he began reading the financial newspapers, for the first time in his life, following the world-wide financial crisis sparked by the Asian currency collapse of the late 1990s. His encounter with the Market God took him by surprise:

> Expecting a terra incognita, I found myself instead in the land of *deja vu*. The lexicon of *The Wall Street Journal* and the business sections of *Time* and *Newsweek* turned out to bear a striking resemblance to Genesis, the Epistle to the Romans, and Saint Augustine's *City of God*. Behind descriptions of market reforms, monetary policy, and the convolutions of the Dow, I gradually made out the pieces of a grand narrative about the inner meaning of human history, why things had gone wrong, and how to put them right. Theologians call these myths of origin, legends of the fall, and doctrines of sin and redemption. But here they were again, and in only thin disguise: chronicles about the creation of wealth, the seductive temptations of statism, captivity to faceless economic cycles, and, ultimately, salvation through the advent of free markets, with a small dose of ascetic belt tightening along the way, especially for the East Asian economies.
>
> The East Asians' troubles, votaries argue, derive from their heretical deviation from free-market orthodoxy—they were practitioners of 'crony capitalism', of 'ethnocapitalism', of 'statist capitalism', not of the one true faith. The East Asian financial panics, the Russian debt repudiations, the Brazilian economic turmoil, and the US stock market's $1.5 trillion 'correction' momentarily shook belief in the new dispensation. But faith is strengthened by adversity, and the Market God is emerging renewed from its trial by financial 'contagion'. Since the argument from design no longer proves its existence, it is fast becoming a post-modern deity—believed in despite the evidence. Alan Greenspan vindicated this tempered faith in testimony before Congress last October. A leading hedge fund had just lost billions of dollars, shaking market confidence and precipitating calls for new federal regulation. Greenspan, usually Delphic in his comments, was decisive. He believed that regulation would only impede these markets, and that they should continue to be self-regulated. True faith, Saint Paul tells us, is the evidence of things unseen.[49]

Cox developed his comparison of the Market God to the Christian God on formal theological principles. For example, he pointed out that both the Market God and the Christian God are credited with omnipotence, omniscience, and benevolence by their followers.[50] In both cases, this produces a need for 'theodicy', that is, an explanation of why such a powerful, wise, all-seeing, all-loving deity would allow so much suffering to occur. Apologists for both gods offer a variety of explanations, but both seem to prefer what theologians call 'process theology', the doctrine that the supreme qualities that are intrinsic to the deity have not yet developed to their full extent so that the full measure of benevolence is yet to come. In other words, things are bound to get better later on if only the faithful keep trusting and believing.[51]

Less-formal parallels between the Market God and Christianity are easily seen, but only a single example, the importance of self-sacrifice, will be summarised here. The Christian God expects the faithful to sacrifice earthly concerns when this becomes necessary in order to do His work. In a similar way, the Market God calls for the faithful to make sacrifices for the market itself. The health of the market may require the faithful to spend beyond their means, to work beyond their capacity, to invest beyond their margin of safety. This message is implicit, for example, in a Canadian news report reprinted from the *Wall Street Journal*:

> Though growth is picking up in the world's major economies outside the United States, consumers in Europe and Japan still aren't pitching in.
>
> That has big implications for the shape of the global economic recovery: The world's growth will continue to rely on debt-laden Americans and their widening trade deficit, making the recovery more vulnerable to a sudden souring of US consumer sentiment …
>
> Not surprisingly, financial officials are exhorting consumers to open their wallets … 'More than ever, euro-area growth has to rely on an improvement in domestic demand', said Julian Callow, European economist with Barclays Capital in London. 'But it's not rising to the challenge'.[52]

Sometimes the exhortation to the faithful to spend recklessly is more fervid and the sacrifice is glossed over. Vancouver's largest daily newspaper sent the following message in its lead editorial on the first day of post-Christmas sales in 2005:

> **Shop til you drop:**
>
> **It's a moral imperative**

> Staying home from Christmas season sales can have a major economic impact, both here and in the developing world, so break out that credit card and support humanity…
>
> If the Christmas season is one in which we are comfortable talking about Prophets and Wise Men, it should also be one in which it's okay to talk about profits and the pleasures inherent in closing out the year by successfully stalking a terrific bargain.
>
> There is, of course, a moral imperative to seasonal shopping, too, although the righteous voices of high-mindedness tend to speak right over it. Think about it this way. What you spend on Christmas gifts and Boxing Day sales will flow benefits to people whom you don't know, will never meet and yet will be grateful for those benefits although they'll likely never thank you …
>
> So eat, drink, be merry, hit those Boxing Day sales. Somebody, somewhere is counting on your generosity—even if it's only to yourself.[53]

As with all religions, there is little factual justification for faith in the Market God. Its ideology does not flow from science or human nature, but is implanted in the population by enormously expensive, sophisticated propaganda.[54] It is not necessary to go beyond mainstream history and the business pages of the newspaper to find abundant evidence of the difference between the ideology and the reality of free-market society. For example, maintaining faith in the Market God requires ignoring the results both of the orthodox economic restructuring imposed on the Third World by the International Monetary Fund[55] and of recent experimental research in economics.[56] To experience free-market society as a deity requires a highly filtered reading of past history and current events. In its extreme form, this can become addiction.

Addictive faith in the Market God

Beyond the everyday faith of millions of believers, many people are *addicted* to free-market orthodoxy (i.e. the Market God). This statement is neither an insult nor a metaphor, but a literal application of the definition of addiction[3].

Many people are heavily addicted to free-market ideology—including entrepreneurs, political leaders, and individuals of modest means and station. Like their counterparts in the Communist Vanguard, they fiercely deny that their economic system has any fundamental faults. They deny that any alternative to it is worth consideration, and impugn the morality and intelligence of all who oppose them. They quickly become tiresome in their single-mindedness and, sometimes, dangerous in their zeal. Like other addicts, they appear immune to all historical evidence and rational argument.[57] Truly inspired fanatics can face direct evidence of environmental, social, and economic catastrophe growing from free-market economics without deviating from their doctrine even slightly.[58] Their logic is sometimes jaw-dropping. For example, it has been seriously claimed that the planet can never run out of usable resources, because the market will always be able to miraculously create new ones.[59] Morris Adelman, a Massachusetts Institute of Technology economist, says straight-forwardly:

> Minerals are inexhaustible and will never be depleted. A stream of investments creates additions to proved reserves, a very large in ground inventory constantly being renewed as it is extracted.... How much was in the ground at the start and how much will be left at the end is unknown and irrelevant.[60]

Addictive faith is also evident in the statements of the people who make it their business to deny the reality of global warming, which, in their minds, simply cannot be caused by human industry because reaching that conclusion that would inhibit the growth of the world's energy markets.[61] When these people run out of plausible arguments, they lash out aggressively, in a way that is reminiscent of those drug addicts who frantically curse everyone within hearing range when they are in the midst of withdrawal. Commenting on a European plan to reduce CO_2 emissions to 20% below 1990 levels, a well-known senior Canadian journalist sensed not only a socialist plot, but a deeper, indefinable evil as well. Here is a snippet:

> At the root of this conceptual mess is hysteria over climate change. The EU's energy policy is intended, according to European Commission President Jose Manuel Barroso, to make Europe the world's 'first post-industrial, low carbon economy.' But isn't Cuba already there?
>
> Sounding, improbably, like a clone of President George W. Bush, Mr. Barroso declared on Wednesday, 'We have an addiction to energy and, like any addiction, it is worse when we are dependent on others to satisfy our addiction.'
>
> Mr. Barroso thus demonized rational self-interest as something pathological. But then this is a very necessary step to justifying the true pathology that climate change injects into policy-making.[62]

This addictive faith can also be seen in the 'irrational exuberance' that kept prices up in the American stock market long beyond any rational justification and in the unstoppable rush to privatisation, mergers, deregulation, and buy-outs whose advocates appear totally unperturbed by calamitous failures in certain domains.[63]

Addictive faith shines through in the unapologetic devotion to immense wealth accumulation by people like Donald Trump and Conrad Black[64] and in the blind imposition of the most extreme free-market structures on the countries of the Third World and the former USSR by international lending agencies, despite repeated economic calamities that have been the result.[65] Free-market fanaticism, like religious fanaticism, totally abandons the law of contradiction. The intellectual task of the true believer is not to identify the error that leads to contradiction, but to show that two contradictory facts can both be true.[66] When normally prudent and intelligent people speak in a way that is patently reckless and foolish, addictive denial would seem a likely explanation.

A book-length illustration of the kind of rhetoric that people addicted to free-market ideology produce is Francis Fukuyama's famous book entitled *The End of History and the Last Man*. Fukuyama laid out the preposterous doctrine that the evolution of free-market capitalism and liberal democracy had brought political history to a halt, as no further changes would ever again be necessary. This book sold well and reviewers found it 'profoundly realistic and important', 'scandalously brilliant', and so forth.[67] Another illustration is a celebrated 2003 May Day article in the *London Times*, which developed the principle that 'global capitalism is the most benign and successful of all human creations'.[68] Another example is the enduring popularity of Ayn Rand's simplistic novel, *Atlas Shrugged*, which still sells well and evokes devotion from very powerful people 50 years after it was first published in 1957.[69]

Naomi Klein captured the essence of addiction to the Market God in the face of the failure of the American plan to create a complete free-market society in Iraq, which resulted instead in a nightmare of death and destruction. She said:

> Iraq was to neocons what Afghanistan was to the Taliban: the one place on Earth where they could force everyone to live by the most literal, unyielding interpretation of their sacred texts. One would think that the bloody results of this experiment would inspire a crisis of faith: in the country where they had absolute free reign, where there was no local government to blame, where economic reforms were introduced at their most shocking and most perfect, they created, instead of a model free market, a failed state no right-thinking investor would touch. And yet the Green Zone neocons and their masters in Washington are no more likely to re-examine their core beliefs than the Taliban mullahs were inclined to search their souls when their Islamic state slid into a debauched Hades of opium and sex slavery. When facts threaten true believers, they simply close their eyes and pray harder.[70]

Eloquent statements of addictive faith in free-market ideology can be found in contemporary mass media and other literature, probably because most of the world's media are owned by huge domestic and transnational corporations that have vested interests in the success of the free-market system.[71] The media can produce a barrage of unquestioning support for free-market ideology because they can hire eloquent 'public intellectuals'[72] who are willing to support it passionately, whether or not they are addicted to it personally.

I meet people occasionally who manifest addiction to the Market God in my neighbourhood, on the bus, at the university. Although they are not as eloquent as the media writers whom they often quote, their passion is intense and it affects their entire lifestyle. For example, it is difficult to have a conversation with them that does not turn to free-market ideology, and it is difficult to remain a friend without acquiescing to their ideology or debating it at every meeting. Debate, however, is always futile, since their faith remains untouched when their arguments are refuted. Addicted believers make up only a fraction of the people who support free-market economics, but their addictive intensity gives them a sense of power, and they are often influential in local public affairs.

Perhaps addiction to the Market God is the most dangerous addiction of all. Survival of this ailing civilisation depends on the ability to perceive the dangers of hypercapitalism, and to subordinate its imperatives to the more essential needs including psychosocial integration, environmental preservation, global peace, social justice, and financial stability.

Fanatical nationalism: addiction to 'American Power'

This chapter was begun early in 2003 amidst the American-led invasion of Iraq. As it is being completed in 2008, the bloody American and British occupation continues, despite proof that all of the public justifications for the invasion were unfounded,[73] including the imagined 'weapons of mass destruction'. This misbegotten war still maintains the unswerving support of millions of people in the Western world in the face of full documentation of its duplicity, cruelty, and incompetence, and despite the continuing harm it does to American moral stature. This section is not meant to portray the United States as a uniquely evil force, but rather as the best current case study of the contribution of addictive nationalism to the history of civilised madness.

The geopolitical aspirations of the United States and the methods it uses to pursue them are neither worse nor better than those of the other so-called 'great powers' of the past two centuries: Great Britain, France, Germany, Japan, Italy, and Russia. Nor are they worse nor better than those of the new great powers emerging in the 21st century: China, India, and Russia.[74] 'Great powers' enhance their power and wealth with complete ruthlessness. When necessary, they resort to slaughter, torture, starvation, spying, censorship, subversion of science, economic exploitation, bold-faced lying, and electoral fraud.[75]

Successive American governments have sought to expand American hegemony and wealth, employing all of the great-power methods when necessary, during the 19th and 20th centuries and into the 21st. The historical record fully documents American employment of the cruellest great-power methods during the Indian Wars of the 19th century, the Spanish American War at the turn of the 20th century, the imposition of American corporate interests in Latin America during the 20th century, the failed attempt to conquer Vietnam after World War II, and the current attempt to impose American power on the Middle East.[76]

Only part of the political support for American power has its origins in addictive dynamics. Some comes from the natural love of American people for their own country, right or wrong. Some comes from American commercial interests that manipulate the perceptions of their patriotic countrymen to make themselves rich. Some comes from thoughtful people from every country who genuinely believe that American domination, with all its flaws, would be a net benefit to a chaotic world.[77] Some comes from people who have decided to accept what they are being told by the mass media uncritically, thus freeing their minds to concentrate on more manageable problems. Some comes from people of every nationality who recognise the realities of American militarism but will not offend the American government for fear of damaging commercial relations.[78] There is no reason to label such people as 'addicted to American power'.

On the other hand, fanatical addiction to American power is a reality. It is widely recognised, both by non-Americans and by those American citizens who are alarmed by the fanatics among them.[79] I recognise people who are addicted to American power by the same criteria that I recognise those who are addicted to alcohol, drugs, gambling, personal power, or anything else. The hallmarks of overwhelming involvement are visible in people who are addicted to American power. Even when American authorities are caught in bold-faced lies or mass torture, addicted people's idealisation of the United States is unshaken. Their friendships are limited to those who can tolerate their railing about American rectitude and the evil of anti-Americanism. Often they regard the present level of American military incursion as too little rather than too much, and urge greater force in the future. Not all of these addicted people gain materially from American geopolitical successes, not all are rich, not all are Americans. Two are generous and intelligent friends of mine who have read this section before it was sent to the publisher.

People addicted to American power do not need to work very hard to justify themselves, because popular media overflows with highly selected news which portrays the United States as the model of moral, political, and economic achievement; the model against which all other countries are to be evaluated; the ultimate defender of freedom of speech, democracy, and human rights; the natural leader of the 'free world'.[80] The unmatched genius and volume of American propaganda[81] provides all of the pre-conceived rationalisations and denial that any addict could need.

A corps of faithful journalists crafts these justifications in all the American mass media (and most of the Canadian mass media as well.) Whether or not such journalists are addicts themselves, they are the equivalent of 'pushers'. Their writings are absorbed with the same avidity with which junkies consume heroin when they are feeling shaky. In the highest potency propaganda, the virtues of the United States acquire a supernatural essence reminiscent of ecstatic descriptions of the 'orgasmic' heroin high. For example, an impassioned article supporting American geopolitical policy in the *Wall Street Journal* said:

> The left, if it is not to condemn itself to become a fantasy ideology, must reconcile itself not only with the reality of America, but with its dialectical necessity—America is the sine qua non of any future progress that mankind can make, no matter what direction that progress may take.[82]

Attempts to refute the mass of documented facts that addicts to American power must overlook are rarely made. Rather, historical documentation is simply ignored in a stupendous act of collective denial. On rare occasions when historical documentation comes to light, fanatical defenders of American policy launch furious invectives against the character and motives of those who reveal it[83] and blindly insist that indefensible American geopolitical actions are undertaken in defence of the highest moral purposes.[84]

The following quote from a well-educated and generous man, a friend of more than four decades, illustrates the views of the people who are addicted to American ideology. He did not write this in the heat of argument, but in a carefully worded personal letter. His words show how addiction to American ideology (like addiction to any ideology) can lead to fatal decisions:

> Here is the bottom line on my Iraqi thought. I have six grandchildren. It is their good fortune and mine that they are American. But if they were Iraqi, and George Bush telephoned me to ask whether he should proceed, advising that two would certainly be killed, as American collateral damage, or as Iraqi shields, or as Hussein murder victims, I would ask Mr. Bush one question. 'Do you intend to stay long enough, so that the net result of the war is not trading an unknown monster for a known monster?' If the answer were affirmative, I would tell him to let slip the dogs of war.
>
> I am proudly a citizen of a superpower nation that is less than perfect, but much less less than perfect than any nation in the history of mankind. With the single exception of Indochina in the 1960s and 1970s, I sincerely believe that every place the American soldier or American factory has 'conquered' has come out better for our having been there. The list specifically includes France taken back from Hitler, post-Hitler Germany, post-Shogun Japan, post-Hiroshima Japan, Marshall plan Europe, the native Americans (10 million starving and killing each other when Columbus arrived, who have become 15 million with Ford pickup trucks), the Philippines, Cuba 1898–1921, Panama before the canal, Panama after Noriega, Taiwan, and even China. Whoops, remembered one more failure—the 1918 intervention in Russia was a flop.

Can addiction to American power be understood as an adaptation to dislocation? Certainly Americans, including the affluent ones, have suffered at least as much from economic dislocation as anyone else because the United States is the current leader in imposing free-market society on the world, including its own citizens. In addition, Erik Erikson pointed out long ago that Americans have grown up with impossibly heightened expectations of personal autonomy and with the expectation that their country will always be free of foreign constraints, as it was for most of the 19th century. Erikson described the devastating effects of frustration of these expectations on American patients in his clinical practice.[85] Could there be a more seductive addiction for people whose dreams of personal and national power have been shattered than an ideology that bestows unlimited power on their country in the belief that it has somehow been selected as the 'world's policeman'?

An addictive complex: Christian moralism, Market God, and American Power

The United States, a country founded upon the 'separation of church and state', is verging on becoming a tri-partite theocracy. A significant minority of its electorate is composed of people who are at once devoted to Christianity, the Market God, and American Power. These people are not typical Christians, typical supporters of free-market capitalism, or typical Americans, but there are millions of them, and they may change the course of history.

The roots of this trinity are very deep. The earliest European settlers in North America were devoted Christians whose personal asceticism and self-sacrifice was commensurate with their pious preaching. In addition to Christian piety, the spirit of the Market God can be detected in the rhetoric of the American revolutionaries of the late 1700s. Who was the 'Creator' who 'endowed men with certain inalienable rights' including 'life, liberty, and the pursuit of happiness' and to whom is it 'self-evident' that 'all men are created equal'? These ringing words from the American Declaration of Independence, signed in 1776, are more inspired by the Market God than the Christian God.[86] St Augustine's God, who was a major inspiration for American Christians, endowed men with equal rights only to seek peace and eternal life in Him. Any pursuit of happiness outside this Christian framework was both futile and sinful. St Augustine's God recognised the importance of social hierarchy: the emperor should rule the people, masters should rule slaves, and Romans should dominate barbarians. Thomas Jefferson, who wrote the famous words from the Declaration of Independence that are quoted above, was an atheist and a student of economics. He believed that Adam Smith's *The Wealth of Nations*, which was also published in 1776, was the 'best book extant' on economics,[87] and cited other European economists who held similar beliefs with approval.

It was the Market God more than the Christian God who led the westward march of the new American nation across the continent, as that economic expansion required the conquest and slaughter of entire nations of indigenous people. While not leading the troops, however, the Christian God was still prominent, offering solace to the survivors. The enormous success of that expansion led to the advent of the third component of the American trinity, adding to the Christian and Market Gods the image of divine American Power itself in the form of 'Manifest Destiny'. More agnostic thinkers have suggested that the phenomenal United States economic successes owe less to the power of the Christian God, the Market God, and Manifest Destiny than to the unprecedented circumstance of a relatively small number of modern settlers laying claim to an entire, previously unexploited continent.[88]

The demands of the three doctrines, Christian, Market, and American, are so internally inconsistent that they defy all rational analysis both by non-believers[89] and by thoughtful believers.[90] The logical incompatibility of the three doctrines requires United States policy makers to invoke holy mysteries such as the necessity of torture to prevent terror, the need to support dictatorships in order to spread democracy,[91] the precise geographical localisation of 'evil' in the nations that resist United States geopolitical ambitions, the American prerogative of disregarding binding international agreements that other nations must follow,[92] and Christian leaders who advocate assassinating uncooperative foreign officials and who apparently ignore the suffering of the poor.[93]

The fact that these three American doctrines cannot be combined without logical contradiction does not prevent the combination from being used as an addictive complex any more than logical considerations could prevent drug users from being simultaneously addicted to 'uppers' and 'downers'; for example, cocaine and heroin.[94] Addictive mixtures of uppers and downers in a single preparation have long been known in the drug world as 'goofballs', although this word has other meanings as well in current-day drug culture.[95] Like people addicted to pharmacological goofballs, many people devote themselves to the ideological goofball of the American trinity with an overwhelming enthusiasm that qualifies as addiction.[96]

There are enough true believers in the American trinity in the United States to fill huge mall-style 'gigachurches' guided by 'pastropreneurs'.[97] The true believers provide an important part of the core electoral support for the American imperial wars. Because of their great political power as a voting bloc in the United States, it now seems conceivable that they may either bring forth a global American theocracy or bring this era of civilisation to nuclear Armageddon.[98]

The current prominence of Americans among the champions of free-market society gives the movement to control hypercapitalism an anti-American colouring at present, but this colouring is not the essential quality of the movement. Anti-Americanism is a natural reaction in 2008 as this is being written, in view of current American foreign policy, but future champions of hypercapitalism are quite likely to have other nationalities. Howsoever history may unfold, current American politics serve to illustrate the role of addictive dynamics in the madness of our era. The next chapter will show that addictive dynamics also have a role in shaping our sanity.

Endnotes

1 Adorno *et al.* (1950). Later scholars investigated other kinds of motives as well (Milgram, 1963; Aly, 2005).

2 Raynes-Goldie (2004).

3 Shepard (1982, as cited in Fish, 2006, pp. 195–196); Suzuki and McConnell (1997); deGraaf *et al.* (2002, Chapter 11); S. Hume (2003a); Dolmetsch (2004); Homer-Dixon (2004); M. Hume (2004b); Mitchell (2004); Radford (2004, 2005); D. Smith (2004); Brethour (2005); D. Jones (2005); Sinaï (2006); Homer-Dixon (2006, Chapters 6 and 7).

4 This is the term given the crime by Hannah Arendt (1965, p. 288).

5 Arendt (1965, pp. 287–288, italics in original).

6 Arendt (1965, p. 25–26).

7 Arendt (1965, p. 22).

8 Arendt (1965, p. 24).

9 For a poignant example of this, see Arendt (1965, pp. 90–95).

10 Arendt (1965, p. 21).

11 Arendt (1965, p. 32).

12 Lifton (1986, pp. 159, 480) and other scholars have argued that Eichmann had a more active role in planning the extermination.

13 In a sensational article in the *Saturday Evening Post*, the trial prosecutor claimed after the trial that Eichmann was insane and sadistic. But Arendt, also present throughout the trial, marshals a great deal of evidence—too much to review here—that he was wrong (Arendt, 1965).

14 Arendt (1965, p. 26).

15 It is more usual to think of these calamities as producing poverty and starvation, which they did, but the dislocation was a prominent source of suffering in the minds of the German people. German nationalist Friedrich Jünger described the dislocation as follows:

> The recent past has destroyed our inherited collective sense of tender intimacy by trying to subvert and weaken all close bonds of community. Everything conspired to speed the disintegration of human ties in state, church, marriage, family, and many other institutions. A mad urge for throwing off all restraints, for dissolution, for unbridled liberty dissolved society into driftwood…

Jünger (1925/2000, p. 155).

16 Arendt (1965, pp. 33–34).

17 Arendt (1965, p. 32).

18 Arendt (1965, pp. 41–42).

19 Milgram (1963); Aly (2005).

20 Arendt (1965, pp. 26–27) makes an argument similar to this when she says: 'Eichmann was indeed normal insofar as he was "no exception within the Nazi regime." However under the conditions of the Third Reich only "exceptions" could be expected to react "normally".' She does not extend the argument to our own era, as I do.

21 Hannah Arendt might well disagree with my generalisations from her biography of Eichmann. She writes (1965, p. 286) disapprovingly of those 'who will not rest until they have discovered "an Eichmann in every one of us"', which is close to what I think I have discovered.

22 Suzuki and McConnell (1997); deGraaf et al. (2002, Chapter 11); Mitchell (2004); D. Smith (2004); Brethour (2005); D. Jones (2005); Radford (2005).

23 Nor does it help for us to condemn ourselves as evil or stupid, forgetting our virtues. Self-mortification cannot explain or change anything, although it can function psychologically to avoid a deeper, more painful understanding.

24 This dilemma is described brilliantly in a recent autobiographical article by Bev Schellenberg (2006).

25 See deGraaf et al. (2002).

26 This couple is a composite of several people whom I have known personally, but it is not an exaggeration. Many social scientists have interpreted contemporary consumer behaviour in a way that is similar to that outlined here. See Homer-Dixon (2006, pp. 193–198) for a brief review of this literature.

27 Johansen (2005).

28 The phrase 'poor in spirit' comes from the Sermon on the Mount where Jesus said, 'Blessed are the poor in spirit, for theirs is the kingdom of heaven …' (Holy Bible, Authorized (King James) Version, 1611/1956, Matthew 5:3). The people who Jesus was addressing in the Sermon on the Mount were Jews suffering under imperial oppression that appeared to dislocate the rich as well as the materially poor.

29 M. Polanyi (2006).

30 Jewish fanaticism has also played an important role in history (Yahya, 1978; Algazy, 1998), but that topic is beyond the scope of this book.

31 Huntington (1996, pp. 97–98); Roy (2002); Belaala (2004); Conesa (2004); Valpy (2004b, c, 2005); Berlinski (2006); Dalrymple (2006b). In addition to studies identifying a specific

connection between social breakdown in Muslim society and fanaticism, like those cited in this endnote, there is extensive documentation of the abrupt social breakdown of Muslim traditions everywhere as a consequence of encroaching free-market society (e.g. Hourcade, 2004; Kristianasen, 2004) and of the connection between social breakdown and fanaticism in non-Muslim societies (e.g. Ramonet, 2002; Camus, 2002; Carrozzo, 2002).

32 Roy (2002, p. 3).

33 Conesa (2004). A similar analysis has been made of the suicide bombers of the London subway in the summer of 2005 (Valpy, 2005; J. Wong and Mills, 2005).

34 B. Hoffman (2003).

35 St Augustine (426 AD/2000, Book 22, Chapter 9); Gibbon (1776/1974); Pagels (1995).

36 Gibbon (1776/1974).

37 Peter Brown (1967, Chapters 19–21).

38 For example, Roth (1937/1964).

39 Homer-Dixon (2006, p. 279) makes a similar point.

40 Lapham (2003); Noble (1997, Chapters 8 and 9).

41 LaHaye and Jenkins (1995).

42 Jarvie (2005).

43 Lapham (2003); M. Polanyi (2006).

44 Normand (1995).

45 Terras (2004).

46 Davis (2006a).

47 Crossman (1950, see pp. 64, 69, 83). See also Dufour (2005, 228–234).

48 Commentators on the religious nature of free-market ideology include the following: Tawney (1926/1947, p. 11); K. Polanyi (1944); Saul (1995, pp. 77, 121); Bourdieu (1998); Herman (2001); McQuaig (2001); Khurana (2002); Stiglitz (2002, pp. 134, 150, 168); Chang (2003); Dufour (2003a, pp. 88–99); Bayly (2004, p. 372); H. Henderson (2005); Beder (2006); Sapir (2006). Among these authors, K. Polanyi (1944, p. 127) dates the origin of this religion most precisely: 'Not until the 1830's did economic liberalism burst forth as a crusading passion, and *laissez faire* become a market creed.' Dufour (2003a, pp. 99, 102) adds the caveat that, in spite of its current popularity, free-market ideology must fail as the basis of a religion in the end because it lacks a creation myth and other transcendent content. I believe Dufour is wrong about this because he has overlooked the fusion of free-market ideology with Christianity (Weber, 1920/1958; Tawney 1926/1947; Posner, 2003). In many ways, Christianity (and other 'world religions') became soul mates to the market in the 19th century (Bayly, 2004, Chapter 9), providing it with abundant transcendental content. China, which leapt into free-market society in the last few decades, has also leapt into Christianity, which is spreading at a phenomenal rate there (G. York, 2004a).

   Einstein (1949/1998), Chossudovsky (1997), Soros (1997), Stiglitz (2002, 2006), Sapir (2006), and many others have shown that the simplistic models of hypercapitalism cannot be considered a validated science.

49 Cox (1999, p. 18).

50 See also Dufour (2005, p. 313).

51 Cox (1999).

52 Rhoads and Moffett (2004, p. B11).

53 *Vancouver Sun* (2005).

54 Beder (2006).

55 Chossudovsky (1997); Stiglitz (2002).

56 Sapir (2006).

57 Stiglitz (2002), Chang (2003), and Klein (2004) have documented this immunity to evidence in its modern form.

58 S. Robinson (2001); Thorsell (2002); Ibbitson (2002b); Saul (2004); Bulard (2005); N. Reynolds (2006a).

59 Homer-Dixon (2006, pp. 83, 201–202).

60 Adelman (1993, p. xi, as cited in Homer-Dixon, 2006, p. 83).

61 Mittelstaedt *et al.* (2007).

62 Foster (2007).

63 Schiller (2003); Drohan (2003c).

64 Halimi (2002); *Globe and Mail* (2002b); Ibbitson (2002a); Houpt (2004); Bower (2006).

65 Stiglitz (2002). Stiglitz has shown that addiction to the Market God provides only part of the explanation for these calamities. The officials of the international lending agencies were also motivated by loyalty to their friends in the financial community and by personal greed (Stiglitz, 2002, pp. 206, 213).

66 Herman (2001, pp. 263–264).

67 These reviewers' comments come from the cover of my paperback edition of Fukuyama (1992).

68 Kaletsky (2003).

69 Rubin (2007).

70 Klein (2004, p. 15).

71 Chang (2003).

72 Maschino (2002); Accardo (2005).

73 There were unpublicised justifications for the invasion as well. These, rather than any kind of addiction, probably provided the motivation for the political leaders who promoted the war. These unpublicised justifications are discussed in Chapter 5 under the heading *The Iraq War*.

74 Dyer (2005).

75 A compact description of the ruthless collusion of 'great powers' in the near annihilation of the tiny, oil-rich country of East Timor within the last decade or so shows the extent of mass murder that great powers are willing to undertake, even today, to achieve their ends (Brière, 2004). The same willingness is shown by the history of great-power support for Saddam Hussein during his years of despicable tyranny. The United States and France both provided substantial support (Despratx and Lando, 2004).

76 There is no end of documentation. I have concentrated on documenting the American use of murder and torture of civilians in the following citations, as that aspect of American use of great-power methodology is sometimes still denied: Tuchman (1966); Zinn (1980); Loewen (1999, esp. Chapters 25 and 78); Burkeman (2004); Crampton (2004); Freeman (2004); Hersh (2004); Klein (2004); N. A. Lewis (2004); N. A. Lewis and Johnston (2004); L. Martin (2004); McCarthy (2004b); Ospina (2004); J. Perkins (2004); Oziewicz (2005, 2006a); Klein (2007). When American troops themselves are caught red-handed at mass murder and torture (Crampton, 2004; Koring, 2004b; N. A. Lewis, 2004; Oziewicz, 2004; Schuman, 2004; Zernike, 2004) the discovery is regarded with pious amazement by American officials, including those who ordered the crimes in the first place (Hersh, 2004; Ramonet, 2004a).

Although the United States carries out extreme violence in some instances, its characteristic approach does not rest as heavily on violence committed by its own troops as on murder and torture inflicted by puppet states and mercenaries. Perhaps the United States' most brilliant marketing achievement in the past few decades has been to have the bulk of its mass murder and torture committed by allied puppet governments (for example, in Argentina, El Salvador, Guatemala, and Honduras) and by private contractors, rather than by troops under the American flag (Hermann and Chomsky, 1988; Mallick, 2004; Klein, 2007, p. 47).

77 K. Dixon (2004); J. Simpson (2004a).

78 Four articles that appeared on different pages of a single issue of the *Globe and Mail* recently (Chase and Fagan, 2004; Ibbitson, 2004; B. McKenna, 2004b; J. Simpson, 2004b), considered together, illustrate Canada's acquiescence to United States militarism and the delicacy with which the motives behind it are discussed.

79 Benjamin (2004); Dreher (2004a).

80 Huntington (1996, pp. 306–307); A. Cohen (2000); L. Martin (2004); Klinenberg (2005).

81 Chomsky (2004).

82 L. Harris (2003, p. 7).

83 Gee (2001); Gove (2003).

84 Gee (2003a, b, 2004a, b); Jeambar (2004, as cited in Cassen, 2004b).

85 Erikson (1959, pp. 73–74).

86 Kenny (1994, pp. 1–34) gives an account of some of the theological controversy surrounding such a 'democratic gospel' even within the post-revolutionary United States.

87 This quote is from a letter that Jefferson wrote in 1790. It is published in a collection of his works (Koch and Peden, 1944, p. 496).

88 K. Polanyi (1944, p. 201).

89 Achcar (2004); Kingwell (2006).

90 McKibben (2005) writes as a mystified American fundamentalist Christian. Canadian mainstream media, which unwaveringly support expansion of free-market society, are occasionally mystified by American inconsistency (*Globe and Mail*, 2005c). T. Friedman (2005) has written as a mystified American champion of the Market God and a supporter of the so-called War on Terror. The articles cited by all three of those sources express bafflement at American policy. See also Achcar (2004), P. Adams (2003), and Gambotto (2005).

91 MacKinnon (2006).

92 *Globe and Mail* (2005c); Golub (2005a); Hurtig (2005).

93 The most publicized recent instance of this is the American Reverend Pat Robertson's public advocacy of assassination of the Venezuelan head of state Hugo Chavez (*Globe and Mail*, 2005d). Christians of the American right have fervently opposed needle exchanges and condoms that could reduce the spread of AIDS in the Third World (Gee, 2005; Trace and Runciman, 2005).

94 Davidson (1964); Fischer *et al.* (2006a).

95 A further linguistic complication is that this mixture is sometimes called a 'speedball' (Fischer *et al.*, 2006a).

96 Combining incompatible ideologies into an addictive complex is by no means only a contemporary American phenomenon. For example, R. H. Tawney (1926/1947, Chapter 4) has shown that many mainstream English Puritans after about 1680 were fervently Christian but

fiercely opposed to charity for the able-bodied, even when they faced starvation. As well, the French pre-Marxist socialism of the 17th and 18th century was generally anti-Christian and materialist, but imbued with the spiritualism of the day, including the deification of 'Art' and medical-spiritual cults like Mesmerism (Dufour, 2005, pp. 221–228).

97 I. Brown (2005a).

98 Hurtig (2004, 2005); Golub (2005b).

Chapter 11

Getting by

Most of my relatives, friends, and acquaintances are not visibly addicted. *But how is this possible?* If dislocation becomes universal as free-market society globalises, and if addiction is the usual way of adapting to dislocation, how could any large number of people escape it? This riddle must be solved before the interaction of addiction and globalising society can be fully understood.

Some people manage to create fulfilling, psychosocially integrated lives, even in the most dislocated of modern societies. Such people seldom, if ever, suffer from depression, addiction, anxiety, loneliness, family dysfunction, boredom, or bitterness, and finish their lives with a palpable sense of contentment and fullness. Unfortunately, I cannot claim membership of this talented and fortunate group myself, although I have the pleasure of knowing a few people who probably can. The larger number of people who manage to live without visible addictions might better be described as 'getting by'. These people—of whom I am one—cope with sustained dislocation less than brilliantly, but still without becoming sufficiently addicted or depressed to breach the limits of toleration of their friends and relatives. Their ways of adapting to sustained dislocation contribute much to the coloration of life in free-market society.

Ways of 'getting by' or coping with a dislocated society are classified into seven types in this chapter: (1) resolute conventionality, (2) resolute unconventionality, (3) participating in a concocted community, (4) political activism, (5) the 'tragically cool', (6) the spiritually sufficient, and (7) the ex-addict. This taxonomy is limited to ways of coping with sustained dislocation that I have observed first-hand, although in many instances the descriptive vocabulary comes from other authors. At the end of the chapter, the role of addiction$_4$ in coping with dislocation is examined briefly.

Resolute conventionality

Many people maintain stable and usually harmonious nuclear families by dint of determination, hard work, and a wise set of priorities, although they are cut off from the support of their extended families and their geographical, ethnic, and religious roots, and are exposed to the full dislocating pressure of 'market forces' in the globalising world. Such families typically compensate for their separation from their roots by travelling 'home' from time to time, often over extraordinary distances, and by devoting large amounts of time to long-distance telephone calls and e-mail. They often compensate for their ethnic dislocation by membership of local societies or by cultivating a pluralistic appreciation of the ethnicities of their neighbours. They often deal with their religious dislocation by choosing among the great variety of spiritual and ethical movements that proselytise everywhere, or by sticking with the old ones with determined enthusiasm. They survive the tumult of modernity by sheer grit and by keeping their priorities straight. The amount of time and money that they expend maintaining a degree of psychosocial integration is large enough that they have little energy for harmful addictions—and little need for them either.

Such families manage to be mutually supportive most of the time. Children, when they leave the nest, have a reasonably strong identity and are ready to take on the task of launching a family of the same sort themselves. Parents, when the children leave, are able to reactivate dormant friendships and interests that maintain their sense of purpose and meaning.

Although families like these are sometimes caricatured as boringly conventional and 'middle class', they remain the ideal to which many of us aspire.[1] Although their lives are conventional in most regards, they are not boring, for their achievement is far from easy. They deal with difficult, unpredictable problems both within the family and within the larger social world. They are aware of the chaos of the world around them, but they are not swept into it. Parents expect to pay an enormous price in time and energy to provide opportunities that will capture the interests of each of their children. Children endure levels of anxiety far higher than those of previous generations.[2] When disaster strikes—a job is lost, serious illness occurs, a family member slides into depression or addiction—they pull together, and the damage is minimized. But they feel the pain and sense the abyss.

It is not easy to maintain a family situation like this, and many people do not quite have the economic resources or the emotional strength to sustain it, so their families finally fracture or fall into dysfunctional strife. Many people, however, do manage to be resolutely conventional and reasonably happy, despite the vortex of dislocation in which they must live. They manage this feat largely by admirable strength of character, with the aid of some good fortune and a little help from their friends.

Resolute unconventionality

Some people find that a conventional lifestyle is not achievable or not adequate to cope with chronic dislocation, and develop unconventional lifestyles that serve a similar purpose. One example is a man of about 40 whom I have known for many years. His home is a sort of refuge in an uninspiring suburb of Vancouver, only a kilometre from Robert Pickton's infamous pig farm. The psychosocial integration of his life is probably just as much the product of his wife's intelligence and courage as his own, but since I do not know her role in it well enough, she has a secondary role in my account.

Both Hogan and Louise have troubled family backgrounds, and both are estranged from their parents and siblings (Hogan completely, Louise not completely). Both originally found inspiration in sports and in university. Hogan had hoped to make a career as a football player, but that did not work out. In the end, both have earned PhDs and are employed as professional psychologists.

Their PhDs were achieved through heroically hard work. Neither of their families of origin provided economic support when Hogan and Louise were in university or graduate school, so they earned their way. Hogan had a series of jobs including a period as a bar 'bouncer', work for which he was well suited by his size and aggressiveness. While attending university, he started a painting contracting company that employed several other workers in its peak periods and provided a good income for the family. Hogan and Louise also worked together, managing an apartment building.

Because neither Hogan nor Louise came from a university-educated family, they worked from a disadvantage that could only be overcome by prodigiously hard work. Hogan's workload was further increased by the fact that he found himself at odds with much of the conventional wisdom in psychology, to the extent that his university assignments sometimes stated controversial positions. He got through by dint of determination, intelligence, and some astute compromising.

Hogan and Louise both wanted children and were deeply distressed when Louise underwent two spontaneous abortions. Finally, their first son was born, followed in a few years by a second. The additions to the family were welcome, but they definitely did not make life easier. The additional workload taxed both of them close to breaking point. Both began to have trouble with physical illnesses, primarily influenza. Yet they insisted that there be ample time for the children and family activities.

Although both children were treated firmly, they were free to express themselves spontaneously and were encouraged to take their own directions. For example, when their first son, big and strong for his age, decided that his main interests lay in dance and music, there was time and money for dancing school and encouragement to persist, although he was often the only boy in the dancing class. Like their more conventional neighbours, Hogan and Louise see the need to engage their children in after-school activities and to get them there, necessarily by car. This was more difficult for Hogan and Louise than for the neighbours, because Hogan and Louise are passionately concerned with the environment and had formerly refused to own a car.

Where does psychological integration come from for a young family where the parents have to work heroically long hours and are estranged from their families of origin? In Hogan and Louise's case, it came primarily from assiduous and successful efforts to organise a stable group of friends—mostly other couples of a wide range of ages—and a series of regular social rituals. An annual Christmas screening of Dr Seuss' *How the Grinch Stole Christmas*, Christmas breakfast for a dozen people, a New Year's Eve Party, an annual party at the streamside home of friends to watch the salmon migration, 'Pie Day' at the peak of blackberry season where berries are picked and pies mass-produced. In addition to rituals, Hogan and Louise help friends with moving, painting, and so on, as the occasions arise.

Psychosocial integration normally has a spiritual component.[3] But Hogan and Louise reject religion, organised and unorganized. However, a clue to the implicit spirituality of their unconventional social world can be drawn from a ritualized musical event that they have hosted regularly for almost 10 years. On 'Disc Night', which occurs about every 6 weeks, about two-dozen friends, many of whom are the same people time after time, attend a musical evening. Many couples arrive with children in tow. People bring food for snacks and wine or beer, marijuana appears for those who want to smoke it, and the evening begins as if it were a party, but ends quite differently. At about 9 o'clock, all gather in the living room facing the fireplace and Hogan's very large speakers, renowned for volume and fidelity. Hogan gives a short introduction to the evening, sometimes followed by another person who specifically introduces the music to be played. For years, the music was predominantly psychedelic rock, particularly Pink Floyd. In recent years, however, the choice has become more eclectic. Classical music or jazz may be played, but it is always music that is important to somebody in the group, who introduces it. There may also be visual art on display or a poetry reading. Sometimes the poems are original.

When the music begins, the atmosphere changes. One must not speak as the music plays; even the children know to be quiet, usually. It is sometimes said that the combination of Pink Floyd music and marijuana can have a spiritual quality in the right setting. In Hogan and Louise's setting, people sit quietly on the floor, facing forward towards the uniquely ornamented fireplace, reverently, it seems to me. Hogan says the fireplace is not an altar, but I say it is.

When the music is finished, people again talk, but quietly; the evening is essentially over. Children are gathered up and families drift away, to their homes.

In the course of this life, Hogan has undergone significant changes. He has gone from being a rebellious student to a mature scholar and a good teacher. He has gone from a distain for 'touchy-feely' psychology to being a good clinician. He has experienced turning points in his own personality. For example, in his work as a prison psychologist at a high-security institution at that time, he dealt with many dangerous men. He felt a certain sense of security in this milieu because of his size and aggressiveness. However, at some point, he realised that he had lost the willingness to hurt people physically, which had served him well during his years as a bouncer. He experienced this change both as an affirmation of his humanity and as placing him in serious danger in the prison, making it important for him to switch jobs.

Is Hogan addicted? Not in the sense of addiction$_3$. He has long smoked marijuana each night, using it as a kind of anti-depressant. Yet he is not overwhelmingly involved with marijuana in any sense. He is no more (or less) addicted than millions of people who take anti-depressants or watch television in a similar way. If prolonged use of marijuana is injuring his health, which is certainly possible, he could be said to be addicted$_2$, but not addicted$_3$.

Hogan and Louise are a unique couple, but there are innumerable other unconventional lifestyles that enable people to live in a world of chronic dislocation without falling into depression or serious addiction. Such lifestyles are a creative response to a dislocated society.

Participating in a concocted community

I lived most of my life in the suburbs of American and Canadian cities spreading across the North American continent between New York City and Vancouver. In 1990, I finally moved from the suburbs of Vancouver into a district of the central city with a distinctive character, where I now live. I could never willingly return to suburban life. It is therefore possible that my account of suburban life is distorted by the zeal of the converted. For simplicity, my account is limited to the North American suburbs that flourished in the baby boom that followed World War II as I was growing up. However, there are indications that it may also apply to a significant degree to the suburbs of today.[4]

At the end of World War II, large tracts of relatively cheap North American farmland were bought up by developers, and houses were built to attract city dwellers with low real-estate prices, built-in appliances, and the gleam of post-war modernity. This formula worked famously in conjunction with the 'baby boom' that was underway. The new cradles were filled and refilled and the population increased geometrically. It became evident quite early in this process that something was wrong with the North American suburban lifestyle, but this 'something' could not be identified precisely at first.

A major part of the 'something' was dislocation. The suburbs could not have been better designed to negate psychosocial integration and maximise dislocation. The custom was for each family to buy the biggest, most expensive house they could afford. The consequence was that neighbours had little in common except the size of their mortgages. Ethnic background, political views, religion, occupation, etc., were shuffled like a deck of cards (except as limited by the racial segregation of that era).

Not only did neighbours have no common cultural roots, they lived in residential aggregations that had no material basis upon which to build a local culture. The only real economic activities were real estate and retail marketing. Most other economic activity took place in the inner city and the outer farmland, so the suburban neighbours 'commuted' to different workplaces each day. People usually did not stay long enough in their suburb to develop roots, because most people worked for large corporations that 'transferred' their employees when their skills were needed elsewhere. Yet it was all-important to fit in at all times. As North American urbanologist Jane Jacobs put it:

> There are people who seemingly can behave like interchangeable statistics and take up in a different place exactly where they left off, but they must belong to one of our fairly homogenous and ingrown nomad societies like … the peripatetic junior executive families of suburbia … [5]

Children formed themselves into more tightly knit groups or gangs, but since the parents knew each other only slightly, if at all, few common cultural norms or traditions could be transmitted from the older generation to the children's groups. Youth gangs generated simpler, sometimes more brutal, norms on their own.

In the absence of culture, adult suburbanites developed a pretence of society. Neighbours were invited 'over'. Drinks were poured, cigarettes lit. Conversation ensued. But topics of general interest were largely limited to real estate, lawns, children, and television, and these were quickly worked through. Cards were then dealt and bridge, canasta, or poker undertaken so that a good time could be had by all. Since there was no real point to any of this, people naturally felt socially adrift. This gave rise to the conspiracy to concoct a community.

The conspiracy was to produce the illusion of a real community or society. One way to participate in the conspiracy was to pretend to be having a good time so convincingly that others would invite you over in the future, so that your convivial presence would help them to convince themselves that they too were having a good time. Another way to participate was to tell jokes that would keep people laughing continuously, since there was little serious to say. The illusion of a real, convivial community was thus created. To reinforce the illusion, the word 'community' was used promiscuously—community chest, community centre, community school, community doctor, community mental health, community police, community standards, community jail.

In fact, there was precious little community, but the illusion was so powerful that many people were able to use it, with jaw-clenching determination and a little drink now and again to sustain themselves. The illusion was further reinforced by televised images of what a model suburban life looked like, by a growing affluence that provided abundant material compensations, by a cultivated sense of superiority over those darker skinned people left behind in deteriorating urban cores, by the exigencies of raising large numbers of children, and by bland suburban churches that never let it be forgotten that the Lord looked favourably upon these arrangements, now and for ever more.[6] Many people were able to find adequate sustenance in suburban living, despite the dislocation that it entailed. It is reasonable, I think, to say that most of these people were not addicted. In fact, some genuine friendships were formed and sometimes suburbs evolved from pseudo-communities to the real thing.

However, when the illusion failed, many people took up addictions to alcohol, drugs, overwork, overspending, overeating, errant sexuality, speculative investment, watching television, and so forth. Yet many people stuck it out in good form and can be counted as having gotten by reasonably well in the modern world.

Political activism

Some popular political movements, like the ecological movement on the political left and the 'family values' movement on the political right, provide participants not only with a sense of moral rectitude and service, but also with a welcoming community of fellow activists. Activist communities are open, since they always need more members to achieve their political ends. They quickly give new members responsibilities and recognition. The awareness of a shared purpose in real and important matters automatically generates friendship.

Even when it fails to achieve its political goals, social activism buffers people against dislocation,[7] reducing the risk of addiction. Naturally, such movements appeal to many people who keenly sense their own dislocation.[8]

A more extensive discussion of the relationship between dislocation produced by the globalisation of free-market society and political activism has been made by Alexandre Dorna, primarily based on the burgeoning populist movements of Europe. Dorna emphasized the distinction between populism and the fanatical nationalism that also has a long history in Europe. Although populism is a way of adapting to dislocation, it cannot be called either fanatical nationalism or addiction. Populists are activists who do not reject society for a hopeless substitute world, but strive in the company of other frustrated people to restore what has been lost. Populism does not take the form of an overwhelming involvement. It does not entail blind obedience to violent religious doctrines and fascism. By contrast, Dorna described fanatical nationalism in this way:

> Fanatical nationalism,[9] like fascism, expresses a singular, rigid, totalizing conception of the world. Within this conception, national identity rests, in the last analysis, upon a racial doctrine and upon a sanctified authority. As well, the bureaucracy and the army are,

especially in the case of fascism, essential aspects of fanatical nationalism and fascism, serving both to lock the masses into a totalizing, patriotic ideology and to impose iron discipline in the name of tradition, of race, or of a deified leader at the top of the formal hierarchy. These doctrines necessarily lead to a belief in the inevitable expansion of the state and of its hegemony. As a consequence, war is viewed spiritually. None of this is found in the populist movement.[10]

Although the distinction between politically beneficial and psychologically supportive activism on the one hand and fanaticism or addiction on the other is very clear, the difference is quantitative rather than qualitative. They are more and less extreme degrees of the same psychological reaction to painful dislocation.

The 'tragically cool'

The anguish of dislocation is now widely recognised, but not everyone believes, as I do, that a societal transformation that would restore psychosocial integration is the only real solution. Many young adults optimistically believe that they can get by quite well in a lifestyle of extreme individualism and dislocation with the aid of high technology and a stoical view of such a life as inevitable and 'cool', if a bit tragic. The autobiographical paper that appeared in Chapter 9 under the heading *A university student* may well illustrate this lifestyle, which can be called 'tragically cool'. However, I am pessimistic about how well these optimistic young adults are really getting by. Both optimistic and pessimistic views of this lifestyle are summarised here.

A study (first introduced in Chapter 5) provides an optimistic view of the tragically cool. Adams and de Panafieu provided a description of young 'cutting-edgers' in nine countries on the basis of extensive questionnaire data and focus-group discussions. Cutting-edgers are employed and affluent; they comprise the 15% of society for whom:

> Nothing is permanent. Everything is in flux. There are no patterns, rituals, or routines. No pithy maxims or words to live by. Nothing is definite, which is why the word 'like' has become for cool youth what the F word is to the underclass. Titles are as irrelevant as the British House of Lords. They search not for a permanent place, but to float above it all, to be cool, to be detached from the things that they cannot control—governments and their policies and social welfare programs, wars, disease, terrorism. They wish instead to be a chameleon that changes with the flow in search of hedonistic little pleasures often in the safety and security of their wired, soon to be wireless homes.
>
> What will replace the state that replaced the church that replaced the warlord? In the minds of our cutting-edgers there is no doubt: The vacuum will be filled by the multinational corporations and institutions that own the technologies that stimulate, alter and extend their intellects and senses.[11]

Cutting-edgers are busy. They use e-mail, cell phones, and BlackBerries to maintain their state of perpetual motion. High-tech aids help them to derive satisfaction from human relationships that cannot last long enough to qualify as psychosocial integration—or even as addiction. For example, cheap, convenient telephoning keeps cutting-edgers in constant contact with the office and with families and friends who also live in perpetual motion;[12] chat rooms and multi-player Internet role-playing games like *Second Life* allow virtually meaningful interactions with strangers;[13]

video games allow intense confrontations of virtual good and evil; 'mass collaboration' with strangers in corporations organised around 'wikinomics' can produce a very good income;[14] Internet-based social-networking systems such as Facebook™ permit economic as well as social interactions;[15] stimulating pharmaceuticals and a bit of esoteric know-how help people to find maximum satisfaction in 'quickie sex'.[16]

A business newspaper article focused this optimism in a slightly different direction. The article identified some young men and women in the business world as 'gamers' (as opposed to 'boomers' of an earlier generation). Brought up with constant access to video games, gamers are presumably infused with expectations of heroism and other aspects of extreme individualism. The authors made the point that such employees are capable of truly heroic attention to the goals of their corporation if correctly motivated and discussed how their talents and personalities can be 'harnessed'.[17]

These lifestyles of the tragically cool fit Erik Erikson's description of 'identity diffusion'.[18] Eriksonian psychologist James Marcia explained identity diffusion as a state in which a person has not made a self-determined commitment to a stable role and belief system and is not in the process of exploring possibilities for these.[19] In his later research, Marcia reported that the percentage of Canadian and American university students who were in a state of identity diffusion doubled in the 1980s, from about 20% to about 40%.[20] Marcia attributed this increase in identity diffusion in part to the social environment generated by extreme free-market economics in Canada and the United States in that decade.[21] He suggested that, whereas some people with diffused identities were in serious psychological difficulty, others whose diffusion afforded them flexibility in the face of rapidly changing circumstances were *better* adapted to free-market society.

Another optimistic view is that the excessiveness and awkwardness of today's tragically cool young adults bespeaks society's evolution to new styles of happiness and grace in the unfolding world of modernity. Philosopher Charles Taylor has argued that the essential task for the present is collectively recognising, developing, and cherishing the sustaining moral core of the new lifestyle that is coming into existence.[22]

Still on the optimistic side, Francis Fukuyama and Joseph Heath have both written brilliant celebrations of the new free-market world that are, indirectly, celebrations of the tragically cool lifestyle as well. Yet, in their exuberance, both of these enthusiasts seemed compelled to include an expression of loss, expressed with unexpected poignancy. Fukuyama's recognition that the modern society that constitutes the end of history has an 'emptiness at the core'[23] was cited earlier. Heath's version of this sentiment goes like this:

> Welcome to the culture of efficiency. It's not perfect, but it's not so bad either.
> This is the compromise at the heart of our society. The world we live in clearly fails to satisfy many of our deeper needs and impulses. And yet any serious attempt to change it seems to entail even greater sacrifice. We may be as close to utopia as we can get ... [24]
> This may not satisfy all of our deeper impulses, but there is very deep wisdom in the realisation that we are unlikely to do any better.[25]

Less optimistic observers perceive the emerging lifestyles as definitely more tragic than cool. A growing number of capable, university-trained young adults in Europe and North America live at home, at the expense of their parents, indefinitely postponing serious commitments to a career and establishing a home of their own, and suffering more than the rest of the population from anxiety, depression, excessive drug use, and compulsive interaction with computer screens. People who live this kind of life have variously been characterized as slackers, underachievers, adultescents, and 'KIPPERS' (Kids In Parents' Pockets Eroding Retirement Savings). Numerous popular books have proposed diverse explanations for this alarming trend.[26] In the context of this book, it would seem that these young adults are reacting to the same dislocated world that cutting-edgers are, but in a less socially acceptable way. When the numbers are eventually tallied, the so-called slackers may provide quantitative evidence that the majority of people cannot live without the support of a stable culture or social group, as cutting-edgers do.

Maschino has decried the damage to society caused by a new generation of French media intellectuals who sound like cutting-edgers in the sense of lacking the staunch commitments of the celebrated French intellectuals of the past. The new generation service their own narcissistic needs adequately, but they harm society in the long run by degrading the quality of public information:

> Playing at being journalists, these caricatures of intellectuals rarely do any actual reporting in wartime (having gone to the scene, they present themselves to the authorities in control, and are taken around, protected by their omnipresent guards, except when they are actually visiting the military itself), and do none of the laborious work of a reporter who takes risks, patiently collects facts, and interviews ordinary citizens as often as politicians and generals. As Pierre Nora says, 'They are not serving any cause but helping themselves to servings of a cause, putting the people's misery at the service of their egos'. And, one might add, at the service of their exorbitant narcissism.[27]

Maschino also argued that the writers he criticizes are essentially indifferent to ideology, maintaining a black-and-white moralism as they shift their political position from one side to the other:

> In the same fashion that they were Stalinists or Maoists, they are now pro-Americans. And in the same manner that they formerly supported internationalism they now support globalisation. They are still black-and-white thinkers, as they always were. And they don't acknowledge that they have changed camps.[28]

Of course, Maschino is a left-winger criticising right wing intellectuals. But his critique applies just as well to some left-wing intellectuals. Many very bright writers, left and right, righteously express a shallow understanding of their position and show no real sign of commitment to it.

Dany-Robert Dufour, whose work was introduced in Chapter 5, provides the most pessimistic view of the tragically cool. He sees such people as extreme manifestations of the personality type that universally grows from post-modern free-market society. He does not dispute their creative abilities, but focuses on their potential for destruction and their vulnerability to madness.[29]

Dufour sees this personality type, which he variously calls 'acritical', 'psychoticising', and 'schizoid', as the inevitable product of a unique period of history following World

War II in which Western society was 'desymbolised'. Desymbolisation means that people came to agree that the great value systems of the past, based on religion, nationalism, and critical intellectuality are no longer tenable, either singly or in combination, in the face of the intimidating achievements of modern science and the awesome power of what Dufour calls 'total capitalism'. Moreover, the free-market system demands ever more flexibility of people to enable the market to keep expanding and changing:

> ... neoliberalism needs to work with a personality that is uncritical and fragmented. In other words, a person who will connect with each new trend, who lacks strong roots, who is infinitely open to the flow of new merchandise and communication technologies, and who always needs more consumer goods: in sum, a precarious person, whose precarious identity is valuable in a market that can use it as a new opening to sell goods that can serve as identity kits or images with which people can identify.[30]

Dufour used the famous writings of Antonin Artaud[31] and Samuel Beckett as the basis of an argument that grotesque, schizoid suffering awaits people who are developing these precarious identities.[32] Despite the madness and misery they describe, these mid-20th-century writers (particularly Artaud) have been seen by some of their followers as glorious exponents of the life of complete freedom and independence. My own young friends who have embraced the lifestyle of the tragically cool do seem to me precocious and vulnerable, although none of them have yet described to me the florid schizoid experiences found in the writings of Artaud and Beckett.

If Dufour's complex argument is pushed to its logical conclusion, it might be said that the cool post-modern personality is deliberately created by a market that must root out all remnants of psychosocial integration in order to supercharge the gross national product. In this nightmare view, free-market society needs people who will work and buy with the abandon that is generated by serial passions rather than any type of settled lifestyle, *even a stable addiction*. Such people must be so fragmented that they can be distracted from their pain by forms of electronic entertainment that can be mass-produced at short notice and at little expense.[33] The final product of such an evolution is a new, post-modern personality, a mélange of spontaneity, madness, depression, and autism. Personalities of this sort are caricatured brilliantly in popular entertainment, particularly in the hugely popular cartoon series about American middle management, *Dilbert*.[34] If Dufour is right, the tragically cool may indeed escape addiction—but at their greater peril.

Is it farfetched to think of the market as an organism that has the foresight to tailor-make personalities with this degree of precision and to use the mystique of the tragically cool as camouflage? I don't know yet. Dufour, however, seems quite certain. He concludes one of his books by saying, 'If there is such a thing as a categorical moral imperative today, it is to resist the implementation of total capitalism.'[35]

The spiritually sufficient

Some people regard conscious resignation to dislocation as a vital component of a spiritual orientation that enables them to live as fully and happily as is possible. This spiritual orientation is often understood as a way of avoiding addiction, as well as other forms of self-destruction. This understanding has been expressed in the language of Christianity[36] and several Asian spiritual traditions.[37]

In general, it is understood that all forms of attachment, including those that make psychosocial integration possible, must be subdued, for all of them lead ultimately to grief. Instead of focusing their lives on cultivating attachments, which are always problematic and often addicting, people can find joy in cultivating the immediate present: a moment of silent affection, a surge of universal love, the serenity of spiritual sufficiency. In prayerful or meditative silence, the unattached seeker finds the ultimate source of all human happiness. In disciplined prayer or meditation, he or she knows aloneness as achievement rather than loss, and the experience of emptiness as victory rather than defeat.

A book by former Catholic monk Thomas Moore, entitled *Care of the Soul: a Guide for Cultivating Depth and Sacredness in Everyday Life*, became a spiritual guidepost for a decade. It was an instant success in the United States and Canada, and by 1994 had been on the *New York Times* best-seller list for 46 weeks. In Moore's form of spiritualism, which can be called neo-Christianity, the 'soul' is not seen as an immortal, immaterial emanation from God that is the object of a 'salvational fantasy', but a god-like aspect of mortal, material life.

In addition to criticizing traditional theology, Moore criticised contemporary psychology, on the grounds that it pays far too little attention to matters of the soul. According to Moore, the soul is the central fact of human nature:

> The great malady of the twentieth century, implicated in all of our troubles and affecting us individually and socially, is 'loss of soul'. When soul is neglected, it doesn't just go away; it appears symptomatically in obsessions, addictions, violence, and loss of meaning. Our temptation is to isolate these symptoms or to try to eradicate them one by one; but the root problem is that we have lost our wisdom about the soul, even our interest in it. We have today few specialists of the soul to advise us when we succumb to moods and emotional pain, or when as a nation we find ourselves confronting a host of threatening evils.[38]

Moore identified himself correctly, I believe, as closely aligned with Roman Epicureanism, ancient philosophy that urged a devotion to the self and inner contemplation but, unlike its Stoic counterpart, did not find it necessary to forsake all material comforts. On the contrary, Epicureanism took enjoyment of wholesome material comforts to be an aid to spiritual development. In Moore's words:

> Tending the things around us and becoming sensitive to the importance of home, daily schedule, and maybe even the clothes we wear, are ways of caring for the soul. When Marsilio Ficino wrote his self-help book, *The Book of Life*, five hundred years ago, he placed emphasis on carefully choosing colors, spices, oils, places to walk, countries to visit—all very concrete decisions of everyday life that day by day either support or disturb the soul.... Ancient psychologists taught that our own souls are inseparable from the world's soul, and that both are found in all the many things that make up nature and culture ...
>
> So, the first point to make about care of the soul is that it is not primarily a method of problem solving. Its goal is not to make life problem-free, but to give ordinary life the depth and value that c[j]ome with soulfulness.[39]

William Pryor, a brilliant writer with a 12-year history of severe heroin addiction and alcoholism who has now been abstinent for 28 years, eloquently described the role of dislocation in the origin of his own addiction.[40] However, he did not attribute his transformation from a degraded drug addict to a successful entrepreneur to re-establishment of psychosocial integration as would be expected from the perspective of the dislocation theory of addiction. Rather, he attributed it to a spiritual awakening inspired by an Eastern guru.

In the course of his transformation, Pryor recognised the inevitability of suffering throughout life[41] and discovered, with the aid of meditation, that this suffering can be converted into creativity rather than addiction. He argued that his own transformation is better understood as a 'discovery' rather than a 'recovery', since he had no salubrious life prior to his addiction that could be recovered, despite being a product of a comfortable, intellectual stratum of English society[42] and a direct descendent of Charles Darwin.

I believe that, in the language of this book, Pryor is revealing that his present prodigious creativity as an entrepreneur has essentially the same roots in dislocation as the destructive drug addiction of his young adulthood. It also seems that, for Pryor, the anguish of dislocation is a component of the most complete kind of life that can realistically be expected in today's painful world. He is getting by through a serene acceptance of unrelenting anguish. Of course, Pryor knows best about his own life, but I will argue in later chapters that it is necessary to find practicable ways of collectively overcoming universal dislocation, in addition to spiritual ways to endure the pain that it brings.

The ex-addict

Many people who are seriously addicted sooner or later build a new life that enables them to leave addiction behind, or at least to switch to a less damaging one.[43] In the most fortunate instances, people overcome addiction completely and achieve an adequate degree of psychosocial integration. Friends, families, and professionals often provide essential help in this crucial transition.

If, however, people who are 'in recovery' from addiction cannot find a sufficient level of psychosocial integration in their post-addict lives, the next most attractive alternative often is to pursue an overwhelming involvement that is not anti-social, but is instead valued by society, and that allows some place for inclusion of family and friends.[44] Quite often, such people find a valuable niche as addiction therapists, devoting themselves to helping others along the difficult road to recovery that they themselves have traversed and serving as living examples that recovery is possible. In such a role, or in other philanthropic roles, formerly addicted persons can earn the sincere admiration of their society. A full-strength overwhelming involvement of this sort would properly be called addiction$_4$ in the language of this book, although it is more polite and less confusing to refer to such a person as a 'crusading former drug user', a 'charismatic therapist', a 'hero', or a 'saint' in the full meaning of these slightly ambivalent terms. One of the founders of Alcoholics Anonymous, Bill W., is a well-known example of addiction$_4$ who is discussed in Chapter 12. Many more addictions in today's world can be classified as addiction$_3$ than as addiction$_4$. This is probably because developing a life of addiction$_4$ is very difficult. Not everybody has the talent or the strength to succeed at it.

Although addiction$_4$ is far less personally destructive than addiction$_3$, and often provides an admirable and important contribution to society, it nonetheless seems to be a way of adapting to dislocation through overwhelming involvement in a narrowed lifestyle. It is properly called 'addiction' in the traditional English meaning of the word.

The role of the devoted ex-addict is well recognised among people who have suffered from addictions to drugs and alcohol, and the dislocation theory would suggest that it is just as likely to occur in the lives of people with addictions to other pursuits. This transformation may become more and more frequent if free-market society continues to expand in the future. At the logical limit, in a complete free-market society everybody would be severely dislocated. Addiction$_3$ would be close to a universal life experience, expanding the possibilities of transforming addiction$_3$ to addiction$_4$. It may be that, in the most extreme and hypothetical case, a world of inescapable dislocation would eventually be populated entirely by saints and sinners. In this grotesque world, a perpetual alternation of addiction$_3$ and addiction$_4$ would be the norm of human existence, and the experience of addiction would become indistinct, or perhaps as invisible as the air we breathe.

Conclusion

This chapter begins with a riddle and ends in dismal speculation. It contains examples of people managing to avoid, or to overcome, severe forms of addiction despite living in a society of severe dislocation. The lives that are described can hardly be seen as joyful and it is difficult to make a clear statement on whether most of the people described in the latter parts of this chapter ought to be considered addicted$_3$ or not. It does not seem likely, however, that any of them are brilliantly fulfilling their human potential. If such descriptions fit many or most people who are getting by in free-market society, where will society turn to find the kind of inspired, fully functioning leaders and workers who will be necessary to pull the world out of its current crises?

As the world moves towards to a global free-market society, everybody must cope with dislocation. Addictive dynamics are always a temptation and frequently a part of life experience for the majority of people who manage to avoid overt addiction. Whereas the word 'addiction' has been used as a medical diagnosis or criminal charge for a form of infrequently occurring social deviance in the past, this soon may no longer be a useful way of speaking. In a world in which addictive dynamics are close to universal, the word 'addicted' loses any sharp edge that could make it useful as a diagnostic label. Nonetheless, the concept of addiction and the dynamic relationship between dislocation and addiction is extremely useful for understanding the temper of our times, including some of its most admirable personal achievements as well as some of its madness.

The experience of ex-addicts leaves a very important question unanswered. Does addiction$_4$ always stem from addiction$_3$? In other words, are there saints who were not formerly sinners? I don't know. This is a spiritual question, however, so it is reasonable to suppose that the answer might emerge from a deeper exploration of spiritual views of dislocation and addiction. This is undertaken in the next chapter.

Endnotes

1 Mahoney (2004b).

2 Dreher (2004b).

3 This point is argued in Chapter 3 under the heading *Psychosocial integration is a necessity*.

4 Mahoney (2005a).

5 J. Jacobs (1961, p. 136, footnote).

6 Apparently, this is still the case. See McKibben (2005).

7 Suzuki and Dressel (2002, pp. 2–4) provided a valuable description of the psychosocial rewards of social activism. Hawken (2007) celebrated the mystique of political activism, which also serves as a buffer against dislocation.

8 Dorna (2003).

9 Dorna used the unmodified word 'nationalism' at this point in his French text. However, the context makes it clear that he referred to a nationalism of a fanatical sort which cannot be translated in Canada simply as 'nationalism'.

10 Dorna (2003, p. 9).

11 M. Adams and de Panafieu (2003, p. A13).

12 Schiller (2005).

13 Avery (2007).

14 Tapscott and Williams (2007).

15 Ticoll (2003); Traves (2006).

16 J. Johnson (2003).

17 Beck and Wade (2005).

18 See Erikson (1959, p. 121). An identity-diffused person would not necessarily live this way, but it is one possibility.

19 Marcia (1966). Marcia (1989, p. 290) wrote 'Their outstanding characteristic is a lack of commitment and a corresponding lack of concern about their committedness.'

20 Marcia (1989).

21 Marcia (1989, p. 292) called that era the 'Reaganized United States'.

22 C. Taylor (1991).

23 Fukuyama (1989). This was cited in Chapter 5 of this book on p. 191.

24 J. Heath (2001, p. 2).

25 J. Heath (2001, p. 39).

26 Shimo (2007).

27 Maschino (2002, p. 28).

28 Maschino (2002, p. 29).

29 J. Wong (2003) has described one Canadian variant on these destructive lifestyles, in an article entitled *Party Animals*.

30 Dufour (2003a, pp. 140–141).

31 Dufour (2005, pp. 247–264).

32 Dufour (2005, pp. 275–297).

33 Dufour (2005, pp. 303–305).

34 S. Adams (2002).

35 Dufour (2003a, p. 251).

36 T. Moore (1992).

37 Das (1998); Pryor (2003).

38 T. Moore (1992, p. xi).

39 T. Moore (1992, p. 4).

40 Pryor (2003).

41 Pryor (2003, pp. 213, 218).

42 Pryor (2003, p. 197).

43 Robins and Murphy (1967); S. Schachter (1982); Koski-Jännes (1998); Granfield and Cloud (1999, 2002); Klingemann *et al.* (2001); Paris and Bradley (2001); Cameron *et al.* (2002); Blomqvist (2004); Öjesjö (2004).

44 For example, William Pryor (2003), described earlier in this chapter as 'getting by' as one of the 'spiritually sufficient', could also be classified as a person who has transformed his addiction from a socially unacceptable one as a heroin addict to a socially acceptable one. He concluded his account of his recovery as follows (p. 225): '… we crave life itself so that we may fulfil our purpose. When we are focussed, all desires get subsumed into that one-pointed purpose.'

Chapter 12

Spiritual Treatment for Addiction: The 'Fifth Pillar'

Every year, I hear gut-wrenching stories of personal and family addiction problems told by university students who are taking my addiction seminar or who just present themselves at my office door.[1] These are not counselling sessions; the students simply want to tell their painful stories to someone who might understand and I want to listen and learn from them. These narratives, which often spread themselves over several meetings, keep me abreast of changing attitudes towards addiction among young adults in my corner of the world. Over the decades, I have witnessed growing despair at the inability of the conventional four pillars of treatment, prevention, law enforcement, and harm reduction[2] to contain the increasing menace of addiction in these students' lives.

As if to offset the despair, more and more of these rational and worldly young adults express bright hopes that some form of spirituality can overcome addiction and other psychological problems that they fear. This fresh upwelling of spirituality is not limited to Christianity. It also springs from a group of traditions that can collectively be called eclectic spirituality. There are, of course, other flourishing spiritual movements in today's world,[3] but these two are the most prominent in my corner of it. Many people are putting their best hopes for doing something about addiction in one or the other. This chapter is about past and present applications of both Christianity and eclectic spirituality to the problem of addiction. It explains why, despite the good they do for many addicted individuals, neither of these spiritual traditions can be expected to bring addiction under control in free-market society.

Although I do not share their spiritual beliefs, I am awed by some of the practitioners of Christian healing and eclectic spirituality. They are as sincere in their work as anyone could be. It feels important and right that they bring their gift of faith and love to people who are suffering from addiction. Sometimes they succeed where conventional interventions fail. Even when spiritual approaches do not overcome addiction, they reframe it as a spiritual story with a deeper meaning. Spiritual interventions constitute a fifth 'pillar' that affirms society's dedication to bringing addiction under control.

The application of these spiritual traditions to the problem of addiction goes back many centuries. Both traditions were clearly recognisable by the late Roman Empire. Their track records of overcoming addiction across the centuries appear to be no worse—but no better—than the four secular pillars. Although these two sources of inspiration can breathe fresh air into today's stale conventional wisdom, they cannot prevent a tidal wave of addiction from engulfing globalising free-market society. The final two chapters of this book propose a very different action plan that affords, I believe, a greater basis for hope than the spiritual traditions that are discussed in this one.

This chapter begins with the classic Christian approach to addiction as originally formulated by St Augustine and proceeds to the radically modernised Christianity of Alcoholics Anonymous. It then considers both classic and modern forms of eclectic spirituality. Nothing in this chapter is intended to disparage spirituality: even though spiritual healing techniques per se cannot overcome today's growing addiction problem, the problem is so enormous that solving it will require many people drawing strength from the deepest wells of their spirits.

Overcoming addiction through Christian conversion: St Augustine revisited

When he described his own youthful addictions[4] in the *Confessions*, St Augustine used the voice of a pathetic sinner, imploring God for help and forgiveness. He deplored his own futile efforts to resist the earthly pleasures and attachments that had made his everyday life a disaster area and blocked the life-saving union with God that he craved.

When he spoke of overcoming addictive sin later in his life, however, St Augustine often used the voice of a powerful Bishop of the Church of Rome, preaching with authority. The tears that drenched the pages of his *Confessions* crystallised into the solid wall with the single narrow gate surrounding the 'City of God' that he described almost three decades later.[5] The stringent orthodoxy and asceticism that Bishop Augustine imposed both upon himself and the people of his diocese are not imposed on everybody who converts to Christianity today. However, St Augustine's model of release from addictive sinfulness by conversion to a life of Christian spirituality remains the conceptual basis of much of today's addiction treatment, secular as well as pastoral.[6]

St Augustine described his personal conversion experience in powerfully religious terms; for example:

> ... I saw with my soul's eye (such as it was) an unchangeable light shining above this eye of my soul and above my mind. It was not the ordinary light which is visible to all flesh, nor something of the same sort, only bigger, as though it might be our ordinary light shining much more brightly and filling everything with its greatness. No, it was not like that; it was different, entirely different from anything of the kind. Nor was it above my mind as oil floats on water or as the heaven is above the earth.... He who knows truth knows that light, and he who knows that light knows eternity. Love knows it. O eternal truth and true love and beloved eternity! You are my God; to you I sigh by day and by night. And when I first knew you, you raised me up so that I could see that there was something to see and that I still lacked the ability to see it.[7]

Following his conversion, St Augustine became celibate and gave up all forms of earthly ambition in favour of monastic poverty and humility. However, he confessed that his old cravings continued to torment him for the rest of his life.

Whereas St Augustine's hope of conquering the entire world's addictive sin by converting it to Roman Catholic Christianity has not been realised, individual conversion still overcomes addiction for some individuals today, as it has for centuries. Many modern people testify to their reclamation from addiction to a life of Christian piety and sobriety in ways that resonate with St Augustine's. They speak with such fullness that it is impossible for me to doubt the truth of what they say. Some of their lives have changed visibly, breaking out of deadly downward spirals.

Although St Augustine fully understood that a politically corrupt world seriously erodes the strength of character needed to resist addiction, he believed that rebelling against any established government, or even working politically to improve it, was an affront to God's judgement in having created things as they are.[8] He urged people to overcome addictive sinfulness by changing themselves rather than by changing society. On the other hand, he believed that Christian society should aggressively increase religious conversion by encouragement, exhortation, and punishment. Thus, St Augustine laid individualistic and moralistic foundation stones for today's conventional wisdom on addiction. To a lesser extent, he laid foundation stones for the medical portion of the conventional wisdom as well. A thousand years before the rise of scientific medicine, he spoke of God as a 'physician'[9] who could heal the addictive 'sicknesses of my soul'.[10]

St Augustine felt that people must supplant every aspect of their addictive sinfulness with strenuous religious devotion. This meant complete abstinence from all worldly pleasures. In addition to obviously destructive practices, like compulsive promiscuity and stealing, St Augustine expected radical curtailment of friendship, family devotion, scientific knowledge, self-esteem, theatre attendance, and much more. He even condemned children's delights in adventure stories and childhood games, and his parents' desire for grandchildren.[11] Although he stressed the importance of a Christian community,[12] he expected its members to work hard at *not* enjoying the musical quality of hymns sung in church and the pleasant tastes of a frugal monastic diet.[13]

Since he advocated supplanting virtually all social involvement and pleasure with devotion to God,[14] St Augustine can be said, in the language of this book, to have endorsed addiction$_4$ to Christian faith as a cure for addiction$_3$. Whereas close study of St Augustine's words in the *Confessions* makes this surprising conclusion inescapable,[15] equating St Augustine's Christian pious life with addiction$_4$ can seem like a deliberate provocation today, no matter how doggedly the word 'addiction' is redefined and no matter how many numerical subscripts may be suspended beneath it. Moreover, equating St Augustine's life as a Christian with addiction$_4$ might seem to imply that all Christian faith is addictive, which of course it is not. Most everyday Christian faith is far from the overwhelming involvement that St Augustine endorsed. Despite the misunderstandings that can arise from acknowledging it, the disquieting fact that St Augustine remedied his addictions$_3$ by adopting a form of addiction$_4$ to God poses important questions about the nature of addiction and society that must be examined further to fulfil the purpose of this book.

Christians have used the word 'addiction' and its synonyms to describe ideal Christian faith from the earliest days of the religion. St Paul urged wayward

Corinthians to emulate those among them who had 'addicted themselves to the ministry of the saints' in the King James translation of the Christian Bible.[16] In the book of Romans, St Paul repeatedly describes himself as a 'slave' or a 'bond slave' of Jesus and urged his fellow Christians to adopt a similar life of voluntary slavery.[17] Chapter 2 showed that voluntary slavery is very close to the root definition of the word 'addiction' in both English and Latin.

The view that Christianity, in its ideal form, calls for a devotion so overwhelming that it fits the traditional definition of addiction and the definition of addiction$_4$[18] is also evident in present-day Christian theology. For example, renowned 20th-century American theologian and monk Thomas Merton described the experience of his own commitment to God as follows:

> Christianity is more than a moral code, more than a philosophy, more than a system of rites … in practice, the integral Christian life is something far more than all this. It is more than a belief; it is a *life*. That is to say, it is a belief that is lived and experienced and expressed in action … In plain words—if you can accept them as plain—Christianity is the life and death and resurrection of Christ going on day after day in the souls of individual men and in the heart of society.[19]

A stronger statement of the addictive nature of ideal Christian faith can be found in the writing of German theologian Dietrich Bonhoeffer who explicitly stated that the 'call to discipleship' requires of those who truly follow Jesus a commitment that is not only total, but also entails unquestioning, immediate abandonment of all previous social and familial ties.[20] Bonhoeffer was a courageous opponent of Hitler in Nazi Germany who was interrogated, imprisoned, and eventually hanged by the Nazis in 1945.

Finally, many forthright young Christians of the Internet era use the word 'addiction' as a capsule description of their own faith. This can be confirmed simply by 'Googling' the phrase 'addicted to Jesus'.[21]

Outside the Christian context as well, addiction$_4$ can be recognised as the salvation of many highly addicted$_3$ people who are unable to restore psychosocial integration. Granfield and Cloud's interview study of 46 people who had recovered from serious drug addictions revealed that many had undergone conversion experiences and subsequently immersed themselves in new lifestyles, some of which were built on Christianity, some on other faiths, and some on various secular bases:

> Whatever activity they chose—whether it was religion, education, community, politics, work, or physical well being—it typically became the focal point of their lives and was fervently performed. Interestingly, our respondent's stories suggest that they had become as deeply involved in these new activities as they had once been in alcohol and drug use during their periods of dependency. Such complete involvement in alternative activities suggests that these pursuits act not merely as substitutes and replacements for addiction, but that they represent avenues to new meaning and epistemologies through which an individual can compose a self in relation to collective life that is incompatible with excessive alcohol and drug use.[22]

Even to a non-Christian like myself, addiction$_4$ to orthodox Christian faith seems far superior to addiction$_3$ because it is socially acceptable and physically harmless, and because it can inspire admirable service to humanity. Nevertheless, I believe that a narrowed life of addiction$_4$ cannot offer the fullness that a life of psychosocial integration can. St Augustine's life seems to confirm this. Even as a full-time member and honoured leader of a vigorous Christian community, he consistently described himself as a resident alien whose true allegiance was to another, holier community called the City of God, a city that is invisible to worldly eyes.[23] In St Augustine's view, being a resident alien was a blessing for it kept him in constant contact with the Holy Spirit. However, as decades passed, he still could not view his life on earth with satisfaction, but as a dutiful submission to torture that would only be relieved in heaven.[24] He spent the last 10 days before his death in solitary prayer and tearful penance,[25] a sad old man alone with his imaginary friend, as it seems to me. In the absence of real evidence, however, the question[26] of whether addiction$_4$, to Christian faith or to anything else, can be an adequate alternative to psychosocial integration remains unsettled in this book, as do other questions about addiction$_4$.

Why St Augustine's solution to addiction works as well as it does

Recovery from addiction through Christian conversion has occurred countless times over many centuries, including the present one. From an orthodox Christian point of view, the direct intervention of God alters the lives of formerly addicted persons, giving them the strength to do what they must, while the presence of the Holy Spirit fills them with joy. If the dislocation theory is an adequate account of addiction, it must be able to provide a secular explanation of why this religious therapy works to the extent that it does.

From the secular view of dislocation theory, Augustinian conversion provides a better lifestyle than addiction$_3$ in several vital ways. Although a lifetime of overwhelming commitment to the Christian God is strenuous to maintain,[27] it is far safer, healthier, and more socially acceptable in the long run than the insalubrious life of addiction$_3$ that it replaces. On a material level, alcohol can damage the liver, syringes can transmit AIDS, computers can cause stress injuries, and even rare cases of water addiction can cause dangerous metabolic imbalance. However, overwhelming involvement with an imaginary being (which I understand God to be) is far less likely to be physically dangerous. Overwhelming involvement with St Augustine's God definitely seems preferable.

Moreover, addiction$_4$ to Christian faith can provide some of the genuine social support and ecstatic experience that addiction$_3$ provides so poorly. Because there is a real and lasting Christian fellowship on earth, religious conversion can provide a closer approach to genuine psychosocial integration than most forms of addiction$_3$. Because Augustinian faith entails rigid self-control, it can provide the identity boost of having overcome a degrading lifestyle through a truly heroic self-transformation.

On a more conceptual level, devotion to Augustine's God can lead to feelings of psychosocial integration with a very large group of Christian neighbours in St Augustine's perfect Christian community on earth.[28] Just as belief in God cannot damage the believer's liver, belief in St Augustine's perfect City of God cannot subject its dwellers to betrayal, social injustice, war, taxes, or parking tickets. St Augustine takes some pains to keep reminding his readers that 'the life of the [City of God] is a social life'.[29] This makes it eminently suitable as a substitute for psychosocial integration, even though the social life only exists because most of the dwellers in this city of Christian perfection are able to imagine the others.

Furthermore, Augustinian doctrine is so intellectually complex that it can keep believers' minds everlastingly occupied and therefore effectively distanced from the pain of worldly dislocation. The Christian God, who by the logic of the present scientific era is an imagined presence (i.e. essentially *nothing*),[30] is, according to St Augustine's Christian theology, more real than anything else: infinite, omnipresent, timeless, omnipotent, and omniscient (i.e. essentially *everything*). In short, to embrace Augustine's faith is to find a way to fully convince oneself that nothing is everything! Could there be a greater intellectual challenge than this? The trinity, and other holy mysteries, present still other formidable intellectual challenges.

Why do so many addicted$_3$ people gravitate to Augustine's addictive$_4$ Christianity, rather than terminating addiction altogether? According to the dislocation theory, addiction can only be fully overcome by establishing psychosocial integration. However, in St Augustine's collapsing Roman Empire and in today's global free-market society, an adequate degree of psychosocial integration is out of reach for a great many people. Therefore, many formerly addicted$_3$ people find it adaptive to establish an overwhelming involvement with Christian faith instead.

Addiction$_4$ can benefit society as a whole as well as addicted$_3$ individuals. In particular, a highly dislocated society has much to gain by encouraging addiction$_4$ to a religious faith, if it does not want to see its social and economic stability undermined by the uncontrolled spread of addiction$_3$.

Why Christian conversion cannot control addiction in free-market society

Despite truly miraculous conversions that occur in every age, and despite the genuine love that is felt by the Christian healers who instigate these life-saving transformations, Christian conversion has proved insufficient to control the continuing spread of addiction in globalizing free-market society. St Augustine recognised in his own time that successful conversion could only occur for a small minority of human sinners.[31] This apparently remains true.

Modern variations of this Christian approach to addiction have been widely accepted and practised for the past two centuries. Jim Orford has shown that, from the 19th century onward, Christian thinking has been the heart of the 'thinly concealed and mostly unacknowledged moral element'[32] that helps to make modern secular treatment work to the extent that it does. But the modern variations of Christian treatment have not been more successful than the classic form. Orford[33] compared the success rates for 19th century Christian temperance meetings at which alcoholics took a public pledge to reform—a powerful conversion experience—with contemporary success rates for the Salvation Army, Alcoholics Anonymous, and various secular forms of treatment. He estimated that all of these have a success rate of around 25–30%. Unfortunately, this does not mean that 25–30% of all alcoholics are helped by these methods, only that 25–30% of the minority of alcoholics who have actually 'taken the pledge' or gone through one of the other forms of treatment have been helped. Many of these would probably have recovered anyway, since there is always a base rate of 'spontaneous remission'. By this reckoning, Christian conversion offers no greater hope of providing an adequate solution for the globalising problem of addiction than any other method of treatment. The single most overtly Christian of the world's developed countries with the greatest reliance on 'faith-based' treatment, the United States, appears to have the worst addiction problems. Although Christian faith does work miracles in some individual cases, it clearly cannot overcome the problem of addiction in free-market society.

The trajectory of globalisation in today's world suggests that healing by traditional forms of Christian conversion is likely to become less, rather than more, successful in the future. Although St Augustine was well aware of the numerous opportunities for addictive sinfulness in ancient Rome, he could not have imagined a world in which addictive pleasures were mass-produced, mass-marketed, and incessantly advertised to the youngest children and the oldest adults. He could not have anticipated powerful corporations whose survival depended on using scientifically developed marketing technologies to draw people ever deeper into addictive consumption and debt. Moreover, he could not have imagined that, in order to maintain the efficiencies of production that such a world requires, free-market economies would create more and more dislocation, even in periods of prosperity. How could globalising free-market society fail to draw ever more dislocated people into addictions?

Just as the ancient Christians could do nothing to mitigate the social and political evils that degraded and corrupted the population of the deteriorating Roman Empire, contemporary Christians cannot hope to control the powerful commercial forces that make sinful addictions more and more attractive in the free-market world. The greatest of Christians have urged the faithful to leave the management of the material world to others. As Jesus said, they must 'give to Caesar what is Caesar's'.[34] St Augustine restated these injunctions more forcefully.[35] And, from the Reformation onward, Protestant sects have found ways to make peace with free-market economic principles.[36]

Finally, there is a hidden risk in replacing addiction$_3$ with addiction$_4$. Although the lives of many pious Christians do honour to the spiritual ideal of Jesus, many others have fallen back into addiction$_3$, this time to Christian faith, with results that have been as destructive as any other form of addiction. Tragic examples can be found in the Catholic Inquisitions, the Protestant witch hunts, the Canadian residential schools, and in the self-destructive lives of some saints.[37] People who find all of their identity in their love of God—like other highly addicted people—have little impetus to moderate their zeal. They are vulnerable to the lure of fanaticism. This potential for faith-based violence is illustrated today in the best-selling *Left Behind* series of novels, currently enjoying huge popularity in the United States.[38]

The radiant humanity of St Augustine's autobiographical writing and his commitment to earthly as well as spiritual charity to the poor[39] suggest that his own devotion to God was a benign instance of addiction$_4$, rather than addiction$_3$.[40] He himself appeared to believe that addiction$_3$ to God was unlikely.[41] Nonetheless, his lengthy descriptions of the burning intensity of his own religious devotion[42] make the potential of dangerous addiction to God in pious Christians seem inescapable. Many contemporary people describe themselves in ways that fit the definition of severe addiction$_3$ to Christian faith. A 12-step organisation called 'Fundamentalists Anonymous' has 40,000 current members and headquarters in New York City.[43]

A modern variant of Christian treatment: Alcoholics Anonymous

How could St Augustine's ancient spiritual doctrine be expected to provide a basis for treatment of addiction in a dislocated, hedonistic, materialistic free-market society? This problem was brilliantly solved by Alcoholics Anonymous (AA). However, in the end, AA doctrine is only a little more successful in controlling addiction than conventional Christianity.

AA is a variant of Christian treatment that provides the closest approximation to a success story in the contemporary field of addictions. Although attempts to document its success quantitatively have proved disappointing, it is impossible to ignore the many people who testify that their lives have been saved. Programmes modelled on AA have spread geographically from the United States, and have extended their scope from alcoholism to myriad other addictions, creating an alphabet soup of new 12-step organisations. Everywhere there are the same testimonials. Everywhere, too, is the recognition that 12-step programmes cost taxpayers nothing, since no expensive professional services or treatment paraphernalia are required.

Although I believe that 12-step programmes, like other derivatives of classic Christianity, are insufficient to control the problem of addiction in free-market society, I have no desire to minimise their accomplishments. The formulaic 12-step literature is easy to stereotype, but the individuals who compose local groups are smart and resourceful—they use the written doctrine for what it is worth, and think beyond it when they need to. Twelve-step groups show amazing patience. People who fail and drop out are always welcome to begin again. Most impressive of all is the human warmth that fills 12-step meeting rooms, even for people who have let down the group by relapsing again. Many lives have been saved, starting with that of Bill W.

The history of William Griffeth Wilson, who called himself 'Bill W' for the purpose of anonymity, shows how St Augustine's doctrine, in a radically modernized form, could bring life-saving abstinence to many thousands of addicts.[44] Bill W.'s recovery is as much a prototype for AA as is St Augustine's conversion for those who minister to addicted people through more conventional Christianity. *Bill's Story* remains Chapter 1 of the *Big Book* of AA to this day.[45]

Prior to becoming alcoholic, Bill W.'s life was a textbook case of dislocation in free-market society. He was born in 1895 in Vermont, a centre of libertarian philosophy and free enterprise since the founding of the United States.[46] When Bill was born, however, Vermont was in a period of economic decline and depopulation due to the ruin of the sheep and granite markets that had made it prosperous for most of the 19th century. Bill W.'s family and neighbours were sharply divided between stern teetotallers on one hand and heavy drinkers on the other. The temperance movement was a major intellectual force in everyday life.

As a child, Bill saw his family fractured by the permanent loss of his hard-working, hard-drinking father to new stone quarries in British Columbia, Canada. Left behind, Bill felt driven by the high standards for success set by his punitive, teetotal mother, who, after obtaining a divorce, moved Bill, aged 10, and his sister, aged 7, into their grandparents' home. She then moved herself to far-away Boston to attend medical school.

Although Bill had a close male friend who was 10 years his senior, he always felt an outcast in his hometown and knew little happiness until he entered a nearby residential high school where, by heroic application, he found scholarly success, athletic prominence, and the girl of his dreams. However, his beloved girlfriend tragically died when he was 17. After this, Bill fell into a long, black depression and a 'nervous breakdown'. Depression recurred throughout his life both before he became alcoholic and after he became sober and co-founded AA.[47]

Bill W.'s severe teenage depression lessened when he met his future wife, Lois, and fell in love again. Following their wedding, the new couple joined Lois's wealthy family in New York City, leaving Bill's early roots behind, although he sometimes visited his teetotal Vermont relatives to 'dry out' as his alcoholism grew.

Despite underconfidence and recurring depression, Bill rose from a successful stint in the American Army in World War I to become a brash, hard-drinking, but successful stock analyst and speculator. While he was flourishing in the heart of the free-market economy of his day—Wall Street during the great bull market of the 1920s—he was falling into severe alcoholism. Alcohol was not Bill's sole addiction. From the perspective of this book, alcoholism was only part of an addictive complex that also included overwhelming involvement with conspicuous consumption, social climbing, heavy smoking, incessant marital infidelity, a co-dependent relationship with his long-suffering wife, and, for a short period, golf.[48]

Bill W.'s alcoholic excesses went from alarming to catastrophic after the 1929 stock market crash brought financial ruin. During the ensuing economic depression, he continued drinking addictively, spending his wife's meagre earnings as a shop clerk and accepting charity from her family. Finally, in 1934, in failing health, he underwent a dramatic conversion experience, which he described in spiritual terms similar to those St Augustine had used 16 centuries earlier:

> Suddenly my room blazed with an indescribably white light. I was seized with an ecstasy beyond description. Every joy I had known was pale by comparison… Then, seen in the mind's eye, there was a mountain. I stood upon its summit where a great wind blew. A wind, not of air but of spirit. In great, clean strength it blew right through me. Then came the blazing thought, 'you are a free man.'[49]

The similarity between this paragraph and St Augustine's earlier quoted description of his own conversion is striking, particularly the vision of an indescribable white light. Bill W. never drank again, although he did not give up his pursuit of riches in the business world until a few years later when he became overwhelmingly involved with AA.

Similarities between Bill W.'s and St Augustine's treatments for addiction

During the year after Bill W.'s conversion experience, he and a few other recovering alcoholics[50] founded AA. Bill W.'s written words in the *Big Book*[51] spelled out AA's approach to alcoholism in a form that was acceptable to the hedonistic, material world of free-market society. Three of the treatment principles that emerge from this 12-step doctrine could have been drawn directly from St Augustine.

1 *Complete individual responsibility.* Addicts are individually responsible for their addiction even when they have endured severe childhood abuse or other events that could cause severe dislocation. If addicted individuals believe that their past misfortunes could explain their addiction, this 'blaming' must be confronted, for others have undergone the same suffering without falling into addiction. Blaming of others must be overcome, for it obscures the arduous work that the addicted individuals must do to change their own lives in order to overcome addiction.

   Alcoholics in AA have nobody to blame for their addictions but themselves, least of all the free-market society of which Bill W. was an unquestioning advocate. Bill W. was a stock speculator as he sank into alcoholism. He renounced alcoholism, but not stock speculation or wealth. He vehemently opposed American President Franklin D. Roosevelt's attempts to end the depression in the United States by softening the stern fundamentals of free-market capitalism that had been established by earlier American governments. Addictive sinfulness has to be confronted on an individual level. AA insists, in the tenth of the '12 Traditions', that it is completely apolitical, thus making it impossible for anyone speaking as an AA member to advocate changes in free-market society. The key to managing alcoholism is between each person and his or her personal 'Higher Power'. As in St Augustine's doctrine, each person must find salvation from addiction individually.

   Similarly, if the treatment fails, it is the addicted individual who is responsible. Usually it is said that the addicted person 'wasn't ready yet' or 'you can't help a person who doesn't want to be helped'. Addicted people learn to acknowledge complete responsibility for their problems both in formal therapy and in self-help groups. Relatives of the addicted person learn not to provide too much sympathy to the suffering addict, lest they be identified as 'co-dependents' who 'enable' the addiction by forestalling the dire but ultimately salubrious experience of 'hitting rock bottom'.

2 *Total abstinence.* Total, lifelong abstinence from addicting practices is necessary for members of AA and other 12-step organisations. The least slip in abstinence restores the addiction to its strongest form, condemning the person to hell on earth, unless he or she repents yet again and starts the recovery process anew. Similarly, St Augustine believed that even a tiny lapse of abstinence quickly re-ensnares the sinner in his or her vice.[52] More importantly, St Augustine believed that God expected *complete* devotion from his people.[53] If they are totally devoted to God, how could they retain even the least interest in earthly pleasure?

3 *The necessity of healing fellowship.* Once people lose control of alcohol or any other earthly pleasure, their well-being can only be restored by the grace of the Higher Power, which entails lifelong attendance at AA meetings in fellowship with others who are recovering by the aid of their own version of the Higher Power. Recovery also entails confessing the exact nature of the alcoholic's wrongs to at least one other person and carrying the message of recovery to other alcoholics. Similarly, Christian life for St Augustine took place in a disciplined Christian community and he showed by his own example that public confession was an essential part of recovery.[54] St Augustine believed that 'the Christian life... could only be a long process of healing'.[55]

AA's modernisation of classic Christianity

Whereas the details of Bill W.'s personal conversion are similar to St Augustine's and the most basic principles of AA are similar to those that St Augustine applied to addiction, the AA philosophy modernises St Augustine's doctrine in at least two important ways: The concept of the Higher Power and the number of earthly pleasures that must be overcome.

The AA Higher Power is not St Augustine's Biblical God. Most of the Higher Power's qualities are determined by recovering alcoholics individually, for themselves alone· Although alcoholics must recognise their powerlessness to control drinking and must follow the steps to recovery laid out by AA, they retain theological independence, as long as it does not infringe on controlling their addiction. Allegiance to St Augustine's Biblical God is not necessary in AA. Jesus is little more than an honoured bystander in the *Big Book*.[56] Because it is theologically eclectic, AA is well suited for the agnosticism and ecumenicalism of a globalising world.

Whereas all earthly pleasures were condemned as fatal distractions from God by St Augustine, each is innocent until proven guilty by AA and other 12-step organisations. A member of a 12-step organisation can enjoy any legal form of pleasure unless he or she goes 'out of control'. There is no reason for people not to drink (unless they are addicted to alcohol), to enjoy sexuality (unless they are addicted to it), or to seek worldly success (unless they are so driven that their ambitions become self-defeating), and so forth. Unlike Augustinian Christianity, there is no essential dissonance between the 12-step philosophy and the hedonistic values of free-market society.

Bill W. felt he had to give up alcohol only after drinking made it impossible for him to support his wife as a respectable contributor to the economy. He did not feel it necessary to curtail the other parts of his addictive complex that did not interfere with his economic role, including his addictive sexuality. Most vitally, he did not feel it necessary to stop smoking cigarettes, even though he was a chain smoker with a cigarette always on the go. 'He didn't just smoke; he sucked in cigarettes, not wanting to miss a puff.'[57] He had a long history of lung disease that seemed to be caused by smoking. By the 1960s, he carried an inhaler in his pocket and, by late in that decade, an oxygen tank by his side—the armaments of his unremitting war with emphysema.[58]

Emphysema won, killing Bill at the age of 76. Although he had officially given up smoking 3 years earlier, he apparently still snuck cigarettes when he had the opportunity.

Smoking proved fatal, but it did not interfere with his productivity until it was too late to matter. Bill hated being dependent on cigarettes,[59] but it was not necessary for him to give them up in order to earn a living or to be the supreme role model of AA.

Early Christian doctrine had a more radically transformative effect than AA does. Christian conversion not only helped Roman Christians overcome their addictive sinfulness but also forged an iron integrity that enabled early Christian martyrs to endure the worst abuses that Roman magistrates, torturers, and executioners could devise, without renouncing their faith. But different versions of the healing message are appropriate at different times in history. If it is important that words like St Augustine's put a flaming sword in the hands of the young church militant, can it be less important that Bill W.'s put a cup of hot coffee in the hands of countless old veterans who would otherwise be swilling beer at the Legion Hall?

A contemporary 12-step organisation called the Augustine Fellowship further illustrates the differences between the approaches of St Augustine and Bill W· The Augustine Fellowship is closely modelled on AA, and it has defined sex and love addiction in a way that fits very closely with descriptions of both St Augustine's and Bill W.'s addictive love lives. Whereas the Augustine Fellowship urges complete abstinence from addictive forms of sexuality, it does not consider celibacy as any part of the solution, but rather cautions against it. One of its websites warns, 'To avoid feeling vulnerable, we may retreat from all intimate involvement, mistaking sexual and emotional anorexia for recovery.'[60]

Thus, AA is best understood as a modernised ritualisation of the ancient Christian drama: the epic struggle to quell the cravings that keep people apart from their God. But, whereas AA helps to quell some of the addictions that keep people apart from St Augustine's Christian God, it ignores many cravings that St Augustine abhorred. Not only does AA accept sexuality, there is nothing in the AA message to prevent its members from taking Viagra®, a drug that is designed specifically to inflame and facilitate sexual lust. How could St Augustine have seen Viagra® as anything other than a hideous blasphemy?

These differences between the two traditions may be the secret of AA's enormous success in this era. In essence, AA does not serve any Higher Power as well as it serves the Market God.[61] Whereas there is no psychological dividing line between the many addictions that are tolerable in the 12-step organisations and the few that require treatment, there is a *religious* dividing line. Within the AA tradition, addictions appear to require treatment primarily if they violate the commandment of the Market God that people must pull their weight as full participants in the free-market economy.

Although the prominence of the Market God in AA revises St Augustine's doctrine substantially, the drama of the struggle against addiction is as heroic for the followers of Bill W. as it is for the followers of St Augustine. It requires great strength for a person who is drowning in a sea of dislocation to honour the commandments of either St Augustine's God or Bill W.'s Higher Power. Nonetheless, many succeed and lives are saved.

Why Bill W.'s solution cannot control addiction in free-market society

The 12-step movement is insufficient to overcome the problem of addiction in the contemporary world. There are two main reasons for this.

First, the 12-step movement does not set out to overcome addiction, but only to manage it. AA members are constantly reminded that an alcoholic who stays sober one day at a time is still an alcoholic. Bill W. insisted on this throughout his decades of sobriety, and inadvertently confirmed it on his deathbed, by begging for whisky over a period of several days, sometimes demanding it belligerently.[62] The Market God is satisfied if an alcoholic stays sober and productive, although from the perspective of the dislocation theory, this is a tragic compromise of the human potential for psychosocial integration.

Bill W. felt he had to control his drinking, but he did not feel he had to control all of the other addictions that impoverished his life. Smoking cigarettes eventually killed him, but his unremitting sexual addiction, an open secret among his friends and colleagues, did untold harm to his wife and, no doubt, to his own self-esteem (although neither he nor she talked about it publicly).[63] Naturally his many friends and admirers disliked this state of affairs, but it made sense within the AA logic that Bill could be the role model of recovery, while the other addictions that were robbing him of the fullness of his life, and literally killing him, could continue.

Many people in 12-step groups gain better control over their addictions than Bill W. did, and some move away from their groups once their addictive crisis has passed, seeking more complete psychosocial integration outside the 12-step community. But in doing this, they are moving away from the 12-step model into new kinds of thinking, because the model insists that addiction is incurable and membership in the group must be forever. Because the 12-step movement has many devoted members and because it does not have a rigid doctrine, it may well be broadening its perspective now.

The second major reason that Bill W.'s solution to the problem of addiction is insufficient is that 12-step programmes do not address the social causes of addiction. Perceiving individuals as the sole cause of their addictive downfall makes sense morally and pragmatically in the 12-step milieu, but it rules out the possibility of social action to ameliorate the dislocating cultural environment. Society is mass-producing both dislocation and the merchandise that makes it easy for people to adapt to that dislocation addictively: addiction cannot be brought under control until this problem is solved.

Twelve-step groups serve important social and spiritual functions for many people and can therefore contribute to the psychosocial integration of some addicted people, even if dislocation is not acknowledged to be a cause of addiction. But the contribution of 12-step groups to psychosocial integration cannot have a serious impact on the immense dislocation that pervades free-market society because both the social and the spiritual impacts of 12-step groups are severely limited. The social function of 12-step groups is officially limited by the 12 Traditions to a self-help function,[64] and each person's spiritual development is kept private so that nobody offends anyone else's interpretation of their Higher Power. Twelve-step groups do not comprise a new culture, but a caring ad hoc group of addicted people employing a common strategy for managing their continuing addictions.

Eclectic spirituality in addiction treatment: Marcus Aurelius, Vipassana meditation, and William R. Miller

In my corner of the world, another faith is at least as influential as Christianity among people struggling to control addictions. I suspect that this faith may become the dominant form of spirituality of the 21st century. Because it has no agreed-upon universal symbol or deity, it is called 'eclectic spirituality' in this book. Eclectic spirituality is at least as ancient as Christianity and there are at least as many versions. Like Christianity, one of its central ideas is universal, compassionate love. Also like Christianity, eclectic spirituality is influential well beyond the field of addiction treatment, since it is accepted as a complete philosophy of life by many serious people.[65]

Eclectic spirituality starts with the belief that one's own serenity is the primary achievable goal in an imperfect world. Serenity comes from accepting life as it is, without judgements or expectations, and from freely sharing compassionate love with all humanity and nature, including oneself. Theology is secondary. Any metaphysical beliefs are acceptable, as long as they do not interfere with serenity, acceptance, and compassionate love.

Eclectic spirituality has its costs. Serenity requires renouncing selfish actions and righteous indignation, even when one's own needs are acute and others are acting offensively. Acceptance requires renouncing political rebellion and competitiveness and learning to be satisfied with the rewards of spirituality. Compassionate love for others and for oneself requires the painful acceptance of personal limitations, including one's own. All of this requires mental discipline, and organised spiritual training can help.

Eclectic spirituality holds that the best means of improving an imperfect world is unceasing improvement of oneself on a spiritual level. By contrast, attempting to directly change the structure of society through social or political action seems arrogant because it implies a moralistic judgement that one's own values are superior to those of others, and because it is aggressive and potentially violent. On the other hand, working towards self-improvement, individually or in spiritually centred communities is seen as contributing to progressive social evolution. Jean Vanier put it this way:

> To be human is to accept ourselves just as we are, with our own history, and to accept others as they are. To be human means to accept history as it is and to work, without fear, towards greater openness, greater understanding, and a greater love of others. To be human is not to be crushed by reality, or to be angry about it or to try to hammer it into what we think it is or should be, but to commit ourselves as individuals, and as a species, to an evolution that will be for the good of all.[66]

In addiction treatment, eclectic spirituality does not put the emphasis on the relationship between the addicted person and God, as in the Christian tradition, or on recovery from addiction, as in AA. Rather, the emphasis is on cultivating the relationship between the addicted person and the infinite cosmos, which is the ultimate home for all beings. Addiction is understood neither as a disease nor as a form of wickedness. Rather, people are seen as turning to addiction and other harmful behaviours because they find so little to fulfil their individual spiritual needs in everyday life. Spiritual helpers do not judge the addicted person morally, nor push for change. Instead, they attempt to share and accept the addicted person's life in the deepest possible way. Through unconditional positive regard and patience, the helper offers balm to the wounded spirit, and cultivates a sense of self-worth and transcendent belonging that will enable the addicted person to overcome addictive cravings—when and if this becomes the right choice for him or her. All people are worthy of respect and freedom, and providing these in abundance will lead people to make the best choices that they possibly can. It is assumed that therapy of this sort will spiritually enrich the spiritual helper at the same time that it improves the life of the addicted person.

This faith does not focus exclusively on addiction and does not necessarily require a spiritual helper. It is often embraced by individuals—addicted or not—who pursue serenity with the aid of self-help or with the inspiration of public speakers and workshops that promulgate eclectic spirituality around the world. The published stories of people's journeys from misery to eclectic spirituality comprise a radiant literature.

This faith is called *eclectic* spirituality in this book because it can be linked to a great variety of spiritual traditions. When expressed in Biblical language, it can be seen as a variety of Christianity,[67] although its ecumenical and non-judgemental character sets it apart from Augustinian forms of Christianity and its self-absorption sets it apart from Christian liberation theology, which is oriented towards intervention in social and political affairs.[68]

Eclectic spirituality is often identified with exotic traditions; for example, Buddhism,[69] Hinduism, Roman Stoicism and Epicureanism,[70] and Existentialism. It is often seen as intrinsically Eastern. It is sometimes portrayed as a flower child born in the hippie upheaval of the 1960s and in the thinking of American humanistic psychologists of that era, especially Abraham Maslow and Carl Rogers.[71] It is sometimes expressed in the terminology of advanced modern science.[72]

Eclectic spirituality has appeared so many times in the course of history that it may qualify as an archetypal way of understanding the world. It seems to be at a peak of influence now, as it was in other historical periods, including the Roman Empire before Christianity became its most important faith. Three forms of eclectic spirituality will be discussed in this section: an ancient Roman form expressed in the *Meditations* of Marcus Aurelius, a current Buddhist form as practised within today's Vipassana meditation, and a contemporary professional psychology form developed by William R. Miller and his colleagues.

Marcus Aurelius

Eclectic spirituality was expressed in a surprisingly modern form in the late Stoic philosophy of the Roman Emperor Marcus Aurelius Antoninus. His book, the *Meditations*,[73] became the basis of the dominant secular philosophy of Rome after its publication in 170 AD.[74] It is still read for inspiration in our own times.[75] A close reading of this ancient book will show that the roots of eclectic spirituality are not necessarily either Eastern or Christian, and are definitely pre-hippie.

In the *Meditations*, Marcus Aurelius lauded 'acceptance' above all other virtues. He preached not only acceptance of the harsh Roman world of war and slavery, but also of one's rank in the social hierarchy, of one's own personal limitations and pain, and of other people just as they are, whatever galling irritations and imperfections they might present.

According to Marcus Aurelius, a life of acceptance produces all the serenity that is possible in an imperfect world, as well as a smooth passage from the inevitable tragedies of earthly life to merciful death. Individual serenity provides the only real and achievable satisfaction in life, whereas more ambitious pursuits are doomed. Marcus Aurelius explained the utter impossibility of achieving happiness through seeking truth, material possessions, or friendship as follows:

> As for truth, it is so veiled in obscurity that many reputable philosophers assert the impossibility of reaching any certain knowledge. Even the stoics admit that its attainment is beset with difficulties, and that all our intellectual conclusions are fallible; for where is the infallible man? Or turn from this to more material things: how transitory, how worthless are these—open to acquisition by every profligate, loose woman, and criminal. Or look at the characters of your associates: even the most agreeable of them are difficult to put up with; and for the matter of that, it is difficult enough to put up with one's own self. In all this murk and mire, then, in all this ceaseless flow of being and time, of changes imposed and changes endured, I can think of nothing that is worth prizing highly or pursuing seriously. No; what a man must do is nerve himself to wait quietly for his dissolution [death]; and meanwhile not to chafe at its delay... [76]

Marcus Aurelius explains the positive value of devoting oneself to self-absorption thus:

> In every action let your own self-approval be the sole aim both of your effort and of your attention; bearing in mind that the event itself which prompted your action is a thing of no consequence to either of them.
>
> Dig within. There lies the well-spring of good: ever dig, and it will ever flow.[77]

> Withdraw into yourself. Our master-reason asks no more than to act justly, and thereby to achieve calm.
>
> Do away with all fancies. Cease to be passion's puppet. Limit time to the present. Learn to recognise every experience for what it is, whether it be your own or another's.... Meditate upon your last hour.[78]

As Emperor of Rome, Marcus Aurelius was chief magistrate of the largest military dictatorship the world had yet known. Slavery, torture, and public execution were routine practices throughout the empire. Marcus Aurelius fulfilled his duty as emperor, military general, and chief magistrate within the normal expectations for a Roman emperor, and was considered more merciful than most. The philosophy that he practised within his own court circle was considered shockingly non-punitive. His behaviour was similar to that of people who work with addicts and criminals in the spirit of eclectic spirituality today. Marcus Aurelius emphasised the importance of accepting the humanity of miscreants of all sorts—certainly including addicted people—despite their objectionable actions. Instead of punishment, he advocated gentle persuasion:

> Teach them better, if you can; if not, remember that kindliness has been given you for moments like these. The gods themselves show kindness to such men; and at times, so indulgent are they, will even aid them in their endeavours to secure health, wealth, or reputation. This you could do… [79]

Vipassana meditation

Vipassana meditation is very similar both to the generalised version of eclectic spirituality described earlier and to the philosophy of Marcus Aurelius. The philosophy of Vipassana meditation is, however, not expressed so much in writing as it is manifested through a formalised meditative technique that is used to 'purify the minds' and 'eradicate the mental defilements' of its practitioners.[80] This powerful technique enables committed practitioners to experience a deep and enduring sense of serenity, acceptance, and universal love, to carry out profound self-examination, to moderate addictive cravings of every sort, and to avoid futile anger.[81] Although this technique draws from the ancient discourses of Gautama Buddha, they have been modernised to serve the globalising world, as have other contemporary 'world religions'.[82] The Vipassana technique has spawned many contemporary organisations; for example, a worldwide non-profit organisation headed by an intellectually impressive and charismatic spiritual leader, S. N. Goenka. Goenka's organisation offers its services in 'Vipassana Meditation Centres' at very low cost[83] to people in about 70 countries today.

Many testimonials confirm the power of this technique for controlling addictive cravings.[84] Personal friends who are devotees of Vipassana meditation have helped me to understand it. In 2006, I participated in a 10-day silent meditation course at a Vipassana Meditation Centre that involved 10.5 hours of disciplined meditation each day plus a daily videotaped lecture of over an hour. I was amazed by the difficulty of this technique, but also by the benefits of the small amount of progress that I personally made. I was deeply impressed by the wisdom and compassion of those who taught it.

People who have not been through a session of this sort may have difficulty appreciating how difficult it is. Sitting in some version of the lotus position without moving or uncrossing one's arms or legs for an hour, several times a day, can be extremely strenuous. It brings serious bodily pain to some participants—definitely including me.[85] The systematic patterns of thought required by the meditation technique evoke memories and feelings that can cause both physical and emotional pain. Not only practitioners but also the leader, S. N. Goenka, acknowledge that pain and anguish are not unusual in the process of learning the technique.[86]

Can the world hope that this highly sophisticated method, or one of the other traditional forms of eclectic spirituality, will bring the problem of addiction and other aspects of modern poverty of the spirit under control? I am convinced that the answer must be 'no', notwithstanding the fact that Vipassana meditation has definitely helped many addicted individuals in the past.

As the globalisation of free-market society continues to increase dislocation everywhere, addictive cravings increase in intensity, making them ever more difficult to overcome simply by individual discipline, especially if the discipline requires real physical and emotional strength and a minimum of 2 hours of daily meditation for the rest of one's life. As people's work hours are extended to keep the economy growing, and as dislocation increases the pressure on families, less and less time can be set aside for practices that are not economically driven. Therefore, I fear that traditional forms of eclectic spirituality cannot bring addiction under control on a large scale. A fuller critique covering all three forms of eclectic spirituality will follow after the final form is introduced.

Beyond its traditional forms, eclectic spirituality is also being applied in professionalised forms within the field of addictions. Its potential for bringing the problem of addiction under control cannot be evaluated fully unless these innovations are taken into account as well.

William R. Miller

Psychologist William R. Miller has brilliantly adapted the ancient message of eclectic spirituality to modern psychological treatment of addiction. Miller noted that people who are part of an organised religious tradition are less likely to have problems with drugs and alcohol and slightly more likely to recover if they do.[87] He described the powerful spiritual components of the 'quantum changes', or conversion experiences, that people frequently and unexpectedly undergo in overcoming addictions.[88] In an extraordinary article entitled 'Rediscovering fire', Miller used compassionate love, or *agape*, to explain a variety of unexpected findings in psychotherapy research, while acknowledging that this explanation would have been unacceptable to mainstream professional psychology of the recent past.

The 'fire' that Miller rediscovered is most precisely labelled *agape*. One of four Greek words for love, *agape* does not refer to sexual or sentimental love of individuals, but to 'a selfless, accepting, sacred form of loving'.[89] Miller pointed out that the healing power of *agape* has been known for millennia, and cited St Paul to document its roots in Christian spirituality. He cited many non-Christian roots of *agape* as a healing technique as well. For example, he drew heavily from the work of 20th-century humanistic psychologist Carl Rogers, who pioneered the use of therapeutic interventions that utilise 'unconditional positive regard', which Miller showed has a great deal in common with *agape*. Miller raised the possibility that the therapeutic application of *agape* can be taught and thereby 'harnessed'[90] in treatment methods of unprecedented efficacy, equivalent in the psychological context to a rediscovery of the oldest successful technology, fire.[91]

Miller's 'working definition of *agape*' translates the traditional spirit of eclectic spirituality into a five-part operational definition in the language of modern psychology:

Patience. The therapist reliably shows patience and endurance, a sense of waiting with the client...

Selflessness. The focus of the therapist's interest and concern is the client. The therapist's own needs and opinions are humbly kept out of the interaction ...

Acceptance. There is an openness to and a curiosity about what really is within the client's life. It encompasses whatever the client experiences. This acceptance extends necessarily to the therapist's own experiencing as well …

Hope. The therapist sees the possibilities in the client, believes in the client, and expects positive change to happen …

Positive Regard. The therapist respects and honours the client as a person of inherent worth. This basic human regard is enduring, and not conditional on what is occurring in the client's life at present …[92]

Although much of Miller's language has the positivistic, managerial style of professional psychology, he simultaneously gives his argument a deeply spiritual quality, for example by quoting theologian Paul Tillich as follows:

It is as though a voice were saying, 'You are accepted, *you are accepted*, accepted by that which is greater than you, and the name of which you do not know. Do not ask for the name now; perhaps you will find it later. Do not try to do anything now; perhaps later you will do much. Do not seek for anything; do not intend anything. Simply accept the fact that you are accepted'.[93]

Miller also pointed out that practising *agape* in therapy is likely to benefit the practitioner as well as the client,[94] again in accord with the expectations of eclectic spirituality.

In parallel with Bill W., William R. Miller may well have succeeded in re-ritualising a kind of ancient wisdom in a form that works well in modern society.[95] If so, his techniques may enhance the healing power of eclectic spirituality in our times, although I am convinced that even the best new techniques cannot overcome its limitations.

Why eclectic spirituality cannot control addiction in free-market society

No matter how sincerely and ingeniously eclectic spirituality is practised, addiction continues to spread in modern society. I hasten to add that some individuals do recover from addictions through the practice of eclectic spirituality, and that acceptance and compassionate love are wonderful gifts, whether they lead to recovery or not. Nonetheless, I predict that neither the three forms of eclectic spirituality described here, nor any other form, will curtail the continuing growth of addiction in free-market society. There are several reasons for this prediction.

1 The causes of dislocation are built into free-market society. As free-market society extends its reach throughout the world, severe dislocation and manufactured products that provide addictive relief from it will continue to proliferate. Acceptance, serenity, and *agape* cannot alter this underlying problem. Major corporations freely add eclectic spirituality to corporate 'wellness programmes',[96] perceiving that it is not incompatible with unlimited economic expansion, which, in turn, inexorably increases dislocation.

2 Spirituality and *agape* work their magic most powerfully when they are embedded in enduring, stable communities. Although solitary spirituality, episodic spirituality within spiritual organisations, and *agape* delivered within established

treatment systems can relieve distress for some individuals, they cannot overcome dislocation in an enduring way. For example, trained therapists can provide acceptance and unconditional positive regard during the therapeutic hour, but they cannot create psychosocial integration for the rest of the week. Achieving psychosocial integration is the project of a lifetime and the product of an enduring community in attunement with an individual.

3 Mainstream professional psychology may have rediscovered the fire of *agape* in 2000 when W. R. Miller's landmark article appeared, but the rest of the world had never lost it. True masters of *agape* have always been found among parents, teachers, coaches, clergymen, siblings, and friends. Many people, including me, can tell stories of how a caring human being, in a special moment, changed their lives forever. Sometimes masters of *agape* are so skilful that one does not realise until years later how great a gift they have given. Fortunately, many psychologists had the good sense to ignore their profession's official scientism and have been compassionately loving other human beings all along. Thus, compassionate love is not an innovation. It is already hard at work among the dislocated people who are vulnerable to addiction, but the tide of addiction has kept rising nonetheless. Teaching more professional psychologists about *agape* in graduate school, while certainly a positive step, can add only a little to the sum total in the world.

4 Although compassionate love is an element of psychosocial integration, it is by no means the whole of it: psychosocial integration includes shared beliefs, differentiated social roles, and economic interdependence as well. It is well known that people who try to substitute intensive romantic love relationships for psychosocial integration are not likely to succeed. In fact, they tend to fall into a sad state that is rightly called 'love addiction'.[97] *Agape* has the same limitation as romantic love—it is only a part of what is missing; it cannot suffice, although in cases where is a person is on the verge of achieving an important life change, it can provide an additional boost that may swing the balance.

There is a place where 'love cannot reach'.[98] Addiction is sometimes the most adaptive alternative that a person has. Eclectic spirituality cannot justifiably ask people to change from a more adaptive to a less adaptive way of living, understanding that they will probably not succeed if they try, and that succeeding would increase their suffering. Something more than eclectic spirituality will be needed to overcome most people's addictions.

5 Within a spiritually pluralistic society, the effectiveness of any kind of spiritual approach is diminished by prejudices that many people automatically have against it. Eclectic spirituality is popular, but so are other religious traditions, and eclectic spirituality itself is divided into competing sects. It cannot offer the powerful reinforcement of universal support. Forming a spiritual community can overcome this problem to some extent, but this requires a kind of isolation from the larger society and thus a new sort of dislocation.

6 There are intrinsic contradictions between the goals of eclectic spiritualism and overcoming dislocation by social action, which, I will argue, is the essential step in

bringing addiction under control. Although some practitioners of eclectic spirituality are among the bravest of social activists,[99] others are drawn to a life of contemplative self-absorption that prevents them from joining in any serious disturbance to the status quo, other than as proponents of their spiritual tradition.

Two important principles of Vipassana meditation, for example, seem especially antithetical to social action to reduce dislocation. First, Vipassana meditation emphasises that addictive cravings result from the human tendency to move automatically from liking particular sensations to craving them addictively. The movement from innocent desire to addictive craving is said to be the natural result of human nature and conditioning.[100] No social or political cause of addictive cravings is even mentioned in Vipassana teaching, to my knowledge.[101] Therefore, social action (other than working to promulgate meditation practise) logically cannot have any influence on the addiction problem. The second principle that seems to stand between practitioners of Vipassana meditation and social or political action is that, like other forms of eclectic spirituality, Vipassana meditation asserts that it is beyond the power of human beings to change society. Vipassana practitioners learn to serve others generously and wholeheartedly, taking 'strong action'[102] when necessary, but this service is focused on promoting meditation and on preventing overt violence, rather than social reorganisation. It is possible that followers of Vipassana meditation and similar traditions might let go of the philosophical principles that seem to militate against social action. However, this seems unlikely in the light of recent political events.[103] Moreover, both of these principles are deeply entrenched in Vipassana meditation and originated in the teachings of Buddha himself, 25 centuries ago.[104]

Could Buddha be wrong about this? Perhaps this is unimaginable, but if he was writing in a world that differed from this one in important ways, these differences could require some reinterpretation of his teachings for the globalising world of today. For example, Buddha's ancient world could have included a high degree of psychosocial integration, in which people did not suffer from universal dislocation but could become dislocated as a consequence of idiosyncratic weaknesses or of the exigencies of life in ancient times—plagues, famines, floods, wars, and so forth. In such a world, there would be no sense in trying to bring addiction under control by changing the structure of society, for the cause would not lie there. Instead, moderating individual desire might have been a more productive way to avoid idiosyncratic instances of dislocation.

But the world of free-market society is profoundly different. If my speculations[105] about the life and times of Buddha are correct, devotees of Vipassana meditation and other forms of eclectic spirituality may find themselves working with advocates of social and political approaches to restore psychosocial integration more and more in the future, without abandoning the essence of their meditative discipline. The recent political protests by Buddhist monks against the military junta in Myanmar may presage the future.[106] I find it intriguing to imagine that Buddha might have approved of such an eventuality had he been able to foresee the present world.

Conclusion

None of this chapter is meant to imply that treatment for addiction based on spirituality or on compassionate love has no place in the future. Obviously, it is important and right for society to give as much spiritual compassion and wisdom as possible to addicted people, and surely this wisdom will help some of them to control or overcome their addictions. However, it is also important not to gratuitously assume that treatment based on spirituality and compassionate love can have any major impact on the problem of addiction, a supposition that is now being defended at the highest political levels in the United States with the movement towards 'faith-based treatment'.[107] Whereas I have no desire to leave spirituality out of society's reaction to the problem of addiction, I believe that a different form of philosophy and spirituality will prove more valuable in the long run. The form of philosophy and spirituality that is proposed in the next chapter has roots that are as ancient as the spiritual traditions that were discussed in this one.

Endnotes

1 I am now retired from the university but teach my addiction course at a community centre. Similar discussions occur there.

2 These four pillars are discussed in Chapter 1 in the special case of Vancouver's Four Pillars Drug Strategy and in generic terms in Chapter 14.

3 Bayly (2004, Chapter 9).

4 Chapter 9 explained why the word 'addiction' can be used to describe St Augustine's lifestyle before his conversion, although he did not use the Latin word 'addictionem' to describe himself.

5 St Augustine (426 AD/2000).

6 Orford (2001a, pp. 332–340).

7 From *Confessions of St. Augustine* by St. Augustine, translated by Rex Warner, copyright © 1963 by Rex Warner, renewed © 1991 by F. C. Warner. Used with permission of Dutton Signet, a division of Penguin Group (USA) Inc. (St Augustine, 397 AD/1963, p. 149.)

8 Although St Augustine was enthusiastic about exhortation and salubrious punishment to save the souls of individuals who fell into sin (St Augustine, 397 AD/1963, Book 13, Chapter 17; St Augustine, 426 AD/2000, Book 19, Chapter 16), and although he advocated ministering to the earthly, as well as the spiritual, needs of the poor (St Augustine, 397 AD/1963, Book 13, Chapter 17), he believed that any attempt to change the social order, such as I will propose in the final chapters of this book, was itself sinful. Because many contemporary Christians may find it difficult to believe that St Augustine actually took this position, it is documented here in his own words.

St Augustine taught that God had created earth and constructed society exactly as he wanted it, including the corrupt, ultra-violent late Roman Empire. Like more recent historians, St Augustine documented the horrible violence and corruption of the late Roman Empire (St Augustine, 426 AD/2000, Book 1, Chapters 5 and 6, Book 19, Chapter 6; Gibbon, 1776/1974; Kiefer, 1934). St Augustine believed that although God recognized all the evils that the Roman Empire would perpetuate, he knowingly established and protected it. St Augustine stated explicitly that God had installed even the worst of imperial Roman regimes, including that of the notorious sadist Nero, as deliberately and wisely as he had created the better emperors and all other earthly kingdoms:

> But he who is a despiser of glory, but is greedy of domination, exceeds the beasts in the vices of cruelty and luxuriousness. Such, indeed, were certain of the Romans … But it was Nero Caesar who was the first to reach the summit, and, as it were, the citadel, of this vice; for so great was his luxuriousness, that one would have thought there was nothing manly to be dreaded in him, and such his cruelty, that, had not the contrary been known, no one would have thought there was anything effeminate in his character. Nevertheless power and domination were not given even to such men save by the providence of the most high God, when He judges that the state of human affairs is worthy of such lords. The divine utterance is clear on this matter; for the Wisdom of God thus speaks: 'By me kings reign, and tyrants possess the land'.

St Augustine (426 AD/2000, p. 172).

Therefore, all who opposed Roman dominance were identified by St Augustine as evil. In this spirit, St Augustine never raised the slightest question about whether any civil or foreign enemy of the established power of Rome might be more just than Rome, even in the periods of Rome's greatest brutality, corruption, and debauchery (St Augustine, 426 AD/2000, Book 2, Chapter 22; Book 5, Chapters 22 and 23). His repudiation of all resistance to established Roman authority included the rebellion led by the Gracchi brothers, whom secular historians of our time, and St Augustine himself (426AD/2000, Book 3, Chapter 24), saw as champions of the poor citizens against arbitrary tyranny. St Augustine urged Roman slaves, generally treated with savage cruelty, to accept their lot:

> This servitude is … penal, and is appointed by that law which enjoins the preservation of the natural order and forbids its disturbance; for if nothing had been done in violation of that law, there would have been nothing to restrain by penal servitude. And therefore the apostle admonishes slaves to be subject to their masters, and to serve them heartily and with good-will …

St Augustine (426 AD/2000, p. 694).

It wasn't only the relative merit of the Romans that won them this divine support—St Augustine urged Christians to support established power in other empires as well:

> And therefore the apostle also admonished the Church to pray for kings and those in authority, assigning as the reason, 'that we may like a quiet and tranquil life in all godliness and love.' And the prophet Jeremiah, when predicting the captivity that was to befall the ancient people of God, and giving them the divine command to go obediently to Babylonia, and thus serve their God, counselled them also to pray for Babylonia, saying, 'In the peace thereof shall ye have peace'—the temporal peace which the good and the wicked enjoy together.

St Augustine (426 AD/2000, p. 707).

See also St Augustine (426 AD/2000, Book 19, Chapter 17).

The only people who could legitimately resist Roman authority, according to St Augustine, were the Christian martyrs, who justly defied the Roman magistrates in service of their greater Lord (St Augustine, 426 AD/2000, Book 19, Chapter 17).

9 St Augustine (397 AD/1963, p. 211).

10 St Augustine (397 AD/1963, p. 237).

11 About his own father's desire for grandchildren, St Augustine said:

> … his pleasure proceeded from that kind of drunkenness in which the world forgets you, its creator, and falls in love with your creature instead of with you; so drugged it is with the invisible wine of a perverse self-will, bent upon the lowest objects.

St Augustine (397 AD/1963, p. 43).

> He treats his mother's desire for grandchildren somewhat more gently, as he describes her after he has taken his oath of celibacy:

> And so you had changed her mourning into joy, a joy much richer than she had desired and much dearer and purer than that which she looked for by having grandchildren of my flesh.

St Augustine (397 AD/1963, p. 183).

> From *Confessions of St. Augustine* by St. Augustine, translated by Rex Warner, copyright © 1963 by Rex Warner, renewed © 1991 by F. C. Warner. Used with permission of Dutton Signet, a division of Penguin Group (USA) Inc.

12 There is a subtlety in St Augustine's expression of this that cannot be fully explored in this short summary. He distinguishes between full participation in the life of the Christian community, which is a holy duty, from an inner life of extreme piety in which no pleasure is allowed unless it comes from God. St Augustine separated the divine from the social, whereas psychosocial integration marries them.

13 St Augustine (397 AD/1963, Book 10, Chapters 31, 33, and 35).

14 For example, he spoke of life in the City of God as involving exclusively Christian emotions, service to fellow Christians by exhorting them to the true faith and punishing their sins, and contemplation of God (St Augustine, 426 AD/2000, Book 14, Chapter 9; Book 19, Chapter 19, including reference to 19:6).

15 Many aspects of St Augustine's meticulous descriptions of his own devotion make it absolutely clear that it fits the definition of addiction$_4$. First, St Augustine was clear that it was his need and desire that his commitment to God be total, leaving nothing left of his life for other interests:

> I fell away and I was in the dark, but even from there, even from there I loved you. I went astray and I remembered you. I heard your voice behind me, calling me back, and I could scarcely hear it for all the noise made by those without your peace. And now, look, I return thirsty and panting to your fountain. Let no one hold me back! I shall drink of it, and I shall live of it. Let me not be my own life! I lived evilly of myself; I have been death to myself; I come back to life in you.

St Augustine (397 AD/1963, p. 290).

> Secondly, St Augustine repeatedly represented his overwhelming involvement with God as a perpetual state of inebriation that would segregate him from the rest of his life:

> OH THAT I might find my rest and peace in you! Oh, that you would come into my heart and so inebriate it that I would forget my own evils and embrace my one and only good, which is you!

St Augustine (397 AD/1963, pp. 19–20, uppercase in original).

Thirdly, St Augustine spoke of his relationship to God as a form of voluntary slavery—the root definition of 'addiction' in the traditional English and Latin sense of the word (see Chapter 2). Describing his own conversion, St Augustine wrote:

> … I was able totally to set my face against what I willed and to will what you willed. But where had this ability been for all those years? And from what profound and secret depth was my free will suddenly called forth in a moment so that I could bow my neck to your *easy yoke* and my shoulders to your *light burden*… Now my mind was free of those gnawing cares that came from ambition and the desire for gain and wallowing in filth and scratching the itching scab of lust. And now I was talking to you easily and simply, my brightness and my riches and my health, my Lord God.

St Augustine (397 AD/1963, pp. 184–185, italics in original).

Fourthly, St Augustine describes his appetite for Christian worship shortly after his conversion as insatiable, as addictions often are:

> In those days I could never have enough of the wonderful sweetness of meditating upon the depth of your counsel for the salvation of the human race. What tears I shed in your hymns and canticles! How deeply was I moved by the voices of your sweet singing Church!

St Augustine (397 AD/1963, pp. 193–194).

From *Confessions of St. Augustine* by St. Augustine, translated by Rex Warner, copyright © 1963 by Rex Warner, renewed © 1991 by F. C. Warner. Used with permission of Dutton Signet, a division of Penguin Group (USA) Inc.

How could an insatiable appetite for voluntary slavery to an inebriating experience that made the rest of life seem repellent not be understood as fitting the definition of addiction; in this case, addiction$_4$?

16 See Chapter 2 under the heading *Traditional meaning of the word 'addiction'*.

17 *Holy Bible, New Living Translation* (1996, Romans 1:1, 6:6–19, 7:14–25).

18 If dislocation is a necessary condition of addiction$_4$, then early Christians would have to have been dislocated. St Augustine recounted the dislocation of people of the late Roman Empire extensively (summarized in Chapter 9). Moreover, he consistently identified Christians as 'pilgrims', even in their own communities and in their own homes. For example, '… they are pilgrims even in their own homes' (St Augustine, 426 AD/2000, p. 21). A pilgrim, in the Christian tradition, is a temporarily or permanently itinerant person who is devoting their existence to godliness (see Bunyan's *The Pilgrim's Progress*, 1678/1985). For St Augustine, home was only to be found following conversion in the 'City of God'. This city was the community of all Catholic Christians on earth (St Augustine, 426 AD/2000, Book 23), regardless of language or ethnicity. (After the second coming of Jesus, its domain is to be extended from earth to heaven, and the City of God would become eternal.) It was not geographically anywhere, but nonetheless provided a real, social community (St Augustine, 426 AD/2000, Book 19, Chapter 17), being densely populated with Christians interacting with each other, with God's angels, with Jesus after the second coming, and with God himself. As in the case of the substitute community that is imagined in some other kinds of addiction$_3$, the City of God is, from my non-Christian point of view, imaginary

19 Merton (1950/2000, p. xvi).

20 Bonhoeffer (1959, Chapter 2).

21 See endnote 49 in Chapter 2.

22 Granfield and Cloud (1999, pp. 86–87).

23 Peter Brown (1967, Chapter 27).

24 Peter Brown (1967, p. 396).

25 Peter Brown (1967, p. 432).

26 Another vital question, introduced in Chapter 9, is whether or not addiction$_4$ exists by itself or always follows addiction$_3$.

27 See Bonhoeffer (1959).

28 Augustine's City of God is a holy mystery. It is an ideal Christian community in which truly faithful Christians dwell with the angels and Jesus Himself while they are on earth, although it is immaterial and has no specific location. As Peter Brown (1967, p. 324) summarised it, 'So the *City of God*, far from being a book about flight from the world, is a book … about being otherworldly in the world.'

29 St Augustine (426 AD/2000, p. 697).

30 By this logic, God is an imagined deity from a middle-eastern legend, akin to countless other tribal deities throughout the ages. Ontologically, He is essentially nothing from this point of view. This is not to say that Christian faith is nothing from this point of view, since its psychological and social impacts are immense.

31 'Not that all who die in Adam shall be members of Christ—for the great majority shall be punished in eternal death' (St Augustine, 426 AD/2000, p. 435).

32 Orford (2001a, p. 339, Chapter 14).

33 Orford (2001a, pp. 334–335). Jesus himself may have had a success rate of around one in four in his own preaching, as suggested by the parable of the seeds (Mark 4:3–9).

34 *Holy Bible, New International Version.* (1984, Matthew 22:21; Mark 12:17; Luke 20:25).

35 See endnote 8, this chapter. See also Bonhoeffer (1959, Chapter 2)

36 Weber (1920/1958); Tawney (1926/1947, Chapter 4).

37 Bell (1987).

38 For example, LaHaye and Jenkins (1995).

39 St Augustine (397 AD/1963, Book 13).

40 However, he skated close to the edge, in my opinion. His violent persecution of the Christian Donatists during his years as Bishop of Hippo may perhaps be overlooked as simply the standard practice of authority in the late Roman Empire, but his heart-wrenching decision to leave his common-law wife, despite their mutual love and faithfulness, because her presence would disrupt his faith, draws me back to the possibility that addiction$_4$ may be as destructive as addiction$_3$.

41 'But if the Creator is truly loved, that is, if He Himself is loved and not another thing in his stead, He cannot be evilly loved; for love itself is to be ordinately loved …' (St Augustine, 426 AD/2000, p. 511).

42 The immoderation of St Augustine's religious devotion is documented by quotations from the *Confessions* in endnote 15 of this chapter. In addition, he described the narrowing of his vision and his intolerance towards unbelievers as his addiction to God grew in the following ways:

> In my own temporal life everything was unsettled and *my heart had to be purged from the old leaven.* The way—the Saviour Himself—pleased me; but I was still reluctant to enter its narrowness.

St Augustine (397 AD/1963, p. 160, italics in original).

HOW AMAZING is the profundity of your utterances! See, they lie before us with a surface that can charm little children. But their profundity is amazing, my God, their profundity is amazing. One cannot look into them without awe and trembling—awe of greatness, trembling of love. *The enemies thereof I hate* with all my strength.

St Augustine (397 AD/1963, p. 294, uppercase and italics in original).

From *Confessions of St. Augustine* by St. Augustine, translated by Rex Warner, copyright © 1963 by Rex Warner, renewed © 1991 by F. C. Warner. Used with permission of Dutton Signet, a division of Penguin Group (USA) Inc.

43 There are many websites on this topic. Search for 'Fundamentalists Anonymous' using Google™.

44 Bill W.'s life has been the subject of intense scholarship. I have here followed *Bill's Story* as told in Alcoholics Anonymous World Services (1976) and Cheever's (2004) biography. The latter is based on Bill W.'s autobiography and other accounts that have been published by AA, as well as independent research by Cheever.

45 Alcoholics Anonymous World Services (1976).

46 Cheever (2004, p. 129) notes that he had 'grown up with Vermont libertarian principles'.

47 These facts are meticulously documented by Cheever (2004) and are confirmed in briefer form in *Bill's Story*, which Bill wrote himself, and is included in the *Big Book* of AA (Alcoholics Anonymous World Services, 1976).

48 The text of *Bill's Story* (Alcoholics Anonymous World Services, 1976, Chapter 1) and of Cheever's (2004) carefully researched biography leave little doubt in my mind that he would be described as addicted to these other pursuits had not they been overshadowed by his much more conspicuous alcoholism. Certainly, St Augustine would have looked at his life as composed almost entirely of addictions.

49 Bill W., quoted by Cheever (2004, p.118).

50 AA was a group project from the first. The official 'cofounder' was 'Dr. Bob', who was quite possibly as important to AA's success as Bill W.

51 Alcoholics Anonymous World Services (1976).

52 St Augustine provides a dramatic illustration of the downfall that can result just from a momentary lapse from abstinence. Similar downfall stories pervade the 12-step literature. St Augustine's example relates to addiction to violent entertainment—the gladiatorial games (St Augustine, 397 AD/1963, Book 6, Chapter 8).

53 St Augustine is uncharacteristically inconsistent on how total religious devotion must be. At some points, he seems to say that some degree of earthly pleasure is acceptable, as long as it is always under control and never comes before God (St Augustine, 397 AD/1963, Book 2, Chapter 5). At his most extreme, he spoke of Christian life (i.e., life in the 'City of God') as involving exclusively Christian emotions and service to fellow Christians by exhorting and punishing to keep them attuned to the true faith and eternal contemplation of God (St Augustine, 426 AD/2000, Book 14, Chapter 9, Book 19, Chapter 19, including reference to 19:6). For example:

… that is not true wisdom which does not direct all its prudent observations, manly actions, virtuous self-restraint, and just arrangements, to that end in which God shall be all and all in a secure eternity and perfect peace.

St Augustine (426 AD/2000, p. 699).

54 Peter Brown (1967, pp. 163–165).

55 Peter Brown (1967, p. 367).

56 See Alcoholics Anonymous World Services (1976, pp. 10–11).

57 Cheever (2004, p. 216).

58 Cheever (2004, Chapter 38).

59 Cheever (2004).

60 The 'characteristics of sex addiction' are summarized in a website of the Greater Cincinnati Area Intergroup of the Augustine Fellowship (http://www.slaacincinnati.org/characteristics.htm).

61 Cheever (2004, pp. 122–123, 235). Cheever and I interpret this theological issue in a similar way, although I do not know if she would give as much weight to the Market God.

62 Cheever (2004, Chapter 38).

63 Cheever (2004, Chapter 35).

64 See Traditions 5, 6, 7, 10, 11, and 12.

65 There is a current fringe of eclectic spirituality that seems to me too fanciful to warrant attention in this book. This fringe is exemplified by a book called *The Secret*. See Whyte (2007).

66 Vanier (1998, p. 15).

67 Vanier (1998), W. R. Miller (1998, 2000).

68 Martín-Baró (1994).

69 This book uses the contemporary Buddhist analysis of S. N. Goenka (1987) as the primary example. See also Das (1998). Buddhism is, of course, a large and diverse religious tradition, some branches of which may not fit within the rubric of 'eclectic spirituality' as defined here.

70 T. Moore (1992) identified eclectic spirituality, as defined here, with Roman Epicureanism. I will identify it in this chapter with the Roman Stoic philosopher Marcus Aurelius. Ellis and Harper (1961, pp. 5, 33) identified it with another Stoic philosopher, Epictetus. Whereas Albert Ellis made himself famous for an abrasive personal style that may seem contrary to eclectic spiritualism, his underlying message fits closely with its message of enlightened self-absorption and acceptance of an irrational world, as can be seen in the following quotation:

> A more irrational world than the one in which we presently live could hardly be conceived. In spite of the enormous advances in technical knowledge made during the last century, and theoretical possibility [of] all of us living in peace and prosperity, we actually exist perilously close to the brink of local strife, world war, economic insecurity, political skulduggery, organized crime, business fraud, sexual violence, racial bigotry, labour and management inefficiency, religious fanaticism, and scores of similar manifestations of idiocy and inhumanity.
>
> On a more personal scale, conditions are equally bad or worse. None of us—no not a single, solitary one of us—can fail to have intimate encounters, almost every day of our lives, with several individuals (be they bosses or employees, husbands or wives, children or parents, friends or enemies) who are stupid, ignorant, ineffective, provocative, frustrating, vicious, or seriously disturbed. Modern life, instead of being just a bowl of cherries, more closely resembles a barrel of prune pits.
>
> Nonetheless: a human being in today's world does not have to be unhappy. Wonderfully enough, along with his being endowed with more than his share of inanity and insanity, man also has a remarkable capacity for straight thinking ...

if he intelligently organizes and disciplines his thinking and his actions, he can live a decidedly self-fulfilling, creative, and emotionally satisfying life even in the highly unsatisfactory world of today.
Ellis and Harper (1961, p. 183).

71 Maslow (1950/1973); Rogers (1957); W. R. Miller (2000).

72 Pert (1997); Wilber (2000).

73 Aurelius (170 AD/1964).

74 Lecky (1911).

75 Staniforth (1967).

76 Aurelius (170 AD/1964, p. 82).

77 Aurelius (170 AD/1964, p. 115).

78 Aurelius (170 AD/1964, p. 110).

79 Aurelius (170 AD/1964, p. 141).

80 Goenka (1987, p. 11).

81 Goenka (1987, 1991).

82 Bayley (2004, Chapter 9).

83 Vipassana meditation is actually taught for nothing, since participants may attend the basic 10-day training course at one of the Vipassana Meditation Centres without paying, even for food and lodging. Although the organisation accepts donations, it exerts no pressure on participants to extract them.

84 Goenka (1991).

85 Some other people report much less discomfort than I experienced. Apart from individual differences in flexibility, there are apparently differences in the degree of postural conformity that is encouraged at different centres.

86 Goenka (1987, p. 43, 1991, Discourse 5).

87 W. R. Miller (1998).

88 W. R. Miller (2004), C'de Baca and Wilbourne (2004).

89 W. R. Miller (2000, p. 12).

90 W. R. Miller (2000, p. 16).

91 W. R. Miller (2000, p. 16).

92 W. R. Miller (2000, p. 13).

93 Paul Tillich (1948, p. 162, as quoted in W. R. Miller, 2000, p. 12, italics in original). Within the paragraph, Tillich is quoting an unidentified universal voice.

94 W. R. Miller (2000, p. 15).

95 Nonetheless, I have steadfastly resisted the temptation to refer to Dr Miller, even once, as 'Bill M.'.

96 Immen (2006). See also the work of Eva Illouz, as analysed by Pieiller (2007, p. 27). Pieiller also points out a structural similarity between eclectic spiritualism and free-market ideology. Both assert that steadfastly working for individual improvement will benefit all of society. In free-market society this happens by intervention of the 'invisible hand'. In eclectic spirituality, the mechanism is not specifically identified.

97 Peele and Brodsky (1975).

98 Miller (2000, p. 15) himself raises the crucial question of 'Where can love not reach?' He would not necessarily answer it as I have.

99 Recent protests by Buddhist monks against the murderous military junta in Myanmar (Mydang, 2007) are an example.

100 Goenka (1987, pp. 45, 53).

101 Goenka (1987, 1991).

102 Goenka (1987, p. 74).

103 Despite the murders of significant numbers of people in Myanmar (including many Buddhist monks) by the military junta in 2007, Vipassana meditation has taken no strong public position that I could find. S. N. Goenka himself grew up in Burma (now Myanmar), although he currently lives in India.

104 Goenka (1987, pp. 47, 53–54).

105 I speculate here, having no specific knowledge of the life and times of Gautama Buddha. All accounts of his life and times are, in fact, ultimately drawn from oral tradition of uncertain veracity.

106 Mydang (2007).

107 Koring (2004a).

Chapter 13

Socrates' 'Master Passions' and *Dikaiosunê*[1]

The dislocation theory of addiction is anything but a new idea. In fact, its essentials appeared in the Socratic dialogues of Plato, written almost 24 centuries ago long before either St Augustine or Marcus Aurelius were born.[2] This chapter begins by revealing the surprising similarity between the lives of today's most notorious addicts and those of the young Athenians who Socrates described as overwhelmed by 'master passions'. It goes on to show the close similarity between the causal analysis of addiction provided by the dislocation theory and the causal analysis of master passions in the *Republic*. These comparisons are intended to establish that the dislocation theory of addiction, like so many important ideas, has its ultimate source in Western civilisation's most fruitful philosophic and spiritual tradition.[3] Finally, this chapter points to implications that emerge from Socrates' dialectical meanderings around the topic of addiction in the *Republic* and *Protagoras*, but are less easily drawn from the more linear presentation of the dislocation theory of addiction in this book.

The *Republic* and *Protagoras*[4] were written by the Athenian philosopher Plato. However, both dialogues were formatted as if they were annotated transcriptions of conversations between Plato's teacher, Socrates, and other Greek thinkers. Following Plato's lead, this chapter attributes all of the important ideas in these dialogues to Socrates, the teacher, rather than Plato, the writer.[5]

Like the Bible, Socratic dialogues can be read in a variety of ways. Each way tends to focus on a particular theme. This chapter focuses on the relationship between addiction and different kinds of society. This reading gives little attention to the concern of some of today's public intellectuals that the *Republic* is dangerously anti-democratic.[6] This issue has little importance here. Little is gained by characterising the vast reaches of Socratic thought in contemporary terms that are as iconic and inconstant in their meaning as 'democratic' or 'anti-democratic'. Socrates says explicitly throughout the *Republic* that he is not creating a blueprint of a utopia, but rather using a hypothetical society as a metaphor to explain the happiest and most temperate way to live.[7]

The first section of this chapter quotes one of Socrates' portrayals of disturbed young men in ancient Greece whose lifestyles closely resembled some of today's most infamous addicts (i.e. 'junkies', 'crack heads', and 'crystal meth addicts'), even though the demon drugs with which these lifestyles are now associated did not exist then.

Addiction in Ancient Greece

In the *Republic*, Socrates' describes people who are overwhelmingly involved with what he called a master passion at some length. For example:

> When a master passion within has absolute control of a man's mind ... life is a round of extravagant feasts and orgies and sex and so on ... So whatever income he has will soon be expended ... and next of course he'll start borrowing and drawing on capital ... when he comes to the end of his father's and mother's resources ... he'll start by burgling a house or holding someone up at night, and go on to clean out a temple. Meanwhile the older beliefs about honour and dishonour, which he was brought up to accept as right, will be overcome by others, once held in restraint but now freed to become the bodyguard of his master passion. While he was still democratically minded ... they only appeared in his dreams; but under the tyranny of his master passion he becomes in his working life what he was once only occasionally in his dreams.... His passion tyrannizes over him, a despot without restraint or law and drives him ... into any venture that will profit itself and its gang.[8]

There can be little doubt that Socrates' depictions of master passions in the *Republic* are similar to contemporary depictions of severe addictions[3]. But why would people behave in this way? Socrates argues that large numbers of people are overcome by master passions only if they are totally lacking in *dikaiosunê* as a consequence of living in a 'tyrannical society'. Although the Greek word *dikaiosunê* is usually translated into English as 'justice', the Greek word itself is used throughout this chapter because, as scholars recognise, the word 'justice' is far too narrow to serve as an adequate translation for *dikaiosunê* in the way that Socrates analysed it in the *Republic*.[9] Socrates also introduced a special way of understanding 'tyrannical society' that will be described later.

Although no everyday English word captures the full scope of the Greek word *dikaiosunê* as Socrates defines it in the *Republic*, the term 'psychosocial integration' as used in this book comes very close. It will require a detailed look at a number of points to establish this equivalence.

The equivalence of *dikaiosunê* and psychosocial integration

Some of the similarities between *dikaiosunê* and psychosocial integration become apparent in the creation myth that is recounted in *Protagoras*,[10] which was written some years before the *Republic*. The god Epimetheus, assigned the task of dispersing unique abilities and physical advantages to each of the animal species at the time of creation, inadvertently overlooks the human species, leaving mankind unhoofed, unfanged, unfurred, unarmoured, and, worst of all, uncooperative. The god Prometheus, seeing the potential tragedy in this, steals the secrets of domestic arts and of fire from other gods and bestows them on mankind. Prometheus is punished terribly for his theft, but, with the aid of the Promethean gifts, mankind learns to speak and to worship the gods and manages to survive, despite its lack of more ordinary animal equipment. However, human beings, still too uncooperative to organise themselves politically, remain dispersed, dangerous to each other, and vulnerable to animal predators.

Zeus, seeing that the human species is still endangered, enlists the aid of Hermes, who gives people the further gifts of mutual respect and custom.[11] With these gifts, human beings finally develop a shared sense of *dikaiosunê* and civic virtue, subdue the predators, and live together harmoniously. Thereafter, the human species thrives.[12] Like *dikaiosunê* in this ancient creation myth, psychosocial integration is essential for human well-being and grows out of respect and custom. Psychosocial integration, like *dikaiosunê* in the myth, is an absolutely essential part of the success story of the human species.

In the *Republic*, Socrates turns to rational argument, rather than mythology, to show that *dikaiosunê* is, at once, the essential feature of a good human society,[13] the source of the greatest possible individual happiness, and a shield against domination by master passions (i.e. addictions.) These same virtues are asserted for psychosocial integration by the dislocation theory (see Chapter 3). The *Republic* differs from *Protagoras* in that *dikaiosunê* is not portrayed just as one of several essential social virtues, but as the central virtue from which of all the other social virtues derive,[14] much like psychosocial integration. Socrates explains in detail how *dikaiosunê* is the font from which the other virtues spring.

In its most elementary meaning, Socrates' defines *dikaiosunê* as the state of people who have a secure role in society to which they are so well suited that they never try to usurp another's. In Socrates' very simplest formulation, '... *dikaiosunê*[15] is keeping what is properly one's own and doing one's own job'.[16]

As Socrates fills out the idea of *dikaiosunê*, it becomes evident, however, that it means much more than a division of labour and pursuit of a career. It defines a hypothetical society in which each individual has not only a secure, respected occupation, but also a reason to identify with everyone else in the society. Diverse individual, family, and class roles are maintained in the ideal society through a complex system of socialisation, education, and indoctrination. For example, rulers are selected and trained with scrupulous care so that they have the abilities and the love for their society as a whole that are essential for them to fulfil their leadership function conscientiously and never oppress those whom they rule.[17] Members of the ruling classes who do not fulfil the criteria of good rulers will be moved to a different class and members of the lowest class will be moved to the ruling classes if they merit it.[18] Therefore, the class system, although hierarchical, serves to organise the ideal society for the benefit of all, rather than to maintain hereditary privilege or to trap people in roles in which they will be exploited.

Because each individual role and each social class is designed to fulfil an essential function of society, all citizens recognize all other citizens as essential to the whole, and each is respected for his or her unique function. Each place in society not only carries responsibilities, but also the rewards that are best suited to people who fulfil the role. Thus, although most of the opportunities for intellectual pursuits and for the exercise of power go to the ruling classes, the members of these classes must live an ascetic life that excludes any contact with wealth or any participation in commerce.[19]

With psychological insight that is not found in the ideology of free-market society, Socrates separates power from both wealth and private property, regarding this separation as necessary to prevent class exploitation and envy. When asked how members of the ruling classes will be happy without personal wealth, Socrates answers that they love intellectual challenge and individual responsibility even more than they love individual wealth. Their happiness will come 'from playing their proper role in making the community thrive'.[20] Most of the society's material wealth apparently goes to public works projects, which benefit the population as a whole, and to the members of the working class, since they have a greater appreciation of material pleasures.

Dikaiosunê not only accords people stability in occupational and family roles, close interdependence, a powerful identification with society as a whole, and a life of moderation and balance, but also social tranquillity. Working-class people naturally regard the ruling classes as fellow citizens, as well as their defenders and protectors. Members of the ruling classes naturally recognise workers as fellow citizens who create their homes and sustenance. All citizens consider ills that befall any other citizen as if they were their own, and gains of any member of society as a cause for celebration.[21]

It can reasonably be argued that this idealised society allows too little latitude for individual development and personal choice. However, it is hard to believe that Socrates, who shows exquisite sensitivity to the complex personalities of the characters in his dialogues, could make the fatal mistake of forgetting the importance of individual autonomy just because he emphasises social belonging. Although he does not emphasise individual accomplishments in *Protagoras* and the *Republic*, he understood that the social roles that he envisioned allowed a great deal of opportunity for individual creativity and autonomy, and that, as contemporary social scientists have shown, people become confused and dismayed in situations where every possible lifestyle is available to them.[22]

After defining *dikaiosunê* on a social level, Socrates defines it as an individual characteristic. Just as the state has three basic social classes—philosophers, other guardians (soldiers and executives), and workers—the individual psyche[23] has three basic parts—the rational intellect, the spirited emotions, and the bodily appetites[24] that closely correspond to the three social classes. *Dikaiosunê* is established on an individual level when each part of the psyche is true to its own nature and simultaneously maintains a proper, respectful relationship to the other parts. This means that the bodily appetites are controlled by reason and spirit, for appetites by themselves are impetuous and insatiable, and therefore cannot lead the person in the best direction. However, reason and spirit must never neglect to provide adequate satisfaction to the various appetites, for the moderate and balanced fulfilment of appetites is a source of health for the person. Thus, addiction, in which one or more appetites overwhelm the entire psyche, is impossible in a state of *dikaiosunê*. Socrates emphasises that a *dikaios* person naturally maintains a state of 'soberness', 'temperance', or 'self-discipline'.[25]

In a state of *dikaiosunê*, society and individuals become stable, people of every social status become as happy and righteous as people can possibly be, and people identify themselves with their society as well as with their own balanced and moderate personalities. There is no room in this picture for addiction. The overlap between the idea of *dikaiosunê* and the idea of psychosocial integration is obvious, and their equivalence grows more and more evident to me each time I revisit the *Republic*. A *dikaios* person is the natural product of a *dikaios* society and a *dikaios* society is the natural product of *dikaios* citizens.[26] Socrates, like Erik Erikson and Karl Polanyi, assumed that a positive identity develops naturally in a well-organised, welcoming society.

However, the society that Socrates outlines in the *Republic* is only hypothetical. It is not real and not a utopian scheme. In fact, Socrates acknowledges that his ideal society would depend for its existence upon an unbroken string of philosopher kings who were completely honest and public-spirited, and upon a sophisticated testing system so that citizens could be assigned functions perfectly suited to their needs—a difficult balancing act indeed.

The most important part of Socrates' argument for this book on addiction is his explanation of why addiction spreads in societies in which *dikaiosunê* has diminished and why addiction becomes universal in societies from which *dikaiosunê* has disappeared. This part of Socrates' argument is important today because, unlike the ideal society, imperfect societies are anything but hypothetical.

Imperfect societies

Towards the end of the *Republic*, Socrates describes at length the sequence in which every society must inevitably deteriorate: from the hypothetical ideal society, to a timarchy,[27] to a commercial oligarchy,[28] to an anarchic democracy,[29] and finally, to tyranny, the lowest form of society. At each stage of deterioration, more and more *dikaiosunê* (i.e. psychosocial integration) is lost, until, in tyranny, there is no *dikaiosunê* left. Therefore, the downward progression also leads to increasing, and finally universal, domination of people by master passions, or addictions.

Socrates argues that every type of society that appears during this progressive loss of *dikaiosunê*, or psychosocial integration, inculcates a characteristic personality in the people who inhabit it. *Dikaios* people are typical in the ideal *dikaios* society, but are found less and less frequently as society declines. Tyranny, as Socrates explains it, is the last stage of deterioration in which *dikaiosunê* no longer exists.[30] Tyranny is the natural habitat of 'tyrannical personalities' (i.e. people who are overwhelmed by one or a few of their basest appetites). Thus, by the end of the *Republic*, Socrates has provided a picture of a society that is plagued with universal addiction, and he has explained this plague as a result of the absence of *dikaiosunê*—in close accord with the dislocation theory of addiction.

Although there are enormous differences between ancient Greek city states and the nation states of the 21st century, Socrates' description of the dynamic relationship between declining society and universal addiction resonates across the centuries. The *Republic* goes a long way towards showing how societies in general can generate epidemic addiction, whether they are free-market societies, conquered tribal people, collapsing civilisations, or modern tyrannies. Each step in societal deterioration has important implications for dislocation and addiction, but, for simplicity, only the most directly relevant of these steps will be discussed in this chapter.

Commercial oligarchy and anarchic democracy

Anarchic democracy arises in reaction to the commercial oligarchy that precedes it in the downward spiral. A commercial oligarchy is ruled by merchants who care about little but money. In order to maximise their own wealth, they deliberately weaken the laws and customs that restrain consumption and give out loans freely, knowing—but not caring—that many of those who accept their subprime loans (as they can now be called)[31] will be ruined when they cannot repay them.[32] In this way, and others, *dikaiosunê* is further reduced.

More and more of the people in a commercial oligarchy become financially ruined and at the same time keenly aware that the ruling commercial class is deliberately luring them into disastrous overconsumption. Realising that the merchants are weak and fat, they rise up against the entire commercial class and form a democracy—of a sort: 'Then democracy originates when the poor win, kill or exile their opponents, and give the rest equal civil rights and opportunities of office…'[33]

As Socrates' description of democracy continues, it becomes clear that, although it corresponds to today's ideal of democracy in some ways (e.g. civil rights), it is antithetical to today's ideal in many other ways. Socrates does not identify the democracy that he describes with an electoral process (since many officials are selected by lot), a constitution that restricts government powers, or a balance of powers between different levels of government. Rather, Socrates emphasises that democracy is popular because of the variety it affords, the minimum of restriction, and the availability of high office to everybody: 'It's an agreeable anarchic form of society, with plenty of variety, which treats all men as equal, whether they are equal or not.'[34]

Socrates describes, however, some of the flaws in this anarchic democracy in a way that may seem strangely familiar:

> … in democracy, there's no compulsion either to exercise authority if you are capable of it, or to submit to authority if you don't want to; you needn't fight if there's a war, or you can wage a private war in peacetime if you don't like peace; and if there's any law that debars you from political or judicial office, you will none the less take either if they come your way. It's a wonderfully pleasant way of carrying on in the short run, isn't it? …
>
> We said that no one who had not exceptional gifts could grow into a good man unless he were brought up from childhood in a good environment and trained in good habits. Democracy with a grandiose gesture sweeps all this away and doesn't mind what the habits and background of its politicians are; provided they profess themselves the people's friends, they are duly honoured.[35]

Although Socrates is not describing anything like the modern ideal of democracy, he has provided a recognisable description of the commercial origins of some apparently democratic values and of the ways in which a democracy can fall to ruin. For example, his description evokes the decadent last days of the democratic Weimar Republic, before the emergence of the Nazi tyranny in the 1930s. Arguably, it might also come close to describing the ruination of democracy in the worst corners of our own free-market world. For example, teachers in some areas of Canada apparently have trouble controlling unruly students in their classrooms or even setting criteria for graduation from high school without being accused of infringing on the rights of individual students.[36] Corporations headquartered in today's most loudly self-proclaimed democracy are carrying on essentially large-scale private wars against people in the Third World to extract the greatest profits that they can.[37] Various sorts of corporate predation have been defended by defining the corporation as a legal person with individual rights.[38]

In the language of the dislocation theory of addiction, the 'democratic character' that Socrates regards as the natural product of this sort of anarchic democratic society is seriously dislocated. Since such people have no reason to respect the authorities in their society, to support classes other than their own, or to accommodate their pleasure-seeking to the needs of other people, they are severely lacking in *dikaiosunê*, or psychosocial integration, although they may still maintain close ties with their parents. Socrates says that such characters are swept away with pleasure-seeking because their families fail to bring them up with a proper sense of self-discipline, leaving them vulnerable to temptation and seductions much of the time. Socrates describes the democratic character as follows:

> ... he lives from day to day, indulging the pleasures of the moment. One day it's wine, women, and song, the next water to drink and a strict diet; one day it's hard physical training, the next indolence and careless ease, and then a period of philosophic study. Often he takes to politics and keeps jumping to his feet and saying or doing whatever comes into his head. Sometimes all his ambitions and efforts are military, sometimes they are all directed to success in business. There's no order or restraint in his life, and he reckons his way of living is pleasant, free and happy, and sticks to it through thick and thin.[39]

In the most extreme form of the anarchic democracy, all restraint is gone. Rulers act like subjects and are unable to exert any control over the increasing madness; citizens act like rulers; parents fear their own children; there is no distinction between citizens and foreigners; the young treat their elders with disrespect 'while their elders try to avoid the reputation of being disagreeable or strict by aping the young and mixing with them on terms of easy good fellowship'.[40] As he warms to his task of mocking extreme, anarchic democracy, Socrates' tone becomes burlesque, elaborating, for example, on the civil rights of horses and donkeys.[41] It seems evident that some people will fall into severe addictions in the dislocated world of anarchic democracies, although Socrates only alludes to this in passing.[42] He reserves his full analysis of addiction for his description of a tyrannical society.

Tyranny and addiction

According to Socrates, anarchic democracy is the breeding ground for a tyrannical society, in which all *dikaiosunê* is lost. He advances a complex explanation for this, based on the anxieties that grow from an ever-increasing excess of personal liberty. People with nothing solid to believe in find refuge in absolutism. They abandon *dikaiosunê* for a singe-minded pursuit of personal pleasure. The most violent and ruthless of these unhappy creatures ultimately takes over as a tyrannical ruler, addicted to personal power and wealth. However, it is not only the ruler of the tyrannical society who is addicted. The tyrannical personality becomes universal as a society moves from democracy to tyranny. In the end, everybody becomes dominated by a master passion.

Whereas the democratic character is captivated by worthy and unworthy desires equally, and is therefore unpredictable, the tyrannical personality is consistently dominated by the very worst kinds of desire. To describe the tyrannical character, Socrates finds it necessary to classify desires into necessary and unnecessary ones. Some of the unnecessary desires are lawless and violent. We know of them mainly through the excesses we commit in dreams where we don't '... shrink from attempting intercourse ... with a mother or anyone else, man, beast, or god, or from murder or eating forbidden food. There is, in fact, no folly or shamelessness it will not commit.'[43]

Unnecessary desires are found in all people, but they become the dominating motivations in the lives of individuals who live in the tyrannical society, producing further destruction of social life. Some of Socrates' descriptions of the tyrannical personality appeared at the start of this chapter under the heading *Addiction in Ancient Greece*.

Some of Socrates' other descriptions of men with tyrannical personalities could serve as descriptions of the inner life of present-day addicts:

> His mind will be burdened with servile restrictions, because the best elements in him will be enslaved and completely controlled by a minority of the lowest and most lunatic impulses ...
>
> So the mind in which there is a tyranny will also be least able to do what, as a whole, it wishes, because it is under the compulsive drive of madness, and so full of confusion and remorse ...
>
> He's clearly far the unhappiest of all men.[44]

Socrates dramatizes the development of the tyrannical personality by imagining the son of still democratically minded parents, who urge him to find a good balance between idle pleasures and disciplined work. This prudential counsel is foiled because, in a tyrannical society, there are many people who would profit by tempting him away from wholesome discipline, and ...

> ... his tempters come in on the other side. And when the wicked wizards who want to make him a tyrant despair of keeping their hold on the young man ... they contrive to implant a master passion in him to control the idle desires that divide his time between them, like a great winged drone.... The other desires buzz round it, loading it with incense and perfume, flowers and wine, and all the pleasures of a dissolute life on which they feed and fatten until at last they produce in it the sting of mania.[45]

Thus, on the crucial question of *why* the tyrannical personality becomes overwhelmingly involved with a master passion, even the immortal Socrates becomes vague and metaphorical. He identifies 'tempters' or 'wicked wizards', who 'implant' a 'master passion' and 'load it with incense and perfume' as the causes of a tyrannical personality (i.e. addiction) in the quotation above, but these metaphors are confusing. Socrates seems to regard the tyrannical personality as 'out of control' in some degree, but just what does that mean? The master passion that controls him is one of *his own* base desires, and the other desires that augment it are also his. But if a person is satisfying his own desire, how is he out of control? Who are the 'wicked wizards'?

Earlier in the *Republic*, Socrates acknowledges this paradox, arguing that such a concept as 'out of control' is a logical absurdity. He points out that saying a person is 'master of himself' (i.e. not out of control) is the same as saying that a person is both his own master and his own subject, although he is only one person.[46] Socrates explains at that point in the *Republic* that it is more correct to say that the better portions of the psyche, particularly the intellect, control the worse portions, in the interest of the whole.[47]

The clearest statement of why the tyrannical personality becomes overwhelmingly involved with a master passion is not a simple statement of cause and effect. The tyrannical personality is engendered in children as they grow up in the tyrannical society, but the tyrannical society exists because the dislocation of anarchic democracy makes it impossible for most people to endure life without developing a tyrannical personality. Addiction is both the cause and the effect of an addicted society. It is perhaps most accurate to say that addiction is intrinsic to the collapse of society.

Although Socrates is somewhat unclear about the cause of addiction in a person that has lost all *dikaiosunê*, he is lucid on the fate of the addict. The tyrannical personality (i.e. addict) will engage in gross excesses of drinking, feasting, and sex. He will turn to crime, first deceiving his parents, and then progress to actual robbery and violence. People like this will fight as mercenaries in any war or, in times of peace, stay home and commit crimes. They live in a continuous state of misery. It is a person like this, probably the worst, who succeeds in becoming a popular leader and ruling tyrant. He will reduce his country to subjection. The tyrant is an example of complete loss of *dikaiosunê* and complete unhappiness. He is unhappy because all parts of his personality except the master passion are forgotten or suppressed. Such a person is able to gather the political support of the poor by plundering the rich and distributing some of the spoils, while keeping most for himself. The temptations of great power and the taste of blood eventually turn the tyrannical ruler into a depraved monster who usurps ever more control in the service of his master passion for power. He stirs up wars to further increase his power and to keep taxes high, so the people must struggle to survive and have no time for revolutions. Completely addicted to power, he must destroy anyone who is wise enough to see what he is doing, even his own parents. He is an extreme form of the political and economic fanaticism discussed in Chapter 10.

Despite the suffering of the addicted people in a tyrannical society, and despite their propensity to harm others, even those they love, Socrates does not argue that they are sick or intrinsically evil.[48] Rather, he sees them as reacting to an impossible social situation in the best way they can. Because they are unable to achieve or even understand *dikaiosunê* in their bizarre society, they seek satisfaction elsewhere, and achieve a shred of satisfaction in their total subjugation to a few, base appetites.

In *Protagoras*, Socrates makes the point explicitly that people always choose the way of the greater good or the lesser evil, provided that they are aware of the consequences of their actions.[49] In other words, people also act as adaptively as possible, within the limits of their knowledge. It follows from this—although Socrates does not take this final, logical step in *Protagoras*—that addicted people are acting adaptively in tyrannical societies and in contemporary society as well. For example, nobody in contemporary society can be unaware of the devastating consequences of severe addiction to heroin, cocaine, and methamphetamine, yet people become addicted to them anyway. Those who adopt these drug addictions, or almost any other addictive habit, know what they are getting into. They do it because it is the lesser evil—that is, because it provides a substitute for an unbearable lack of psychosocial integration, or *dikaiosunê*.

Socrates' tyrannical society was definitely not dominated by free-market practices and principles, which Socrates could not even have imagined, since the few free markets that existed in ancient Greece never dominated society.[50] However, Socrates' tyrannical society is similar to free-market society in precisely the attribute that is most likely to cause addiction.

Free-market society, like Socrates' anarchic democracy, breaks down traditions and legitimate authority, so that people can participate in the market as individual economic actors. The corporations that exercise political control of free-market society use the mass media to glorify a sense of individual freedom that enables people to devote themselves to buying and consuming whatever products of the free-market system they desire for their individual happiness—to the profit of the corporations themselves. Socrates' descriptions of the inconstancy of the democratic personality type are reminiscent of frantic consumers in the shopping centres and are reflected in the ubiquitous portrayals of scatterbrained (but loveable) people in the popular media.

Although this condition of society has not usually led to the tyranny of a single depraved leader, modern life is redolent with the scent of tyranny. In a society that idolises democracy, people speak incessantly of behind-the-scenes tyranny of materialism, the corporations, the profit motive, the military-industrial complex, 'the rich', the free-market ideology, the new 'anti-terrorist' laws,[51] and so forth. They 'rage against the machine'.[52] Their statements are often exaggerations, but they are not empty talk. Free-market society with its hypercapitalism has reached a state of single-mindedness so extreme that it can qualify as tyranny, in Socrates' sense.

In our world, overwhelming involvement of the sort that Socrates called a master passion—and this book calls addiction—is more and more common among ordinary people as well as corporate and political elites. Therefore, the dislocation theory of addiction may best be understood as a specific application to free-market society of Socrates' more encompassing analysis of the effects of tyrannical society on personality and addiction. Earlier chapters of this book use the language of economic determinism, but the essence of the dislocation theory of addiction would stand whether the root cause of individual dislocation in society was the tyranny of a particular economic system or any other drastic constriction of the full range of human potential.

It should by now be crystal clear why addiction is spinning out of control in the modern world. Addiction is a predictable way of adapting to the dislocation that is built into unbalanced societies, of which free-market society is a current exemplar.

Socrates' final puzzle

At the beginning of the *Republic*, Socrates agrees to demonstrate two principles. First, that life based on *dikaiosunê* is the happiest way to live and, secondly, that his Athenian listeners can attain this happiness for themselves. He proceeds to define *dikaiosunê*, showing from many different angles that it is the happiest way for human beings to live, thus fulfilling his first undertaking completely. However, by portraying *dikaiosunê* as a way of life that is not engendered by imperfect societies, he seems to put a life of *dikaiosunê* out of reach for people who do not live in an ideal society, which Athens of his day definitely was not. Athens was in a state of terminal decline after a long golden age, and sometimes fell into periods of anarchic democracy and tyranny of the sort that Socrates had shown to be antithetical to the development of *dikaiosunê* in individuals.

Nonetheless, Socrates manages to demonstrate his second principle too, although less consistently than the first. By the end of the *Republic*, he has offered his listeners two different ways to achieve a life of *dikaiosunê* in an imperfect society. The first is a secular way. He counsels his listeners that they will suffer more if they abandon themselves to self-indulgence and corruption than if they strive to achieve as much *dikaiosunê* as possible in their own, imperfect society.[53] Maximising *dikaiosunê* would entail making sure that all of their actions are guided by reason, but always in a way that provides a reasonable degree of satisfaction for their instinctive and irrational needs, as well as their rational ones. Here Socrates' bedrock philosophy, which has come to be called 'rationalism', shines through. Rationalism holds that the rational quest for truth, fairness, and balance, more than the battle for wealth or power, is the path to individual and social well-being. The rationalistic path to truth entails study and disciplined conversation. Rationalism provides no guarantee of success, for individuals and civilisations will continue to rise and fall, but it guarantees that its followers will be doing the best that they can.

By contrast, Socrates' second solution to the problem of attaining a life of *dikaiosunê* while living in an imperfect society is based on otherworldly mysticism and reincarnation.[54] This last-minute leap into mysticism changes the nature of the *Republic*, because Socrates' argument up until that point had been fundamentally naturalistic, even though he had invoked the gods from time to time and based his logic on a rationalist dualism of material objects and immaterial forms.

In his second ending of the *Republic*, however, Socrates discusses the psyche (here translated as 'soul') in an entirely different way, flabbergasting his most avid listener, Glaucon:

> 'Don't you know,' I [Socrates] asked, 'that our soul is immortal and never perishes?
>
> He [Glaucon] looked at me in astonishment, and exclaimed, 'Good Lord, no! Are you prepared to maintain that it is?'[55]

Continuing in this mystical vein, Socrates makes *dikaiosunê* achievable in a spiritual sense by proposing that a person could keep *dikaiosunê* in his heart after death and in his long preparation for reincarnation in the next life. Following a period of purgatory, which could last 1000 years, the soul will be allowed to choose a new life, and that choice can be made wisely if guided by an understanding of *dikaiosunê*,[56] although some people will still make the wrong choice and be condemned to live another earthly life without *dikaiosunê*.

Like Glaucon, I am astonished by Socrates' last minute shift into otherworldly mysticism. I believe that the *Republic* would have been more consistent, and ultimately more valuable, if he had concluded rationalistically *and politically*, arguing that people can understand *dikaiosunê* and work together to create a society that fosters it. Yet, Socrates did not even discuss the possibility of actively promoting social change in the *Republic*. In fact, he explicitly states that a person should not participate in politics in an imperfect society.[57]

This mystical second ending of the *Republic* seems out of character on many levels. Socrates started his discourse near the beginning of the *Republic* with the example of a simple agrarian society in which *dikaiosunê* apparently was achieved without any need for otherworldly mysticism, since the agrarian society did not have to deal with the perils of war and wealth that faced the affluent, warlike ideal society that is described in the remainder of the *Republic*.[58] Why did he not extend that agrarian example to show that *dikaiosunê* can be achieved in a large society, provided it can find a way to achieve the balance of a simpler life? In his description of the psyche early in the *Republic*, Socrates identified it as the conjunction of reason, spirit, and appetite[59] in the same naturalistic way that Freud, 24 centuries later, would speak of the mind as the conjunction of id, ego, and superego. This kind of a psyche does not seem well suited for life after death and reincarnation, as Socrates himself pointed out.[60] Moreover, in *Protagoras*, Socrates ultimately recognised that *dikaiosunê* and other aspects of virtue can be achieved through the best kind of secular education.[61] Why does he abandon his faith in education at the end of the *Republic*? Finally, Socrates' swerve into otherworldly mysticism and reincarnation at the end of the *Republic* is inconsistent with his position in another dialogue, the *Apology*, where he states that it is unwise for anybody to claim to know what happens after death. He says there that it is just as likely that death is like an eternal dreamless sleep as that any kind of supernatural events occur in the underworld.[62] Historically, his swerve into mysticism and reincarnation in the *Republic* weakened the force of his secular rationalism and provided part of the basis for the obscurities of Neoplatonism and Augustinian Christianity.[63]

Perhaps it was simply too politically dangerous in Athens for even Socrates to carry his naturalistic, rationalistic argument to its natural conclusion. After all, he was eventually executed for vaguely defined crimes, and he may well have been toeing the line as much as he could before that fatal time. Alternatively, Plato, the actual writer of the dialogue, may have been worrying about his own skin in the still-dangerous Greek political world of his own day.

On the other hand, it may be that Socrates, the wisest of human beings, saw a deeper truth. Perhaps he realised that, whereas human beings absolutely must have *dikaiosunê*, or psychosocial integration, civilisation was evolving in directions that would more and more rule it out. Perhaps he concluded that the best solution to this problem is transforming *dikaiosunê* from an achievable social principle to a mystical inner experience that could get people through their lives and hold society together for as long as possible. Perhaps Socrates believed that rationalism, powerful as it is, is not powerful enough to halt an event with as much momentum as the decline and fall of a civilisation, just as all our modern technical knowledge of celestial mechanics is insufficient to stop the eventual burn-out of the sun, or slow it by a single iota.

Perhaps Socrates was as wise in his turn to mysticism as he was about everything else. Perhaps, therefore, *dikaiosunê*, or psychosocial integration, should be understood as achievable only on a spiritual plane and, consequently, widespread addiction must be regarded as inevitable in the globalising world of today. However, I cannot accept this conclusion. Because I find Socrates' secular rationalism persuasive at the deepest level, I cannot accept his late-breaking mysticism at the end of the *Republic*. The final chapters of this book follow the trajectory of Socrates' rationalism rather than that of his mysticism.

Obviously, it is not for the likes of me to improve on Socrates. But surely, now, as globalising civilisation teeters on the brink of self-destruction, rationalism of the sort that Socrates practised, with its powerful combination of rationality, naturalism, compassion, and psychological insight, provides the last, best chance of drawing us back from the precipice—even if the wisest of human beings, Socrates himself, did not follow this path to the end. The last two chapters of this book will map out the rationalistic path that Socrates pointed to, but did not follow to the end of the *Republic*.

Endnotes

1 Special thanks to Ethan Alexander-Davey, whose knowledge of ancient Greek and whose good sense improved this chapter greatly. All publication dates given for Plato's writings are educated guesses.

2 This is not to imply that all ancient accounts of addiction directly support the dislocation theory, as Socrates' does. For example, Aristotle's (*c.* 330 BC/1925) account of *akrasia* in the *Nichomachean Ethics* does not. On the other hand, the essentials of the dislocation theory can be drawn from some other ancient writings, including those of the Buddha.

3 It is not always recognised that the Socratic dialogues have a spiritual content as well as a rational, philosophical content. In addition to the spiritual passages that are cited at the end of this chapter, the *Republic* is based on a radical dualism in which the normal world of the senses is far less real than the world of the forms, which exists beyond normal space and time. People can find truth only by somehow gaining access to the world of the forms in a mystical experience that Socrates describes as follows:

> … our true lover of knowledge naturally strives for reality, and will not rest content with each set of particulars which opinion takes for reality, but soars with undimmed and unwearied passion till he grasps the nature of each thing as it is, with the mental faculty fitted to do so, that is, with the faculty which is akin to reality, which approaches and unites with it, and begets intelligence and truth as children, and is only released from travail when it has thus attained knowledge and true life and fulfilment…

From *The Republic* by Plato (*c.* 360 BC), 490b, translated with an introduction by Desmond Lee. Harmondsworth, UK: Penguin Classics 1955, second revised edition 1987. Copyright © H. D. P. Lee, 1953, 1974, 1987. Reproduced by permission of Penguin Books Ltd.

Another illustration of the spiritual content of the Socratic dialogues is Socrates' equation of the highest intellectual attainments with the experience of immortality in the *Symposium* (Plato, *c.* 385 BC/2005, pp. 45–62, 201d–209a).

4 There are many translations of these two dialogues. The quotations from the *Republic* in this chapter are from Desmond Lee's modern English translation (Plato, *c*. 360 BC/1987) because the language is reader-friendly. When different translations of the *Republic* conflict, I have relied on Phillip Shorey's (Plato, *c*. 360 BC/1930) as the final arbiter, because it is said to be the most literal translation, although its language is sometimes tedious. For *Protagoras*, I have relied on W. K. C. Guthrie's translation (Plato, *c*. 388 BC/1956) and to a much lesser extent on Lowell's 1871 translation.

5 Some scholars argue endlessly about which of these ideas belong to Plato and which to Socrates. None of that is relevant here, because the body of ideas stands together as a pillar of Western thought, regardless of which ideas are attributed to Plato and which to Socrates. Where there are inconsistencies in the dialogues, I find it useful to understand these as conflicting ramifications of a single line of thinking, rather than trying to sort out which belong to Plato and which to Socrates.

6 Stone (1988); Vlastos (1992); Saul (1995, pp. 55–59); Drury (2005); Kingwell (2006).

7 Plato (*c*. 360 BC/1987, 366d–369b).

8 From *The Republic* by Plato (*c*. 360 BC), 573d–575a, translated with an introduction by Desmond Lee. Harmondsworth, UK: Penguin Classics 1955, second revised edition 1987. Copyright © H. D. P. Lee, 1953, 1974, 1987. Reproduced by permission of Penguin Books Ltd. This quotation is a condensation of a dialogue between Socrates and Glaucon. I have reduced it to a monologue by leaving out Socrates' questions to Glaucon, Glaucon's responses, and some redundant content.

9 For a discussion of problems with using 'justice' as a translation of *dikaiosunê*, see translator Desmond Lee's comments in Plato's *Republic* (*c*. 360 BC/1987, p. 7, footnote 1). Socrates explains the essence of *dikaiosunê* in a way that includes the normal legalistic meanings of 'justice', both as usually understood by his ancient Greek audience and by modern readers, but goes far beyond those meanings. Socrates' meaning of *dikaiosunê* encompasses the necessary basis both for a happy and successful individual life and for a wise, courageous, and temperate society in which addiction and other forms of social deviance would be rarities. In *Protagoras*, Socrates shows that all of the social virtues, including *dikaiosunê* as well as wisdom, courage, knowledge, temperance, and holiness, are intermeshed and inseparable, despite the claim of Sophists that they can teach each of them as if they were separate courses in school. This is part of a long, rambling argument that begins at 329d in Plato (*c*. 388 BC/1956).

10 In *Protagoras* (Plato, *c*. 388 BC/1956), the myth is spoken and interpreted by the sophist Protagoras, rather than Socrates. Socrates does not dispute Protagoras's version of the story, including the origin that it portrays for *dikaiosunê* in mutual respect and custom, although he turns the topic of discussion away from the myth to the question of whether Protagoras understands virtue well enough to teach it to others.

11 (Plato, *c*. 388 BC/1956, 322c). I use the word 'custom' here, although the Desmond Lee translation that I have cited uses the word 'justice'. The original Greek word is not *dikaiosunê* but *dikê*, which is ordinarily translated as 'custom', 'tradition', or 'right', although it has secondary meanings that make 'justice' a possible translation in this context. When this same translation uses the word 'justice' later (Plato, *c*. 388 BC/1956, 323a), the original Greek word is *dikaiosunê*, as indicated in the text above.

12 Plato (*c*. 388 BC/1956, 320c–323b). See also Dufour (2005, pp. 21–23).

13 Socrates' argument takes the form of a lengthy description of a hypothetical, perfect society. In our times, this ideal 'Republic' is sometimes viewed disapprovingly for its overt censorship of literature and the arts, for its control of population levels by infanticide, and for

other unappealing practices. However, Socrates was speaking to an ancient world in which such practices were commonplace, and there is no sign that he surprised his critical listeners by advocating them. Moreover, these now-shocking practices (which served the same functions as media propaganda and birth control techniques in our own day) were not essential features of the hypothetical society he was describing. Its defining feature was *dikaiosunê*.

14 Plato (*c.* 360 BC/1987, 427d–434d, 441c–444e).

15 The original word *dikaiosunê* from the Greek text is inserted in this quotation in place of the word 'justice' that was actually written in the English translation.

16 From *The Republic* by Plato (*c.* 360 BC), 434a, translated with an introduction by Desmond Lee. Harmondsworth, UK: Penguin Classics 1955, second revised edition 1987. Copyright © H. D. P. Lee, 1953, 1974, 1987. Reproduced by permission of Penguin Books Ltd.

17 Plato (*c.* 360 BC/1987, 412b-414a).

18 Plato (*c.* 360 BC/1987, 415a-415c).

19 Plato (*c.* 360 BC/1987, 417a).

20 Plato (*c.* 360 BC/1987, 419a-421c).

21 Plato (*c.* 360 BC/1987, 462a-466d).

22 B. Schwartz (2004).

23 The Greek word that is transliterated as 'psyche' is usually translated into English as 'soul', but that seems inappropriate at this stage of the *Republic*, where Socrates is making all of the gross bodily appetites that are not normally associated with 'soul' in the Western Christian tradition part of it. Later in the *Republic*, and in the *Phaedo*, Socrates uses the word 'psyche' in a way that corresponds more naturally with 'soul' in the familiar Western sense, introducing a spiritual element into the discussion that was not evident at this early stage.

24 Plato (*c.* 360 BC/1987, 435c–441c).

25 Plato (*c.* 360 BC/1987, 430e–431b, 442c–442d). See also Plato (*c.* 360 BC/1930, 430e–431b, 442c–-442d) for a more literal translation of these complex passages.

26 Socrates makes his assumption of a close linkage between culture and personality explicit at various points in the text of the *Republic*. See, for example, Plato (*c.* 360 BC/1987, 435e–436a).

27 Timarchy is a stage in the decline of society where the rulers are too unwise to see the necessity for *dikaiosunê* and allow the ruling classes to accumulate private property and wealth, reducing the working class to poverty and serfdom. Although timarchy is characterised by greed, unintelligence, and pugnacity, the people at least retain their rigor and ambition.

28 The normal English translation is simply 'oligarchy'. I call it commercial oligarchy to distinguish it from other types of oligarchy that are conceivable to modern readers, for example, a theocratic oligarchy.

29 The normal English translation is simply 'democracy'. I call it anarchic democracy here to distinguish it from the modern ideal of a representative democracy, which is far from the anarchic state that Socrates was describing.

30 Plato (*c.* 360 BC/1987, 576d).

31 The phrase 'subprime loans' is now often restricted to home mortgages, but it is used here in a general sense to apply to any debt that is likely to be defaulted.

32 Plato (*c.* 360 BC/1987, 555).

33 From *The Republic* by Plato (*c.* 360 BC), 557a, translated with an introduction by Desmond Lee. Harmondsworth, UK: Penguin Classics 1955, second revised edition 1987.

Copyright © H. D. P. Lee, 1953, 1974, 1987. Reproduced by permission of Penguin Books Ltd.

34 From *The Republic* by Plato (*c.* 360 BC), 558c, translated with an introduction by Desmond Lee. Harmondsworth, UK: Penguin Classics 1955, second revised edition 1987. Copyright © H. D. P. Lee, 1953, 1974, 1987. Reproduced by permission of Penguin Books Ltd.

35 From *The Republic* by Plato (*c.* 360 BC), 557–558, translated with an introduction by Desmond Lee. Harmondsworth, UK: Penguin Classics 1955, second revised edition 1987. Copyright © H. D. P. Lee, 1953, 1974, 1987. Reproduced by permission of Penguin Books Ltd. In this quotation and some others, I am leaving out some material that is partly redundant and am leaving out all of Glaucon's responses to Socrates' statements, which, in this portion of the *Republic*, are simply agreements or minor amplifications of Socrates' points.

36 Wente (2004).

37 Drohan (2003a, b).

38 Bakan (2004, pp. 16–17).

39 This description of the democratic character is preceded by an explanation of how the democratic character is a natural product of the democratic society:

> [Unworthy desires gain control of his mind,] having discovered that the young man's mind is devoid of sound knowledge and practices and true principles, the most effective safeguards the mind of man can be blessed with…. And back he goes to live with the Lotus-eaters. If his family sends help to the economical element in him, the pretentious invaders shut the gates of the citadel, and will not admit the relieving force, nor will they listen to the individual representations of old and trusted friends. They make themselves masters by force of arms, they call shame silliness and drive it into disgrace and exile; they call self-control cowardice and expel it with abuse; and they call on a lot of useless desires to help them banish economy and moderation, which they maintain are mere provincial parsimony…. They expel the lot and leave the soul of their victim swept clean, ready for the great initiation that follows, when they lead in a splendid garlanded procession of insolence, license, extravagance, and shamelessness. They praise them all extravagantly and call insolence good breeding, license liberty, extravagance generosity, and shamelessness courage…. For the rest of his life he spends as much money, time and trouble on the unnecessary desires as on the necessary. If he's lucky and doesn't get carried to extremes, the tumult will subside as he gets older, some of the exiles will be received back, and the invaders won't have it all their own way. He'll establish a kind of equality of pleasures, and will give the pleasure of the moment its turn of complete control till it is satisfied, and then move on to another, so that none is underprivileged and all have their fair share of encouragement…. If anyone tells him that some pleasures, because they spring from good desires, are to be encouraged and approved, and others, springing from evil desires, to be disciplined and repressed, he won't listen or open his citadel's doors to the truth, but shakes his head and says all pleasures are equal and should have equal rights …

> From *The Republic* by Plato (c. 360 BC), 560b–561d, translated with an introduction by Desmond Lee. Harmondsworth, UK: Penguin Classics 1955, second revised edition 1987. Copyright © H. D. P. Lee, 1953, 1974, 1987. Reproduced by permission of Penguin Books Ltd.

40 Plato (*c.* 360 BC/1987, 563b).

41 [Glaucon says], Let's have the whole story while we're at it....

> Right, [says Socrates] you shall. You would never believe—unless you had seen it for your-
> self—how much more liberty the domestic animals have in a democracy. The dog comes
> to resemble its mistress, as the proverb has it, and the same is true of the horses and don-
> keys as well. They are in the habit of walking about the streets with a grand freedom, and
> bump into people they meet if they don't get out of their way. Everything is full of this
> spirit of liberty.
> You're telling me [says Glaucon]. I've often suffered from it on my way out of town.
> What it all adds up to is this [says Socrates]. You find that the minds of the citizens
> become so sensitive that the least vestige of restraint is resented as intolerable, till finally,
> as you know, in their determination to have no master they disregard all laws, written and
> unwritten.... Well, this is the root from which tyranny springs... a fine and vigorous
> beginning.

From *The Republic* by Plato (c. 360 BC), 563c–563e, translated with an introduction by
Desmond Lee. Harmondsworth, UK: Penguin Classics 1955, second revised edition 1987.
Copyright © H. D. P. Lee, 1953, 1974, 1987. Reproduced by permission of Penguin
Books Ltd.

42 Plato (*c.* 360 BC/1987, 561a–561b).

43 From *The Republic* by Plato (*c.* 360 BC), 571d, translated with an introduction by
Desmond Lee. Harmondsworth, UK: Penguin Classics 1955, second revised edition 1987.
Copyright © H. D. P. Lee, 1953, 1974, 1987. Reproduced by permission of Penguin
Books Ltd.

44 From *The Republic* by Plato (*c.* 360 BC), 577d–578b, translated with an introduction by
Desmond Lee. Harmondsworth, UK: Penguin Classics 1955, second revised edition 1987.
Copyright © H. D. P. Lee, 1953, 1974, 1987. Reproduced by permission of Penguin
Books Ltd.

45 From *The Republic* by Plato (*c.* 360 BC), 572e–573a, translated with an introduction by
Desmond Lee. Harmondsworth, UK: Penguin Classics 1955, second revised edition 1987.
Copyright © H. D. P. Lee, 1953, 1974, 1987. Reproduced by permission of Penguin
Books Ltd.

46 Socrates stated this conundrum as follows:

> Self-discipline... is surely a kind of order, a control of certain desires and appetites. So
> people use 'being master of oneself'... and similar phrases as indications of it.... But
> 'master of oneself' is an absurd phrase. For if you're master of yourself you're presumably
> also subject *to* yourself, and so *both* master *and* subject. For there is only one person in
> question throughout.... What the expression is intended to mean, I think, is that there is a
> better and a worse element in the personality of each individual and that when the natu-
> rally better element controls the worse then the man is said to be 'master of himself', as a
> term of praise ...

From *The Republic* by Plato (*c.* 360 BC), 430e–431a, translated with an introduction by
Desmond Lee. Harmondsworth, UK: Penguin Classics 1955, second revised edition 1987.
Copyright © H. D. P. Lee, 1953, 1974, 1987. Reproduced by permission of Penguin
Books Ltd.

47 Plato (*c.* 360 BC/1987, 430e–431b).

48 Plato (*c.* 360 BC/1987, 571b–571c).

49 Plato (c. 388 BC/1956, 358c–358d).

50 Although Athenian society contained some elements of capitalism, including loans for commercial ships that plied the Mediterranean and the famous agora, a free market in which any
person could exchange coins for food, there was nothing that even approached
a free-market society; that is, a society dominated by free-market principles and practices
(K. Polanyi et al., 1957, Chapter 5).

51 The observation of tyranny wrapped in the illusion of democracy is not only made in informal conversation. It appears in the work of excellent thinkers, including Nobel Prize winner
José Saramago. See Globe and Mail (2004b) and Saramago (2004).

52 Rage Against the Machine is the name of a very popular American 'Rapcore' band.

53 Plato (c. 360 BC/1987, 588b–592b)

54 Plato (c. 360 BC/1987, 613e–621d)

55 From The Republic by Plato (c. 360 BC), 608d, translated with an introduction by
Desmond Lee. Harmondsworth, UK: Penguin Classics 1955, second revised edition 1987.
Copyright © H. D. P. Lee, 1953, 1974, 1987. Reproduced by permission of Penguin
Books Ltd. A more literal translation of 'Good Lord, no!' is 'No, by Zeus' (Plato, c. 360
BC/1930, 608d).

56 Plato (c. 360 BC/1987, 618c–619b).

57 Plato (c. 360 BC/1987, 592a–592b).

58 Plato (c. 360 BC/1987, 368e–372d). Unfortunately, Socrates was interrupted before he got
very far with his description of the agrarian society, so it is hard to be sure how it would have
ended. It is clear, however, that the need for mysticism in the Republic arises from
contradictions in society that were not present in the agrarian society.

59 Plato (c. 360 BC/1987, 435c–441c).

60 Plato (c. 360 BC/1987, 611b).

61 In Protagoras, Socrates takes on the question of why some people appear to be so overcome
with short-term pleasure that they knowingly and consistently do evil to society and to
themselves (i.e. addiction$_3$, or something close to it). It would follow from his analysis of this
question that the key to all virtues, including dikaiosunê is knowledge, which can be inculcated through education, although Socrates clearly suggests that sophists like Protagoras do
not understand virtue well enough to teach it. The conclusion that virtue is teachable is
summarised briefly in (Plato, c. 388 BC/1956, 361a–361c)

62 Plato (c. 387 BC/1967, 29b-29c, 40c–41d). Socrates offered a more mystical account of death
on the day of his execution as described in Phaedo, but he preceded this mystical account
with a statement that it is a mythical representation of what he believes about his impending
death (Plato, c. 388/1941, 61d).

63 Peter Brown (1967, Chapter 9).

From Blindness and Paralysis to Action

Ancient wisdom, modern history, and common sense all point towards the same conclusion. Addiction is one of the major ways that people adapt to dislocation. As free-market society spreads dislocation around the globe, the dark shadow of addiction will keep pace.

Although this realisation goes far beyond the conventional wisdom on addiction, it does not, by itself, solve any problems. It remains difficult to see all the intricate connections between addiction, dislocation, and free-market society. Even when connections are seen, it is hard to take action. This chapter first undertakes to show why it is so natural *not* to see and *not* to act upon the connections between addiction, dislocation, and free-market society. Then, it shows that it is nonetheless absolutely necessary to discern these many connections and to act on them. Finally, it outlines three practicable levels of action: personal, professional, and social. Personal action involves people coping with their own addictions and those of their family members and friends. Professional action involves people working as practitioners in the field of addictions. Social action involves people acting in groups to change the social structures that spread dislocation—and thereby addiction—in globalising free-market society. Action is already underway at all three levels, of course, but each requires rethinking in the context of this book.

The third level of action—social action to change the structures that spread dislocation—is the most difficult. It is, however, the most important at this time in history. Social action will become the central topic by the end of this chapter. Chapter 15 will provide specific examples. Showing how social action can be practicable will require working through two highly contentious issues before this chapter is done. One is the charge of naiveté that arises whenever people attempt social change that deviates from the presumed natural domination of the modern world by 'market forces'. The other is the precise meaning of the troublesome pronoun 'we', which will be used with increasing frequency as the chapter progresses.

Although this chapter is not based on Christianity, or on eclectic spirituality, or on the otherworldly Greek mysticism that crops up at the end of the *Republic*, it grows from an equally ancient faith, which, like Greek mysticism, is rooted in the Socratic dialogues. This is the faith that human beings, reasoning together in a rigorous way, are capable of reaching understandings that are not merely intelligent, but also practicable, effective, and spiritually uplifting.[1] This faith was bequeathed to the world by Socrates himself,[2] and its importance has been reaffirmed by the greatest of modern thinkers.[3] My belief is that Socratic rationalism, far from being a dry intellectual exercise, has been the source of the most brilliant magic of Western civilisation[4] and that we can look to it again now.

Socratic rationalism holds that human beings, reasoning together, are capable of seeing the highest truths and of acting well when they do. However, people cannot accomplish this when they are blind or paralysed.

Civilised blindness

Every society carefully protects its foundational beliefs because they give it stability and meaning. As free-market society becomes globalised, therefore, it carefully obscures the connections between free markets, mass dislocation, and addictive misery because seeing them would undermine its foundational belief in the magnanimity of free markets. Obscuring the connections between free markets, dislocation, and addiction has made it almost impossible to understand the current spread of addiction.[5]

By contrast, it is not in the least threatening to attribute addictive misery to demonic drugs, neurochemical deficiencies, genetic defects, individual immorality, or original sin, for these attributions do not undermine the foundational beliefs of free-market society. That is probably why there are hundreds of inconclusive theories of addiction within the conventional wisdom, rather than a single useful one. This multitude of theories is the product of an exhaustive search for the underlying cause of addiction everywhere, except where it is. These theories, colourfully projected on the globalised cave wall[6] by sophisticated communication technologies, protect society from an understanding of addiction that would create unbearable tension. *This is blindness.*

Mass media and political leaders cultivate this blindness, celebrating the achievements of markets, competition, and innovation with dazzling fireworks and deafening fanfare, while labelling those who point out side effects of free-market society as 'cynical', or worse.[7] Governments resolutely insist both on expanding the sway of free-market economics and on bringing addiction under control. They seem unaware that their first imperative countermands the second.[8] Some left-wing thinkers appear as blind to this dilemma as those on the political right.[9] In particular, those who advocate the so-called 'Third Way' or 'efficient society' seem to believe that the dislocating effects of hypercapitalism can be obviated by enhancing welfare programmes, minority rights, and individualism.[10] Meanwhile, destructive addictions—from alcoholism to zealotry—continue to multiply everywhere.

Blinded, the institutions of free-market society confront the problem of addiction in the dark. For example, research institutions that might unearth the social roots of addiction are lured into research on outmoded disease theories of addiction by the gleam of government and industry research money.[11] Politicians who might warn the public of the dangers of dislocation instead terrify it with more tales about fiendishly addictive drugs and the all-powerful drug lords and gang members who purvey them. Investigative journalists who might learn of the connection between dislocation and addiction from the people around them instead interview distant scientists about new neurochemical theories of addiction so esoteric that they cannot be comprehended by anybody without an advanced degree.[12] Television stations soberly admonish their audiences—between flashy advertisements—to adopt a healthy lifestyle and 'just say no' to drugs. Schools pump the conventional wisdom about addiction into the minds of the students, reserving critical analysis for topics of less importance.

In the second half of the 20th century, blindness about addiction broke into a so-called War on Drugs, a bizarre spectacle of sightless, murderous flailing. Today, this misbegotten war still retains the moral support of the United Nations through its International Narcotics Control Board,[13] the imprimatur of the American government, and, arguably, the support of the current British and Canadian national governments.[14] The War on Drugs still provides official justification for American political and military incursions in Latin America, most obviously in Colombia at the present time.[15] For many years, even failure on an enormous scale[16] did not open most people's eyes to the futility of a war that so perfectly shielded free-market society from painful self-examination.

Civilised paralysis

Collective blindness about the connections between free-market society, dislocation, and addiction has diminished somewhat in the last decade because most of the glittering promises that were made about the new post-Cold War globalised world have failed to materialise. Society owes its clearer view of addiction and other side effects of globalisation to eye-opening disasters that made it possible to think again about the pros and cons of hypercapitalism. These disasters include the abject failure of economic 'shock therapy' in Russia after the fall of the USSR;[17] the East Asian currency collapse of 1997; the bursting of the 'bubble stock market' in 2002; the exposure of devastating corruption in superstar transnational corporations like Bre-X, Enron, Tyco, Worldcom, Hollinger, and Parmalat; the exposure of the ruthless behaviour of the worldwide pharmaceutical industry;[18] the insidious impoverishment of middle- and working-class people in the richest countries relative to their compatriots in the boardrooms and executive offices;[19] famine and epidemics in numerous Third-World countries that have accepted the free-market 'reforms' of the International Monetary Fund and World Bank;[20] and the increasingly apparent slaughter of Third-World people by corporate[21] as well as national armies spreading free-market society.[22] Most of all, we may owe our diminished blindness to the shocking spectacle of the mighty United States unwilling to rescue its own citizens after a major hurricane struck the city of New Orleans in 2005, unable to establish peace in Iraq after crushing it militarily,[23] and, quite possibly, unable to maintain its economic domination of the world after the 'credit crisis' that began in 2007.[24] Dark stains show through even on the whitewashed daily news.[25]

Although the harmful consequences of free-market society on dislocation and addiction are more easily seen now that the euphoria that accompanied the current wave of hypercapitalism has passed, it still feels impossible to do anything about them. The world economy and the global media remain under the domination of multinational corporations, private equity funds, and economic experts who cling to free-market ideology with an iron death grip.[26]

The failure of collective social action cannot be blamed entirely on the vested interests that maintain the economic status quo. Multitudes of people have come to recognise the ravages of globalisation in mass dislocation, as well as ecological destruction, social injustice, financial instability, and the growing risk of nuclear war—but that is where solidarity ends. Collectively, the citizens of the wealthy nations have the power to impose effective controls on the unrestrained globalisation of free-market society, yet do not act together. Most people live in a haze most of the time, apparently still hoping to find satisfaction in the glittering baubles that free-market society showers down upon the affluent world, and still dreaming that the future will somehow take care of itself. *This is paralysis.*

This paralysis does not result from lack of information, for the facts are available to anyone who knows how to use Google™. Nor does the paralysis result from lack of courage, for people act bravely in their personal crises. The paralysis results most of all from bewilderment.[27] Free-market society has been the nursery of our understanding. Our minds stand alone and afraid without the comforts of its intellectual pap and swaddling. Malnourished on a diet of marketbabble from infancy, we struggle weakly to discern what is important and to act well.[28] Sensible ideas, mocked and distorted by corporatised media, appear no more substantial than the great puffball slogans that dominate mass culture. Those who dream of a better world await a unifying symbol, an incontrovertible syllogism, a prophet, Godot.[29]

Addictive dynamics exacerbate this paralysis. Addictions to work and wasteful consumption give people a feeling of status and membership in free-market society, even as they provoke catastrophe. Foreign wars and shameless alliances bring countries recognition from the superpower, which swells nationalistic pride, temporarily mitigating dislocation. Although feeling deep unease about free-market society, most people do not study the critical literature or vote for candidates who propose real alternatives—somehow those naysayers seem like aliens.[30]

The spiritual traditions that people rely on for identity and membership, including most forms of Christianity and of eclectic spirituality, hold as articles of faith that it is impossible to change society and arrogant even to try.[31] Therefore, they inadvertently protect free-market society, even while they decry its materialistic values. Faith in the Market God goes further still. It confidently promises that no matter how catastrophic things seem, the market's invisible hand will put them right, bestowing abundance and contentment on an unlimited population, if people can only be patient and believe.[32]

The need for action on addiction

Dislocation and addiction must be confronted, because they are among the very worst of the threats facing global civilisation, even in this era of multiple catastrophes. Dislocation and addiction are close to the top of the list of threats, in part because they multiply the others. As shown in Chapter 10, severely dislocated people can be seduced into Eichmann-like bureaucratic excess, grossly wasteful consumption, political and religious fanaticism, and financial recklessness. Social changes that do not reduce the dislocation that spawns addictive dynamics are unlikely to eliminate the other crises that face modern civilisation.

Even more importantly, dislocation and addiction top the list of threats because the soul—whether defined naturalistically as in this book[33] or in a more mystical way—is at least as central to human well-being as are ecosystems, social justice, financial stability, and safety. Dislocation is at the core of modern poverty of the spirit. Addiction is artificial filler material packed in where the living soul should be.[34] A 'brave new world' where people live in a state of perpetual dislocation and intermittent addiction would hardly be worth preserving, even if it could solve its other problems.

I believe that the problem of dislocation is *more* urgent than the more publicised ecological, social, military, and financial threats that terrorise the contemporary world. However, there is no need to argue priorities of urgency, since all of these problems must be solved.

There is a dismal possibility that any serious action about dislocation and addiction must await a seismic catastrophe in global civilisation, such as might be precipitated by a cascading environmental disaster, a global economic collapse, a bloody uprising of the poor, or a nuclear war.[35] Any of these unthinkable events would surely clear the minds of those people who had the good fortune to survive, and would open the door to a new stage of civilisation.[36] However, such events have consequences that can only be contemplated with fear and trembling. Moreover, the collapse of global free-market society, or any civilisation, would be an event of such unfathomable complexity[37] that no human being can hope to anticipate what will follow. I do not feel qualified even to guess.

Therefore, this chapter assumes that a seismic catastrophe of global society does not lie in the near future—that the teetering house of cards can still be rebuilt on a more solid framework. Under these assumptions, a practical approach to dealing with the problem of addiction in the still-globalising world must begin with an effort to transcend blindness and paralysis as much as possible, hoping to see the roots of addiction clearly and to act constructively within the still-globalising civilisation of the early 21st century. This action starts on a personal and professional level, but, if it is to succeed, it must be expanded to the social and political level as well.

From blindness and paralysis to personal action

Effective action on addiction at a personal level can only be achieved by people who have, to some degree, overcome their own blindness and paralysis. For most of us, overcoming blindness and paralysis does not begin with academic study, but with reflection on the struggles with addiction that we observe in family members and friends or in ourselves. Recognising that the highly publicised suffering of junkies and alcoholics is essentially the same as the addictive miseries that we observe in our personal worlds can begin this reflection. The next step may be simply overcoming the denial that shields an intimate's or one's own drug or alcohol addiction from conscious understanding. More likely, however, the next step requires the more complex recognition of addictive dynamics that are not connected to drugs and alcohol and thus are camouflaged in free-market society. These addictive dynamics may involve love, food, work, fantasy, narcissistic self-absorption, shopping, gambling, ideology, television, video games, or any of the myriad new addictive possibilities that free-market society provides.

Awareness of addiction in oneself or in one's family or friends is acutely painful because it means acknowledging serious, sometimes irremediable harm that the addicted person has done to other people and to his or her own life. It also means acknowledging the depth of the dislocation that has made the person vulnerable to addiction. Facing up to one's own addiction and dislocation can be excruciating, but it does not need to provoke incapacitating despair. It can provoke action instead.

Addictive problems in one's personal world need not provoke despair because they are not manifestations of mental illness or malice, but of a struggle to survive. Nor are they abnormal. Many, perhaps most, of our compatriots in the new global civilisation live with addictive dynamics of some degree. Like us, they are neither diseased nor evil at heart. Like us, they find themselves unable to endure the lack of psychosocial integration without becoming, at times, overwhelmingly involved with habits that partially substitute for it. Like us, they sometimes act badly, wastefully, recklessly, but without evil intent. There is no reason for despair over dislocation either, because it does not grow from a lack of personal worth or human appeal, but from a fragmented society. Becoming aware of one's own addictive dynamics and dislocation, and those of one's intimates, can be an enormous personal relief. It brings the joy of discovering a common humanity with others who bear similar burdens.

Making others aware of one's own addictive lifestyle also brings relief. The liberating effects of voluntary confession were discovered long ago by many of the world's religions. A similar discovery of many contemporary people has been that describing one's own addictive experience in a self-help group—definitely a type of confession—has a wonderfully liberating effect, even though it is done outside a religious context.[38] Through the centuries, three participants in the confessional were envisioned by Christian theology: the person confessing, the priest, and the Holy Spirit.[39] The great revelation of more recent times is that confession in the presence of another person is therapeutically powerful, whether or not the Holy Spirit attends.

Listening to others' descriptions of their addictive experiences is as important as revealing one's own. The world is full of people who are dying to tell their addiction stories. No professional qualifications are required of a listener. All that is needed is willingness to share a familiar human experience with a modicum of compassion.

Unfortunately, facing up to an addictive problem in oneself, a friend, or a family member does not, by itself, bring it to an end. There is no easy way out of addiction in a dislocated world, but many people get out nonetheless. Although personal strength and courage are absolutely necessary, the way out is not simply suppressing an addictive habit with iron will-power, for this often precipitates other kinds of social problems or different addictions, which can be worse.

The best way out of addiction is overcoming dislocation by finding a secure place in a real community. People sometimes work their way out of dislocation by rejoining their previous world of family, friends, and society, with an enhanced appreciation of its importance. Sometimes, however, this familiar world is too fragmented or dys-functional, and people must create communities with others who have likewise been forced to build their communities anew. The description of Hogan and Louise in Chapter 11 of this book is an example. Of course, newly created communities are more fragile than old, established ones. However, when someone slips into addiction or another type of problem, common sense interventions taken within a calm and thoughtful group can work wonders, even if the group is a new, fragile one. When both a person's natal society and their social circle are too dysfunctional to serve as a basis of psychosocial integration, people can often find the psychosocial integration that they need in spiritual communities and self-help groups. These sometimes work wonders too. Sometimes people cannot achieve full psychosocial integration there, but can shift from a more dangerous addiction to a less dangerous one; for example, from alcoholism to compulsive attendance at meetings of a self-help group. Although the addiction problem remains, the shift to a less harmful addiction can set the stage for a further transition later on.

Addicted people need help in overcoming dislocation. Helpers need not be professional practitioners or another person with a visible addiction, because addiction is a common human problem. Every person who has achieved some level of maturity in a dislocated world is qualified to listen and to offer advice and encouragement. Of course, action at this informal, personal level does not always succeed. Sometimes professional helpers are essential, and, in some devastated societies, restoring psychosocial integration will be the work of more than a single generation.

Sometimes, discovering one's own addiction leads to an unending lifelong preoccupation with recovery. However, most people eventually put their personal recoveries behind them and find that they can use their hard-won experience to help others. People who have mostly recovered from their own addictions form a sizeable proportion of those who help others overcome addictions, and their personal experiences give them unique insights that may be helpful to others, as long as they can resist the temptation to generalise from themselves too dogmatically.

From blindness and paralysis to professional action

Most professional practice in the addictions field can be categorised as treatment, prevention, law enforcement, or harm reduction. However, these 'four pillars',[40] as they are often called, are primarily concerned with addiction$_2$ rather than addiction$_3$. The primary purpose of prevention and law enforcement, for example, is to keep people from using illegal drugs, whether they are addicted$_3$ or not. Prevention and law enforcement are rarely directed towards addictions$_3$ that do not involve drugs. Treatment is often evaluated by its effectiveness in reducing the amount of drugs or alcohol that a person *uses,* whether or not the person remains addicted to the drug or to a larger addictive complex. Harm reduction is most fundamentally a way of attempting to protect intravenous drug users from infectious diseases, regardless of whether they are addicted or not.

Nonetheless, a reconceptualised four pillars can provide a useful architecture for controlling addiction$_3$. Moreover, this reconceptualisation of the four pillars is already well underway. Each of the four pillars is considered in turn here.

Treatment

Professional counsellors and psychotherapists around the world offer the gifts of genuine understanding and wise counsel to people suffering from addiction.

Treatment professionals differ from each other in that each wraps his or her gift in words and images derived from a particular school of professional training. Whether or not these heartfelt gifts enable addicted clients to overcome their addictions successfully, their value can never be discounted.

The dislocation theory predicts that treatment will become more effective when it is oriented towards achieving or restoring psychosocial integration, because addiction itself is never the primary problem, but rather a way of adapting to painful, underlying dislocation. There is no point in cajoling a person to control an addictive lifestyle unless some better lifestyle is made feasible.

Douglas Cameron has pointed out that there are many kinds of identity transformations by which a person can overcome addiction in a pluralistic society, and that all such transformations require social support. Some, but not all, of the possible identity transformations are supported by existing therapeutic institutions. Twelve-step treatment, for example, supports a particular kind of identity transformation that helps *some* people to overcome addiction but is repellent to other people, including many people from non-Western cultural traditions. Cameron suggests the creation of diverse new social institutions to support other kinds of identity transformations.[41] Similarly, Jim Orford and his colleagues have pointed out that Australian aboriginal families can be helped to assist alcoholic relatives more effectively, especially if interventions can be devised that are aligned with aboriginal traditions[42]—a fact that is also recognised by native healers.

Counsellors cannot force psychosocial integration upon addicted people. They can only help to set the stage upon which it can flourish. Setting the stage includes making people aware that recovery occurs frequently with or without treatment, that people have taken diverse recovery paths successfully, and that these paths usually entail achieving some form of psychosocial integration. Jan Blomqvist has summed this up succinctly as follows: 'Effective help to substance misusers is best conceived as a means of evoking, facilitating, and/or strengthening their own efforts to change.'[43] Something close to this logic seems to lie behind the impressive efficacy of motivational interviewing and community reinforcement relative to other types of treatment for addictions.[44]

Addiction treatment professionals can contribute at least as much in the role of public educators as in the role of therapists. Through their daily work, counsellors become uniquely knowledgeable about addiction. Their expert knowledge and their professional credentials give them the credibility to raise the level of public knowledge above the conventional wisdom, and some of them take that opportunity. For example, Dr Gabor Maté is an admirable Canadian practitioner of public education,[45] as well as addiction medicine.

By speaking out, either as qualified experts or through their professional associations, therapists can help the public see why the myth of demon drugs and the rest of the conventional wisdom on addiction are not incontrovertible 'scientific knowledge' but part of an incapacitating blindness. They can also let the public know that the power of the treatment that they themselves do is often seriously exaggerated by governments and media as a way of distracting attention from the more costly interventions that are needed to overcome dislocation. In the end, professionals have the most to lose when their professional prowess is oversold.

Prevention

The word 'prevention' has two quite different meanings that have run together in the past, causing confusion. The first meaning is preventing all use of alcohol and intoxicating drugs. The second meaning is preventing addiction. At one time, these two meanings could be merged into one, because people seriously believed that any use of alcohol and illegal drugs inevitably caused addiction. These meanings can be recognised as distinct now that the myth of demon drugs has been disproved.[46]

The first kind of prevention is about enforcing an abstemious moral belief that is hard to justify in a materialistic, pluralistic society. Why, for example, would it be more important to prevent youthful drug experimentation than to prevent any other form of youthful experimentation that can lead to addictive problems? Other risky forms of experimentation include kissing, dieting, exercising, betting, shopping, driving motor vehicles, playing video games, using the Internet, and practising religion.[47] Would it not be more important in each case to offer mature guidance on safe ways to experiment? Although drug experimentation is no less risky than the others, it can, like them, have genuine benefits as well. For example, membership in a group of adventurous classmates who sometimes experiment with illegal drugs probably saves students in some cultural milieux from solitude and exclusion, *increasing* their psychosocial integration and quality of life.[48] In a pluralistic society, many cultural and religious traditions are valid. Some European cultures introduce children to small quantities of alcohol with their meals from a young age. Moreover, moderate use of cannabis is acceptable in some East Indian societies. In both cases, moderate drug use plays a positive role in cultural life.

The word 'prevention' in the first abstemious meaning has sometimes served to justify terrifying school children about any experimentation they may undertake with alcohol and illegal drugs to the consternation of more reflective advocates of prevention.[49] Scare tactics, including the DARE (Drug Abuse Resistance Education) programme in the United States and Canada, seem at best marginally effective in preventing drug use by children both while they are in school and after leaving.[50] How could drug experimentation by children ever be prevented by occasional jolts of fear when popular media and pharmaceutical advertising incessantly attribute miraculous powers to mind-altering drugs?[51]

A realistic educational programme built on preventing addiction would honestly acknowledge both the attractions of drugs and various drugless ways of having similar experiences. It would explain the real risks of hazardous drug use, overdose, and addiction. It would make the people aware of both shared and divergent values of their community on the topic of drugs, whatever they may be. It would debunk both the myth of 'addictive' drugs with demonic powers and the commercial myths that portray currently legal drugs as panaceas and magic bullets. These myths crowd out useful information that could help people to make the choices they will face in the future.

Education is also important in preventing addiction to practices other than drug use. On aggregate, these other practices present a far greater addictive hazard to people than drugs and alcohol. People need to understand the wide range of practices to which severe addictions occur and the causal relationship between dislocation and addiction. Although the actual cause of addiction cannot be explained in the simplistic and dramatic way that the myth of demon drugs has been, children and adults can understand it readily. Realistic discussion of dislocation and addiction can give them insight into their own motivations in a dislocated world, reducing the likelihood of addiction.

It is now apparent that neither drug use nor addiction can be prevented in a free-market society. Nonetheless, the prevalence of addiction$_3$ to drug use and to other pursuits can be reduced, by reducing dislocation. *The most promising way of controlling addiction is not prevention of experimentation, but prevention of dislocation.*

Building on this use of the word 'prevention', addiction professionals can work to enhance psychosocial integration by supporting schools, affordable housing, services for needy parents, employment and local businesses, community centres, celebrations and festivals, neighbourhood crime control, medical and disability insurance, local art and culture, and welfare services for the unemployed. Prevention of dislocation in these ways requires not only financial support, but also insightful administration. Public services and public housing in the past have sometimes been administered in ways that destroy psychosocial integration rather than enhancing it.[52] In the most basic terms, good public services of all sorts can be a bulwark against addiction, whereas poor public services can increase it.

The Four Pillars Coalition in Vancouver[53] has proposed some particularly insightful prevention measures for the Hastings Corridor of the Downtown Eastside, emphasising construction of new affordable housing units for homeless people in accord with a 'housing first' movement in many localities in North America.[54] Vancouver's Portland Hotel Society led the way in this direction, with its implementation of 'no-eviction' policies in its rental facilities years ago.[55] More recently, this same non-profit society has gone beyond housing by opening a medical clinic, a credit union, a life-skills centre, and, wondrously, an art gallery in the Hastings Corridor. Although this kind of social innovation seems to be at odds with the more familiar first meaning of 'prevention', a recent city document on prevention takes a bold step towards redefinition.[56] Unfortunately, the provision of subsidized housing in Vancouver has become more controversial recently with the election of free-market-oriented governments in the city, the province, and the nation.[57]

Profit-making corporations can have an important role in prevention of addiction. For example, in Vancouver a local telephone company has expressed interest in helping to prevent addiction and has contributed money to support the cause in visible ways. However, rather than sponsoring expensive seminars, the telephone company could make sure that functioning public telephones were readily available in the poor sections of the city where people rarely have telephones in their homes and only drug dealers can afford cell phones. A telephone company could provide an extremely valuable service by sponsoring an inexpensive, accessible long-distance phone service to enable poor, dislocated people to keep in touch with distant relatives. On another note, the telephone company may have eased the problem of sex addiction when it yielded to public pressure to reverse its earlier decision to introduce new pornography services on its cell phone screens. Real-estate developers can work together to make sure that their highly profitable gentrification of poor neighbourhoods does not destroy but instead enhances the housing of the stable community that is already there.

Professionals in the area of prevention can solicit corporate involvement in prevention, broadly defined, through their agencies and their positions on civic committees.

Law enforcement

For the past century, police have been burdened with the impossible assignment of eliminating crime by stopping the flow of 'addictive' drugs. The worldwide War on Drugs proved that no amount of flogging, imprisonment, or capital punishment of people for drug crimes could eliminate either drugs or crime. There was never any hope that the drug wars could have any impact on addiction because most addictions are not centred on drugs. Terrorising people out of one kind of addiction inevitably increases the attractiveness of other kinds. The dislocation theory of addiction implies that the prevalence of severe addiction would remain essentially unchanged if every single 'addictive' drug were miraculously eliminated from the face of the earth.

Striving to enforce an unachievable and pointless abstinence has done great harm. Spectacular, highly publicised seizures of drugs by police around the world and billion-dollar campaigns that kill and terrorise peasant producers of poppies and coca in the Third World have no measurable impact on the supply of drugs to illicit users. They do not even drive up the price![58] Arrests and violent searches of drug users in Vancouver over the decades have injured many people and killed some, with no apparent benefit.[59] Moreover, police have been called upon to bring anti-drug scare tactics to classrooms, making themselves objects of ridicule to many students by the time they reach university. LEAP (Law Enforcement Against Prohibition) is an organisation of police professionals who are willing to speak out publicly against the futility and harmfulness of the drug war in which they have served as foot soldiers.[60] Yet sweeping, punitive drug laws remain in place in most countries and the only alternative appears to be sweeping legalisation. A legal alternative that fits better with the dislocation theory of addiction is suggested in Chapter 15.

Many police are now concentrating their attention on functions that are more constructive.[61] For example, police can carefully enforce closing-hour laws, drunk-serving laws, and age restrictions for bars and can manage after-hours crowds to reduce the mayhem.[62] Police can publicise drug information that is strictly accurate, but still cautionary, when contaminated drugs are found on the street.[63] As genuine authority figures, police can give stern but sympathetic advice to young people who they see becoming addicted to street drugs. Police can use existing drug laws judiciously to get sick street addicts into prison where they will be well fed and allowed to recover their health for a time.

Perhaps most important, police can take the time to seriously investigate and prosecute the blight of small-scale burglaries and car thefts that are often perpetrated by illicit drug users. 'Petty crime' is anything but petty to economically stressed families who must make up the losses. If a family car, even one with little market value, is stolen, how do the parents get themselves to work and the kids to hockey practice? Petty crime is a cause as well as an effect of dislocation. Effective police work, in conjunction with a programme of restorative justice can nourish psychosocial integration. Yet the sort of glamourless, painstaking police work that can control petty crime is scarcely being pursued in the residential areas of my city now.[64]

Harm reduction

Well-known harm-reduction measures, such as methadone and heroin maintenance, needle exchanges, and safe-injection sites (also known as drug-consumption rooms) can lower the death rate from disease, overdose, and criminal involvement among injecting drug addicts.[65] New forms of harm reduction now appearing around the world can extend this success.[66] Beyond saving lives, harm reduction measures can show addicted people that others care about their plight, serving as an invitation back to mainstream society when they are able. Although harm reduction cannot be expected to reduce the prevalence of addiction per se, harm-reduction measures can provide a basis for more integrative subcultures for addicted people. For example, an addict subculture sometimes forms in methadone programmes or needle-exchange programmes in which participants identify themselves as an association of medical patients rather than as criminal junkies.[67]

Harm reduction innovations abound. Agencies in the UK are experimenting with 'wet day centres' where alcoholics, traditionally required to abstain in order to receive treatment, can continue to drink but still have access to counselling and other services.[68] Scientists are developing ever safer and more attractive ways of delivering nicotine as alternatives to cigarettes.[69] Vancouver is expanding its innovative housing and community services for injecting drug users.[70] Legal oral stimulants may soon be provided to injecting stimulant users and crack smokers in Vancouver to protect their health and keep them out of jail.[71]

An inspiring harm-reduction innovation in Vancouver targets pregnant women who are either drinking heavily or taking drugs.[72] An earlier policy of apprehending these women's babies at birth backfired, creating a situation where drug-addicted women were so fearful of losing their babies that they would seek neither prenatal services nor addiction counselling. The cruelty of turning pitiably abused and demoralised women into fugitives because they wanted to care for their babies became evident. New harm-reduction counselling initiatives give these women respectful assurance that their babies will not be seized merely because they have used drugs during pregnancy. Rather than instilling shame, these initiatives build on the women's natural desire to bear healthy children and to recover from their addictions.[73]

Taxation can serve as a kind of harm reduction for alcohol addiction. Alcohol should not become so inexpensive that people are drawn into bars by the irresistible prospect of bargain shopping at 'happy hour'. Fine tuning of tax laws can exert a degree of control on alcoholic drinking.[74]

The philosophy of harm reduction can be adapted to non-drug addictions as well. Whereas many dislocated people will become addicted no matter what the consequences, they can be encouraged to move from more dangerous to less dangerous addictions. For example, efforts to move violent gang members into the somewhat safer world of aggressive sports have long been made, and some lives have certainly been saved. On my visit to the North American gambling mecca, Las Vegas, about 20 years ago, I discovered the great popularity of the so-called 'penny slots'. These are fully fledged slot machines that sit in the casinos amidst the same irresistible ambiance as all the other one-armed bandits, yet do less harm. Nobody can possibly lose a fortune there. At the time of my visit, there were only a few penny slots in the Las Vegas casinos, and they were always in use with other people waiting their turns. Why are casinos not required to devote more of their floor space to penny slots in the interest of harm reduction? (Maybe, with inflation, 'penny slots' have become 'nickel slots'.) Could small-denomination slot machines function as methadone for some gambling addicts? Similarly, although there is no reasonable justification for prohibiting video games, surely the most hateful and sadistic of them should be banned or taxed into disuse. Although efforts like these are not usually understood as harm reduction, the concept fits, and other kinds of methadone-like substitutes might well be developed for other kinds of addictions.

From blindness and paralysis to social action

Although personal and professional efforts by people who have overcome blindness and paralysis sometimes work wonders, neither personal nor professional action can stem the rising tide of addiction₃ in the 21st century any more than they were able to cure the so-called disease of addiction in the past.[75] The four pillars cannot control the addiction problem because they address neither its full domain, of which drug and alcohol addiction are merely a small portion, nor its root cause, which is the ever-increasing dislocation that is built into free-market society. Some addiction professionals describe their work metaphorically as pulling drowning people out of a river and putting them on the bank, hoping that some will dry out and walk away from the river. However, they add that their work cannot have any substantial effect if people are being swept into the water upstream at an ever-increasing rate.[76]

When the pain of dislocation and addiction becomes unbearable—as I believe it already has—society must be changed to reduce dislocation. There is no easier solution. Addiction can only be brought under control when citizens reach a level of concern and exasperation that makes them ready to restructure free-market society. This does not mean overthrowing capitalism, but it does require energetic actions to domesticate it in diverse ways that will be illustrated in the final chapter of this book.

Effective action on the social level begins with an even more painful self-examination than that required for individual or professional action.[77] Social action requires expanding the focus of self-examination from seeing ourselves as victims of dislocation, to also seeing ourselves as part of the cause. This painful self-scrutiny is unavoidable because reducing dislocation requires not only improving 'their' behaviour (e.g. politicians, corporate executives, and mindless consumers) but 'ours' as well. More importantly, examining our own role in the policies that perpetuate dislocation rewards us with a clearer understanding of the multifarious forms such policies may take.

This kind of self-examination entails dropping precious defence mechanisms, and facing the painful reality that they have concealed. For instance, we must face the degree to which we have been seduced by the flimsy reassurances of free-market ideology, and the ways that we have personally contributed to various kinds of dislocation in occupational roles ('Just doing my job'), political inaction ('It's just too depressing'), and so on. The most painful realisation is that of having been more a part of the problem than a part of the solution.

At the beginning of the 21st century, the required self-examination is easiest to illustrate in the context of global warming. Although global warming has diverse causes in economic structure, political malfeasance, and corporate greed, a major cause is gross overconsumption of goods and energy by the good citizens of developed countries, like my own. Canada, in fact, has the highest per capita energy consumption of any country on the planet by some measures, higher even than that of the United States and far higher than China's.[78] Recycling some of the residue of our wastefulness makes hardly any difference at all. The environmental crises that afflict the planet cannot be resolved without major changes in the lifestyles of people who are consuming the resources and producing the toxic wastes. I know few people—certainly not myself—who stand immune to this indictment.

Our roles as perpetrators of dislocation and addiction are just as important as our roles as perpetrators of global warming, although they are less publicised. Here are two current examples from my country, but there are innumerable other examples, everywhere.

A major part of Canadian national wealth comes from the displacement of aboriginal societies, leaving their land, trees, animals, fish, ore, and oil for the European settlers. Remnants of plundered tribal groups now dwell on the outskirts of mainstream society, often in a state of perennial dislocation and epidemic addiction. This tragedy is more than a shameful relic of historical conquest. It is a crime that is re-enacted—with visible augmentation of dislocation and addiction—every time a native band is moved or their resources taken or despoiled in order to increase the wealth of free-market society. This happens regularly today; for example, when native people's territories are flooded for hydroelectric projects, toxified by the tailings from mining operations or fish farms, deforested by clear-cut logging, or made uninhabitable by industrial development, military training exercises, or garbage dumping.[79] When this continuing assault on native culture is publicly acknowledged, it is generally described in terms of economic exploitation rather than dislocation, but material poverty is the smaller portion of the damage. Generally speaking, subsistence for native people is provided by a government dole when necessary, so the destruction of native resources does not produce new economic privation. However, the additional dislocation is devastating to the psychosocial integration of people who are already struggling to recover from earlier cultural destruction.[80] No amount of economic compensation or addiction treatment can undo it.

It is reassuring to blame this continuing dislocation of native people on politicians and greedy corporations. However, politicians will cease these practices if they perceive that they will not be re-elected if they continue. Corporations will stop if people do not buy their products. Yet governments and corporations are confident that most people are still more concerned with keeping down taxes and prices and increasing their affluence, so the dislocation continues for exactly the same reasons that it did in past centuries. Most people are willingly blind to it, most of the time.

Gambling provides a second example of the public role in the continuing dislocation produced by free-market society. We allow our elected representatives to spread convenient high-stakes gambling attractions throughout our cities and towns. Glittering casinos and ubiquitous lottery ticket outlets are designed to entice players to risk as much money as possible, sometimes 24 hours a day.[81] Some players become addicted gamblers to the apparent advantage of the rest of us whose taxes stay low because huge revenues flow from heavy gamblers to government coffers. Some of this revenue is spent to diagnose and treat gambling addicts and their families, as if that could compensate for the exploitation. But neither treatment nor any of the other three pillars can undo the damage.

Gambling addicts and their families are harmed by socially approved gambling promotion, but so are the supposed beneficiaries. How can it not degrade people's self-respect and identity to see—however dimly—that their taxes are low because they allow gambling establishments to prey on the addictive vulnerabilities of their more susceptible neighbours? Psychosocial integration requires, among its other components, a sense of pride in belonging to an honourable society.

A dozen other current examples of the role of the citizenry in perpetuating dislocation and addiction could be documented in my city alone. These would include allowing repeated cuts to tax-supported services that ameliorate the dislocation of the poor, such as day care for the children of poor people and single parents;[82] allowing government to enter into international and interprovincial agreements that essentially void laws that protect the environment and human welfare;[83] allowing and participating in speculative real-estate bubbles that make housing unaffordable for the young and ruin many people economically in the long run; allowing taxation policies that increase the gap between the rich and the poor and thus foster a corrosive sense of social injustice; and allowing governments to undertake megaprojects that support big business at the expense of degrading urban neighbourhoods and rural communities.[84]

Many people are already working on an individual level to reduce the damage. They recycle. They consume less. They cast their votes for politicians who promise to protect native communities and limit casino development. But these efforts cannot suffice.

Although virtuous individual actions can slow the increase in dislocation somewhat, they cannot stop or reverse it. They depend upon individuals swimming heroically against the full flood of a globalising free-market society that is impelled by all the institutions of social power. We are not raising enough heroes to reverse the flow. Overcoming dislocation and the other side effects of free-market society requires structural changes in the institutions that propagate them. Ultimately, structural change must be embedded in law, policy, and a new collective vision that guides the institutions of society. Structural change of this magnitude can only come about through collective, political action of an aroused citizenry, since most corporations and governments are dead set to increase, rather than decrease, hypercapitalism.[85]

This situation is dangerous and complex, but it is not hopeless. The next and final chapter of this book describes social actions that are being taken now and others that can be undertaken in the near future. However, it is first necessary to defang the charge of naiveté that such talk inevitably provokes. After that, it will be necessary to address another sticky side issue, which is the meaning of the pronoun 'we' that will crop up more and more as the book approaches its end. By confronting these sticky issues, the chapter moves towards the arena of Socratic rationalism. Socrates' famous 'myth of the cave' insists that an essential reality exists behind even the most mystified social images, and that people are capable of learning what it is. Working towards this essential knowledge requires ignoring the propaganda that is so colourfully projected on the global cave wall and turning instead towards a brighter reality. The light of day ultimately outshines the glow of pixelated screens.[86]

Naiveté

The four paragraphs that follow could have been considered the sheerest naiveté at one time, but no longer. I will explain why.

If globalised civilisation survives its current crises, it will emerge neither as a socialist utopia nor as a free-market paradise, but as a true global society. Global society means much more than a planetary marketplace. Like any society, a global society will engender a sense of belonging and meaning in its members, along with respect for individual initiative and freedom. People will defend it and protect its resources for posterity because they know it to be their home. In the economy of the new global society, markets will serve to facilitate innovation and the production of material wealth, but will always be overseen and supplemented by institutions that put the deeper interests of society first. Market autonomy will be subordinated to the needs for psychosocial integration, social justice, planetary ecology, economic stability, and peace. If the economic religion of the Market God survives, it will be recognised as one of many faiths tolerated by a pluralistic society, rather than an absolute truth. Hypercapitalism, which currently subordinates all other institutions of society to the needs of the economy, will be remembered in history books as a preliminary stage that civilisation tried and outgrew, like feudalism and slavery. Reduced addiction will be only one among many life-preserving consequences of these structural changes.

For the most part, the emerging global society will be densely populated, urban, and highly technologised.[87] Nonetheless, it will shepherd its resources to support both urban and rural families, protecting them from the economic pressures and volatility that currently reduce their capacity to nurture children, empower adults, honour elders, and maintain close, supportive contact between family members. Moreover, the emerging society will provide welcoming schools and community centres with adequate resources for communities to pass on the skills they consider essential and the values they cherish. The new global society will protect city neighbourhoods and rural settlements from destructive market forces whether they take the form of environmental destruction, artificial real estate bubbles, encroaching freeways, homogenising retail franchises, industrial waste contamination, or abrupt relocation of essential industries.

At the same time that the emerging global society supports families, communities, and the natural environment, it will recognise that social institutions inevitably change and that gradual, reflective change benefits society. It will welcome new institutions and social forms that foster psychosocial integration and individual accomplishment when the old ones become insufficient. It is impossible to know what new institutions will evolve, although many are now being tried. Some new institutions will utilize the Internet and other technological marvels; some will work through direct human contact. The emerging global society will consciously maintain a balance between stability and change, between

*social belonging and individual freedom. It cannot be expected to work miracles, because
the march of human folly will follow any route that it may embark upon. However, it will
achieve the best balance that can be found for each time and place.*

*Local communities and nation states in the emerging world society will maintain rela-
tionships that are fair to both sides. Relationships between countries will be controlled so
that ruinous wars and devastating economic exploitation are prevented. At the outset,
this requires a redistribution of wealth between rich and poor countries and between rich
and poor individuals because today's obscene inequalities[88] must appal any human being
who is not blind or paralysed. In the long run, peace requires stable international institutions with the power to adjudicate international conflicts that could lead to war and to
maintain a decent distribution of wealth.*

Not long ago, the previous four paragraphs would have been laughably naive.
However, that hopeless time has passed. In the 21st century, a truly global society has
become a real possibility, as well as a matter of 'do or die'. A true global society is now
a real possibility because, for the first time, two-way global communication technology exists that makes it possible in principle for every citizen to be in contact with
each other. The Internet, or some successor to it, creates the basis for radically
enlarged interpersonal communication. The benevolent global society has become a
matter of 'do or die' because the accumulated evidence of planetary ecological
destruction is alone sufficient to show that structural change—both economic and
political—is absolutely essential to the survival of civilisation. Ecological destruction
is not limited to global warming caused by increasing greenhouse gases, but also
includes loss of vital marine species that feed the planet, depletion of irreplaceable
mineral resources, loss of fresh water, desertification of productive land, loss of irreplaceable species and biodiversity, severe perturbations in the essential flow pattern of
the Gulf Stream, and on and on. Most qualified scholars, scientists, and scientific
associations of the world are convinced that the ecological consequences will lead
from regional breakdowns to irreversible, cascading collapse of vital ecosystems if
change is not initiated before it is too late.[89]

Many scholars recognise, and the general public senses, that the interests of multinational corporations and political leaders who defend hypercapitalism stand
squarely in the way of real solutions to the ecological crisis.[90] Under these conditions,
it is simple to convince oneself that society cannot impose structural change on
its own corporations, governments, and economic system in order to survive. But
to think in that pessimistic way is to give up all earthly hope. It is also to ignore the
history of the last two centuries during which aroused popular movements
forced society into substantial changes: from the abolition of slavery to the disman-
tling of the Soviet Union, and countless more local examples. Naomi Klein has
documented important 21st-century examples in Lebanon, Thailand, and New
Orleans, USA.[91]

As an example, the anti-slavery movement began with the concerns of a few isolated
individuals in England and eventually inspired mass protests in Europe and North
America. In the late 1700s and early 1800s, at least 300,000 British men, women,
and children boycotted sugar produced by slaves and many boycotted the stores
that sold it, with a major impact on the slave-powered sugar industry and on the

British parliament.[92] Later in the 1800s, American soldiers sang of freeing slaves around the 'watch-fires of a hundred circling camps'[93] during their great Civil War of 1861–1865. Naturally, defenders of the huge, enormously profitable free market in human slaves fought back fiercely in all the ways that the defenders of today's free-market society do, including expensive advertising, the pronouncements of tame public intellectuals, and physical violence.[94] Paul Hawken summarised the situation that the early English anti-slavery activists faced as follows:

> They were reviled and dismissed by businessmen and politicians. It was argued that their crackpot ideas would bring down the English economy, eliminate growth and jobs, cost too much money, and lower the standard of living.[95]

Nonetheless, over the course of a century and at great cost, the aroused citizens of the anti-slavery movements on two continents were able to bring legal slavery in Europe and the Americas to an end.[96] Similarly, citizens of all classes created a labour movement that was eventually able to regulate the free market in paid labour by enacting legal restrictions against child labour, grossly unsafe working conditions, starvation wages, and other unjust and dislocating excesses.[97] Large groups of aroused citizens carried the day, although some of their gains are being eroded in the current phase of hypercapitalism.

Paul Hawken argues, with contagious optimism, that as many as one million separate grass-roots organisations make today's ecology and social justice movements larger and potentially more powerful than any that have existed in the past.[98] We can hope that these organisations are large and resolute enough, or that they soon will be. We can also hope that these organisations perceive the importance of psychosocial integration as clearly as they perceive the more visible problems of environmental protection and social justice.[99] On the other hand, it would be too much to hope that domestication of free-market capitalism can be achieved without some ugly confrontations and violence. The history of past social movements indicates that fierce opposition will arise, and that we must be ready to act bravely and forcefully when it does.

Some scientists still do not accept the reality of today's ecological crisis. Once, their scientific scepticism served the important function of provoking critical debate. However, that issue has now been decided. Although science, by its nature, never reaches unanimity, societies survive by taking action on a reasonable balance of evidence, without waiting for the absolute certainty that only fatal disaster can bring. It is now imprudent to devote much time to the never-ending objections of a few scientific dissenters puffed up by their indefatigable publicists in governments and the media. They are distractions in a time of genuine crisis.

Beyond the few dissident scientists, there are public intellectuals as well as ordinary citizens who would rather perish than give up their sustaining faith in free-market ideology. However, the rest of us cannot be expected to see our world ruined to indulge their overpowering needs. Let them shout! Sometimes it is kinder to leave addicts raging for their drug than to indulge them.

Of the genuine terrors the world must face, the ecological crisis constitutes the most immediate threat. However, it cannot be solved independently. The other crises must be addressed simultaneously because they too are manifestations of hypercapitalism and are, thus, inextricably connected. This book is about dislocation and addiction, which are crucially important psychological aspects of this many-headed beast.[100]

Significantly reducing the problem of addiction and the dislocation that causes it requires nothing less than increasing psychosocial integration for society as a whole.[101] Increasing psychosocial integration, much like solving the ecological crisis, requires nothing less than rebalancing the lopsided priorities of free-market society. This will be a wrenching change. In some instances, rebalancing priorities will reduce profits, growth, consumer choice, and the so-called 'standard of living', especially for wealthier people and countries. However, it is not naïve to propose that all of this will happen. The truly widespread naiveté of our era lies in supposing that any less substantial form of action could ever bring the problem of addiction, or any of the other devastating effects of free-market society, under control. The greatest naiveté of all would be to imagine that we still have plenty of time.[102]

The stark choice is between structural change and global cataclysm. Because structural change will not be initiated by the people at the highest echelons of power, it is anything but naive, in view of the history of civilisation, to expect structural change to be instigated by an aroused populace in the near future. But *who* will constitute this aroused populace?

We will.

Defining 'we'

I have found it impossible to finish this book without increasing recourse to the word 'we'. 'We' naturally implies the existence of 'they'. But who actually constitutes these opposing forces? The distinction between 'we' and 'they' is very real and important, but it is not as simple as it may seem. As I have grown older, I have learned that 'we' sometimes fall into the same excesses of consumption, the same failures of empathy, the same reliance on propaganda, and the same uncritical acceptance of portions of free-market ideology that 'they' do. Moreover, I have relearned that 'they' also care about the injustices and cruelties of the world, and that 'they' honestly believe (or conscientiously struggle to believe) that these problems will be solved by more 'wealth creation', 'productivity', 'trickle-down', 'economic growth', and so forth. In fact, many people flip back and forth, being 'we' in some parts of their lives and 'they' in others. A great many people in free-market society are neither 'we' nor 'they' most of the time, because they are struggling too hard just to get by—no energy is left for broader issues. *Despite all this, the conflict between 'we' and 'they' is absolutely real and it is essential that 'we' prevail.*

The conflict is not between simple absolutes like good people and bad people, left and right, rich and poor, or masculine and feminine. Rather it is between two overarching world views, both of which abide, at some level of consciousness, within most people in the globalising world. The tension between 'we' and 'they' expresses itself as much in inner conflict as in outer confrontation.

'We' see that the needs for individual wealth, achievement, and power are dangerously overvalued in current society and that collective survival requires that these needs be balanced by the need for psychosocial integration as well as the needs of global ecology, social justice, peace, and financial stability. This requires a radical rebalancing of the institutions of society.

'They' believe that the marvellous powers of the market economy and material abundance can solve society's problems, if only people will act with enough individual strength and resourcefulness. 'They' believe that only the market economy is true to human nature, because people's most fundamental need is to develop their individual capacities to the fullest—too much reliance on the community can only make people weak and dependent.[103] Therefore, 'they' believe that individual wealth, achievement, and power together with corporate competitiveness, growth, and productivity must take precedence over other needs on most occasions.

Having now been defined, 'we' and 'they' and 'us' and 'them' will be used henceforth without quotation marks.

The conflict is essentially between a pluralistic world view and a singular, free-market world view.[104] The good news is that our world view is spreading quickly[105] after a couple of forlorn decades at the end of the 20th century when their view seemed so incontrovertible that it was possible for them to celebrate 'the end of history'. Now it is again thinkable that the balance will tip resoundingly, and it is essential that it does.

The outer conflict between us and them usually takes the form of forceful confrontations between groups of people contesting a social issue. Such confrontations decide important matters. But the inner conflict is more important because there will always be another public confrontation, and the same people may appear on opposite sides in the next confrontation or may conclude that it is too much trouble to participate at all—depending on the outcome of the inner conflict. Thus, the inner conflict is more crucial to tipping the balance than the outer conflict, for it alone can multiply the public support that we need to win outer conflicts in the future. They listen so much more attentively when we visibly outnumber them.

I believe that the inner conflict is the primordial struggle of human existence—the struggle for dominance of the wisest vision within us when action is most urgently needed. Joining with us in helping the wisest vision to prevail entails adopting a lifestyle other than that of the consumer idiots that we have all been educated to be, and still, at times, are. This lifestyle change frees energy from the rat race and from the mind-fogging mass media that can then be directed to restructuring the current system.

Joining with us also means avoiding the many intellectual land mines that could cripple us. The ten that I have come to see as the most incapacitating are:

1 The dream that free-market society can be saved by more of the same: more growth, more production, more cheap energy, more free markets, more innovative technology, more economic freedom, more police, more privacy, more surveillance, more tolerance, more security, more war on the official enemies.[106]

2 The intellectually suicidal idea that people are incapable of grasping social reality, and must, therefore, dither forever in post-modern uncertainty.

3 The lure of secure professionalism in which educated people can speak with assured authority about their own fields of specialisation, but must forever plead ignorance about larger issues.[107]

4 The fear of expressing valuable social critique because it will be labelled as a 'conspiracy theory'.[108]

5 The fantasy of creating a better world by always 'thinking positively', maintaining 'civil society', and finding 'win–win solutions', thus tacitly accepting destructive actions that must, instead, be exposed, discredited, and stopped.[109]

6 The wishful hope of eclectic spirituality that a person can save the world simply by seeking his or her own spiritual enlightenment.

7 The sophisticated muddiness of the 'Third Way', 'pink conservatism', and the *Euston Manifesto*, which discourse eloquently about the miseries of the world but ignore the role of free-market society in their creation, condoning unlimited expansion of free-market economics and Western military domination.[110]

8 The fantasies of 'green politicians' who argue that we can protect our environment while expanding corporate profits and driving gas-guzzlers.

9 The so-called identity politics that suppose that the only people really suffering from the current situation are poor, non-white, female, or homosexual.

10 Two forms of moral absolutism that make a balanced society difficult to achieve. One can perceive only intolerable danger in capitalism and the other can perceive only intolerable danger in socialism.

Finally, joining with us entails study. They have every advantage, save one, in the outer conflict. We can rely on the truth that our global free-market society is causing a multi-level disaster, whereas they must rely on vague slogans and humbug to argue that it is not.[111] Using the truth requires taking the time to find it. Finding the truth includes arduous tasks like unearthing and reporting significant facts that are not reported in the mainstream media. It also requires learning history to avoid the fate of repeating it. It requires learning economics so as to separate the small amount of knowledge that can be drawn from this politicised discipline from the large amount of humbug. It requires carefully investigating claims that the market must have its way for the common good, for it is important not to be obstructive in those cases where this claim is actually true. Nobody can learn all of the truth single-handedly, so finding it entails working with other people in a scholarly way. It means sharing information, but more importantly, criticising and enhancing conclusions that are drawn from it. The intellect of a single human being never amounts to much, but truth-seeking groups can become very smart indeed.

Naturally, we cannot devote ourselves to full-time scholarship rather than action, for this is yet another intellectual land mine. We must act bravely and decisively—and we must also allow time for dancing and singing as well. Ultimately, we are all about restoring psychosocial integration to its proper place in society.

The next, and final, chapter of this book gives examples of social actions designed to control dislocation and addiction that are underway in Vancouver and various other regions of the globe. It also includes some that exist only in my imagination.

Endnotes

1 The spiritual qualities of Socratic rationalism are sometimes overlooked. Socratic spirituality is explained at length in the *Republic* (Plato, *c.* 360 BC/1987, 474b–497a) and is discussed in endnote 3 of Chapter 13.

2 His secular rationalism is stated in its most compact form in the early and middle sections of Plato's *Republic* (*c.* 360 BC/1987). However, the final section of the *Republic* swerves into otherworldly mysticism in its consideration of human immortality, as shown in Chapter 13 of this book. Socrates' secular rationalism is more evident in his treatment of the experience of immortality in Plato's *Symposium* (*c.* 385 BC/2005, pp. 45–62, 201d–209a). The present book grows from my faith in secular rationalism (without otherworldly mysticism) both as epistemology and as a spiritual discipline.

3 I believe this list would include Albert Einstein (1949/1998), Noam Chomsky (2003b), Karl Kraus (see Accardo, 2005), and William James (1907/1981), each of whom I see as essentially a rationalist. I single these rationalists out because, in my view, their essential rationalism was not only fiercely rigorous, but also deeply humanistic, spiritual, and action-oriented. I believe that when the final reckoning is done for our era, each of these thinkers will be seen to have moved mountains. Speaking from a slightly less exalted platform, addiction researcher Jerome Jaffe expressed his own rationalism in a 1999 interview (Jaffe, 1999, p. 29).

4 For example, the mysteries of Catholic Christianity can be traced to Plotinus and Neoplatonism. The magic of modern science can be traced to mathematical essentialism.

5 Addiction is by no means the only instance of this civilised blindness. For example, Karl Polanyi (1944, pp. 89–92) showed how the cause of the rise of 'pauperism' in the late 18th century was invisible to an English gentry that was infatuated with self-regulating markets and international trade.

6 Socrates' famous 'myth of the cave' (Plato, *c.* 360 BC/1987) likens society to people who live their entire lives in the darkness of a cave. They have no knowledge of the outer world, and, therefore, believe that the shadows projected by the fire onto the cave wall are the whole of reality.

7 Beder (2006) documented that many billions of dollars have been devoted to this effort in the United States by the major corporations, beginning in the 1930s. She reviews records showing that the effort was conscious, organised, and—at first—resisted by the American government.

8 Matas (2005a).

9 The goal of expanding free-market society, disregarding its effect on dislocation, is currently accepted—either enthusiastically, grudgingly, or unconsciously—by many of those who wear the label 'left', 'radical', 'labour', 'intellectual', 'Third Way', or 'liberal' (in the American sense of the term) on the political spectrum (Giddens, 1998, pp. 64–68, 99–100; Goytisolo and Grass, 1999; K. Dixon, 2000; J. Heath, 2001; Lordon, 2003, 2004; Duhaime, 2004; Sader, 2005; Uchitelle, 2006; Bricmont, 2007).

10 Giddens, for example, has written eloquently on the devastating effect of modernity on psychosocial integration (Giddens, 1991). Yet he is a leading theoretician for the 'Third Way', a political movement that is based on strong support for expanding globalisation of free-market society (Giddens, 1998, pp. 99–100). He writes of the need to 'recreate social solidarity' as if this goal could be attained along with ever-increasing dominance of free-market society (Giddens, 1998, p. 67), but he does not explain how this is possible in any way that I can take seriously. For example, he speaks of replacing 'the lost forms of social

solidarity' with 'civil society', 'social and material refurbishment', 'cosmopolitan values', and 'philosophical conservatism' (Giddens, 1998, pp. 67, 79). He speaks of solving the problem of people 'abandoned to sink or swim in an economic whirlpool' (Giddens, 1998, p. 99) with 'the social investment state' (Giddens, 1998, p. 99) and an 'inclusive society' (Giddens, 1998, p. 105). Words like these ring hollow to me as solutions to the problem of dislocation, even when he explains them at length (Giddens, 1998, Chapters 3 and 4). One does not have to look too far in contemporary England to find evidence that the ideal of civil society is not being achieved (Renzetti, 2005a; Newland, 2007) and that heroin addiction is spreading like wildfire (Dalrymple, 2006a, p. 16; Reuter and Stevens, 2007, p. 7). The government of 'Lula' in Brazil seems to have adopted a logic that is similar to the 'Third Way' (Sader, 2005), as has the political left in France (Bricmont, 2007).

Economist Frédéric Lordon captures the essence of the left-wing embrace of free-market ideology in his description of the collapse of France Télécom:

> ... the problem of France Telecom resides probably less in the innate curse of public ownership [as certain French neoliberals have charged] than in the aberration of a public owner acting exactly like private owners.

Lordon (2003, p. 45).

11 Szasz (1975); Alexander (1992); Healy (2003); Fowlie (2004); Motluk (2004); Lippman (2005); DeGrandpre (2006, Chapter 1). Government manipulations of science in general have recently been dramatically documented in the United States (Union of Concerned Scientists, 2004).

12 P. Taylor (2005); Ubelacker (2005a); Carey (2006); Denizet-Lewis (2006).

13 International Narcotics Control Board (2004).

14 It is rare to hear the phrase War on Drugs used by politicians now. However, the American 'National Drug Control Strategy', which includes most of the activities that people refer to as the War on Drugs, was budgeted to receive more than US$12 billion in 2004 and in 2005 (White House, 2004). British drug strategy under the Blair government was widely regarded to have assumed the proportions of a War on Drugs (Rolles et al., 2004; Jenkins, 2006). The current Conservative government in Canada seems determined to restart the War on Drugs (Mickleburgh and Galloway, 2007).

15 Lemoine (2000, 2001); Ospina (2003, 2004).

16 Many people have contributed to the mountain of evidence about the futility and illogic of the War on Drugs. My own book on this topic may be as comprehensive as any (Alexander, 1990).

17 Stiglitz (2002).

18 See Healy (1997, 2003), Marsa (1997), Alphonso (2003), Motluk (2004), Lippman (2005), Picard (2005d), Priest (2005), DeGrandpre (2006, Chapter 2), and Meier (2007) on unscrupulous marketing and the subversion of science by American drug companies in the interest of profits.

19 Bouillon (2005); Homer-Dixon (2005); Howlett (2005); Dash (2006); Halimi (2006).

20 Conference des Nations unies sur le commerce et le dévelopement (2004, as cited in Harribey, 2004); Homer-Dixon (2005); Vasagar (2005).

21 Drohan (2003a, 2004b).

22 Abramovici (2004).

23 Cohn (2005); Mallick (2005); Roberts (2005).

24 Evans-Pritchard (2007a, b).

25 Economist Todd Hirsh (2005) expressed this observation poignantly in a newspaper article.

26 Stiglitz (2002, Chapters 8 and 9); Halimi (2005); Chase (2007).

27 The greatest of contemporary thinkers dissect the failures of free-market society and propose fundamental changes with great hope. However, their diagnoses are more convincing than their prescriptions. How will enlightened national governments overcome the dislocation and other problems that are built into the very foundations of free-market economics? How will citizens' movements that are so terribly difficult to arouse and coordinate ever prevail against the armies of well-paid public-relations experts, journalists, police, and soldiers working for multinational corporations and governments? The answers that have been proposed to these questions are too vague to be credible (Glendinning, 1994, Chapter 15; Giddens, 1998, Chapters 3 and 4; J. Heath, 2001; Suzuki and Dressel, 2002; Albala, 2003; Dobbin, 2003, Chapter 7; Dufour, 2003a, pp. 249–251; Feixa, 2003; Latouche, 2003; Sader, 2003; Bulard, 2004; Jacquard, 2004; Poupeau, 2004; Homer-Dixon, 2006). To the degree that their proposed solutions are specific in their details, they conflict sharply from one scholar to another. Compare, for example, the solutions of Glendinning (1994, Chapter 15), Giddens (1998, Chapter 3), Sader (2003), Feixa (2003), and Poupeau (2004).

28 K. Polanyi (1944, p. 3); Ellul (1965); Brune (2004); Judith Warner (2005); Beder (2006); Homer-Dixon (2006, pp. 214–219).

29 Godot is a famous character who never appears in the play, *Waiting for Godot*, throughout which the other characters anticipate his arrival (Beckett, 1965).

30 For example, Mel Hurtig (National Party) in Canada or Ralph Nader (Green Party) in the United States.

31 Many Christians and followers of eclectic spirituality are effective social activists. Nonetheless, as Chapter 12 documents, basic writings of their doctrines contend that this is futile.

32 See Chapter 10 under the heading *Faith in the 'Market God'*, as well as Nickson (2007).

33 See Chapter 3 under the heading *Psychosocial integration is a necessity*.

34 This is true whether 'soul' is meant in the way that St Augustine used the word in the *Confessions* (St Augustine, 397 AD/1963; see also Chapter 9 of this book), the way that Karl Polanyi used the word in *The Essence of Fascism* (K. Polanyi, 1935, p. 370), or in the way that Socrates described the just 'psyche', normally translated 'soul', in the *Republic* (Plato, c. 360 BC/1987, 441c–444e; see also Chapter 13 of this book).

35 Serious scholars are now raising alarms about the possibility of a nuclear world war in the short term (e.g. Golub, 2005a, b; Hurtig, 2005).

36 Under these conditions, we might discover that our inspiring prophet had already arrived. Who in the blind and paralysed multitude would have recognized him or her?

37 Toynbee (1948).

38 Confession has long been valued in such religions as Christianity, Buddhism, Hinduism, and Islam, as well as in several North and South American native cultures apart from any influence of early missionaries (Pennebaker, 1997). Self-disclosure, as a form of confession, in contemporary psychotherapy, counselling, and many self-help groups has also been shown to be beneficial. See Shelton (2003) for a review of the history and benefits of self-disclosure in secular contexts.

39 Saul (1995, p. 79).

40 When written in lower case, 'four pillars' refers simply to treatment, prevention, law enforcement, and harm reduction, rather than to Vancouver's 'Four Pillars Drug Strategy',

which, although it has the same four categories of intervention, is a more specifically defined programme applied in a single city.

41 Cameron (2004).

42 Orford *et al.* (2000).

43 Blomqvist (2004, p. 157).

44 For a discussion of motivational interviewing, see W. R. Miller (1989; 2000, p. 9) and Yahne *et al.* (2002). Motivational interviewing is designed to inculcate motivation for change in subtle ways, but one of its principles is that the therapist enters into a supportive relationship even with clients who are not interested in giving up their addictions. For the 'Community Reinforcement Approach', see Chapter 7 of this book under the heading *Psychosocial integration makes recovery from addiction possible.*

45 See Maté (2000, 2005a, b, 2008).

46 See Chapter 8 of this book.

47 In each case, most children engage in harmless forms of the activity, but sizeable numbers of participants progress to the 'hard stuff' (i.e. fully fledged addiction₃ or physically dangerous or illegal behaviours).

48 Shedler and Block (1990) and others have provided statistical evidence that students who completely abstain from drugs and alcohol in some parts of the world are less sociable and emotionally stable on average than those who use drugs moderately. (Students who use drugs heavily are the least well off.) Recent research on this controversial topic is inconsistent, but even those who failed to replicate the earlier finding (e.g. Walton and Roberts, 2004) found little average difference in psychological characteristics between abstainers and moderate users, providing a quantitative basis for the observation that some moderate drug users function better than some abstainers.

49 More reflective practitioners of prevention conceptualise their field far more broadly (Steinmann, 2004).

50 Alexander (1990, Chapter 2); Ennett *et al.* (1994); Granfield and Cloud (1999, pp. 200–202); Room (2003); S. L. West and O'Neal (2004); Wibberly (2005). There are, of course, some conflicting results, but the overall trend is quite clear.

51 Motluk (2004); Picard (2004c); DeGrandpre (2006).

52 J. Jacobs (1961, pp. 137–138); Giddens (1998, p. 36).

53 Four Pillars Coalition (2005).

54 Scott (2006).

55 Gurstein and Small (2005).

56 MacPherson *et al.* (2005, pp. 1–4, 13–15).

57 M. Hume (2006a, b).

58 Sanger and Forero (2004); Otis (2006).

59 Alexander (1990, Chapter 2); E. Wood *et al.* (2004b).

60 See Wikipedia entry 'Law Enforcement Against Prohibition', at http://en.wikipedia.org/wiki/Law_Enforcement_Against_Prohibition.

61 For example, Puder (1998).

62 Plant and Plant (2006, Chapter 7).

63 J. Woodward (2005).

64 People whose houses have been burgled in Vancouver frequently report that the police investigation was cursory at best. Sometimes police do not even find the time to attend the scene of a household burglary. When my own house was burgled of thousands of dollars of

computer equipment, the burglar cut himself as he broke in and left a trail of blood throughout the house. The attending police officer did not take a blood sample (which would surely have been strong evidence for a conviction) because it was 'too expensive to use blood as evidence except in a major offence'.

65 See Chapter 1, endnotes 28, 30, and 31. See also Laurance (2007).

66 Stimson (2007).

67 See Alexander and Tsou (2001). It may help if drug addicts adopt the role of medical patients in maintenance programmes, even though drug addiction is not literally a disease.

68 Crane and Warnes (2005).

69 Sweanor *et al.* (2007).

70 PHS Community Services Society (2005). Some of the innovations of this dynamic agency were discussed earlier in this chapter under the heading *Prevention*.

71 Alexander and Tsou (2001); *Vancouver Sun* (2007).

72 This one is not connected with the Portland Hotel Society.

73 Poole and Isaac (2001); Poole and Urquhart (2007).

74 Plant and Plant (2006, Chapter 7).

75 Historical documentation for this conclusion is summarised in endnote 9 of Chapter 1 of this book.

76 I borrowed this metaphor from Robert Derkson who borrowed it from Ricks *et al.* (1999).

77 L. Wong (1990).

78 International Atomic Energy Agency (2005).

79 See Chapter 6 of this book under the heading entitled *Canadian Aboriginal Peoples*.

80 There are two very current examples. One is the Innu people of Labrador and northern Quebec whose story has been written by Samson (2003). The other is the Kwadacha people of northern British Columbia whose story will be recounted in Chapter 15.

81 In 2007, some, but not all, casinos were open 24 hours a day, every day.

82 Coalition of Child Care Advocates of BC (2007); Lee (2007).

83 Barlow and Clarke (2001, pp. 22–25); Patrick Brown (2006, p. 2); E. Gould (2006–2007); J. Hill (2006); Island Tides (2007a); Bates (2007). The first of these citations concerns the Multilateral Agreement on Investment (MAI), which was ultimately defeated. The last five concern the Trade, Investment and Labour Mobility Agreement Between British Columbia and Alberta (TILMA) in Canada that came into effect on 1 April 2007 (see Governments of British Columbia and Alberta, 2006).

84 A current example in British Columbia is the so-called 'Gateway Program' (Bates and Kromka, 2007; Dodds, 2007). See also Greater Vancouver Gateway Council (2003); Livable Region Coalition (2004); Ministry of Small Business and Economic Development and Ministry of Transportation (2005).

85 John Ralston Saul (1995, pp. 175–190) has argued this point powerfully.

86 Socrates' 'myth of the cave' appears in the *Republic* (Plato, *c.* 360 BC/1987, 514a–517a).

87 Most people now live in cities of this sort and this trend will continue in the foreseeable future (J. Jacobs, 1961, pp. 218–221; Davis, 2006b).

88 Oziewicz (2006b).

89 Homer-Dixon (2006, Chapters 6 and 7) provides a fully documented, up-to-date review of this literature.

90 Homer-Dixon (2006, Chapters 6 and 7, pp. 219, 293, 305) has reviewed the relevant literature at length and stated this conclusion unequivocally, but he is only one voice among many. See also Gross (1980), Shepard (1982, as cited in Fish, 2006, pp. 195–196), Suzuki and McConnell (1997), deGraaf *et al.* (2002, Chapter 11), S. Hume (2003a), Dolmetsch (2004), Homer-Dixon (2004), M. Hume (2004b), Mitchell (2004), D. Smith (2004), Radford (2004, 2005), Brethour (2005), D. Jones (2005), Sinaï (2006), Hawken (2007, pp. 51–68), and Mittelstaedt (2007a). A recent report by Sir Nicholas Stern may change this somewhat, but this story is still emerging as this manuscript is being submitted (Mittelstaedt, 2007b).

91 Klein (2007, pp. 553–561).

92 McKitrick (1963); Hochschild (2005, pp. 192–196); Jensen (2006, p.107).

93 These words are from the American *Battle Hymn of the Republic* (Howe, 1862), a beautiful and militant anti-slavery anthem.

94 Hochschild (2005, pp. 154, 159–160, 187).

95 Hawken (2007, p. 24). Of course, there were other lines of argument in favour of slavery as well, including those based on law, tradition, and racial inferiority of blacks (McKitrick, 1963).

96 Hawken (2007, pp. 24, 77). Slavery continued elsewhere, and British bankers continued to finance it and British industry continued to use slave-grown cotton (Ankomah, 2007).

97 Polanyi (1944).

98 Hawken (2007).

99 McKibben (2007, Chapter 3) is a well-known American social activist who eloquently argues for the importance of psychosocial integration.

100 The reasons that dislocation and addiction are as least as important as the others are summarised earlier in this chapter under the heading *The need for action on addiction.*

101 Erik Erikson cautioned against simply bolstering people's self-esteem as a way of dealing with their identity fragmentation:

['Ego bolstering' is] socially dangerous, because its employment implies that the cause of the strain (i.e. 'modern living') is perpetually beyond the individual's or his society's control—a state of affairs which would postpone indefinitely the revision of conditions which are apt to weaken the infantile ego.

Erikson (1959, pp. 47–48).

102 J. Williams (2007).

103 A person can also become a part of an ideologically opposite 'them' by believing that the collective must take precedence over the pursuit of individual enterprise and achievement on virtually every occasion, another intoxicatingly simple formula.

104 At a more fundamental level, it is tempting to compare the difference between what I am calling a pluralistic world view and a singular world view to the difference between polytheism and monotheism. This comparison goes too far afield for this book, however.

105 Hawken (2007, pp. 1–26).

106 The essential structural change is not a matter of more (or less). It is qualitative, rather than quantitative. It is a creative rebalancing of power between competitive markets and cooperative social institutions.

107 This idea is the antithesis of democracy in which the widest and deepest intellectual visions come from encompassing thinkers rather than narrow technicians.

108 Labelling social critique as a 'conspiracy theory' in no way demonstrates its falsity. Such labels should be ignored. The essential question is whether or not the institutions and practices of free-market society are doing unsustainable harm and must be changed. Whether or not the people involved are involved in any sort of conscious conspiracy makes little difference. In most instances, they probably are not.

109 In the history of Western civilisation, protest, rebellion, and uprising have been the sources of the rights and traditions that we now cherish (see Robert, 2006; Garnier, 2007). Why would this be different now?

110 Contradictions in the ideology of the 'Third Way' are discussed in this chapter under the heading *Civilised blindness*.

The *Euston Manifesto* has a distinctly muddy logic (*Euston Manifesto*, n.d.; Glavin, 2006). The writers of the manifesto express their concern for human welfare and for universal application of the United Nations' Universal Declaration of Human Rights. Yet they are silent on the role of free-market society in abrogating many of these rights for multitudes of people. They vehemently oppose Anti-Americanism, although they acknowledge that the United States, as militant champion of free-market economics, has proved itself the most potent enemy of many of these rights for many peoples. The *Euston Manifesto* largely restricts itself to condemning the violation of these rights by non-free-market societies and enemies of the United States.

111 This is not to say that they do tell the truth when it serves their purpose, but true statements must always be embedded in a larger pattern of deception because their basic claims are false.

Chapter 15

Social Actions to Control Addiction: Question Period

Each time I finish delivering a public lecture on addiction, someone in the audience brings my lofty abstractions down to earth by asking some form of the question, 'What can I do about addiction from the perspective of the dislocation theory?' To my ever-lasting frustration, this very personal question cannot be answered well in the rush of a short question period. The short answer is that whereas 'I'—one person alone—can help a few individuals at best, we[1] have the knowledge and power to bring addiction under control, by acting together. Concerted social action can domesticate today's globalising free-market society, bringing dislocation to heel. Indeed, we must succeed at this if our children and grandchildren are to endure the world of the future without needing ever more addictive solace. However, much more than this must be said.

A fuller answer to the question is laid out in this final chapter. It begins with the acknowledgement that we pursue social actions that are intended to rebalance free-market society not so much because of their prospects for success, but because of who we are. We are not the self-absorbed, insatiable consumer idiots that we have been conditioned to be,[2] even if we still act that way in weak moments. Rather, we are human beings whose qualities of reason, compassion, and courage come to the fore in times of crisis, such as these.

The bulk of this chapter consists of detailed examples of social actions that can help to domesticate free-market society. These actions are not oriented towards preventing or treating addiction directly like those described in the first sections of Chapter 14, but towards controlling it indirectly by reducing dislocation. Moreover, these social actions do not bear *exclusively* on dislocation. Dislocation and addiction are inextricably intertwined with other adverse effects of free-market society.[3] Although dislocation and addiction remain the central topics in this chapter, limiting social actions to those intended to reduce them alone would be impracticable, and would nourish the mistaken belief that addiction can be controlled without confronting the multifaceted crisis of hypercapitalism.

Restructuring society through social action is anything but a new idea. Throughout the 19th and 20th centuries, powerful mass movements arose to introduce change when they were most needed,[4] including the 19th-century anti-slavery movement described in Chapter 14, as well as more recent movements that helped to end apartheid in South Africa and the Soviet imperialism in Eastern Europe. As these great social transformations fade into history, it is easy to forget how much power was wielded by groups of aroused citizens and how unlikely it is that the vital changes would have occurred without them.

Professionals in the field of addictions have a central role to play in the social actions that must be undertaken to bring dislocation and addiction under control. Professionals can see from close range that controlling addiction requires going beyond individual and professional interventions. Professionals can also see why social action designed to control addiction cannot be entirely focused on material poverty and social injustice, vitally important as these are. Addiction professionals have seen the power of dislocation to make powerful and privileged people addicted, and therefore know that the dangers of dislocation are not limited to the poor and homeless. By their dedication, addiction professionals have earned the credibility to convince people that social change must counteract poverty of the spirit as well as material poverty.

The first section of this chapter describes some specific social actions that can increase psychosocial integration on local and national levels. The second, more ambitious section describes some social actions with a global scope.

Social action at local and national levels

Many of the examples in this section are drawn from my own corner of the world. This is partly because I know the situations and the people involved well enough to describe them in detail. More importantly, Vancouver provides an excellent prototype of a city that is actively struggling with the side effects of free-market society. It is a hub of global trade, a major destination point for human migration, and an established centre of addiction.[5] In today's era of unprecedented urbanisation and migration, hundreds of young cities with similar characteristics house a major portion of the world's population. In 2008, for the first time in human history, half of the world's population lives in cities. The urban proportion of the population will continue to grow rapidly as new cities continue to come into existence and old cities expand.[6] In 2007, the United Nations Population Fund singled out Vancouver as an example to show that the social problems of 21st-century urbanisation, such as homelessness, strike rich cities as well as poor, Third-World cities.[7] Actions that can reduce addiction in Vancouver may well be useful in other cities of the globalising world as well.

'What can I do about addiction from the perspective of the dislocation theory?' The most powerful thing you can do is to join with your neighbours in social actions like those described in this chapter. Your participation will be welcomed warmly, because the people already involved need your help. The first, and arguably the most pressing, example is the struggle to overcome the devastating effects of today's mass media.

Overcoming indoctrination

Mass-crculation newspapers, radio stations, television channels, and Internet news sources[8] create formidable barriers to psychosocial integration by tirelessly weaving free-market ideology and values into the news and entertainment that shape people's world view. The mass media indoctrinate us from earliest childhood with individualistic, competitive, and acquisitive values that undermine psychosocial integration.[9] They ignore or distort news events that could reflect badly on free-market society.[10] They prepare us to accept the psychosocial and environmental sacrifices that are necessary to nourish 'the market' or 'the economy'.[11] They mock alternative ideas as naive and unsophisticated.

Beyond trumpeting the ideology and values of free-market society, the mass media obscure its side effects. They reassure us with images of people deftly mastering their dislocation and stress without falling into depression or addiction. They distract us by lavishing attention on a few grotesque scandals, while virtually ignoring the mundane, grinding devastation that grows from free-market society everywhere. For example, the four leading French dailies devoted 344 stories between 5 May and 5 July 2004 to sexual abuse of several children in the French town of Outreau. By the end of the media circus, 14 of the 18 accused were completely exonerated and most of the alleged crimes were proven to be imaginary.[12] During the same period, the same four dailies devoted a total of three stories to research produced by the World Health Organisation showing that 3 million children die each year from air pollution, water pollution, and other environmental hazards. Of course, child sexual abuse is intolerable. However, the media circus surrounding the Outreau affair not only distracted public attention from much more widespread harm to children, but also devastated the lives of 14 innocent adults, one of whom committed suicide in detention.[13]

Beyond misrepresenting reality, the conventional news media also blatantly misrepresent themselves as bastions of 'balanced reporting' and 'objectivity'. Any small deviation from free-market ideology is said to reveal the machinations of the dreaded 'left-wing media', to which the sacred ideals of balanced reporting and objectivity are supposedly unknown.[14] However, rather than shining exemplars of objectivity, today's conventional news media constitute a formidable indoctrination system for hypercapitalism.[15]

Like all businesses, mass media operate in the interests of their owners and investors who are, for the most part, executives of huge multinational corporations with vested interests in expanding the reach of free-market society, no matter how much devastation it causes.[16] In Vancouver—perhaps an extreme example—three of the four major daily newspapers, 12 free community newspapers, and nine analogue and digital television stations are owned by a single corporation that rigidly requires its reporters to support free-market values and American foreign policy.[17] Most of the remaining media are owned by other large corporations or by a national government currently committed to free-market society. Individual television shows, newspapers, movies, and so forth are sponsored by other corporations with similar interests.

It is very difficult for the few independent news sources to compete with the dazzling production standards, graphics, and special effects of the mass media indoctrination system, which are so expensive that they cannot usually be produced without rich subsidies from the advertising revenues from multinational corporations.[18] Canada once maintained a high-quality public broadcasting system, the Canadian Broadcasting Corporation (CBC). However, the CBC has been so starved of public funds by successive Liberal and Conservative governments[19] that it no longer provides an effective alternative to the mainstream English-language media in Canada, although it still manages to air a few excellent programmes.

Largely because of this mass-media indoctrination system, the ideas and values that legitimatise free-market society have come to seem obvious, natural, and unquestionable to many people. The myth of demon drugs discussed in Chapter 8 is a single example, among countless others, of a manufactured belief that blinds people to the roots of social problems in free-market society.

The indoctrination system is formidable, but not impregnable. Today, people are breaching its defences on many sides. Some people contribute their talents to independent newspapers and radio stations, often without pay, because independent media must operate without subsidies from corporate advertising. People who work for independent media strive to help others to see through the highly selected and distorted 'news' that the indoctrination system promulgates. The independents, like all media, approach the news from a particular angle, but many of them are scrupulously factual in their reporting.[20] At the other extreme, some independents are as unconcerned with factual reporting as the most propagandistic of the conventional mass media, although their biases take them in different directions.

Many independent media are small or medium-sized, but provide an excellent service nonetheless. In the Vancouver area, *The Tyee, Island Tides, The Republic of East Vancouver*, and *The Georgia Straight* newspapers, *Adbusters* magazine, the Canadian Centre for Policy Alternatives think tank, and Co-op Radio are among the best. My favourite international reference, and a major information source for this book, is *Le Monde diplomatique*, published monthly in Paris. *Le Monde diplomatique* is written in French and each issue is translated into 25 languages for worldwide distribution. It is famous for high-quality writing and scrupulous factuality.

Some people counteract the mass media indoctrination system by writing books, often published by university presses with high scholarly standards. Their books compile the information that conventional news media systematically ignore or distort. Dozens of works of this sort are cited in the bibliography of this book. Other people contribute their talents by diligently circulating information that does not appear in the propaganda apparatus on websites, Internet mailing lists, documentary film, and printed articles. Still others film live events that are normally overlooked by the media and bring them to public attention through YouTube and other Internet services.

The mass media ignore all of these efforts whenever possible. They publicly react only when an item influences people on a large scale, as have recent documentary films by Al Gore and Michael Moore for example. When some basis can be found, the offenders are subjected to legal challenges that can cripple them financially, even if no libel or slander is actually proven. Even if there is no basis for legal action, outrageous slurs on the personal character of those who publicise independent thinking flood the conventional news media.[21] The relentless intensity of these attacks chills the enthusiasms of onlookers who might otherwise contribute their talents to the independent media.

Some people work politically to reduce the concentration of mass media ownership in the hands of powerful corporations through political channels. Governments are occasionally forced to respond.[22] The continuing struggle of independent media against the indoctrination apparatus must be won before psychosocial integration can be restored and addiction can be brought under control. 'What can I do about addiction from the perspective of the dislocation theory?' You can help to provide an alternative to the mass media indoctrination system. New helpers are always welcomed by the independent media and their supporters, and it is critical that they fulfil their mission.

But what about children and the media? Commercial television's methods of moulding children appear to be especially powerful.[23] Children are easily seduced by glittery toys, breakfast cereals, superheroes, and free-market symbolism. They are thereby distracted from the far less glittery but actually attainable pleasures of family and neighbourhood life and of independent thought. Moreover, some advertisers sabotage family relationships by providing children with role models in their commercials for aggressively hassling their parents to buy them the toys they are led to desire.[24] How could this manipulation of children not increase the dislocation of free-market society?[25]

Manipulation of children by the media can be brought under control politically when citizens become sufficiently aroused to motivate their governments to the task. Sweden and some other countries have achieved partial victories in this regard. Beginning in 1991, the Swedish government banned all television advertising that targets children under 12 years of age, all advertising directed at adults in time slots immediately before or after children's programmes, and all advertising featuring characters that play a conspicuous role in children's programming. A poll taken in 2001, 10 years after the bans were introduced, showed that 88% of Swedish people supported them.[26] Similar bans are in place in Norway, in the Flemish-speaking region of Belgium, and in the French-speaking Canadian province of Québec. Québec appears to be the world leader in this regard, having instituted its ban in 1980. Less severe regulations on television advertising for children have been instituted in Denmark, The Netherlands, Greece, Luxembourg, and Portugal.[27] New European Union (EU) controls may be in the works in light of recent discoveries about the relationship between rampant childhood obesity and fast-food advertising directed at children.[28]

Nevertheless, the majority of other nations have not yet enacted initiatives to protect children from manipulation by television advertisers. In addition, shrill attacks have been made on such initiatives in the European mass media, which have labelled them 'extremist' and 'anti-economic'. The Swedish initiative has been deliberately subverted by a British television channel that has begun broadcasting Swedish language programmes into Sweden. Nonetheless, Sweden has maintained its position and a small battle against the propaganda apparatus has been won.

Prohibiting specific abuses is only a first step towards replacing the indoctrination system with communications media that foster psychosocial integration. However, this first step shows that the media can be brought under control by an aroused citizenry. It also shows that the conventional media will use their economic and political resources to fight back fiercely and that national controls are not sufficient by themselves, since many television shows cross national frontiers.

In the future, the news media can serve a totally different function than they presently do, as was envisioned early in the 20th century when they came into existence.[29] Early 20th-century thinkers envisioned local radio and television stations strengthening democratic government and local communities by providing a low-cost way of circulating ideas on locally important topics. The experience of local media, including Canada's CBC before it was starved by underfunding, shows that talented media professionals are enthusiastic about serving this function.

A simple change in licensing policy for stations could bring this about now. Some of the licences now apportioned to commercial stations could be made available for local exchange of ideas and debate through local organisations, churches, ethnic groups, and schools. Taxes on commercial stations could provide enough money to enable non-commercial stations to produce shows with attractive production values. Laws could prevent the concentrated ownership that enables huge corporations to build their strength as institutions of mass indoctrination.

Video games present a new kind of media challenge. Like children's television, many of them indoctrinate players into a hypercapitalistic view of the world. Some may also incite some children to real-life violence.[30] For these reasons and because they sometimes become objects of severe addictions themselves, they pose a genuine danger to the children who are growing up with them and to society in general.[31] The regulatory regime that is needed to control video games will require careful thought as the problem continues to expand and change in the future. Implementing any regulatory regime will require concerted social action, because the video game industry will certainly oppose any regulations that threaten its immense profits, and the free-market machinery will not willingly give up such a powerful vehicle for propaganda. On the other hand, it is important for those who see the dangers built into the explosive spread of video games not to lapse into the frantic, prohibitionistic thinking of the earlier temperance and anti-drug movements. Instead, it is necessary to move towards a regulatory regime that recognises the educational and entertainment values of video games,[32] while minimising the harm that they do. The creative challenge is to devise attractive video games that promote, rather than undermine, psychosocial integration.

In sum, the dazzling technology that underlies today's mass media can and should be used to facilitate psychosocial integration, rather than to undermine it. Citizens have the power to bring this about by supporting existing and creating new independent media, as well as by joining pressure groups to make mass media a political issue that government cannot afford to ignore. Overcoming the powerful vested interests that support the present mass media indoctrination system is a huge task, but it is not larger than overcoming the vested interests that supported the vast system of industrial slavery that existed two centuries ago, or overcoming the repressive regime of the former Soviet Union. Obviously, the problem of dislocation in free-market society cannot be solved completely by restructuring the mass media, crucially important though that task is. Many other forms of social action will also have to be undertaken.

Reclaiming real estate

From its earliest beginnings, free-market society has required the movement of land from the control of communities and traditional society to the control of the persons with the largest amounts of money to spend in real-estate markets. These transactions have been financed by banks and, more recently, international financial institutions. The results have been devastating in many cases. Two examples may suffice to show how people can reduce dislocation by reclaiming land from real estate markets.

Native land claims

The attempt to wholly assimilate Canada's native people into free-market society has failed. Whereas some people of native descent are now fully at home in the cosmopolitan world of cities and towns, the majority continue to identify with their own tribal groups and a substantial number continue to live with their own people on remnants of their former tribal lands that have been set aside as 'reserves'. Many native people remain severely dislocated, and native people comprise a grossly disproportionate number of those afflicted by addiction, family violence, HIV/AIDS, mental illness, and criminality.[33]

The problem of addiction in Canada and in other nations with a similar history cannot be solved without reducing the appalling dislocation of today's native people. In part, this requires providing suitable environments for those who continue living in aboriginal tribal groups. Providing suitable environments, in turn, requires resolving the fearsomely complex issue of native 'land claims'. In a more abstract sense, the essential issue underlying 'land claims' goes beyond native groups to the population as a whole.

Although native land was seized everywhere in Canada, British Columbia, in its mad dash for expansion and prosperity late in the 19th century, paid the least attention to the legal nicety of signing treaties. In most cases, the province simply expropriated whatever land it wanted. However, a landmark decision of the Supreme Court of Canada in 1997 has recognised the long-suppressed right of native tribes whose lands were taken without a treaty to press their land claims in court[34] as legally recognised 'First Nations'. If native people did not have this right, the government would appear simply to have stolen their land.

In reality, Canada *did*, in many senses of the word, steal the land of all the native peoples who had lived in its current territories prior to European invasion.[35] However, this was done following the prevailing colonial practices of that time and—in most provinces—at least negotiating treaties with a few representatives of each tribal group.

This continental-scale land seizure cannot be undone now without committing an even greater seizure, because the millions of people who occupy the former aboriginal land purchased it (or the logging or mineral rights to it) in good faith in a market that was legitimatised by the governments and churches they trusted. Moreover, virtually all nations—not just white ones, but also Asian, African, and Aboriginal ones—have committed similar land seizures in the past or are doing so currently.[36]

Complete social justice is not an option under these conditions.[37] However, the effects of past seizures can be mitigated by quickly settling native land claims that are now stuck in limbo. Only then can aboriginal people re-establish whatever portions of their native heritages are still recoverable and get on with life in a stable and predictable environment.[38]

The British Columbian provincial government now faces very large numbers of legally recognised claims. Since claims by different tribal groups overlap, the total area that has been claimed is greater than the total area of the province.[39] In response to this legal dilemma, the government has perfected the art of delay. Although there have been a few settlements recently, most 19th- and 20th-century claims remain unsettled in the 21st century.

The depth of this problem is illustrated by the history of the Nisga'a Treaty in northwestern British Columbia, finally signed and enacted in the year 2000 after more than a century of tortuous delays and negotiations.[40] The Nisga'a people's struggle for justice first entered the history books in 1887, when tribal chiefs took it upon them-selves to travel about 800 km from their land to the provincial capital in Victoria to present their claim. When this claim was not recognised, they directly petitioned the Privy Council in London in 1913. Serious negotiations did not begin until 1990. A settlement was eventually reached, but, although many Nisga'a people are pleased with it, others remain profoundly dissatisfied.[41] The Nisga'a treaty remains one of a very small number of settlements in recent years, and no quick solution to the rest of this enormous problem appears to be on the horizon.

Land-claims settlements are more than real-estate deals. Native people must know which land is theirs in order to function as secure individuals within a viable culture. Moreover, legitimate claims cannot be delayed for decades or a century without pul-verising the claimants psychologically, since government delay tactics allegedly recog-nise but actually ignore their identities. Could there be a better formula for exacerbating dislocation?

The native land claims dilemma provides another opportunity for citizens to do something substantial about addiction. Concerned citizens have the power to force governments to settle native land claims with dispatch because of the dislocation and addiction that is produced by continuing uncertainty. Settlements might never be reached without resolute agitation by aroused citizens because provincial and federal governments appear to be content with the present situation—despite their rhetoric. The present situation serves the interests of the corporations that want to draw the province's natural resources into the free market.[42] Untangling this mess lies far beyond the reach of this book, but it is well within reach for a properly constituted citizen's commission, and people have the power to force their governments to convene one.[43]

Non-native land claims

As this chapter was being written, a different kind of land claim was being made in my own neighbourhood. A 66 × 125 ft parcel of land on Salsbury Street in Vancouver was purchased by a developer with the intent of replacing two very small single-family homes with two large duplexes with attached garages. Three-fifths of the land was, however, occupied by a park-like garden that had been started in 1907 and was set off from the surrounding cityscape by dense bushes and the highest trees in that quarter of the city. The garden, which became known as Salsbury Garden, also contained a tiny 'cob house' built of natural materials. At night, the renters of the two homes on the property encouraged use of the cob house and garden for neighbourhood gather-ings. During the day, it was frequently used by neighbours as a refuge from the nearby clamorous commercial neighbourhood.

When a group of neighbours protested the impending redevelopment of the prop-erty, the city Parks Board offered to buy it from the developer at full market value—more than he had paid. He refused the offer and proceeded with his plans to build the two large duplexes, which would obliterate Salsbury Garden.[44] The Vancouver City Planner approved the developer's plans, which required variance of local zoning restric-tions. The neighbourhood group then launched a last-ditch appeal to Vancouver's Board of Variance, a city panel that rules on exceptions to building and zoning by-laws.

The neighbourhood group prepared an elaborate presentation to the Board of Variance, which included a mock-up of the garden, including each tree and bush made to scale, and a mock-up of the proposed duplexes. The main thrusts of the group's claim were that the garden served as an important refuge for the neighbourhood, that the garden played an important role in the aesthetic and social integrity of the immediate area, and that the two small 1907 vintage homes on the property should be protected as heritage sites. Technical arguments about specific by-laws were also advanced.

After a long hearing, the Board of Variance denied the developer the right to proceed with his plan by a three-to-one vote, to the surprise and delight of the 50 or so neighbours who had stuffed themselves into the municipal meeting room. This decision appeared to leave the developer little option but to sell his property to the city at market value. The neighbours began preparing proposals for the future of this parcel of land that the city would soon own. On a tiny scale, a group of non-native people had successfully made what could be called a 'land claim' on the basis of the land's historic role in the psychosocial integration in their neighbourhood.[45]

This story is reminiscent of many other heartening accounts of local people in the developed world finding a way to draw land out of the control of the market. People often find that they can make their own decisions and provide for their needs better outside the reach of profit-oriented developers and market forces. Not only are their needs met, but their psychosocial integration is enhanced.[46]. However, it is naïve to expect developers and corporations always to wave goodbye to profits without a fight. Quite often, laws and procedures have been changed to reinforce real estate markets against legitimate land claims by the people. When this happens, people must be prepared to persevere.

Shortly after this successful land claim in Vancouver, the city council fired the entire Board of Variance.[47] On appeal from the developer, the British Columbia Supreme Court reversed the decision of the previous Board of Variance and ruled that it had exceeded its jurisdiction to hear third-party appeals; that is, appeals from anyone other than the land's legal owner, in this case, the developer. This legal decision removed an avenue for appealing development that had become well established in the city over 40 years.[48]

Shocked that their attempt to save Salsbury Garden had resulted in removal of an avenue for appealing urban development for the entire city, the group of neighbours has now brought a legal action to the Court of Appeals, which in British Columbia can overturn Supreme Court decisions. The group, which calls itself Reinstate Third-Party Appeals, formerly known as Friends of Salsbury Garden, is able to go to court because of a lawyer who is contributing his time, and because of cash donations from other citizens. There is no hope of saving Salsbury Garden now—it was excavated to build the new duplexes—but there is a reasonable hope of preserving the right of citizens in the future to petition the Board of Variance to protect their neighbourhoods from the ravages of profit-driven urban development.

As this book goes to press, the Court of Appeals has not yet ruled on the neighbours' petition. It has instead adjourned to consider a procedural motion from the developer's legal staff to the effect that the neighbourhood group did not have the legal standing to petition because it had failed to fill out some required documents before the case came to court. Ironically, it appears that the main blockade to non-native land claims, as was the case prior to 1997 with native claims, is not the issue of justice but the technicalities over whether a claim *can even be made* in court.

Clearly, the law governing native and non-native land claims is structured and interpreted to serve the interests of the free-market rather than those of local communities. We have the power to change this situation by concerted action, but the experience of the Nisga'a and the Reinstate Third-Party Appeals group show how much effort will be required.

Reviving community art

The arts are more than just entertainment. They also provide a necessary part of the imagery that holds communities together, contributing to people's sense of identity and shared meaning. Artists from local communities played a major role in psychosocial integration before their function was largely usurped by mass-produced entertainment, with its glossy professionalism, instant availability, and its eerie capacity to create the illusion of local reality—people often discuss media personalities as if they were neighbours. Like the news media, mass-produced entertainment is richly subsidised by commercial advertisers. Community art struggles to compete with those high-budget production standards.

If dislocation is to be brought under control, community art must assume its central function again, enriching people's awareness of their real neighbours and their own local issues. At the beginning of the 21st century, successful community art projects are being launched in many areas of the world with this aim in mind.[49] Local granting agencies provide funds to support these ventures and local people participate enthusiastically.

Community art is not art therapy.[50] It is art integrated with community interests and concerns, leading to productions and events that celebrate, commemorate, and educate. Unlike art therapy, it does not put people into the roles of providers and consumers of psychotherapy, but into the role of community members who nourish important ideas and social connections through the medium of each other's creativity.

The emerging role of community art in Vancouver's Downtown Eastside provides an example. Although it contains the highly publicised Hastings Corridor with its open-air drug and sex markets, most of the Downtown Eastside is made up of ordinary residential areas, stores, and light industry.[51] The Downtown Eastside is the oldest area of the city, situated near the waterfront where the first permanent European residents settled in 1862. It has a rich aboriginal, immigrant, and working-class history, although many of its residents are poor and it has long been a dumping ground for the city's problems.[52] Threatened with extinction by a major freeway and urban renewal project in the 1960s,[53] the area united in political protest and defeated the proposal. The great majority of people in the Downtown Eastside would not think of patronising the notorious drug and sex markets of the Hastings Corridor.

The Downtown Eastside is a safe and friendly urban area for the most part, although the Hastings Corridor runs through it and people sometimes find used needles and condoms on the nearby streets and school yards.[54] Dislocation in the Downtown Eastside has increased in recent decades as the gap between rich and poor has widened and as gentrification has demolished community landmarks and affordable housing. Homelessness is increasingly visible.[55] Sensationalised publicity about the Hastings Corridor stigmatises the entire Downtown Eastside.

A series of community art initiatives have been carried out in recent years in the Downtown Eastside for and by local residents with support from professional artists and community organisations.[56] Public performances, art and media projects, and festivals foster community solidarity and draw the Downtown Eastside into the larger cultural life of the city. Art galleries are currently flourishing in the Downtown Eastside, which has the advantage of low commercial rents.

There has been a discernible shift in the ambiance of the Downtown Eastside and even—to my amazement—in the Hastings Corridor. While addictive misery, poverty, and open-air drug and sex markets still dominate several city blocks, many Hastings Corridor residents are now enjoying—and producing—community art, as well as participating in forums, classes, and social activism. Although addictive misery has certainly not disappeared from the Hastings Corridor, community art seems to be supplanting some of the dislocation that underlies it.[57]

Vancouver Moving Theatre provides one example of this artistic development. A successful theatre company founded in 1983 by Terry Hunter and Savannah Walling, Vancouver Moving Theatre turned its attention from international touring to community art in the mid 1990s when it began producing a neighbourhood festival.[58] It then proved that theatrical art could flourish on a larger scale by co-producing[59] a community play, *In the Heart of a City*, with the participation of a variety of arts professionals and granting agencies. This 2003 play was inspired by stories from the Downtown Eastside and was performed by over 80 people involved in the area, most of whom had never performed before. Some of the performers were either drug-addicted or undergoing recovery as they rehearsed and performed. Over 2000 volunteers were involved in every aspect of play creation, including research and skill-building workshops, working backstage, building sets, writing, and performing. *In the Heart of a City* played to sold-out houses for eight performances and left the performers and the audiences—including the city's mayor—amazed at what had occurred.[60]

Since 2003, four annual Heart of the City Festivals followed,[61] with interactive events, performances, and workshops spread over several days. By 2006, this annual festival had grown to include 95 events at 28 locations over a 2-week period.

Following *In the Heart of a City* in 2003, some cast members proposed doing a play about addiction. With this and other inspirations,[62] Vancouver Moving Theatre and its partner organisations undertook the project. The eventual result was a spectacular shadow-theatre play about addiction called *We're All in This Together*[63] that ran for eight performances in April 2007. A shadow screen 5 m high and 6 m wide presented the central images of the play as moving shadow pictures (see Figure 15.1 here and in the colour section). The actors performed and sang at the front of the stage or behind the screen so that their enlarged, projected shadows formed part of the moving images. The overall effect of this staging was quite magical.[64]

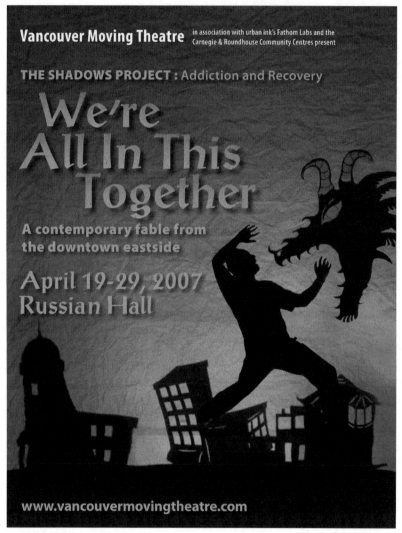

Figure. 15.1 Programme cover for *We're All in This Together*. (Courtesy of Vancouver Moving Theatre. Image conception: John Endo Greenaway and Terry Hunter. Graphic design and photography: John Endo Greenaway. Shadow images: Tamara Unroe. Actor: Michael McNeeley.)

In front of the shadow screen, audiences learned about addiction and recovery from the viewpoint of people from the Downtown Eastside. Personal addiction problems were linked to cultural history and dislocation. At points, the imagery was violent, such as when a local politician, a boss drug dealer, and a pharmaceutical manufacturer smacked their lips over a metaphorical barbecue of human flesh. At other points it was gentle, such as when the recovering mother of a fractured family sang a lullaby to her little girl who had been frightened by the addictive dragons lurking in the basement of their home—and the mother sang herself to sleep as well.[65] The original music was sophisticated, the professional musicians were excellent, and the amateur singing was entrancing.[66]

Developing the play over a 3-year period involved frequent meetings between writers, performers, and back-stage crew; workshops on various skills, including avant-garde shadow-theatre techniques, writing, and digital media; public previews and forums as the play was coming together; and a collaborative effort to produce a 24-page souvenir programme, the cover of which appears in Figure 15.1. Behind the scenes, the professional producers worked constantly on funding, advertising, casting, interpersonal conflicts, and shadow-theatre technology.

Serious obstacles and challenges might be expected in such a situation, and they did arise. Key professionals, including the original director, stage manager, and composer, eventually left the project for other commitments. The project lost some cast members who were overwhelmed by troubling memories unearthed by the play. A lead singer left a week before opening night and was hurriedly replaced. Sometimes cultural differences, communication difficulties, and jealousies erupted. Some of the participants were on medications or illegal drugs, some were in recovery, some had serious trouble being on time.

Talking circles, rehearsal rules created by the participants, advice from staff and counsellors, and the shared sense of mission helped the troupe contain these problems. Meanwhile, the time that was needed for producing an extremely complex show was running out.[67] There were several points in the 3-year development of the play when it might have died, but the importance of the project and the enthusiasm of the participants brought it to completion.

In spite of its hurdles, the play was a resounding success. As the word spread, audiences kept increasing until the final four performances were sold out, with some extra patrons sitting in the aisles while others had to be turned away at the door. Enthusiastic reviews appeared in the theatre sections of most Vancouver newspapers and on theatrical websites.

It is impossible to measure the effects of the play on psychosocial integration in the Downtown Eastside, but something amazing definitely had occurred. Participants, some of whose lives had been extremely chaotic, found the discipline to perform with dedication, passion, and conviction. Some found new friendships and a renewed sense of belonging in the community and of their own strength. Within the 3 months following the play, some of the troupe joined other theatrical projects, applied for arts-related jobs, created new arts projects, published poems, or became involved in community activism.

The psychosocial impact appears to have reached beyond the Downtown Eastside. Whereas some audience members from outside the area experienced a view of addiction that surprised them, others found a mirror of their own past, affirming the strengths as well as the weaknesses of addicted people. Normal social markers seemed to dissolve in the discussion circles of performers and audience members that were organised after each performance. It was as if the people had forgotten the conventional distinction of addicted versus non-addicted. Rather, they spoke as citizens of a distressed city with shared concerns and ideas to work over together.

The best data on the effect of the show on psychosocial integration came from audience feedback forms. Analysis of these forms left no doubt that audiences were seeing the performers empathetically and were listening, as neighbours do, to each other's ideas about shared concerns.[68]

Cultural fusion

Vancouver can never return to the 'good old days' of cultural solidarity that are imaginable in some other localities, because it has never had a deeply rooted culture. In its century and a half of existence, it has always been an immigrant city. Even today, few Vancouverites were actually born in Vancouver.[69] Vancouver's (and Canada's) self-concept in recent decades has been that of a multicultural society in which each ethnic group preserves its particular heritage, with the collection of diverse ethnicities forming a harmonious polity.[70]

However, although multiculturalism gives Vancouver a wonderfully tolerant, cosmopolitan atmosphere, it has not controlled dislocation, in part because all ethnic traditions break down rapidly in free-market society. People need secure places in a stable, integrated society, not just respectable ethnic identities at school, work, and the shopping centres.

Multiculturalism needs to be augmented by new cultural forms that reinforce and ultimately replace the older ethnic traditions that are breaking down. Present-day Vancouver offers an amazing array of opportunities for cultural fusion. There are community centres, cooperatives, block parties, neighbourhood festivals, sports teams, unions, churches, and on and on. There is little ethnic discrimination to keep people from participating. The ultimate antidote to widespread dislocation could turn out to be a unique Vancouver cultural blend comprising dozens of ethnicities, religions, and races, none of which predominates·

On the first sunny day in May a few years ago, walking through my multicultural neighbourhood in East Vancouver, I came upon a group of early teenage girls demonstrating cultural fusion in full flower. The tallest and most striking of the girls was African, a couple of others were Asian, one was white, and the remaining three or four, possibly children of mixed marriages, filled out the spectrum of human skin tones. This group had no shared history. It was a mixture of mixtures. Yet in the warmth of new sunshine after the usual sodden Vancouver winter, the girls were playing and joking with each other in a relaxed and quite hilarious way, as if they had belonged together for generations.

I felt sure in that vivid moment that human culture cannot be annihilated by any degree of dislocation, repression, or heterogeneity whatsoever, because it regenerates itself anew in a way that is as irrepressible as springtime. Cultural history should be honoured and preserved, but the roots of culture do not lie only in the past. They lie in the future as well, as long as they can be allowed to propagate freely. It may be that only new cultural creations can crowd out the roots of addiction in multicultural societies.

Cultural fusion in Fort Ware

Although settling native land claims must have high priority for dealing with the horrendous problem of native dislocation and addiction, as discussed earlier in this chapter, no native culture can be restored to what it was because the social milieu and the earth itself have changed in the last century. Fort Ware, also known as Kwadacha, is a remote Indian reserve that is home to about 300 Sekani and Kaska people. It serves as a case study of how native people can both preserve elements of their former way of life and benefit from cultural fusion. Although Fort Ware is remote, it is economically linked at the most fundamental level with metropolitan Vancouver.

The nomadic ancestors of the people who now live in Fort Ware hunted, fished, trapped, camped, and buried their dead in the northern river valleys for uncounted centuries. Far from Vancouver and other European settlements, those who lived in the Finlay and Parsnip River valleys maintained something close to their traditional way of life until the middle of the 20th century. They exchanged furs for supplies with white traders and sometimes worked in logging and mining industries during the short summers. They spent the long, subarctic winters with their families, on their land, re-assembling in larger tribal groups each spring. Their problems increased in the 1930s when non-native outsiders infiltrated their valleys to survive the Great Depression by trapping, and increased further between 1940 and 1970 when many children were forced to attend residential schools, returning transformed. In the meantime, fur prices fell sharply. The situation collapsed between 1968 and 1971 when a major part of the lands where these native people had lived were permanently flooded by Williston Lake Reservoir, the largest hydroelectric reservoir in the world at the time of its construction.

The native people who lived in these areas were not consulted about the construction of the dam, and many could not comprehend that their land would be permanently flooded.[71] When the rivers overflowed their previous banks and kept on coming, the people had to move to higher ground. There was at least one drowning and several near drownings in the new, debris-filled lake.

The inexpensive electricity from the Bennett Dam at the foot of the enormous Williston Lake Reservoir now keeps the electrical gadgets in Vancouver homes humming and whirring, and the city's businesses competitive. Much of it is sold in international markets far to the south, enriching California as well as British Columbia. Although large areas of the people's land were not flooded by Williston Lake Reservoir, this remainder has been exploited by extensive clear-cut logging, mining, and commercial big-game hunting. Although the land still holds great symbolic meaning for these formerly nomadic people, they no longer live on it. Many now reside permanently in Fort Ware and a few other widely scattered reserves. Like other reserves, Fort Ware suffers from chronic alcoholism and domestic violence and the native people are badly demoralised much of the time. The children speak English and show limited enthusiasm for their own native language.

At present, the village of Fort Ware struggles to enforce alcohol and drug prohibition. Bootlegged liquor must travel 420 km over unpaved logging roads from the nearest highway, but it gets through. The dedicated principal[72] and teachers of the Aatse Davie School are having better success as they work to keep the children in class. Some native women and men from the reserve, including Victor McCook, a son of the long-time chief,[73] work in the classrooms alongside university-trained teachers, who are either white or native people from other places. The teachers find ways to teach reading and writing, although many of their students' lives are regularly interrupted by family dysfunction and violence.[74] The first graduate of the school, Angie Hocken, completed grade 12 on 21 June 2006, National Aboriginal Day in Canada. The following June there were three graduates.

Beyond the school, other endeavours have been introduced to Fort Ware in an effort to honour the people's connection to the land. Despite strong opposition from the provincial Ministry of Forests, Donald Gordon, a builder and community activist from Vancouver, was able to access conservation funding in 1996–1997 to survey and restore a network of communally owned cabins and 140 km of trails through the land, with the aid of native people who remembered the traditions. The Fort Ware school provides funds for an annual 'Sudze K'anusta [I am looking into my heart] Rediscovery Project', in which Sekani elders and guides and youth from the school make extended backpacking trips into the land on the forest trails, literally walking in the footsteps of their ancestors. Both elders and youth participate enthusiastically, feeling their personal strength during long days on the trails and sharing ideas around nightly campfires. This project has now run every year since 1997.

On my first visit to Fort Ware in 2005, I witnessed a startling fusion of aboriginal and Korean culture. The Kwadacha Dene Taekwon-Do club was established in Fort Ware in September 2002 by Robert Derkson,[75] a psychological counsellor who grew up in the suburbs of Vancouver. It was led until a year ago by Derkson and by another black-belt, Gerald MacIsaac, who lives on another reserve. Having sweated through a few years of martial arts training myself as a younger man, I was able to appreciate the skills of the youths who I saw leaping, punching, kicking, and responding to verbal commands in English and Korean. Four of the students, including one who dropped out of elementary school at an early age, have been awarded black belts by the Canadian Taekwon-Do Federation, even though they had been training for little more than 3 years at the time they took the test in the city of Prince George. Fourteen students attended their first competition against other clubs away from the reserve in 2003 at the Western Canada Taekwon-Do Championships. The 14 students brought home 17 medals, five of them gold! The students have since attended several other prestigious tournaments and each time brought home more than their share of medals.[76] People in the village have supported the Taekwon-Do Club wholeheartedly. The students practise at home with diligence, sometimes amusing their parents who tease them about all the huffing and puffing.

Taekwon-Do is much more than a technique for winning fights. Much of the training involves formalised movements that require intense personal discipline and regular practice outside of class. Some of the moves involve feats of strength and agility that cannot be accomplished without intense physical conditioning. Most importantly, perhaps, Taekwon-Do requires a social and spiritual commitment as well as physical discipline. Students who have attended tournaments have received recognition and praise from the officials present for their discipline as well as their outstanding performances. The ideal that the students are learning is formalised in the official Taekwon-Do Student Oath, which the students recite, loud and clear, during each training session. The oath recognises virtues of courtesy, integrity, perseverance, self-control, spirit, and respect.

Since 2005, other projects that embody cultural fusion have been established. For example, several of the students have taken advantage of new electronic technology to become involved with film-making under the guidance of a talented artist who teaches in the school.[77] Several adults belong to a historical discussion group organised by a white scholar who taught adult education classes at the reserve school years earlier and is now married to a local band member. There is a hope of putting together a definitive version of a complex past that fuses history written in the Western traditions with oral history that extends much further back.[78] Of course, none of this makes much difference if the people of Fort Ware cannot find a sustainable basis for individual and cultural survival. This basis can only come from confronting the corporate and political interests that have thus far felt little compunction about devastating their land. Political action will be required that can draw its power from a functioning native community, the larger aboriginal movements in Canada, and … us.

What will the future look like in Fort Ware? This question cannot be answered now. But there is room for hope that it will be led by visionaries who understand the dangers of dislocation, backed by a government that knows it must be as concerned with its people as with its gross domestic product, inspired by arts with diverse ethnic origins, and embedded in history carefully preserved by people who were once in danger of forgetting it.

Rewriting drug laws

Some people passionately believe that stringent prohibition of illicit drugs protects society from moral collapse, whereas others believe with equal passion that some form of 'legalisation'[79] is long overdue because the existing regime of drug prohibition affronts human rights and dignity. The perennial, high-tension conflict between these two positions has generated far more heat than light.

The prohibition versus legalisation conflict was characterised in Chapter 3 of this book as a false dichotomy.[80] I did not mean to trivialise the truly important issues that underlay the conflict or to impugn the sincerity of the participants. The dichotomy becomes false, however, when prohibition and legalisation are rhetorically puffed up into rival ways of controlling addiction, since, in fact, neither can have much effect on the addiction problem. As Chapters 2 and 3 showed, drug addiction is only a small corner of the addiction$_3$ problem. Moreover, imposing and repealing prohibition has repeatedly been shown to have little effect on overall levels of drug consumption.[81] Finally, since the demon-possession myth about drugs is false, occasional successes in legally preventing drug experimentation in children are unlikely to have any effect on whether or not the children grow up to be addicted. In sum, none of the prohibition and legalisation policies that are now so hotly debated have the power to deter the globalisation of addiction.

There is, however, at least one way of resolving the conflict over prohibition and legalisation that could foster psychosocial integration and might thereby ameliorate the problem of addiction to some extent and solve some other problems. The current debate over marijuana legalisation in Canada and the history of the 1878 Canada Temperance Act will provide the main examples.

The marijuana prohibition debate cannot be resolved in Canada because the general population is about evenly split on this issue.[82] Moreover, the topic is not really a debatable one. The health arguments that are typically advanced on both sides seem little more than overworked debating rituals. The competing values, tastes, and metaphysics that underlie and energise the debate are rarely mentioned, and could not be resolved rationally if they were. The conflict is more akin to a holy war than to a rational discussion. It has been going on since the 1960s.

A model for resolving this problem can be found in the Canada Temperance Act of 1878.[83] This resolution is sometimes called 'local option'. The Canada Temperance Act was introduced in an era when conflict was as deep and fierce over liquor as it currently is over marijuana. The Act empowered counties and municipalities to prohibit alcohol consumption by majority vote. After prohibition had been in force for 3 years, it could be upheld or rescinded by another referendum.[84] Many referenda were held under the Act in the 19th and early 20th centuries. Sometimes prohibition was enacted, sometimes not. Often prohibition was tried for a while and then rescinded by a later referendum. In general, prohibition was more likely to be imposed in the eastern Maritime Provinces and in rural areas and was less likely to be imposed in the west and in the large cities.[85]

When prohibition was established under the rubric of the Canada Temperance Act, it usually did not have the violent qualities of current drug legislation.[86] For example, the Act provided that, wherever alcohol was prohibited, alcoholic products could still be distributed legally for medicinal, sacramental, and industrial purposes through a pharmacist designated for this purpose, with the number of such pharmacists to be limited.[87]

Allowing medicinal, sacramental, and industrial use of alcohol obviously made it possible for a highly motivated person to obtain alcohol for recreational and addictive purposes. There were other loopholes as well. For example, the Act allowed people within a locality that had imposed prohibition to manufacture wine and sell it to others who were taking it out of that jurisdiction for consumption elsewhere.[88] Nonetheless, all indications are that alcohol prohibition, where it was introduced, helped to establish a clear definition of the prevailing community standards and might have reduced the amount of alcohol consumption that took place to some extent. That is to say, prohibition under the Canada Temperance Act was about as effective as prohibition under the War on Drugs, but less violent.

It took almost a century after the introduction of the Act for the alcohol situation to finally stabilise in Canada. In the meantime, Canada saw alcohol prohibition come and go in many municipalities, counties, and provinces. There was no national prohibition except for a single year during World War I when it was introduced to conserve grain for the war effort.[89] Today, every city and province allows consumption of alcohol, although some native reserves and other isolated areas still maintain alcohol prohibition. The rules by which alcohol use is controlled have become fairly standard but there are still some local variations.

Introducing a modern form of the Canada Temperance Act for marijuana would require Canada to disregard international pressure to continue imposing an unenforceable total prohibition.[90] Equally importantly, it would enable Canada to avoid the backlash that national legalisation of marijuana would inevitably produce, since a major proportion of the population is passionately opposed to any form of drug legalisation.

A modern form of the Act applied to marijuana would provide local communities with a legal framework that would enable communities to debate this divisive social issue meaningfully and to experiment with a variety of regulatory structures. Although a Canada Temperance Act for marijuana would undoubtedly see prohibition enacted in some, or perhaps most, localities, it would have nothing in common with a war on drugs. Where prohibition was enacted, the medicinal uses of marijuana would be exempted. This exemption is required by natural justice, because of the proven necessity of marijuana treatment for certain serious conditions, including glaucoma and nausea induced by chemotherapy. Sacramental and educational uses of marijuana would also be exempted, if they can be justified.[91] Marijuana prohibition laws would not have harsh penalties or mandatory minimum sentences. They would draw their legitimacy from local communities, rather than from a distant federal or global bureaucracy. And, if a locality rethought the issue, it could change its law through another referendum.

The final outcome of local option over marijuana laws cannot be foreseen. Perhaps different localities would gradually establish a patchwork of local traditions of tolerance or prohibition, and people with strong feelings on the issue could gravitate to communities with marijuana laws that suited them. The majority of people for whom marijuana laws are a matter of little concern would continue to live comfortably both in communities that prohibited and in those that legalised it. Alternatively, Canada might, in the end, establish a consensus somewhere between prohibition and legalisation that would be embedded in encompassing federal legislation. Whatever the outcome, the process would be democratic and the ability of localities to function as political units would be strengthened.

It could be argued that a small town that decided to impose marijuana prohibition under this legal regime would have no possibility of enforcing it if the surrounding jurisdictions did not, but this argument overlooks an essential point. Marijuana laws are not enforceable now, nor have they been in the past, even where people are subjected to very severe penalties. For example, marijuana use was virtually unknown in Canada in 1923 when it was first made illegal. It established a place in Canadian society only after it was banned. The current high levels of consumption first occurred after 1961 when marijuana was subjected to the same draconian and vigorously enforced laws as heroin and cocaine under the Narcotic Control Act, including life sentences for marijuana trafficking.[92] At the other extreme, the essential decriminalisation of marijuana use in England in 2004 did not lead to an increase in marijuana use, but to a small decline.[93]

Although drug prohibition laws are not enforceable, they can nonetheless serve an important social purpose. Prohibition laws are a way that a village, city, county, or province can express a consensus about its values that it espouses to its children and to those who respect its standards.[94] Perhaps recognising this symbolic function, penalties specified by the Canada Temperance Act for jurisdictions that imposed alcohol prohibition were mild. Under the Act, the maximum penalty for trafficking in alcohol, which could be imposed only on a third or subsequent offence, was no more than 2 months in prison.[95] This law was not part of a war on drugs, but an instrument for managing a deep social conflict in a way that was attuned to ethnic and temperamental diversity. It facilitated the evolution of a national consensus about the way alcohol should be regulated.

'What can I do about addiction from the perspective of the dislocation theory?' You can refuse to be distracted by the shouting match over prohibition and legalisation of drugs, particularly marijuana, and instead respect the legitimacy of people's opposing feelings and beliefs about drugs. Where the pubic divisions over drugs are deep and symbolic, you can look for a way to accommodate both sides. Drugs are not important enough in the larger addiction problem to be the object of a holy war. Instead, they are simply one powerful technology among many that modern society must learn to use and regulate wisely.

Reclaiming Christianity

Ever since the American Christian right discovered that Jesus loves the American Way of Life and hates Communism, its flamboyant and highly publicised actions have reinforced the impression that Christian faith is linked to free-market zealotry. For example, it seemed somehow natural in 2005 that prominent televangelist and presidential candidate Pat Robertson urged the assassination of Hugo Chavez, President of Venezuela and friend of Fidel Castro, by American covert operatives. (Later, under pressure from the world press, Robertson retracted his statement, explaining that he had spoken out of 'frustration'.[96])

Despite the visibility of the American Christian right, however, the great majority of Christians are addicted neither to American power nor to the Market God. On the contrary, some of the people who are most involved in domesticating free-market society are pious Christians.[97] Their mission finds at least as much support in the Christian Bible as does the mission of the Christian right.

Because Christianity is globalizing almost as quickly as free-market society, Christians who work to domesticate free-market society and to re-establish Christianity as a religion of compassion and fellowship have an especially important role to play. 'What can I do about addiction as viewed from the perspective of the dislocation theory?' If you are a Christian, you can work with a variety of Christian organisations to reclaim your faith from those who would make it a tool of a skewed economic system that destroys human fellowship.

The Bible is politically ambiguous because it is not a political document, but a spiritual one. In the years before World War II, there were important organisations of Christian Social Democrats, Christian Socialists, and Christian Fascists, in addition to the Christian supporters of hypercapitalism.[98] In today's world, the citizen's movement for curtailing the excesses of free-market society includes many Catholic and Protestant Christian groups, some of them evangelical.[99]

Ignacio Martín-Baró, an influential Jesuit priest and a psychologist, took a strong position against hypercapitalism that is diametrically opposite to that of the Christian right. Martín-Baró studied theology in Spain, but served most of his priesthood in El Salvador until his death in 1989. He was a devout Roman Catholic who joined the Latin American movement called 'liberation theology'. He was also a prolific writer, although most of his work is available only in Spanish.[100] Martín-Baró's formulation of liberation theology sets a high standard for Christians who want to do something about addiction.

Like the people that St Augustine served in ancient Rome, the poor *campesinos* that Martín-Baró served in El Salvador were suffering under a brutal, imperial regime. The imperial oppression that Martín-Baró confronted was imposed by national governments in El Salvador and elsewhere in Central and South America that derived their power from American financial support and military force. These governments used their power to impose free-market economics and to enable American corporations to exploit local oil and gas, minerals, oil, bananas, coffee, and labour.[101]

The misery that free-market colonialism caused for *campesinos* during Martín-Baró's lifetime was multifaceted, but, in the context of this book, the most important facet was the dislocation. Martín-Baró himself argued at some points that dislocation was the most harmful aspect of the oppression that surrounded him, even though it was less visibly gruesome than the murder, torture, and starvation.[102]

Dislocation had many causes in Martín-Baró's world: protracted rebellions, systematic dispossession of *campesinos* whose land had become commercially valuable, destruction of coca and marijuana crops in support of the American War on Drugs, and desperate migrations to distant urban slums or other countries. Beyond actual displacement from their homes, people became dislocated as their rural traditions were overwhelmed by urban and foreign institutions, including North American evangelical churches that competed successfully with the existing mixture of Roman Catholicism and folk religion.[103]

Dislocated *campesinos* suffered from diverse addiction problems, including alcoholism, drug addiction, religious zealotry, and political fanaticism.[104] Although Martín-Baró mentioned addiction problems often, they were not his sole concern. He recognised addiction as one of several psychological problems caused by the oppression of the *campesinos*.[105]

Like Polanyi, Martín-Baró directed his attention to the misery caused by the imposition of free-market society on rural people. Whereas Polanyi analysed the problem from the viewpoint of an economic theorist working to reform the world economic system, Martín-Baró approached the problem as a priest and a psychologist. He focused his attention on local people struggling to find collective strength to resist the oppression that afflicted them. Rather than trying to rebalance or domesticate free-market society, Martín-Baró left the form of the new world that he dreamed of to the collective instincts of ordinary people, once the burden of oppression was lifted.

Martín-Baró's theology differed from that of the American Christian right and from St Augustine's in several profound ways. First, Martín-Baró's liberation theology put the primary emphasis on ordinary earthly existence, rather than the bliss of heaven or of the City of God. As Martín-Baró put it:

> The object of Christian faith is a God of life and, therefore ... a Christian must accept the promotion of life as his or her primordial religious task. From this Christian perspective, what is opposed to faith in God is not atheism but rather idolatry; that is, the belief in false gods, gods which produce death.[106]

Like the other liberation theologists, Martín-Baró emphasised the 'preferential option for the poor'. He believed that Jesus was intensely concerned with the suffering of the poor and that the fullest Christian experience comes only through working amongst the poor:

> The theology of liberation affirms that one has to look for God among the poor and marginalized, and with them and from them live the life of faith. There are multiple reasons for this option. In the first place, that was, concretely, the option of Jesus. Second, the poor constitute the majority of our peoples. But third, it is only the poor who offer the objective and subjective conditions for opening up to the other, and above all, to the radically other. The option for the poor is not opposed to universal salvation, but it recognizes that the community of the poor is the theological place *par excellence* for achieving the task of salvation, the construction of the Kingdom of God.[107]

The 'preferential option for the poor' is a very different concept from 'Christian charity'. Beyond helping people to find their individual sources of faith and morality, Martín-Baró stood with the poor in their collective efforts to relieve the oppression imposed on them by governments and corporations dominated by other sorts of Christians. He intended to persuade those who oppressed the poor where possible, but to resist those who would not be persuaded with all the political power that aroused citizens could muster. He believed that these efforts would ultimately benefit the oppressors as much as the oppressed.

Unlike St Augustine, Martín-Baró did not conceive of sin only in terms of personal weakness and failure, but also as a consequence of social injustice. He identified social injustice itself as a sin:

> The Christian faith in a God of life ... demands a first step of liberating the structures— the social structures first, and next the personal ones—that maintain a situation of sin; that is, of the mortal oppression of the majority of the people.[108]

Martín-Baró's formulation of liberation theology emphasized social action over personal piety:

> Actions are more important than affirmations in liberation theology, and what one does is more expressive of faith than what one says. Therefore, the truth of faith must be shown in historical achievements that give evidence of and make credible the existence of a God of life. In this context, everything becomes meaningful that mediates the possibility of people's liberation from the structures that oppress and impede their life and human development.[109]

Martín-Baró had a radically different view of pride and self-confidence than St Augustine. Where St Augustine railed against his own pride as the worst of sins, Martín-Baró saw the loss of pride and self-confidence among the *campesinos* as a state that is caused by, and sustains, social injustice. He sought to restore wholesome pride:

> The predominantly negative image that the average Latin American has of himself or herself when compared with other people ... indicates the internalisation of oppression, its incorporation into the spirit itself; fertile soil for conformist fatalism, and so very convenient for the established order.[110]

In sum, both St Augustine and Martín-Baró were horrified by the poverty of the spirit that they saw in worlds dominated by decadent, corrupt empires. Although both were pious Christians, their responses to the horrors were dramatically different. St Augustine saw the Roman Empire as so powerful that it must be a manifestation of God, and believed that people could only find happiness through escape from mundane life into otherworldly godliness. Martín-Baró, by contrast, concluded that nothing as cruel as the exploitation that he witnessed could possibly be the will of God. Therefore, he believed that God would approve the struggle to relieve the oppression of the poor, and, although he remained a priest and a university professor, he joined in the struggle himself.

Unfortunately, he was destroyed before his mission was complete. The university residence that was shared by Martín-Baró, five other Jesuit professors, a female housekeeper, and the housekeeper's daughter at the campus of the Central American University was invaded by a Salvadorian death squad on 16 November 1989. All eight residents were shot to death. At the time, Martín-Baró, then aged 47, was Chairman of the Psychology Department and Vice Rector for academic affairs at the university.[111] The death squad was formally known as the Atlacatl Battalion, an elite Salvadorian unit that had been created, trained, and equipped at the US Army School of Special Forces, beginning in 1981.[112]

Liberation theology did not die with Martín-Baró or with its other martyrs. In 2007, on the eve of a visit to Brazil by Pope Benedict XVI, an outspoken opponent of liberation theology throughout his career, a *New York Times* reporter investigated the current status of liberation theology in Brazil. He discovered that there are about 80,000 liberation theology 'base communities' in present-day Brazil, despite the opposition of many current Brazilian bishops. Base communities are the grass-roots building blocks of the liberation theology movement. They meet in poor areas to hold religious ceremonies, to plan demonstrations and petitions, to pressure local governments for adequate sanitation facilities in their neighbourhoods, to cooperate with labour unions, and to develop Christian anti-neoliberal philosophy. In addition to the base communities, there are about a million 'Bible circles' in Brazil that meet regularly to discuss scripture from the viewpoint of liberation theology. A liberation theology activist explained their activities this way:

> We believe in merging the questions of faith and social action ... We advise groups and social movements, mobilize the unemployed, and work with unions and parties, always from a perspective based on the Gospel.[113]

In South America, joining liberation theology is as simple as locating the nearest active group. Christianity in the rich countries has perhaps not yet risen to challenge free-market society as often as it has in the poor countries. Perhaps this is because the problem is more subtle in the rich countries. Poverty of the spirit in the rich countries is clearly not restricted to the poor and oppressed, so the simple rhetoric of social class is not as helpful. Moreover, the major Christian religions seem to be controlled by those who will not support social action against the causes of dislocation, although they support Christian charity. It is not for me to offer advice to Christians of rich countries on resolving these dilemmas. If their God is truly benevolent, there is a solution, and they know how and where to look for inspiration.

Outflanking the university

I write these critical thoughts on universities with some anxiety. It might seem that I have forgotten the kindnesses that my old friends and colleagues at Simon Fraser University, some now dead, showed me over the 35 years I worked there, and continue to show me now. But, I can never forget these gifts. I offer this critique to my university and my colleagues with affection and respect.

Arthur Erickson, architect of the Vancouver university where I worked for 35 years, dreamed of a community of scholars atop a small mountain in the rain forest. Because of the climate, he designed the whole university as a single sprawling building that would allow anybody on campus to visit anybody else, without getting soaked in the long winter drizzle. Faculty offices were not to be segregated by department, but rather interspersed to facilitate interdisciplinary exchange. He understood that high-level scholarship requires social interchange as well as solitary exertion.[114]

The dream has faded since his building opened in 1965. As times changed, the university strove harder and harder to fulfil its designated market function by graduating the maximum number of employable experts and conducting profit-oriented research in collaboration with high-tech corporations.[115] These activities occurred under the management of a business-oriented board of directors and ever more market-oriented administrations.[116] University funds from government and business produced a 'research park', set away from the main campus, for proprietary researchers to work in partnership with industry but out of sight of their colleagues. Faculty and students learned to segregate themselves in the pursuit of ever more intensive specialisation, despite the unitized campus.

The university's endowment lands are now being developed as a small city of condominiums, most of which will be sold at market prices to the highest bidders, whether or not they have any connection to the university, while most students must commute up and down the mountain each day in jam-packed busses.[117] Professors are hired less and less for their ability as teachers and scholars, and more and more for their ability to 'attract money' from government and corporate funding agencies. Students are registered for classes with an online programme that rigidifies the system. Class sizes grow steadily, so that the university can graduate more students per unit of professor and teaching-assistant time. This makes it ever more difficult for students to experience the forms of university education that are labour-intensive; for example, dialectical discussion and coaching in writing. These market-oriented lines of development are intended to conserve money for the university, offsetting the continuing reduction in government funding that originally provided financial security.

Simon Fraser now ranks high among middle-sized Canadian universities in number of faculty research grants, student awards, and per capita support for students received from government.[118] The cost of attracting money at this pace can be judged from the students' attitudes. In a 2004 national poll of university students conducted at every university in Canada, Simon Fraser University's students rated it slightly below the median in educational quality (10th out of 17 medium-sized Canadian Universities) and abysmally (17th out of 17) in student services.[119] In more recent polls, Simon Fraser has moved closer to the bottom on measures of student satisfaction.[120]

All this could be changed. The university could be rededicated to the development of a scholarly community that would foster collaborative intellectuality within a campus community. Fees at the university could be kept low enough that entry could be based on talent and motivation, rather than the ability of parents to buy their offspring a ticket to a promising career. Degrees could be awarded for serious study of the foundational ideas of Western culture,[121] in addition to specialized training for a particular line of work. Students could be encouraged to share their knowledge and learn from each other rather than to compete ruthlessly for grades and scholarships. The complex of grades and credits—an academic piecework system—could be discarded. Education cannot be dispensed in independent packages like merchandise. Academic research at the university could be shaped by the needs of local, national, and global society, rather than by professional journals, academic publishers striving to maximise profit,[122] honorary 'chairs' funded by multinational corporations, or grants from governments and corporations whose main concern is economic growth.

The vision of a university proposed here stands on the other side of a chasm from the view of education that grows from free-market ideology. If there is any doubt about the depth of this chasm, it will be removed by a look at economist and Nobel Laureate Milton Friedman's views on education.[123] Because the vision proposed here opposes the vision that derives from free-market ideology, it naturally evokes opposition from the champions of free-market society. In fact, it is probably too late to turn my university from its present course, because its marketised direction has been gradually reinforcing itself for a generation. There is little significant opposition to it left, even among the faculty.

If universities like mine cannot be induced to change their ways substantially, the best strategy to restore balance in higher education may be, I fear, to abandon them to the service of the Market God and to find new venues for high-level scholarship that promote the common interest and psychosocial integration. Although taking over the intellectual and social functions of modern universities without a multimillion-dollar budget may not sound like stark realism, I believe it may be the best alternative, under the prevailing circumstances. Moreover, society can be expected in the long run to recognise the importance of intellectuality that stands outside the strictures of hyper-capitalism and to make sure that efforts to foster the larger form of intellectuality are adequately supported.

Vancouver is the home of a wonderful group of independent scholars, journalists, publishers, photojournalists, political activists, and documentary filmmakers. Together, they constitute a sprawling intellectual bazaar that functions outside the constraints of universities and free-market ideology. Some of the media and organisations within this intellectual community were mentioned earlier in this chapter, and there are many more. Although I might have overrepresented left-wing organisations in that list, this is simply a reflection of my previous associations rather than a deliberate intent. The political left has no patent on intellectual community. A viable intellectual community must welcome the most diverse opinions and must replace the bland apoliticism of universities with impassioned intellectual engagement. A unique resource for Vancouver is scholars who have risen from the large native community, and whose work is both intellectually rigorous and culturally rich in a way that is rare outside the indigenous culture.

Local scholars and institutions such as these produce intellectuality at a level that is, in my experience, often higher and more independent than that of university academics. I think it is a small step from talent like this to a useful institutional structure that could offer critical, non-market-oriented educational programmes at a price that people could afford in a socially integrative setting where words like 'intellectual community' would be more than buzzwords. Naturally, such educational opportunities would be free of credits and grades and other academic impediments. My colleagues Terry Patten, Frank Harris, and I are conducting our own modest experiments on non-market-oriented educational collaboration in the Commercial Drive district of Vancouver with the support of the Britannia Community Centre.

Social action at the global level

The system of government that is wishfully called 'liberal democracy' is failing at the global level even more spectacularly than at local and national levels. Individual people have scant understanding of, or influence on, the international trade agreements, treaties, and military exploits that dislocate their existence and devastate their global environment. The kinds of social action proposed up to this point directly confront these problems, but they cannot turn the tide until many more people participate actively. We cannot politely vote our way out of global dislocation or any of the other disasters that have arisen from free-market society. We cannot petition our way out of them either—who actually cares how many signatures appear on our petitions or how many people join the next protest march? In the language of an overworked phrase, there is no point in 'talking truth to power' when power has a vested interest in blindness and paralysis.[124] However, citizen activists can talk power to power on a global level and, thereby, change the course of events.[125]

Just as the current political system cannot control global dislocation and other crises that face modern civilisation, the economic system cannot solve them either. Since hypercapitalism is the fundamental cause of our worst crises, the belief that 'market solutions', 'voluntary regulations' of corporations, or the charity of billionaires can relieve the crises is bound to be disappointed. Even free-market society functioning at its very best cannot control dislocation. In particular, the welfare state policies that structured much of the Western world between the Great Depression of the 1930s and the 1970s manifested an admirable concern for social justice, but did not address the problems of mass dislocation. Some well-intentioned welfare state policies were as dislocating to their own citizens as current policies of free-market society.[126] Moreover, they generated their own forms of bureaucratic over-control and ideological rigidity.[127] The most pertinent example of the failure of welfare states to cope with dislocation is that many of their governments, led by the United States, reacted to the alarming growth of drug addiction after World War II with moralistic punitiveness. This way of reacting later became known as the War on Drugs.[128]

The structural changes that are needed to rebalance society at the global level do not require political revolution, but they must be very deep. Since neither the current political system nor the free-market economic system is up to the task, they must be forced into a better state of balance by an aroused citizenry. There is no other realistic hope.

Examples of rebalancing that have already occurred in the arena of national and international politics provide beacons of hope for the future. The examples described here are not widely known because they are scarcely reported in the mainstream media. The essential rebalancing may be well underway in Latin America and Europe before it receives any serious attention from conventional news media in countries like Canada.

Political changes in Latin America provide the most dramatic example. Latin America has been politically dominated and exploited for more than a century by the United States, and in earlier centuries by Spain and other European countries. The imposition of dictatorships espousing hypercapitalism accelerated dramatically in the early 1980s with the 'dirty wars' in Chile, Argentina, Uruguay, and Nicaragua, and with the imposition of free-market economics by the International Monetary Fund (IMF) and World Bank. This system enriched transnational corporations and locked the Latin American underclass in a state of escalating destitution. But it is now being overturned.

American 'unilateralism', as it is now being called, was challenged by the Cuban revolution and further disrupted by popular socialist governments in Chile and Nicaragua that were eventually crushed by American military and political intervention. More recently, however, despite huge expenditures and bloodletting, the United States and its domestic allies within Colombia have failed to crush a popular uprising led by workers and indigenous organisations. At the same time, popular movements have helped to establish independent governments in many countries, most visibly Venezuela, Argentina, Brazil, Bolivia, Uruguay, Ecuador, and Nicaragua. Smaller-scale uprisings have succeeded in gaining real political power in Mexico, most famously in the Zapatista movement in Chiapas. These are not orthodox Communist revolutions, but popular, pragmatic movements that are willing to work with capitalist institutions some of the time to achieve their goals. At the highest bureaucratic level, the United States appears to have lost its political control of the Organisation of American States,[129] and six Latin American states have formed a new Bank of the South to replace the ideologically governed IMF and the World Bank.[130]

This vast movement in Latin America finds popular expression in the World Social Forums that have taken place every year since they began in 2001 in Porto Allegro, Brazil. The goals of the diverse groups that participate are sometimes moral, sometimes ecological, sometimes social, sometimes political, sometimes psychological, and sometimes spiritual. The overarching purpose is easily recognisable, however.[131] They seek to domesticate free-market economics. It is quite possible that the leadership in global political change in the 21st century will come from Latin America.[132]

The EU, which had been increasingly dominated by free-market economic policies, appears to have shifted course significantly. In 2005, the proposed new European constitution was defeated in binding referenda, first in France, then in The Netherlands. The defeated constitution was a formula for dislocation, because it made inadequate provision for meaningful democratic representation, social protection, individual dignity, and the maintenance of national traditions.[133] Nevertheless, it was supported by every government in the EU and by all of the major media. This popular refusal of an onerous structural change was brought about by aroused citizens who were informed by small groups of intellectual and professional activists working through the Internet. Only a small number of independent magazines and newspapers publicly argued that social values should take precedence over free-market orthodoxy. This was by no means the first reaction against free-market orthodoxy in the EU, but it was the first time that the opposition had coalesced sufficiently to exert decisive political power. The free-market steamroller was momentarily halted.

Some global actions of the Canadian government during the last decade also show the power of citizen involvement, albeit at a lower level of accomplishment. These include Canada's rejection of the Multilateral Agreement on Investment; refusal to participate in the latest invasion of Iraq with the Americans, British, and Australians; and refusal to overtly participate in the American Ballistic Missile Defense system. Each of these Canadian rejections of free-market policy was influenced by large citizen groups who petitioned the government and took to the streets—and to the Internet—by the thousands. I am proud to have played a tiny role, and I plan to play a larger role in the future, for other struggles are lining up fast. Unfortunately, none of these achievements were final victories and all are reactive, rather than proactive, in character; that is, nothing was accomplished other than slowing further encroachments of a free-market society that has already fragmented every aspect of social life. Yet there is joy in baby steps, for they can mature into firmer strides.

It is urgently necessary to take larger steps at the global level soon. It is not difficult to envision what some of these steps must be, although it will be extremely difficult to achieve them. As with the previous discussion of local and national actions, the problem is not that there are too few answers to the question, 'What can I do about addiction as viewed from the perspective of the dislocation theory?' The problem is that there are too many to fit in this chapter.

The Tobin Tax is one global-level example that can be explained in a brief way. The Tobin Tax is a global tax on all international currency exchange. Global currency exchange amounts to about US$2 trillion in transactions each day, about 80% of which is purely speculative. As currently proposed, the tax rate would not be prohibitive. In fact, it would be extremely low, less than 0.25% of each transaction. Nobel Prize-winning economist James Tobin originally conceived the idea of the tax in 1972 as a measure to reduce the volatility of exchange-rate fluctuations caused by speculative currency trading, which sometimes results in currency crises that impoverish and dislocate people en masse. An influential article by Ignacio Ramonet in 1997 pointed out that implementing the Tobin Tax would have major additional effects. It would assert the authority of world society over the nearly independent free markets in currency. Moreover, the huge tax revenue, more than US$100 billion each year, could be put in the service of reducing social inequalities and dislocation.[134] An international citizens' organisation devoted to implementing the Tobin Tax was established in 1998 and currently has branches operating in about 40 countries.[135] Other organisations and economists have put the Tobin Tax high on their agendas. Economists generally agree that the tax can be implemented with existing technology. Although the Tobin

Tax has many public supporters, including billionaire financier George Soros,[136] it has still not been enacted 10 years after it became a major public issue. However, it can be enacted with additional citizen involvement and pressure.

Additional tax measures have been suggested. For example, global media can be taxed heavily enough to fund high-quality non-commercial radio and television stations that would give voice to concerns other than those of multinational corporations that are rich enough to fund their own global media outlets. Imagine the usefulness of a high-quality global media source that publicised the work of Amnesty International, Doctors Without Borders, the Red Cross, and the World Health Organisation, rather than the merchandise of multinational corporations.

Administrative changes are also possible. Structural changes that reorient the work of the IMF and other international lending agencies could reduce the social dislocation and impoverishment of weak countries by strong ones. Such changes have been proposed in a popular book by Joseph Stiglitz, former chief economist of the World Bank.[137] Administrative changes in international treaties like the North American Free Trade Agreement could remove all provisions that penalise public initiatives and co-operatives if they threaten the profits of multinational corporations or investors.[138] In fact, the value of international trade agreements per se needs careful re-examination, as does the march towards privatisation. The continuation of publicly owned institutions in many areas, for example health care, not only saves money, but also gives people a shared sense of ownership in their essential services. Administrative changes in the extra-parliamentary powers of elected governments could protect people in the western hemisphere from being unknowingly locked into military alliances with the United States that will eventually bring them disrepute.[139] Acting as an American puppet state not only makes today's Canadians accomplices to American imperial depredations, it also robs us of a shared sense of national sovereignty, thus contributing to our dislocation.

The power of citizen boycotts is large. As discussed in Chapter 14, one major weapon of the British abolitionists who succeeded in banning slavery in the British Empire by 1838 was a boycott of sugar produced by slaves, which had a major economic impact on the slave-powered sugar industry of the West Indies.[140] More recent boycotts have also been effective.[141] It seems only a matter of time until global boycotts are organised to domesticate hypercapitalism. French political scientist Paul Ariès proposed a 'general strike in consuming' for this purpose,[142] although it is not yet clear what form this would actually take. Perhaps a general strike in consuming would be a powerful enough force to stop the participation of Western nations in the never ending, exploitative wars that shatter and dislocate the Third World.

The action required to achieve structural changes at the global level will not be solitary, because citizen involvement is growing fast.[143] Moreover, joining this effort is not difficult. Countless grass-roots organisations that operate on an international level in every corner of the globe are eager to put volunteers to work. New organisations can be formed and find themselves welcomed by the existing ones. Such organisations are not competing with each other, but working together. They are tightly connected by shared concerns, if still uncoordinated in their actions. In Western countries, joining the struggle against hypercapitalism is not even dangerous in comparison with Third-World countries where success must so often be bought with blood. Protest organisations and dissident professionals are accepted as legitimate within the political process in Western nations.

This final chapter has discussed social actions on the local, national, and global levels that can have a real impact on dislocation and addiction as well as the many other side effects of free-market society. Many of these social actions are underway, although some still exist only in the imagination. Actions like these can bring dislocation and addiction under control.

The missing, magical piece of the puzzle

A crucially important issue has not yet been mentioned, because it cannot be resolved in this book. Getting beyond the first steps of social action described here requires a global transformation in world view. The world view that underlies a civilisation is the source both of its greatest strengths and its greatest weaknesses. When its weaknesses become catastrophic, the world view must change or the civilisation risks destroying itself. Western civilisation, which has now become the basis of global civilisation, appears to be in exactly that precarious position at the beginning of the 21st century. Its defining philosophy, which can be described from an economic point of view as free-market ideology, is leading to catastrophe on several levels at once. Widespread addiction is just one of these. The kinds of social change that are needed to avert a rising tide of addiction and the other catastrophes cannot be achieved fast enough to save the day until the underlying philosophy changes in the minds of the great majority of people.

Already, huge numbers of people are profoundly cynical about the conventional world view that they have absorbed from birth, but the global tipping point requires something more than cynicism and something more too than the words and actions of those people described in this chapter who are currently devoting themselves to bringing about social change one step at a time. World society will change at a gallop when its world view changes, but its world view will not change until a galvanising alternative philosophy appears, together with images, ceremonies, music and metaphysics that can give it life in human hearts and minds. The ability to create these magical pieces of the puzzle lies miles beyond the prosaic imaginations of rationalistic academics like myself. The talented people who can produce them intuitively will materialise, as others have in previous eras of despair and confusion. We can only hope that they will appear sooner rather than later and that we are able to recognise them when they do.

In the meantime, idle hoping not enough—determined social action is the task of the hour.

Endnotes

1 The word 'we' is used in the same meaning in this chapter as in the previous one, without quotation marks.

2 Many people are recognising the situation in terms similar to the ones I have used. See, for example, Wheatley (2005). Simultaneously, the proponents of free-market society strive unrelentingly to convince us that we are little more than irredeemable consumer idiots (e.g. J. Heath, 2001, Chapter 11).

3 This intertwining is described at length in Chapter 10.

4 Polanyi (1944); Glendinning (1994); Nikonoff (2004); Hawken (2007). I write this paragraph with a conviction that would have been impossible in past years, in part because the shared enthusiasm for social action along these lines has become so powerful in the people around me, as well as in the people whose works I read. Some of the impetus comes from professional community psychologists (e.g. Jason and Kobayashi, 1995), but most comes from people acting in the non-professional capacity of concerned citizens.

5 All of these points are documented in Chapter 1 of this book.

6 Davis (2006b, Chapter 1); United Nations Population Fund (2007).

7 Drake (2007); Leidl (2007).

8 The mass media are normally taken to include newspapers, radio, television, and cinema. However, it is becoming clear that video games, because they too comprise multi-billion dollar industries whose products are universally accessible, belong in this discussion of the mass media propaganda apparatus. In one genre of video games that has recently been reviewed (Fortin, 2007), players are enlisted as agents fighting against the enemies of the current world order and the United States. The enemies to be killed to restore domination of the world by normal market forces and the United States include Muslim fighters (labelled 'terrorists'), Cubans, Venezuelans, and Russians. No complex ideological arguments are advanced to justify slaughtering these enemies. Rather they are portrayed as incarnations of pure evil and the players who overcome them are portrayed as killing—and sometimes tor-turing—to preserve 'freedom'. As Tony Fortin describes these colourful and adventurous games, they 'struggle desperately to reenchant an ideology that has contributed so much to disenchanting the world' (Fortin, 2007).

9 deGraaf et al. (2002).

10 Hersh (2007). The extent of this distortion is almost impossible to believe until it is witnessed first-hand. For example, thousands of Canadians and Americans learned of it by attending the 1999 protests against the World Trade Organisation meetings in Seattle, Washington, and then viewing the grossly distorted coverage in the media (Hawken, 2007, pp 117–138). Increasingly, the news media derive the information that they promulgate from the public-relations wings of multinational corporations and from government rather than from the direct observations of reporters (Hermann and Chomsky, 1988); they cannot report news events factually because they do not in fact know what has occurred!

11 Ellul (1965); Hermann and Chomsky (1988).

12 Balbastre (2004); C. S. Smith (2005).

13 Balbastre (2004).

14 There are films, newspapers, and books that deviate substantially from the party line of the propaganda apparatus. However, these are very small, in large part because they do not receive the massive corporate subsidies in the form of advertising revenues that accrue to the media that constitute the propaganda apparatus.

15 Hermann and Chomsky (1988); Chomsky (2007).

16 Bower (2006); Bénilde (2007); G. Williams (2007).

17 Gutstein (2005); Condon (2007); Robertson (2007).

18 There are rare exceptions. *Adbusters* magazine manages to achieve dazzling production stan-dards without any subsidies.

19 J. Simpson (2005).

20 The most scrupulously factual independent source that I know at the global level is *Le Monde diplomatique*. The most factual that I know at the local level in the Vancouver area

are the *Tyee* and *Island Tides* newspapers and the articles circulated by the Canadian Centre for Policy Alternatives.

21 Krugman (2007).

22 See Your Media (2007) for a list of Canadian and international organisations that are pursuing this goal. Citizens groups, professional groups, and advocacy publications appear on this list.

23 Jacobsson (2002).

24 deGraaf *et al.* (2002, Chapter 7).

25 Alphonso (2005).

26 Brune (2004).

27 Jacobsson (2002); Brune (2004); Caraher *et al.* (2006). Many other countries have what are optimistically called 'voluntary regulations', which have no important effect.

28 Froguel and Smadja (2004); Caraher *et al.* (2006).

29 Smythe (1981).

30 Anderson and Dill (2000).

31 The hypercapitalistic perspective and addictive dangers of video games were discussed and documented in Chapter 7 under the heading *Imaginary or virtual community*. See Fortin (2007) for a more specific discussion of their ideological content.

32 G. Dixon (2007).

33 Native Indians constitute at most 5% of the British Columbian population. However, they constitute more than 50% of the children in institutions or foster homes (Olsen, 2005, p. 24).The year 2004 brought an unprecedented demographic 'flip' in the Canadian province of Saskatchewan. It was the first time in recent history that the aboriginal population of a Canadian province has gone from a minority to a majority. At the same time, Saskatchewan is racing into the high-tech free-market world. The aboriginal population of Saskatchewan has been severely dislocated for over a century, and has suffered from much violent racism, at least by Canadian standards. As Saskatchewan's native population rises, it threatens to become the leading Canadian province for both alcoholism and murder (MacGregor, 2004). See also *Globe and Mail* (2006b, p. A14).

34 This right is established in the landmark decision in the Delgamuukw appeal of 1997. See Samson (2003, Chapter 1) and Shields (2007).

35 This history is reviewed in Chapter 6 under the heading *Canadian Aboriginal Peoples*. For a single authoritative source, see Tennant (1990).

36 Bayly (2004, Chapter 12).

37 The reason that this is so is spelled out vividly by Samson (2003, especially Chapters 1 and 2).

38 The pragmatic outlook recommended here is controversial among natives and non-natives in Canada. Many native people have committed themselves wholeheartedly to the process of legally settling land claims. However, other eloquent native voices continue to argue that the land claims process is unjust and unacceptable (Bobb, n.d.; Manuel, 2007). I have come to believe that no more just solution than settling land claims will be forthcoming, and that an unjust settlement is less devastating to people than continuing to live in limbo.

39 This is because the claims of various tribal groups overlap with each other, as well as with land title held by others.

40 A. Rose (2000, especially Chapters 8–10). See also Indian and Northern Affairs Canada (2004).

41 *BC Treaty Negotiating Times* (2007).

42 G. Hill (2007); Hunter (2007).

43 British Columbia experimented with a Citizen's Commission on Electoral Reform. The commission was composed of 160 randomly selected citizens who met for a limited period to formulate a new electoral system that was then submitted to the voters in a referendum. The results were impressive (Wilcocks, 2007).

44 O'Connor (2005).

45 Potvin (2005a, b).

46 McKibben (2007, Chapters 2–4)

47 Apparently, the Salsbury Garden decision was only one Board of Variance decision to which the city council objected (Boei, 2006a).

48 Bula (2006); Reinstate Third-Party Appeals (2007).

49 Cleveland (2005).

50 Although community art performances are definitely not meant to be art therapy, they sometimes have therapeutic effects on troubled individuals, as in the case of a Vancouver blues singer, Dalannah Bowen, who was a homeless cocaine user with a wrecked career at the time she signed up to perform in the play *In the Heart of a City* in 2003. She subsequently turned her life around and summed up the experience of performing in the play by saying it was:

> … integral to my healing. After that it was, 'Oh, I remember who I am now.' That started the process, it allowed me to connect with my spirit again … I think art is one of the great underrated tools with connecting to the spirit and when you're lost … it's a direct avenue.

Quoted in J. P. McLaughlin (2006).

More usually, the effects of community art performances are not understood in the language of healing, but in the language of individual and community growth and well-being. There are many testimonials of this sort as well (Harris, 2006).

51 The term 'Downtown Eastside' is quite often used in Vancouver to refer to what is being called the 'Hasting Corridor' in this book. However, 'Downtown Eastside' actually refers to a much larger area, including Chinatown, Strathcona, and Oppenheimer Park.

52 Prostitutes are not allowed to ply their trade openly in most of the city, but they are in the Hastings Corridor and a few other areas, effectively dumping the prostitution problem in these areas. Mental patients who were 'deinstitutionalised' in large numbers in past decades often migrated to the Hastings Corridor, where the rents are relatively cheap.

53 Sommers and Bromley (2002, p. 35).

54 Richardson (2005).

55 N. Smith and Derksen (2002); Sommers and Bromley (2002); Drake (2007); Leidl (2007).

56 The one with which I am the most familiar is the Community Arts Council of Vancouver, an organisation with a six-decade history of successfully promoting arts in the city (O'Kiely, 1996) and now concentrating its attention on the Downtown Eastside through the work of the Downtown Eastside Community Arts Network. Others include the City of Vancouver itself, the Carnegie Community Centre Association, the Downtown Eastside Community Arts Trust, the Association of United Ukrainian Canadians, the Firehall Arts Centre, Gallery Gachet, des media, Coop Radio, and Theatre in the Raw.

57 A Vancouver reporter at the 2006 Heart of the City Festival put it this way:

> It's in need of some major surgery, but the heart of our city can indeed be found beating strongly on the Downtown Eastside. The third annual Heart of the City Festival

> reminds Vancouver that for every negative aspect of life at our core, proof of a dynamic community working hard to deal with its problems is also much in evidence.

Birnie (2006, p. C1).

58 The Strathcona Artist at Home Festival, 1999–2004.

59 The other co-producer was the Carnegie Community Centre, located in the heart of the Hastings Corridor. This play was the culminating event of celebrations commemorating the Carnegie building's 100th anniversary.

60 Terry Hunter and Savannah Walling (personal communication, May 2007). The city's mayor wrote, 'The community play is a shining example of how arts and culture are making an impact in this community' (L. Campbell, 2003). See also Walling (2007b).

61 These were produced with the cooperation of the Downtown Eastside Community Arts Network, the Community Arts Council of Vancouver, and the Carnegie Community Centre.

62 Another inspiration was the play *Enough is Enough*, a community shadow play about addiction produced in Enderby, British Columbia, in 2004 by Runaway Moon Theatre Arts Society and the Spallumcheen Band Health Department.

63 *We're All in This Together*—The Shadows Project: Addiction and Recovery was written by Rosemary Georgeson and Savannah Walling with Sheila Baxter, Wendy Chew, Paul Decarie, Mary Duffy, Melissa Eror, Patrick Foley, Leith Harris, Stephen Lytton, Muriel Williams, and contributions from Larry Reed, James Fagan Tait and members of the cast. The play was directed by Kim Collier, with original music by Ya-wen V. Wang and Joelysa Pankanea. Shadow designs by Tamara Unroe and lighting design by Adrian Muir. Stage Manager, Robin Bancroft-Wilson; Community Liaison and Host, Rosemary Georgeson; Artistic Director, Savannah Walling; Producer, Terry Hunter. Shadow-theatre technique introduced by James Fagen Tait and David Chantler (Trickster Theatre, Calgary) and elaborated by Larry Reed (Shadowlight Productions, San Francisco). Produced in Vancouver's Russian Hall by Vancouver Moving Theatre in association with Urban Ink's Fathom Labs and the Carnegie and Roundhouse Community Centres.

64 Wasserman (2007).

65 Georgeson *et al.* (2007).

66 Marie (2007).

67 Walling (2007a).

68 Marie (2007).

69 Mahoney (2005b).

70 Friesen (2005).

71 Fong (2006).

72 Andreas Rohrbach is the principal. See McMullen and Rohrbach (2003).

73 Victor McCook's father, Emil McCook, was chief until 2006. The new chief is Donnie vanSomer.

74 Reid *et al.* (2006).

75 With the support of Curt Ottesen, International Examiner, Freedom Taekwon-Do, Prince George, British Columbia.

76 This account is based on my own observations in Fort Ware, British Columbia, on interviews with Robert Derkson and Mary Reid in Fort Ware, and on information provided by historian Susan McCook in Prince George, British Columbia. It is partially documented by short news items and by various letters of support and recognition provided by Robert Derkson, and by a conference presentation by Reid *et al.* (2006).

77 Thanks to Maria Constantineau for a report on this project.

78 Thanks to Susan McCook for a report on this project and for help in getting the historical facts correct.

79 As explained in Chapter 3 under the heading *False dichotomy 4: drug prohibition or legalisation?*, the word 'legalisation' will be used broadly in this book to refer to any regime that makes drugs accessible to consumers more or less in the way that other commodities are. Thus, the word 'legalisation' in this book includes the drug control regime that is sometimes called 'decriminalisation', as well as the introduction of a 'regulated market'.

80 See Chapter 3 under the heading *False dichotomy 4: drug prohibition or legalisation?*

81 J. Kaplan (1983, p. 198); Alexander (1990, Chapter 2); Single *et al.* (2000); Sanger and Forero (2004); Reinarman *et al.* (2004); Otis (2006); Reuter and Stevens (2007, p. 51).

82 Armstrong (2004d); Angus Reid Strategies (2007, p. 6).

83 The best-known form of this legislation, the Canada Temperance Act (Government of Canada, 1878), was actually preceded by the less well-known Dunkin Act, also known as the Temperance Act of 1864 (Government of Canada, 1864), which served a similar function.

84 Government of Canada (1878, section 97).

85 Smart and Ogborne (1996); Dupré (2004).

86 There were violent exceptions, however. See Alexander (1990, pp. 27–28).

87 Government of Canada (1878, section 99.3–4).

88 Government of Canada (1878, section 99.6–9).

89 Hallowell (1985).

90 C. Clark (2004); Alisa Smith (2004); Bolan (2005); Matas (2005b); Mickleburgh (2005).

91 It is not clear yet what the sacramental and educational uses might be. There are claims of sacramental and educational use that need to be carefully investigated. See Tupper (2002) for a convincing argument about the potential uses of 'entheogens' in education. Also, see Stolaroff (1997), for a convincing argument that many 'psychedelic' drugs, possibly including marijuana, may have important functions to play in psychotherapy.

92 J. Kaplan (1983, p. 198); Alexander (1990, pp. 52–54).

93 Reuter and Stevens (2007, p. 51). For further documentation of the unenforceability of marijuana prohibition laws, see Single *et al.* (2000); and Reinarman *et al.* (2004).

94 The book, *Symbolic Crusade*, by Gusfield (1963) explored the symbolic nature of drug prohibition in the case of the alcohol prohibition movement in the United States.

95 Government of Canada (1878, Section 100).

96 *Globe and Mail* (2005d); *WorldNetDaily.com* (2005).

97 McLeod and McLeod (1987, Chapter 2); Martín-Baró (1994); McKibben (2005, 2007).

98 K. Polanyi (1935); Lewis *et al.* (1935).

99 DiNicola (2005); T. Stanton (2005).

100 See Martín-Baró (1994) for English translations of some of his articles.

101 Martín-Baró (1994, Chapter 2); Chavez (2003a, 2003b).

102 See Martín-Baró (1994).

103 Roman Catholicism overwhelmed South American aboriginal traditions when it was imposed under Spanish and Portuguese colonial rule, causing massive dislocation. Eventually, it became entrenched in aboriginal culture in many places.

104 Huntington (1996, p. 99).

105 Martín-Baró (1994).

106 Martín-Baró (1994, p. 26).

107 Martín-Baró (1994, p. 26, italics in original).

108 Martín-Baró (1994, p. 26).

109 Martín-Baró (1994, p. 26).

110 Martín-Baró (1994, p. 30).

111 Marín (1991).

112 Chomsky (1993, Part 2 Chapter 2).

113 Rohter (2007).

114 The architect was Arthur Erickson. The educational concept was conceived by him and was accepted by the university along with his architectural design (Johnston, 2005).

115 Fowlie (2004); Scofield (2006); C. Smith (2006a).

116 J. Woodward (2006).

117 Larsen (2007).

118 *Maclean's* (2004).

119 Alphonso (2004). In the 2005 survey, the university moved up to 7th place out of 17 in 'education' and 14th out of 17 in 'student services'. It ranked 17th out of 17 in 'atmosphere', meaning the degree to which students feel comfortable on the campus (*Globe and Mail*, 2005e).

120 *Maclean's* (2004, p. 34); *Globe and Mail* (2006c, p. 35; 2007b).

121 As a student in the 1960s, I absorbed the arguments against a curriculum based on the classic writings of the 'dead white males'. I did not read any of their writings as a student in my haste to become a professional psychologist, but in the decades that followed, I read many of them at my leisure. I can now join with those who testify that the wisdom and creativity found in these treasures of Western culture make a mockery of those who, like me, thought we would learn more from avant-garde textbooks.

122 A. Schwartz (2006).

123 M. Friedman and Friedman (1979, Chapter 6).

124 Homer-Dixon (2006, pp. 218–219).

125 This is recognised by insiders in the current power structure. For example, Joseph Stiglitz, former chief economist of the World Bank and Nobel Prize winner, makes this point throughout his recent book (Stiglitz, 2002).

126 J. Jacobs (1961, pp. 137–138); Giddens (1998, p. 36).

127 K. Polanyi (1944, pp. 254–258A); M. Friedman and Friedman (1979).

128 Musto (1987); Alexander (1990, pp. 8–15); Alexander *et al.* (1996).

129 Lemoine (2005) is a single, compact source for most of the facts in this paragraph. See also Chomsky (1993), Blore (2005), Forero (2005), Frankel (2005), Raimbeau (2005), Veltmeyer (2005), Castañeda (2006), and Boyer (2007).

130 Toussaint and Millet (2007).

131 Amin and Houtart (2006). The Charter of Principles published by the World Social Forum is available on the Internet (World Social Forum, 2006).

132 Bobb (2005).

133 Ramonet (2005); Robert (2005, 2006); Van den Brink (2005). The interpretation of the European constitution that these authors outline is contested. For example, former British Prime Minister Tony Blair interpreted the constitution and its defeat quite differently (Ghafour, 2005; *Globe and Mail*, 2005b).

134 Ramonet (1997).

135 Association pour la Taxation des Transactions pour l'Aide aux Citoyens (2002).

136 Islam (2001).

136 Stiglitz (2002, p. 226).

138 Partridge (2007).

139 Hurtig (2004).

140 Hochschild (2005, pp. 192–196).

141 Diamond (2005, pp. 556–557).

142 Ariès (2006).

143 Cassen (2005).

References

Aaron, P. and Musto, D. (1981) Temperance and prohibition in America: a historical overview. In M. H. Moore and D. R. Gerstein (eds), *Alcohol and Public Policy: Beyond the Shadow of Prohibition*, pp. 125–181. Washington, DC: National Academy Press.

Abley, M. (2004, 3 April) Where's the rage when you need it? [Review of the book *The Defiant Imagination: Why Culture Matters.*] *Globe and Mail*, p. D4.

Abraham, C. (2005, 19 February) FDA panel narrowly allows Vioxx sales to resume: regulator imposes strict warnings and patients must sign consent forms. *Globe and Mail*, p. A1.

Abramovici, P. (2004, July) Activisme militaire de Washington en Afrique. *Le Monde diplomatique*, pp. 14–15.

Accardo, A. (2005, August) Karl Kraus, contre l'empire de la bêtise: un appel à resister. *Le Monde diplomatique*, p. 23.

Achcar, G. (2004, April) Le nouveau masque de la politique Américaine au Proche Orient. *Le Monde diplomatique*, pp. 14–15.

Adams, M. and de Panafieu, C. (2003, 16 June) God is dead? 'Whatever'. *Globe and Mail*, p. A13.

Adams, P. (2003, 24 June) U.S. adds trade to Mideast road map. *Globe and Mail*, p. B8.

Adams, S. (2002) *All Dressed Down And Nowhere To Go*. Kansas City, KS: Andrews McMeel.

Addiction Science Network (1998) *The biological basis of addiction*. Addiction Research Unit, University of Buffalo, Buffalo, NY. Retrieved 7 April 2007, from http://www.addictionscience.net/ASNbiological.htm

Addiction Science Network (2000) *A primer on drug addiction*. Addiction Research Unit, University of Buffalo, Buffalo, NY. Retrieved 7 April 2007, from http://www.addictionscience.net/ASNbiological.htm

Adelman, M. (1993) *The Economics of Petroleum Supply*. Cambridge, MA: MIT Press.

Adler, A. (1954) *Social Interest: a Challenge To Mankind*. London, UK: Faber and Faber. (Original work published 1934.)

Adorno, T. W., Frenkel-Brunswick, E., Levinson, D. J., and Sanford, R. N. (1950) *The Authoritarian Personality*. New York, NY: Harper.

Agar, H. (1999) Introduction. In H. Agar and A. Tate (eds), *Who Owns America: a New Declaration Of Independence*, pp. 1–5. Wilmington, DE: ISI Books. (Original work published 1936.)

Albala, N. (2003, December) Crimes économique impunis. *Le Monde diplomatique*, p. A3.

Albee, G. W. (1986) Toward a just society: lessons from observants in the primary prevention of psychopathology. *American Psychologist*, **41**, 891–898.

Alcohol and Drug Services of British Columbia (1996) *The Biopsychosocial Theory: a Comprehensive Descriptive Perspective On Addiction*. Victoria, BC: Government of British Columbia.

Alcoholics Anonymous World Services (1976) *Alcoholics Anonymous: the Story of How Thousands of Men and Women have Recovered from Alcoholism*, 3rd edn. New York, NY: published by the author.

Alexander, B. K. (1982) James M. Barrie and the expanding definition of addiction. *Journal of Drug Issues*, **11**, 77–91.

Alexander, B. K. (1990) *Peaceful Measures: Canada's Way Out of the 'War on Drugs'.* Toronto, ON: University of Toronto Press.

Alexander, B. K. (1992) Impact of research on drug use: putting cocaine in perspective. In P. Vamos and P. J. Corriveau (eds), *Drugs of Society to the Year 2000: Proceedings of the XIV World Conference of Therapeutic Communities*, pp. 296–306. Montreal, QC: Portage.

Alexander, B. K. (1994) L'héroïne et la cocaïne provoquent-elles la dépendance? Au carrefour de la science et des dogmes établis. In P. Brisson (ed.), *L'usage des Drogues et la Toxicomanie*, pp. 3–30. Montreal, QC: Gaëtan Morin.

Alexander, B. K. (2000) The globalisation of addiction. *Addiction Research*, **8**, 501–526.

Alexander, B. K. (2001) *The roots of addiction in free-market society*. Occasional paper of the Canadian Centre for Policy Analysis, Vancouver, BC, Canada. Available at http://www.policyalternatives.ca/index.cfm?act=newsandcall=224anddo=articleandpA=BB736455

Alexander, B. K. (2003a, 20 February) In conversation with a human shield. *Republic of East Vancouver*, p. 1.

Alexander, B. K. (2003b, 11 December) Bidden to Bagdad. *Republic of East Vancouver*, p. 11.

Alexander, B. K. (2004) A historical analysis of addiction. In P. Rosenqvist, J. Blomqvist, A. Koski-Jännes and L. Öjesjö (eds), *Addiction and Life Course*, pp. 11–27. Helsinki, Finland: Nordic Council for Alcohol and Drug Research.

Alexander, B. K. (2006) Beyond Vancouver's 'Four Pillars'. *International Journal of Drug Policy*, **17**, 118–123.

Alexander, B. K. and Dibb, G. S. (1975) Opiate addicts and their parents. *Family Process*, **14**, 499–514.

Alexander, B. K. and Dibb, G. S. (1977) Interpersonal perception in addict-families. *Family Process*, **16**, 17–26.

Alexander, B. K. and Schweighofer, A. R. F. (1988) Defining 'addiction'. *Canadian Psychology*, **29**, 151–162.

Alexander, B. K. and Tsou, J. Y. (2001) Prospects for stimulant maintenance in Vancouver, Canada. *Addiction Research and Theory*, **9**, 97–132.

Alexander, B. K., Beyerstein, B. L., Hadaway, P. F., and Coambs, R. B. (1981) The effect of early and later colony housing on oral ingestion of morphine in rats. *Pharmacology, Biochemistry, and Behavior*, **15**, 571–576.

Alexander, B. K., Peele, S., Hadaway, P. F., Morse, S. J., Brodsky, A., and Beyerstein, B. L. (1985) Adult, infant and animal addiction. In S. Peele (ed.), *The Meaning of Addiction: Compulsive Experience and its Interpretation*, pp. 73–96. Lexington, MA: DC Heath.

Alexander, B. K., Schweighofer, A. R.F., and Dawes, G. A. (1996) American and Canadian drug policy: a Canadian perspective. In W. K. Bikel and R. J. DeGrandpre (eds), *Drug Policy and Human Nature: Psychological Perspectives on the Control, Prevention, and Treatment of Illicit Drug Use*, pp. 251–278. New York, NY: Plenum.

Alexander, B. K., Dawes, G. A., van de Wijngaart, G. F., Ossebaard, H. C., and Maraun, M. D. (1998) The 'temperance mentality': a comparison of university students in seven countries. *Journal of Drug Issues*, **28**, 265–282.

Alexander-Davey, E. (2005) Russkaya natsional'naya ideya v kontseptsii Aleksandra Sergeevicha Panarina. [The Russian national idea in the concept of Aleksandra Sergeevich Panarin.] *Politicheskaya Ekspertiza*, **2**, 50–73.

Alfred, T. (1999) *Peace, Power, Righteousness: an Indigenous Manifesto*. Oxford, UK: Oxford University Press.

Algazy, J. (1998, February) En Israël, l'irrestistible ascension des 'hommes en noir': le gouvernement de droite, otage des partis religieux orthodoxes. *Le Monde diplomatique*, pp. 14–15.

Allen, R. S. (1992) *His Majesty's Indian Allies: British Indian Policy in the Defence of Canada, 1774–1815*. Toronto, ON: Dundern.

Alphonso, C. (2003, 30 May) Drug tests favour sponsor's product, study says. *Globe and Mail*, p. A8.

Alphonso, C. (2004, 13 October) University report card: why it's back to school for profs. *Globe and Mail*, p. A15.

Alphonso, C. (2005, 2 September) Whining for back to school loot at fever pitch. *Globe and Mail*, p. A3.

Alsop, S. (1974, August) The right to die with dignity. *Good Housekeeping*, **69**, 130–132.

Aly, G. (2005, May) Ainsi Hitler achata les Allemands. *Le Monde diplomatique*, 22–23.

American Psychiatric Association (1994) *Diagnostic and Statistical Manual of Mental Disorders (DSM-IV)*, 4th edn. Washington, DC: published by the author.

American Psychiatric Association (2000) *Diagnostic and Statistical Manual of the Mental Disorders (DSM-IV-TR)*, 4th edn. Washington, DC: published by the author.

Amin, S. and Houtart, F. (2006, May) Trois défis pour les Forums sociaux. *Le Monde diplomatique*, p. 31.

Anderson, C. A. and Dill, K. E. (2000) Video games and aggressive thoughts, feelings, and behavior in the laboratory and in life. *Journal of Personality and Social Psychology*, **78**, 772–790.

Anderssen, E. (2004a, 9 October) Come on, get happy. *Globe and Mail*, pp. F1, F7.

Anderssen, E. (2004b, 18 December) They know when you are sleeping, they know when you're awake—and whether you like sushi. *Globe and Mail*, pp. F1, F8.

Andrews, M. (2004, 17 September) New dance combo offered for online dating: TangoPersonals.com gives clients option of live, voice connection. *Vancouver Sun*, pp. G1, G2.

Angus Reid Strategies (2007) *National public opinion poll: illegal drugs*. Retrieved 29 June 2007, from http://www.angus-reid.com/admin/collateral/pdfs/polls/ARS_Drugs.pdf

Ankomah, B. (2007, October) Slavery abolition: how Britain deceived the world. *New African*, pp. 12–19.

Anon. (1986) *Sex and Love Addicts Anonymous*. San Antonio, TX: The Augustine Fellowship, Sex and Love Addicts Anonymous, Fellowship-Wide Services.

Ansbacher, H. (1999) Alfred Adler's concepts of community feeling and social interest and the relevance of community feeling for old age. In *Adlerian Year Book 1999*, pp. 5–19. London, UK: Adlerian Society of the United Kingdom and the Institute for Individual Psychology.

Ansberry, C. (2002, 25 June) 'Just-in-time' deliveries slow down U.S. recovery: orders from manufacturers are smaller, more rushed as economic anxiety lingers. *Globe and Mail*, p. B13.

Anthony, J. C., Warner, L. A., and Kessler, R. C. (1994) Comparative epidemiology of dependence on tobacco, alcohol, controlled substances and inhalants: basic findings from the national comorbidity study. *Experimental and Clinical Psychopharmacology*, **2**, 244–268.

Arendt, H. (1965) *Eichmann in Jerusalem: a Report on the Banality of Evil* (rev. edn). Harmondsworth, UK: Penguin.

Ariès, P. (2006, 10 October) Manifeste pour une grève générale de la consommation. [Extract from P. Aries, 2006, *No Conso*, Editions Golias.] Retrieved 24 August 2007, from http://paul-aries.fr/index.php/2006/10/10/8-manifeste-pour-une-greve-generale-de-la-consommation

Aristotle (1925) *The Nichomachean Ethics* (D. Ross, trans.). Oxford, UK: Oxford University Press. (Original work published *c.* 330 BC.)

Armstrong, J. (2003a, 10 May) For many, the goal is never leaving Las Vegas: the Nevada oasis of gambling and illusion draws hundreds of runaways every month … *Globe and Mail*, p. A3.

Armstrong, J. (2003b, 11 June) Police abusive on Eastside, groups say: Mayor rejects charges Vancouver force brutalizes city's downtrodden residents. *Globe and Mail*, p. A11.

Armstrong, J. (2003c, 24 July) Pickton's elusive brother describes a 'nightmare'. *Globe and Mail*, pp. A1, A6.

Armstrong, J. (2003d, 24 July) Pickton to stand trial for deaths of women. *Globe and Mail*, p. A6.

Armstrong, J. (2004a, 2 January) Bank's closing a blow to troubled area: Four Corners Bank lent dignity to poor in Vancouver's Downtown Eastside. *Globe and Mail*, p. A10.

Armstrong, J. (2004b, 10 January) Crystal meth is sweeping BC. Police, youth workers and health authorities are alarmed and afraid: toxic drug causes lasting damage to brain. *Globe and Mail*, pp. A1, A7.

Armstrong, J. (2004c, 21 February) Once a hunter … Tales of torture and mass murder have made sex offenders a national concern. Now the fastest-growing segment of the federal prison population, they all seek treatment when they're caught … *Globe and Mail*, pp. F1, F8.

Armstrong, J. (2004d, 25 November) Pot—it's not just for bohemians anymore. *Globe and Mail*, p. A3.

Arnett, C. (1999) *The Terror of the Coast: Land Alienation and Colonial War on Vancouver Island and the Gulf Islands, 1849–1863*. Burnaby, BC: Talonbooks.

Arterburn, S. and Felton, J. (1991) *Toxic Faith: Understanding and Overcoming Religious Addiction*. Nashville, TN: Oliver Nelson.

Ashby, T. (2004, 29 September) Nigerian rebels demand that firms shut off oil taps. *Globe and Mail*, p. A13.

Associated Press (2003, 13 November) French executives sentenced. *Globe and Mail*, p. B9.

Association pour la Taxation des Transactions pour l'Aide aux Citoyens (2002, 21 June) *Plateform Attac*. Montreuil-sous-Bois, France: published by the author. Retrieved 20 August 2007, from http://www.france.attac.org/spip/php?article7. Also available in English as *Platform of the Association Attac* at http://www.france.attac.org/spip.php?article2737

Atkins, R. C. (2002) *Dr Atkins New Diet Revolution: Completely Updated*. New York, NY: Avon.

Atlas, R. D. and Walsh, M. W. (2005, 27 November) Pension officers putting billions into hedge funds: question raised on risk. *New York Times*, pp. A1, A27.

Attané, I. (2006, July) L'asie manque de femmes. *Le Monde diplomatique*, pp. 1, 16–17.

Aurelius, Marcus (1964) *Meditations* (M. Staniforth, trans.). New York, NY: Penguin Books. (Original work published 170 AD.)

Austin, G. A. (1985) *Alcohol in Western Society from Antiquity to 1800: a Chronological History*. Santa Barbara, CA: ABC-Clio Information Services.

Avery, S. (2007, 27 February) Virtual world 'more than a geeky escape'. *Globe and Mail*, p. B3.

Babineau, G. (2004, 12 February–19 February) The business of romance. *Georgia Straight*, pp. 21–23.

Babor, T., Caetano, R., Casswell, S., *et al.* (2003) *Alcohol: No Ordinary Commodity*. New York, NY: Oxford University Press.

Bailey, S. and Elliot, L. (2003, 23 February) New numbers link gambling, suicide: 10% of victims in Alberta gambled: betting's social cost in spotlight. *Toronto Star*, p. A01.

Bakan, J. (2004) *The Corporation: the Pathological Pursuit of Profit and Power*. New York, NY: Free Press.

Balbastre, G. (2004, December) Les faits divers, ou le tribunal implacable des médias. *Le Monde diplomatique*, pp. 14–15.

Baran, P. A. and Sweezy, P. M. (1966) *Monopoly Capital: an Essay on the American Economic and Social Order*. New York, NY: Monthly Review Press.

Barlow, M. and Clark, T. (2001) *Global Showdown: How the New Activists are Fighting Global Corporate Rule*. Toronto, ON: Stoddard.

Barlow, M. and Winter, J. (1997) *The Big Black Book: the Essential Views of Conrad and Barbara Amiel Black*. Toronto, ON: Stoddard.

Barman, J. (2005) *Stanley Park's Secret: the Forgotten Families of Whoi Whoi, Kanaka Ranch, and Brockton Point*. Madeira Park, BC: Harbour Publishing.

Barrie, J. M. (1892) *My Lady Nicotine*, 4th edn. London, UK: Hodder and Stoughton.

Barrie, J. M. (1928) *Peter Pan, or the Boy Who Would Not Grow Up*. London, UK: Hodder and Stoughton.

Barrie, J. M. (1929) *Tommy and Grizel*. New York, NY: Charles Scribner's Sons. (Original work published 1900.)

Barrie, J. M. (1937) *The Greenwood Hat*. London, UK: Peter Davies.

Barron, J. (2003, 11 October) In show, Limbaugh tells of pill habit; plans to enter clinic. *New York Times*, p. A1.

Barry, G. and Lombardi, M. (2004, 3 June) Medicare's deadly numbers game: we grossly underspent our way into this health-care mess with its dangerous waiting lists. *Globe and Mail*, p. A17.

Bates, D. (2007, 15 March–28 March) TILMA: NAFTA's filthy offspring. *Republic of East Vancouver*, p. 7.

Bates, D. and Kromka, B. (2007, 15 March–28 March) The façade of choice. *Republic of East Vancouver*, 'Roadkill' Supplement, p. 3.

Bayly, C. A. (2004) *The Birth Of The Modern World, 1780–1914*. Oxford, UK: Blackwell.

BC Treaty Negotiating Times (2007, Summer). Nisga'a now. *BC Treaty Negotiating Times*, pp. 1, 3.

Beaud, S. and Pialoux, M. (2000, January) Cette casse délibérée des solidarités militante: des ouvriers sans classe. *Le Monde diplomatique*, pp. 10–11.

Beck, J. C. and Wade, M. (2005, 7 January) Harness talents of gamer generation. *Globe and Mail*, pp. C1, C7.

Becker, D. (2007, 12 April 2002) When games stop being fun. c|net News.com. Retrieved 22 July 2007, from http://news.com.com/2100–1040–881673.html

Beckett, S. (1965) *Waiting For Godot: a Tragicomedy In Two Acts*. London, UK: Faber and Faber.

Beder, S. (2006) *Free Market Missionaries: the Corporate Manipulation of Community Values*. London, UK: Earthscan.

Beecher, H. K. (1959) *The Measurement of Subjective Responses: Quantitative Effects of Drugs.* New York, NY: Oxford University Press.

Belaala, S. (2004, November) Misère et djihad au Maroc. *Le Monde diplomatique*, pp. 1, 16–17.

Bell, R. M. (1987) *Holy Anorexia.* Chicago, IL: University of Chicago Press.

Beniger, J. R. (1986) *The Control Revolution: Technical and Economic Origins of the Information Society.* Cambridge, MA: Harvard University Press.

Bénilde, M. (2007, August) Predateurs de presse et marchands d'influence. *Le Monde diplomatique*, p. 24.

Benjamin, D. (2004, 23 January) The terrorism 'experts' and the White House whistle blower [Review of the book *An End to Evil: How to Win the War on Terror.*] *Globe and Mail*, p. D8.

Bennett, R., Batenhorst, R., Graves, D., *et al.* (1982) Morphine titration in postoperative laparotomy patients using patient-controlled analgesia. *Current Therapeutic Research*, **32**, 45–51.

Berger, J. (2003, February) Où sommes-nous? 'Au sein du chaos le plus tyrannique'. *Le Monde diplomatique*, p. 15.

Berlinski, C. (2006, 9 September) Mere anarchy is loosed upon the world. [Review of the book *Murder in Amsterdam: the Death of Theo van Gogh and the Limits of Tolerance.*] *Globe and Mail*, pp. D7, D8.

Berman, M. (1982) *All That iIs Solid Melts into Air: the Experience of Modernity.* New York, NY: Simon and Schuster.

Berridge, V. and Edwards, G. (1987) *Opium and the People: Opiate Use in Nineteenth Century England.* London, UK: Allan Lane.

Berton, P. (1990) *The Great Depression 1929–1939.* Toronto, ON: McClelland & Stewart.

Beyerstein, B. L. and Alexander, B. K. (1985) Why treat doctors like pushers? *Canadian Medical Association Journal*, **132**, 337–341.

Beyerstein, B. L. and Hadaway, P. F. (1990) On avoiding folly. *Journal of Drug Issues*, **20**, 689–700.

Bianco, L. (1971) *Origins of the Chinese Revolution, 1915–1949.* Stanford, CA: Stanford University Press.

Biernacki, P. (1986) *Pathways from Heroin Addiction: Recovery Without Treatment.* Philadelphia, PA: Temple University Press.

Birkin, A. (1979) *J. M. Barrie and the Lost Boys.* London, UK: Constable.

Birnie, P. (2006) Dynamic talent beats at the heart of the city. *Vancouver Sun*, p. C1.

Black, W. A. (1991) An existential approach to self-control in the addictive behaviors. In N. Heather, W. R. Miller, and J. Greely (eds), *Self-control and the Addictive Behaviours*, pp. 262–279. Sydney, Australia: Maxwell-MacMillan Publishing.

Blackwell, J. S. (1982) Drifting, controlling, and overcoming: opiate users who avoid becoming chronically dependent. *Journal of Drug Issues*, **13**, 219–235.

Blackwell, R. (2003a, 3 October) Corus banking on 'Kidfluence'. *Globe and Mail*, pp. B1, B10.

Blackwell, R. (2003b, 15 November) Hollinger admits to 'inaccuracies'. *Globe and Mail*, pp. B1, B5.

Blackwell, R. (2003c, 18 November) Black's darkest hour: Hollinger scandal forces him out as CEO. *Globe and Mail*, pp. A1, A6.

Blackwell, R. (2004, 30 August) Hollinger directors to come under fire. *Globe and Mail*, pp. B1, B9.

Blackwell, R. (2005, 19 August) Radler charged with fraud. *Globe and Mail*, p. A1.

Blackwell, R. and Waldie, P. (2005, 12 September) Radler writes new chapter on Conrad Black, Hollinger. *Globe and Mail*, pp. B1, B6.

Blatchford, C. (2004, 18 June) Heart of darkness: the Holly Jones case: as child-porn aficionado Michael Briere gets life for killing the little Toronto girl, the chilling tale of evil sparks calls for an Internet crackdown. *Globe and Mail*, p. A1.

Blomqvist, J. (2004) Sweden's 'War on Drugs' in the light of addict's experience. In P. Rosenqvist, J. Blomqvist, A. Koski-Jännes, and L. Öjesjö (eds), *Addiction and Life Course*, pp. 139–171. Helsinki, Finland: Nordic Council for Alcohol and Drug Research.

Blore, S. (2005, 28 June) Despite the calm, reform pressures challenge Bolivia. *Globe and Mail*, p. A12.

Blum, K., Cull, J. G., Braverman, E. R., and Comings, D. E. (1996, March–April) Reward deficiency syndrome. *American Scientist*, **84**, 132–145.

Boal, I. (in press) *The Long Theft: New Enclosures and the Case of Biotechnology*. San Francisco: City Lights Press.

Bobb, R. (n.d.) *The Treaty Process and Indian Nationalism*. Unpublished manuscript.

Bobb, R. (2005) *Toward a Strategy for Native Indian Sovereigntists*. Unpublished manuscript.

Bock, D. (2006, 6 May) Journey to the end of Roth [Review of the book *Everyman*.] *Globe and Mail*, p. D6.

Bock, W. J. (1980) The definition and recognition of biological adaptation. *American Zoologist*, **20**, 217–227.

Boei, W. (2006a, 1 July) Council fires board of variance: panel had blocked plan for a luxury marina in False Creek. *Vancouver Sun*, p. B1.

Boei, W. (2006b, 26 August) Two cities, two mayors, one big problem. *Vancouver Sun*, pp. A1, A3.

Bolan, K. (2005, 20 August) The long arm of Uncle Sam. A growing number of U.S. crime-busters are operating in BC in a cross-border crackdown. *Vancouver Sun*, pp. A1, A4.

Bonelli, L. (2003, February) Une vision policière de la société. *Le Monde diplomatique*, p. 3.

Bonhoeffer, D. (1959) *The Cost of Discipleship*, 2nd edn (R. H. Fuller, trans.). New York, NY: Macmillan.

Booth, M. (1996) *Opium: a History*. New York, NY: St Martin's Press.

Bouffartigue, P. (2002, May) Fracture chez les cols blancs. *Le Monde diplomatique*, pp. 8–9.

Bouillon, F. (2005, October) Le squat, un lieu de résistance. *Le Monde diplomatique*, p. 3.

Bourdieu, P. (1998, March) L'essence du néolibéralisme. *Le Monde diplomatique*, p. 3.

Bourdieu, P. (2003, June) Ce terrible repos qui est celui de la mort sociale. *Le Monde diplomatique*, p. 5. (Original work published 1981.)

Bourgois, P. (1997) In search of Horatio Alger: culture and ideology in the crack economy. In C. Reinarman and H. G. Levine (eds), *Crack in America: Demon Drugs and Social Justice*, pp. 57–76. Berkeley, CA: University of California Press.

Bower, T. (2006) *Conrad and Lady Black: Dancing on the Edge*. London, UK: Harper-Collins.

Boyd, N. (1984) The origins of Canadian narcotics legislation: the process of criminalisation in historical context. *Dalhousie Law Journal*, **8**, 102–136.

Boyd, R. (1994) Smallpox in the Pacific Northwest: the first epidemics. *BC Studies*, **101**, 5–40.

Boyd, R. (1996) Commentary on early contact-era smallpox in the Pacific Northwest. *Ethnohistory*, **43**, 307–328.

Boyd, R. (1999) *The Coming of the Spirit of Pestilence: Introduced Infectious Diseases and Population Decline among Northwest Coast Indians, 1774–1874*. Seattle, WA: University of Washington Press.

Boyer, J.-F. (2007, April) Une gauche mexicaine en desordre de bataille. *Le Monde diplomatique*, pp. 10–11.

Bozarth, M. A., Murray, A., and Wise, R. A. (1989) Influence of housing conditions on the acquisition of intravenous heroin and cocaine self-administration in rats. *Pharmacology, Biochemistry, and Behavior*, **33**, 903–907.

Braucht, G. N., Brakarsh, D., Follingstad, D., and Berry, K. L. (1973) Deviant drug use in adolescence: a review of the psychosocial correlates. *Psychological Bulletin*, **79**, 92–106.

Brauman, R. (2005, September) Mission civilisatrice, ingérence humanitaire: inconsient colonial. *Le Monde diplomatique*, p. 3.

Brecher, E. M. (1972) *Licit and Illicit Drugs*. Boston, MA: Little, Brown.

Breggin, P. R. (1994) *Talking Back to Prozac*. New York, NY: St Martin's Press.

Brethour, P. (2005, 8 November) There's still lots of oil—at a price: IEA. *Globe and Mail*, p. B11.

Bricmont, J. (2007, August) An 01 de la gauche, on arrête tout, on en réfléchit. *Le Monde diplomatique*, pp. 6–7.

Brière, E. (2004) *East Timor: Testimony*. Toronto, ON: Between the Lines.

British American Security Information Council (2006) *Escaping the subsidy trap: why arms exports are bad for Britain*. Retrieved 17 April 2006, from http://www.basicint.org/pubs/subsidy.htm

Bronfenbrenner, U., McClelland, P., Wethington, E., Moen, P., and Ceci, S. J. (1996) *The State of Americans: this Generation and the Next*. New York, NY: Free Press.

Brook, T. and Wakabayashi, B. T. (eds) (2000) *Opium Regimes: China, Britain, and Japan, 1839–1952*. Berkeley, CA: University of California Press.

Brown, I. (2005a, 5 March) Supersize thee. *Globe and Mail*. pp. F1, 4–5.

Brown, I. (2005b, 1 October) Look and see. *Globe and Mail*, pp. F1, 6–7.

Brown, J. H. S. (1988, February–March) A parcel of upstart Scotchmen. *Beaver*, pp. 4–11.

Brown, Peter (1967) *Augustine of Hippo*. Berkeley, CA: University of California Press.

Brown, Patrick (2006, 14 December) TILMA: the Trojan horse. *Island Tides*, pp. 1–3, 7.

Brown-Bowers, A. (2007, 11 April) Working under the influence. *Globe and Mail*, pp. C1, C2.

Browne, A. and Finkelhor, D. (1986) Impact of child sexual abuse: a review of the research. *Psychological Bulletin*, **99**, 66–77.

Brune, F. (2004, September) De l'enfant-roi à l'enfant-proie. *Le Monde diplomatique*, p. 3.

Bry, B. H., McKeon, P., and Pandina, R. J. (1982) Extent of drug use as a function of number of risk factors. *Journal of Abnormal Psychology*, **91**, 273–279.

Buckner, D. (2003, 15 November) A corporate heart of darkness. *Globe and Mail*, pp. D6, D7.

Bula, F. (2006, 23 September) Neighbours lose long-held right to challenge developers: Vancouver residents can't appeal decisions of the city's planning department. *Vancouver Sun*, p. A1.

Bula, F. and Ward, D. (2000, 3 March) Vancouver envy: why the world is beating a path here to learn how to fix its broken cities. *Vancouver Sun*, pp. A1, A8-A9.

Bulard, M. (2004, March) Etat d'urgence sociale. *Le Monde diplomatique*, p. 3.

Bulard, M. (2005, January) Les fourberies de M. Camdessus. *Le Monde diplomatique*, pp. 1, 10–11.

Bulkeley, W. M. (2004, 19 January) 'Off-shoring' peek given: IBM documents reveal expected savings. *Globe and Mail*, p. B11.

Bulych, T. and Beyerstein, B. L. (1989) Facing the real problems: authoritarianism and misinformation as sources of support for the War on Drugs. In A. S. Trebach and K. B. Zeese (eds), *New Frontiers in Drug Policy*, pp. 137–149. Washington, DC: The Drug Policy Foundation.

Bunyan, J. (1985) *The Pilgrim's Progress*. Urichsville, OH: Barbour. (Original work published 1678.)

Burchfield, R. W. (ed.) (1972) *A Supplement to the Oxford English Dictionary*. Oxford, UK: Clarendon Press.

Burke, E. L. (1978) Some evidence for Erikson's concept of negative identity in delinquent adolescent drug abusers. *Comprehensive Psychiatry*, **19**, 141–152.

Burke, M. (2002, 1 June) What were they fighting for? For those who recall the war against Vietnam's Communists, there's a sad irony in that country's pursuit of U.S. style capitalism. *Globe and Mail*, p. A17.

Burkeman, O. (2004, 15 September) Rumsfeld ignored evidence of abuse in 2002, book says. *Globe and Mail*, pp. A1, A11.

Burley, E. I. (1997) *Servants of the Honourable Company: Work, Discipline, and Conflict in the Hudson's Bay Company, 1770–1879*. Don Mills, ON: Oxford University Press.

Burroughs, W. S. (1967, July) Kicking drugs: a very personal story. *Harper's*, **235**, 39–42.

Byck, R. (ed.) (1974) *Cocaine Papers by Sigmund Freud*. New York, NY: Stonehill.

Cameron, D. (2004) Reshaping drinkers' identities? In P. Rosenqvist, J. Blomqvist, A. Koski-Jännes, and L. Öjesjö (eds), *Addiction and Life Course*, pp. 173–184. Helsinki, Finland: Nordic Council for Alcohol and Drug Research.

Cameron, D., Manik, G., Bird, R., and Sinorwalia, A. (2002) What may we be learning from so-called spontaneous remission in ethnic minorities? *Addiction Research and Theory*, **10**, 175–182.

Campbell, L. (2003, December) A vision for the heart of the city. *Four Pillars News*, **1**, 11.

Campbell, M., Keenan, G., and Tuck, S. (2004, 14 April) Ontario to lure leading-edge plants. *Globe and Mail*, pp. B1, B5.

Camus, J.-Y. (2002, May) Métamorphoses de l'extrême droite en Europe: Du fascisme au national-populisme. *Le Monde diplomatique*, p. 3.

Canadian Centre on Substance Abuse (2004) Canadian addiction survey: a national survey of Canadians' use of alcohol and other drugs: prevalence of use and related harms. Ottawa, ON: published by the author.

Caplan, G. (2005, 22 June) Live 8: thumbs down on hypocritical 'aid'. *Globe and Mail*, p. A13.

Caraher, M., Landon, J., and Dalmeny, K. (2006) Television advertising and children: lessons from policy development. *Public Health Nutrition*, **9**, 596–605.

Carey, B. (2006, 4 April) Living on impulse: researchers are beginning to identify why one person's spontaneity is another's descent into self-destruction. *New York Times*, pp. D1, D6.

Carlson, K. T. (ed.) (1997) You are asked to witness: the Stó:lo in Canada's Pacific Coast history. Chilliwack, BC: Stó:lo Heritage Trust.

Carrigg, D. (2004, 10 October) Slow change: despite reported successes, cops like Sgt. Greg McCullough face frustration and abuse as they tackle the Downtown Eastside. *Vancouver Courier*, pp. 1, 4–6.

Carrozzo, S. (2002, May) Le sort contrasté des 'frères' belges du Front national. *Le Monde diplomatique*, pp. 4–5.

Carstairs, C. (2004, September) *Drug hysteria and the end of maintenance.* Paper presented at the meeting Moving Forward: Improving Treatment for Heroin Addiction, Vancouver, BC, Canada.

Carstairs, C. (2006) *Jailed for Possession: Illegal Drug Use, Regulation, and Power in Canada, 1920–1961.* Toronto: University of Toronto Press.

Cassen, B. (2004a, January) Une constitution pour sanctuariser la loi du marché. *Le Monde diplomatique*, pp. 6, 7.

Cassen, B. (2004b, September) L'apparent affrontement transatlantique. *Le Monde diplomatique*, pp. 30–31.

Cassen, B. (2005, December) Marchandage sur la marchandisation. *Le Monde diplomatique*, p. 5.

Castañeda, J. G. (2006, May/June) Latin America's left turn. *Foreign Affairs*, 23–48. Retrieved 1 June 2006, from http://www.foreignaffairs.org/20060501faessay85302/jorge-g-castaneda/latin-america-s-left-turn.html?mode=print

C'de Baca, J. and Wilbourne, P. (2004) Quantum change: ten years later. *Journal of Clinical Psychology: In Session*, **60**, 531–541.

Célérier, P. (2004, March) Shanhaï sans toits ni lois: la Chine en mutation. *Le Monde diplomatique*, pp. 16–17.

Centers for Disease Control and Prevention (2005) *Chronic fatigue syndrome: what is CFS?* Retrieved 3 June 2005, from http://www.cdc.gov/ncidod/diseases/cfs/about/what.htm

Cernetig, M. (1999, 23 June) China's painful blast from the past: outlawed for decades, the rickshaw is back, as are porn, prostitutes, and even opium. 'Mao would not be happy.' *Globe and Mail*, pp. A1, A11.

Chaker, A. M. (2003, 4 January) Can't stop shopping? Here's a pill. *Globe and Mail*, p. F7.

Champagne, P. (2003, April) Quand les paysans servent de cobayes. *Le Monde diplomatique*, p. 8.

Chandler, C. (2006, 5 May) NIDA director delivers spirit lecture. *NIH Record*, **58**. Retrieved 6 October 2007, from http://nihrecord.od.nih.gov/newsletters/2006/05_05_2006/story06.htm

Chandler, M. J. and Lalonde, C. (1998) Cultural continuity as a hedge against suicide in Canada's First Nations. *Transcultural Psychiatry*, **35**, 191–219.

Chandler, M. J., Lalonde, C. E., Sokol, B. W., and Hallett, D. (2003) *Personal Persistence, Identity Development, and Suicide: a Study of Native and Non-native North American Adolescents.* Monographs of the Society for Research in Child Development, vol. 68, no. 2.

Chaney, L. (2005) *Hide-and-seek with Angels: a Life of J. M. Barrie.* London, UK: Hutchinson.

Chang, H.-J. (2003, June) De protectionnisme au libre-échangisme, une conversion opportuniste. *Le Monde diplomatique*, pp. 26–27.

Chappell, B. (2006) Petros Roukas—blessed are the poor in spirit. *byFaith Online*. Retrieved 24 April 2006, from http://www.byfaithonline.com/partner/Article_Display_Page/0,,PTID323422%CCHID664022%7CCIID1882538,00.html

Chase, S. (2002, 15 August) Canada, U.S. undercutting green gains, UN study says: North American consumer culture blamed for eroding progress made on environment. *Globe and Mail*, p. A5.

Chase, S. (2007, 19 April) Ottawa rolls out 'validators' to bolster anti-Kyoto stand. *Globe and Mail*, pp. A1, A6.

Chase, S. and Fagen, D. (2004, 30 April) Decision to join missile shield already made, opposition says. *Globe and Mail*, p. A6.

Chavez, W. (2003a, May) Eruption annoncée du volcan bolivien. *Le Monde diplomatique*, pp. 12, 13.

Chavez, W. (2003b, May) Une nouvelle gauche à l'offensive. *Le Monde diplomatique*, p. 12.

Cheever, S. (2004) *My Name is Bill: Bill Wilson—His Life and the Creation of Alcoholics Anonymous.* New York, NY: Simon & Schuster.

Chein, I., Gerard, D. L., Lee, R. S., and Rosenfeld, E. (1964) *The Road to H: Narcotics, Delinquency, and Social Policy.* New York, NY: Basic Books.

Chen, J. (1975) *Inside the Cultural Revolution.* New York, NY: Macmillan.

Chenery, E. (1890) *Alcohol Inside Out From Bottom Principles: Facts for the Millions*, 2nd edn. Boston, MA: published by the author.

Chepesiuk, R. (2001, May) Colombia's oil war: the U'wa battle Occidental over 'the blood of mother earth'. *Toward Freedom Online Magazine.* Retrieved 24 November 2004, from http://www.towardfreedom.com/2001/may01/ colombia_oil.htm

Chomsky, N. (1993) *What Uncle Sam Really Wants.* Retrieved 28 October 2005, from http://www.zmag.org/chomsky/sam/sam-contents.html

Chomsky, N. (1998, April) The drug war industrial complex: Noam Chomsky interviewed by John Veit. *High Times.* Retrieved 13 August 2007, from http://www.chomsky.info/interviews/199804-.htm

Chomsky, N. (2003a, August) Le meillure des mondes selon Washington: sans le droit et par la force. *Le Monde diplomatique*, pp. 1, 8–9.

Chomsky, N. (2003b) *Hegemony or Survival: America's Quest for Global Dominance.* New York, NY: Henry Holt.

Chomsky, N. (2004) Western complicity in the Indonesian invasion of East Timor. In E. Brière (ed.), *East Timor Testimony*, pp. 48–53. Toronto, ON: Between the Lines.

Chomsky, N. (2007, August) Le lavage de cerveaux en liberté. *Le Monde diplomatique*, pp. 1, 8–9.

Chossudovsky, M. (1997) *The Globalisation of Poverty: Impacts of IMF and World Bank Reforms.* London, UK: Zed Books.

Chrisjohn, R. and Young, S. (with Maraun, M.) (1997) *The Circle Game: Shadows and Substance in the Indian Residential School Experience in Canada.* Penticton, BC: Theytus Books.

Chu, H. (2000, 1 August) China keeping its executioners busy. *San Francisco Chronicle.* Retrieved 8 April 2007, from http://www.commondreams.org/headlines/080100–03.htm

Church, E. (1999, 14 May) Corporate executives suffer too. *Globe and Mail*, p. M1.

Clark, C. (2004, 8 May) Liberals prepared to allow marijuana bill to die. *Globe and Mail*, pp. A1, A4.

Clark, T. (2004, 3 June) Spitzer sues Glaxo for allegedly suppressing study data: safety for use in treating children, teens questioned. *Globe and Mail*, p. B19.

Clarke, A. (1997) *The Origin of Waves.* Toronto, ON: McClelland and Stuart.

Clerc, D. (2007, January–February) Ordre social et dictature du marché. *Manière de voir*, **91**, 10–13.

Cleveland, W. (2005) *Making Exact Change: how U.S. Arts-based Programs have Made a Significant and Sustained Impact on their Communities.* Saxapahaw, NC: Art in the Public Interest. Retrieved 23 May 2007, from http://www.communityarts.net/readingroom/archive/mec/exactchange4.pdf

Clinton, W. (1997, 21 May) *Remarks by the President at the U.S. Conference of Mayors Breakfast.* Washington, DC: The White House, Office of the Press Secretary. Retrieved from http://www.iprc.indiana.edu/prevention/clinton.html

Cloud, W. and Granfield, R. (2004) Life course perspective on exiting addiction: the relevance of recovery capital in treatment. In P. Rosenqvist, J. Blomqvist, A. Koski-Jännes, and L. Öjesjö (eds), *Addiction and life course*, pp. 185–202. Helsinki, Finland: Nordic Council for Alcohol and Drug Research.

Cloward, R. A. and Ohlin, L. E. (1960) *Delinquency and Opportunity: a Theory of Delinquent Gangs*. New York, NY: Free Press.

Coalition of Child Care Advocates of BC (2007) *Minister Reid—Resign!* Retrieved 19 February 2007, from http://www.cccabc.bc.ca/res/pdf/ResignRestoreBuild.pdf

Cohen, A. (2000, 4 July) 224 years old and in really great shape: with their usual gusto, Americans celebrate Independence Day knowing their lives, and their country, have never been better. *Globe and Mail*, p. A7.

Cohen, P. (2004, 4–5 March) *Bewitched, bedevilled, possessed, addicted. Dissecting historic constructions of suffering and exorcism.* Presentation at the London UKHR Conference, London, UK. Retrieved from http://www.cedro-uva.org/lib/cohen.bewitched.html

Cohen, P. and Sas, A. (1993) *Ten Years of Cocaine: a Follow-up Study of 64 Cocaine Users in Amsterdam.* Amsterdam: University of Amsterdam.

Cohn, M. (2005) The two Americas. *Truthout.* Retrieved 8 September 2005, from http://www.truthout.org/docs_2005/090305Y.shtml

Coleman, A. M. (2001) *A Dictionary of Psychology (Oxford paperback reference).* Oxford, UK: Oxford University Press.

Condon, S. (2007, September–October) The death of Canadian journalism. *Adbusters*, **73**, 24–30.

Conesa, P. (2004, June) Aux origines des attentats suicides: Sri Lanka, Irak, Tchétchénie, Israël … *Le Monde diplomatique*, pp. 14–15.

Cook, D. R. (1987) Self-identified addictions and emotional disturbances in a sample of college students. *Psychology of Addictive Behaviours*, **1**, 55–61.

Cook, D. R. (1991) Shame, attachment, and addictions: implications for family therapists. *Contemporary Family Therapy*, **13**, 405–419.

Coomber, R. and South, N. (2004) *Drug Use and Cultural Contexts Beyond the West.* London, UK: Free Association Books.

Coombs, R. H. (1981) Drug abuse as a career. *Journal of Drug Issues*, **11**, 369–387.

Copes, P. (2005, 8 February) *Aboriginal fishing in British Columbia.* Presentation to Retirees Association, Simon Fraser University, Burnaby, BC, Canada.

Cordonnier, L. (2006, December) Guerre aux chômeurs! Des experts aux idées fracassantes. *Le Monde diplomatique.* pp. **1**, 4,5.

Coupland, D. (2006) *jPod.* Toronto, ON: Random House Canada.

Courtwright, D. T. (1982) *Dark Paradise: Opiate Addiction in America Before 1940.* Cambridge, MA: Harvard University Press.

Courtwright, D. T. (2002) The roads to H: the emergence of the American heroin complex, 1898–1956. In D. F. Musto (ed.), *One Hundred Years of Heroin*, pp. 3–19. Westport, CT: Auburn House.

Courtwright, D. T., Joseph, H., and Desjarlais, D. (1989) *Addicts who Survived: an Oral History of Narcotic Use in America, 1923–1965.* Knoxville, TN: University of Tennessee Press.

Covington, S. S. (1982) *Sexual experience, dysfunction, and abuse: a descriptive study of alcoholic and nonalcoholic women.* Unpublished doctoral dissertation, Union Graduate School, Union Institute and University, Cincinnati, OH, USA.

Cox, H. (1999, March) The market as God. *Atlantic Monthly*, pp. 18–23.

Coyhis, D. and White, W. L. (2002) Addiction and recovery in Native America: lost history, enduring lessons. *Counselor*, **3**, 16–20.

Craib, K. J. P., Spittal, P. M., Wood, E., *et al.* (2003) Risk factors for elevated HIV incidence among Aboriginal injection drug users in Vancouver. *Canadian Medical Association Journal*, **168**, 1–6.

Crampton, T. (2004, 26 August) U.S. intelligence officers involved in prison abuse: probe in Abu Ghraib scandal confirms more involvement than was made public. *Globe and Mail*, p. A12.

Crane, M. and Warnes, A. (2005, November) Wet day centres in Britain. *Drug and Alcohol Findings*, **12**, 24–29. Retrieved 3 November 2005, from http://www.drugandalcohol findings.org.uk

Crosbie, L. (2003a, 22 February) From superstar to superfreak. *Globe and Mail*, p. R8.

Crosbie, L. (2003b, 1 November) Courtney Love's rags to ditches story. *Globe and Mail*, p. R2.

Crossman, R. (ed.) (1950) *The God that Failed: Six Studies in Communism*. London, UK: Hamish Hamilton.

Cross-National Collaborative Group (1992) The changing rate of major depression: cross-national comparisons. *Journal of the American Medical Association*, **268**, 3098–3105.

Crozier, L. and Lane, P. (eds) (2001) *Addicted: Notes from the Belly of the Beast*. Vancouver, BC: Greystone Books.

Cruise, D. and Griffiths, A. (2003) *Vancouver*. Toronto, ON: HarperCollins, Canada.

Crumbaugh, J. C. and Maholick, L. T. (1964) An experimental study in existentialism: the psychometric approach to Frankl's concept of noogenic neurosis. *Journal of Clinical Psychology*, **20**, 200–207.

Csillag, R. (2003, 31 March) Scholar was 'hooked' on religion: Willard Oxtoby, 1933–2003. *Globe and Mail*, p. R5.

Culbert, L. (2004a) Liberal fundraiser's home was searched: brother of Deputy Premier Christy Clark active in federal party. *Vancouver Sun*, pp. B1, B5.

Culbert, L. (2004b, 24 February) Vancouver is Canada's drug 'warehouse-distribution centre'. *Vancouver Sun*, pp. A1, A5.

Cushman, P. (1995) *Constructing the Self, Constructing America: a Cultural History of Psychology*. Reading, MA: Addison-Wesley.

Dalgarno, P. and Shewan, D. (2005) Reducing the risks of drug use: the case for set and setting. *Addiction Research and Theory*, **13**, 259–265.

Dalrymple, T. (2006a) *Romancing Opiates: Pharmacological Lies and the Addiction Bureaucracy*. New York, NY; Encounter Books.

Dalrymple, T. (2006b, 20 August) When educated idealists—think bomb plots—go bad. *Globe and Mail*, p. A13.

Danziger, K. (1990) *Constructing the Subject: the Historical Origins of Psychological Research*. Cambridge, UK: Cambridge University Press.

Darwin, C. (1958a) *The Origin of Species*. New York, NY: New American Library of World Literature. (Original work published 1859.)

Darwin, C. (1958b) *The Autobiography of Charles Darwin, 1809–1882* (Nora Barlow, ed.). New York, NY: W. W. Norton and Company. (Original work published 1887).

Darwin, C. (1981) *The Descent of Man, and Selection in Relation to Sex*, 1st edn. Princeton, NJ: Princeton University Press. (Original work published 1871.)

Das, Lama S. (1998) *Awakening the Buddha Within: Eight Steps to Enlightenment: Tibetan Wisdom for the Western World.* New York, NY: Bantam Doubleday Dell.

Dash, E. (2006, 9 April) Off to the races again, leaving many behind. *New York Times, Sunday Business,* pp. 1, 5.

Davidson, H. A. (1964) Confessions of a goofball addict. *American Journal of Psychiatry,* **120,** 750–756.

Davies, J. B. (1992) *The Myth of Addiction: an Application of the Psychological Theory of Attribution to Illicit Drug Use.* London, UK: Routledge.

Davies, J. B. (1997) *Drugspeak: the Analysis of Drug Discourse.* Amsterdam: Overseas Publishers Association, Harwood.

Davies, P. J., Hughes, J., and Tett, G. (2007, 13 September) So what is it worth? Financiers and accountants wrangle over credit pricing. *Financial Times,* p. 13.

Davis, M. (2003, April) Les famines coloniales, gènocide oublié: aux origines du tiers-monde. *Le Monde diplomatique,* p. 3.

Davis, M. (2005, October) Capitalisme de catastrophe. *Le Monde diplomatique,* pp. 1, 4–5.

Davis, M. (2006a, September) Les petits sorciers de Kinshasa: de l'explosion urbaine au bidonville global. *Le Monde diplomatique,* p. 24.

Davis, M. (2006b) *Planet of Slums.* London, UK: Verso.

Dawkins, R. (1989) *The Selfish Gene* (rev. edn). New York, NY: Oxford University Press.

Dawson, D. A., Grant, B. F., Stinson, F. S., Chou, P. S., Huang, B., and Ruan, J. (2005) Recovery from DSM-IV alcohol dependence: United States 2001–2002. *Addiction,* **100,** 281–292.

Dawson, M. (2003) *The Consumer Trap: Big Business Marketing in American Life.* Champagne, IL: University of Illinois Press.

De-Angelis, D., Hickman, M. and Yang, S. (2004) Estimating long term trends in the prevalence of opiate use/injecting drug use and the number of former users: backcross calculation methods and overdose deaths. *American Journal of Epidemiology,* **160,** 994–1004.

de Dianous, S. (2004, September) Les damnés de la terre du Cambodge. *Le Monde diplomatique,* pp. 20–21.

deGraaf, J., Wann, D., and Naylor, T. H. (2002) *Affluenza: the All-consuming Epidemic.* San Francisco, CA: Barrett-Koehler.

DeGrandpre, R. (1999) *Ritalin Nation: Rapid-fire Consciousness and the Transformation of Human Consciousness.* New York, NY: Norton.

DeGrandpre, R. (2006) *The Cult of Pharmacology: How America Became the World's Most Troubled Drug Culture.* Durham, NC: Duke University Press.

Denizet-Lewis, B. (2006, 25 June) An anti-addiction pill? *New York Times Magazine,* pp. 48–53.

Desjardins, N. and Hotton, T. (2004) Trends in drug offences and the role of alcohol and drugs in crime. *Juristat: Canadian Centre for Justice Statistics,* **24,** 1–23 (Statistics Canada, catalogue no. 85-002-XPE).

Desmond, A. and Moore, J. (1991) *Darwin.* New York, NY: Warner Books.

Despratx, M. and Lando, B. (2004, November) Notre ami Saddam. *Le Monde diplomatique.* pp. 12–13.

Dewey, J. (1922) *Human Nature and Conduct.* New York, NY: Modern Library.

Deyken, E. Y., Levy, J. C. and Wells, V. (1987) Adolescent depression, alcohol and drug abuse. *American Journal of Public Health,* **77,** 178–181.

Diamond, J. (2005) *Collapse: How Societies Choose to Succeed or Fail.* London, UK: Penguin.

Dickens, C. (1994) Gin shops. In M. Slater (ed.), *The Dent Uniform Edition of Dickens' Journalism: Sketches by Boz and Other Early Papers, 1833–1835*, pp. 180–185. London, UK: J. M. Dent. (Original work published 1833–1835.)

Dikötter, F., Laamann, L., and Xun, Z. (2004) *Narcotic Culture: a History of Drugs in China.* Chicago, IL: University of Chicago Press.

Dineen, T. (1998) *Manufacturing Victims: What the Psychology Industry is Doing to People*, 2nd edn. Montreal, QC: Robert Davies.

DiNicola, M. (2005, 14–16 October) *A Polanyian analysis of the Catholic social justice tradition's critique of laissez-faire capitalism.* Paper presented at the 10th International Conference of the Karl Polanyi Institute, Istanbul, Turkey.

Dixon, G. (2007, 11 August) A healthy way to spend your summer? *Globe and Mail*, pp. R1, R7.

Dixon, K. (2000, January) Dans les soutes du 'blairisme': la troisiéme voie, version britannique. *Le Monde diplomatique*, p. 3.

Dixon, K. (2004, September) Sainte alliance Londres–Washington. *Le Monde diplomatique*, pp. 30–31.

Dizard, J. (2004, 3 September) Invitation to a Titanic sinking? *Globe and Mail*, p. A11.

Dobbin, M. (1998) *The Myth of the Good Corporate Citizen: Democracy Under the Rule of Big Business.* Toronto, ON: Stoddard.

Dobbin, M. (2003) *Paul Martin: CEO for Canada?* Toronto, ON: Lorimer.

Dobson, J. (1995) *Life on the Edge.* Nashville, TN: Word Publishing.

Dodds, T. (2007, 15 March–28 March) Greenwashing the smokescreen: Government says more cars mean less emissions. *Republic of East Vancouver*, 'Roadkill' Supplement, p. 1.

Dolmetsch, C. (2004, 10 June) Human impact could further slow Earth's next ice age, study finds. *Globe and Mail*, p. A14.

Donahue, K. C. (2007, 29 January) Tanzanite: commodity fiction or commodity nightmare? *Social Science Research Network*. Retrieved March 2007 from http://ssrn.com/abstract=960814

Donnachie, I. (2000) *Robert Owen: Social Visionary.* Edinburgh, UK: John Donald.

Dorna, A. (2003, November) Faut-il avoir peur du populisme? *Le Monde diplomatique*, pp. 8–9.

Doucet, C. (2005, 26 February) Ethnic cleansing the Canadian way. [Review of the book *A Great and Noble Scheme: the Expulsion of French Acadians.*] *Globe and Mail*, p. D6.

Drake, L. (2007, 28 June) Downtown Eastside cause for concern, UN says. *Globe and Mail*, p. S1.

Dreher, C. (2004a, 21 February) Is there a cure for 'superpower syndrome'? For decades, psychiatrist Robert Jay Lifton has been analyzing the mental dynamics of world conflict and crisis. Now, he's put the White House on the couch and Bush loyalists won't like his diagnosis. *Globe and Mail*, p. F6.

Dreher, C. (2004b, 25 September) Are hip tots heading for trouble? *Globe and Mail*, p. F8.

Drohan, M. (2003a) *Making a Killing: How and Why Corporations use Armed Forces to do Business.* Toronto, ON: Random House Canada.

Drohan, M. (2003b, 29 July) We are risking a collapse. *Globe and Mail*, p. A13.

Drohan, M. (2003c, 6 August) Now they tell us: privatisation is no panacea. *Globe and Mail*, p. A13.

Drohan, M. (2004a, 26 January) It could and did happen here. The idea that American executives have a corner on vice is, to use a polite word, balderdash … We're quickly becoming a nation of dupes. *Globe and Mail*, p. A15.

Drohan, M. (2004b, 5 July) Alien torts: U.S. resolve, our hypocrisy. *Globe and Mail*, p. A13.

Drohan, M. (2004c, 17 August) How we can help Africa (without spending a cent). *Globe and Mail*, p. A13.

Drug Free America Foundation (2007) *Heroin*. Retrieved 17 April 2007, from http://www.dfaf.org/drugfacts/heroin.php

Drury, S. (2005) *The Political Ideas of Leo Strauss* (updated edn). New York, NY: Palgrave Macmillan.

Dube, S. R., Anda, R. F., Felitti, V. J., Edwards, V. J., and Croft, J. B. (2002) Adverse childhood experiences and personal alcohol abuse as an adult. *Addictive Behaviors*, **27**, 713–725.

Dube, S. R., Felitti, V. J., Dong, M., Chapman, D. P., Giles, W. H., and Anda, R. F. (2003) Childhood abuse, neglect, and household dysfunction and the risk of illicit drug use: the adverse childhood experiences study. *Pediatrics*, **111**, 564–572.

Duclos, D. (2002, August) Patrons fraudeurs et tueurs fous. *Le Monde diplomatique*, pp. 4–5.

Dufour, D.-R. (2001, February) Les désarrois de l'individu-sujet. *Le Monde diplomatique*, pp. 16–17.

Dufour, D.-R. (2003a) *L'Art de Réduire les Têtes: sur la Nouvelle Servitude de l'Homme Libéré à l'Ere du Capitalisme Total*. Paris: Éditions Denoël.

Dufour, D.-R. (2003b, October) Servitude de l'homme libéré: a l'heure du capitalisme total. *Le Monde diplomatique*, p. 3.

Dufour, D.-R. (2005) *On achève bien les hommes: des conséquences actuelle et future de la mort de Dieu*. Paris: Denoël.

Duhaime, G. (2004, July) Offensive contre l'Etat social au Québec. *Le Monde diplomatique*, pp. 16–17.

Dunbar, J. (1970) *J. M. Barrie: the Man Behind the Image*. Boston, MA: Houghton, Mifflin.

Dupré, R. (2004, September–October) *The prohibition of alcohol revisited: the U.S. case in international perspective*. Paper prepared for the International Society for New Institutional Economics Conference, Tucson, AZ, USA.

Duran, E. and Duran, B. (1995) *Native American Postcolonial Psychology*. Albany, NY: State University of New York Press.

Durkheim, E. (1951) *Suicide: a Study in Sociology* (J. A. Spaulding and G. Simpson, trans.). Glenco, IL: Free Press. (Original work published 1897.)

Dyer, G. (2005, 11 January) The global giant trips up: Washington's real agenda, retaining America's global dominance, has been ill-served by its recent tactics … *Globe and Mail*, p. A15.

Eckersley, R. M. (2005) 'Cultural fraud': the role of culture in drug abuse. *Drug and Alcohol Review*, **24**, 157–163.

Edgar, P. (2003a, 17 May) Trying to break the cycle of natives and the law. *Vancouver Sun*, p. B1.

Edgar, P. (2003b, 17 May) Red Road Warrior steers the young from addiction: going straight: culture is treatment, says Willard Cooke, who laid off the drugs and beer in 2002. *Vancouver Sun*, p. B5.

Edwards, B. and Foley, M. (1998) Civil society and social capital beyond Putnam. *American Behavioral Scientist*, **42**, 124–140.

Edwards, J. (1847) *Temperance Manual*. New York, NY: American Tract Society.

Einstein, A. (1998, May) Why socialism? *Monthly Review*, **50**. (Reprinted from *Monthly Review*, **1**, May 1949.) Retrieved from http://www.monthlyreview.org/598einst.htm

Elie, M.-P. (2007, May) Fini les lendemains de veille! *Québec Science*, **45**, 16–22.

Ellis, A. and Harper, R. A. (1961) *A Guide to Rational Living*. North Hollywood, CA: Wiltshire Books.

Ellul, J. (1965) *Propaganda: the Formation of Men's Attitudes*. New York, NY: Knopf.

Engels, F. (1966) Introduction to K. Marx. In *Travail Salarié et Capital*, pp. 1–12. Beijing, China: Editions en Langues Étrangères. (Original work published 1891.)

Ennett, S. T., Tobler, N. S., Ringwalt, C. L. and Flewelling, R. L. (1994) How effective is Drug Abuse Resistance Education? A meta-analysis of Project DARE outcome evaluations. *American Journal of Public Health*, **84**, 1394–1401.

Erdman, B. (2007, 2 January) Private equity rules as buyout kings. *Globe and Mail*, pp. B1, B8.

Erickson, P. G. and Alexander, B. K. (1989) Cocaine and addictive liability. *Social Pharmacology*, **3**, 249–270.

Erickson, P. G., Adlaf, E. M., Smart, R. G., and Murray, G. F. (eds) (1994) *The Steel Drug: Cocaine and Crack in Perspective*, 2nd edn. New York, NY: Lexington Books.

Erikson, E. H. (1946) Ego development and historical change. *Psychoanalytic Study of the Child*, **2**, 359–396.

Erikson, E. H. (1959) Identity and the life cycle. Selected papers (Monograph). *Psychological Issues*, **1**, 1–171.

Erikson, E. H. (1963) *Childhood and Society*, 2nd edn. New York, NY: Norton.

Erikson, E. H. (1968) *Identity, Youth and Crisis*. New York, NY: Norton.

Eurchuk, R. (2003, 27 November) Don't believe everything you read. *Republic of East Vancouver*, pp. **1**, 7.

Euston Manifesto (n.d.) Retrieved 3 June 2006, from http://eustonmanifesto.org/joomla/index.php?option=com_contentandtask=viewandid=12andItemid=38

Evans-Pritchard, A. (2007a, 10 August) China threatens 'nuclear option' of dollar sales. *Daily Telegraph*. Retrieved 21 September 2007, from http://www.telegraph.co.uk/money/main.jhtml?xml=/money/2007/08/07/bcnchina107a.xml

Evans-Pritchard, A. (2007b, 20 September) Fears of dollar collapse as Saudis take fright. *Daily Telegraph*, p. 5.

EverQuest Widows (2007) *EverQuest Widows Unite!* Retrieved 22 July 2007, from http://health.groups.yahoo.com/group/everquest-widows

Faiola, A. (2006, 27 May) When escape seems just a mouse-click away. *Washington Post*, p. AO1. Retrieved 29 May 2006, from http://www.washingtonpost.com/wp-dyn/content/article/2006/05/26/AR2006052601960_pf.html

Fawcett, B. (2004, 3 April) Saving culture from the market. [Review of the book *Blockbusters and Trade Wars: Popular Culture in a Globalized World*.] *Globe and Mail*, p. D5.

Feixa, T. (2003, November) Ces libertaires qui luttent contre la technoscience. *Le Monde diplomatique*, pp. 18–19.

Felitti, V. (2003) The origins of addiction: evidence from the Adverse Childhood Experiences Study. English manuscript version of an article published only in German [Ursprünge des Suchtverhaltens—Evidenzen aus einer Studie zu belastenden Kindheitserfahrungen.] *Praxis der Kinderpsychologie und Kinderpsychiatrie*, **52**, 547–559.

Fenwick, M. (2004, 14 June) Couch potato plea. [Letter to the editor.] *Globe and Mail*, p. A12.

Ferron, J. (1993) *Contes*. Montreal, QC: Biblioteque nationale de Québec. (Original work published 1968.)

Fingarette, H. (1988) *Heavy Drinking: the Myth of Alcoholism as a Disease*. Berkeley, CA: University of California Press.

Fischer, B., Chin, A. T., Kuo, I., Kirst, M., and Vlahov, D. (2002) Canadian illicit opiate users' views on methadone and other opiate prescription treatment: an exploratory qualitative study. *Substance Use and Misuse*, **37**, 495–522.

Fischer, B., Cruz, M. F., and Rehm, J. (2006a) Illicit opioid use and its key characteristics: a select overview and evidence from a Canadian multisite cohort of illicit opioid abusers (OPICAN). *Canadian Journal of Psychiatry*, **51**, 624–634.

Fischer, B., Rehm, J., Patra, J., and Cruz, M. F. (2006b) Changes in illicit opioid use across Canada. *Canadian Medical Association Journal*, **175**, 1385–1387.

Fish, L. M. (2004) *Sin, Debauchery, Moral Degeneration, Genetic Disease, or Social Failing: What is Addiction?* Unpublished manuscript.

Fish, L. M. (2006) *Nature, culture, and abnormal appetites: an ecopsychological analysis of addiction.* Unpublished doctoral dissertation, Union Institute and University, Cincinnati, OH.

Fisher, R. (1992) *Contact and Conflict: Indian-European Relations in British Columbia, 1774–1890*, 2nd edn. Vancouver, BC: University of British Columbia Press.

Flood, C. (2002) *Making a Stone of the Heart*. Toronto, ON: Key Porter.

Fong, P. (2005, 4 October) Vancouver named most liveable. *Globe and Mail*, pp. S1, S3.

Fong, P. (2006, 13 December) Province, natives settle claim over flooding caused by dam. *Globe and Mail*, p. S3.

Forero, J. (2005, 26 November) Advocate for coca legalisation leads in Bolivian race. *New York Times*, p. A3.

Fortin, T. (2007, July) Guerres à la portée de tous. *Le Monde diplomatique*, p. 27.

Foster, P. (2007, 12 January) Europe's masterplan. *National Post*. Retrieved 29 January 2007, from http://www.canada.com/nationalpost/columnists/story.html?id=d96478ed-e3bc-49f1-8dc4-d8641f6e6518andp=1

Four Pillars Coalition (2005) *Four Pillars, Four Years. Where to Now?* Vancouver, BC: Drug Policy Program, City of Vancouver, BC, Canada.

Four Worlds International Institute (n.d.) The Alkali Lake community story. In *Social Security Reform: Part IV—Case Studies*, pp. 135–149. Lethbridge, AB: published by the author. Retrieved from http://www.4worlds.org/4w/ssr/Partiv.htm

Fowlie, J. (2004, 13 November) Universities get $194 million to lure top researchers: Economic spinoff: move to help Canada compete in global economy. *Vancouver Sun*, pp. G1, G11.

Frank, R. and Cherney, E. (2003, 3 December) More Hollinger deals raise independence questions: helped fund conservative magazine linked to directors Perle and Kissinger. *Globe and Mail*, p. B9.

Frank, R. and Cherney, E. (2004, 27 September) Hollinger board of directors emerge as particularly passive: allowed Lord Black and colleagues to siphon more than $400-million from firm. *Globe and Mail*, p. B10.

Frankel, K. (2005, 28 June) The man who would be president. *Globe and Mail*, p. A15.

Freeman, A. (2004, 10 June) Bush government blasted over memo advising on torture. *Globe and Mail*, p. A13.

Freeman, A. (2006, 30 October) $7-trillion warning on global warming. *Globe and Mail*, pp. A1, A14.

Freud, S. (1929) *Civilisation and its Discontents*. Chicago, IL: Great Books.

Friedman, M. and Friedman, R. (1979) *Free to Choose: a Personal Statement*. San Diego, CA: Harcourt Brace Jovanovich.

Friedman, S. R. (2002) Sociopharmacology of drug use: initial thoughts. *International Journal of Drug Policy*, **13**, 341–347.

Friedman, T. (2000) *The Lexus and the Olive Tree* (rev. edn). New York, NY: Farrar, Strauss and Giroux.

Friedman, T. (2005, 29 May) Times come to close Guantanamo Bay site. *GrandForksHerald.com*. Retrieved 12 August 2005, from http://www.grandforks.com/mld/grandforks/news/opinion/11766221.htm?template=conte ntModules/printstory.jsp

Friesen, J. (2004, 15 September) Adbusters suing networks for not airing its TV spots. *Globe and Mail*, pp. A1, A8.

Friesen, J. (2005, 20 August) Blame Canada (for multiculturalism)? *Globe and Mail*, p. F8.

Fritz, M. (2005, 23 August) Not enough babies: report fingers new threat to economy. *Globe and Mail*, p. B12.

Froguel, P. and Smadja, C. (2004, December) L'obésité au bout du repas. *Le Monde diplomatique*, p. 13.

Fromm, E. (1941) *Escape from Freedom*. New York, NY: Avon Books.

Fu, B. (2003, March) Les silence diplomatique de la Chine. *Le Monde diplomatique*, p. 26.

Fukuyama, F. (1989, Summer) The end of history. *National Interest*. Available at http://www.wesjones.com/eoh.htm

Fukuyama, F. (1992) *The End of History and the Last Man*. New York, NY: Avon.

Furness, E. (2004) Cycles of history in plateau sociopolitical organisation: reflections on the nature of indigenous band societies. *Ethnohistory*, **51**, 137–170.

Galbraith, J. K. (1985) *The Scotch*. Toronto, ON: Macmillan of Canada.

Galloni, A. and Mollenkamp, C. (2004, 1 January) The Parmalat scandal: how it happened. *Globe and Mail*, pp. B1, B4.

Galloway, G. (2004, 2 February) Depression hits harder in older teenage girls. *Globe and Mail*, pp. A1, A2.

Galt, V. (2004a, 17 February) Workplace stress exacting heavy toll, group says. *Globe and Mail*, pp. B1, B2.

Galt, V. (2004b, 27 July) Software helps ease pain for cubicle dwellers. *Globe and Mail*, pp. A1, A8.

Galt, V. (2004c, 29 July) Rising workloads, stress seen taking toll on productivity. *Globe and Mail*, p. B60.

Galt, V. (2004d, 31 July) Disengagement said 'common' in workplace. *Globe and Mail*, p. B7.

Galt, V. (2005, 12 April) Business's next challenge: tackling mental health in the workplace. *Globe and Mail*, pp. B1, B20.

Galt, V. (2007, 11 April) Issues from home found to create pitfalls on the job. *Globe and Mail*, pp. C1, C7.

Gambotto, A. (2005, 27 August) Error in the name of God. [Review of the book *The Sins of Scripture: Exposing the Bible's Texts of Hate to Reveal the God of Love*.] Globe and Mail, p. D10.

Ganguly, K. (2004) Opium use in Rajasthan India: a socio-cultural perspective. In R. Coomber and N. South (eds), *Drug Use and Cultural Contexts Beyond the West*, pp. 83–100. London, UK: Free Association Books.

Garnier, J.-P. (2007, October) Des chercheurs au secours de l'ordre établi. *Le Monde diplomatique*, p. 3.

Gartner, Z. (2003, 24 May) Poor little hungry girl. [Review of the book *Appetites: Why Women Want.*] *Globe and Mail*, p. D16.

Gawin, F. H. (1991) Cocaine addiction: psychology and neurophysiology. *Science*, **251**, 1580–1586.

Gay, G. R., Senay, E. C., and Newmeyer, J. A. (1974) The pseudo junkie: evolution of the heroin lifestyle in the non-addicted individual. *Anesthesia and Analgesia*, **53**, 241–247.

Gee, M. (2001, 1 December) Anti-Semitism and anti-Americanism: blood brothers of hate. *Globe and Mail*, p. A21.

Gee, M. (2003a, 30 April) Bush puts corrupt regimes on notice. *Globe and Mail*, p. A9.

Gee, M. (2003b, 20 June) So the United States and Britain lied to the world. So what? *Globe and Mail*, p. A13.

Gee, M. (2004a, 6 February) The onus was on Saddam to show he had no WMD. *Globe and Mail*, p. A13.

Gee, M. (2004b, 9 June) He was right about one thing. *Globe and Mail*, p. A25.

Gee, M. (2005, 7 September) Saying no to condoms still a killer. *Globe and Mail*, p. A23.

Genet, J. (1963) *Our Lady of the Flowers*. New York, NY: Grove Press. (Original work published 1943.)

Georgeson, R., Walling, S., Baxter, S., *et al.* (2007, 9 March) *The Shadows Project: We're All in this Together* (rehearsal draft). Vancouver, BC: Vancouver Moving Theatre.

Ghafour, H. (2003, 3 December) Guns, ballots and hope in the new Afghanistan. *Globe and Mail*, pp. A1, A15.

Ghafour, H. (2005, 24 June) EU must modernize or suffer, Blair says. *Globe and Mail*, p. A12.

Gibb-Clark, M. (1999, 31 May) Retreat probes mid-life malaise. *Globe and Mail*, p. M1.

Gibbon, E. (1974) *The Decline and Fall of the Roman Empire*, vol. 1. New York, NY: Random House. (Original work published in 1776.)

Gibson, J. R. (1982–1983) Smallpox on the Northwest Coast, 1835–1838. *BC Studies*, **56**, 61–81.

Giddens, A. (1990) *The Consequences of Modernity*. Cambridge, UK: Polity Press.

Giddens, A. (1991) *Modernity and Self-identity: Self and Society in the Late Modern Age*. Stanford, CA: Stanford University Press.

Giddens, A. (1994) Living in a post-traditional society. In U. Beck, A. Giddens and S. Lash (eds), *Reflexive Modernisation*, pp. 56–109. Cambridge, UK: Polity Press.

Giddens, A. (1998) *The Third Way*. Cambridge, UK: Polity Press.

Ginisty, B. (1999, December) La spiritualité au risque des idoles. *Le Monde diplomatique*, p. 32.

Gittings, J. (1973) *A Chinese View of China*. New York, NY: Pantheon.

Gittings, J. (2005) *The Changing Face of China: from Mao to Market*. Oxford, UK: Oxford University Press.

Glaser, F. B., Heather, N., Drummond, D. C., *et al.* (1999) Comments on Project MATCH: matching alcohol treatments to client heterogeneity. *Addiction*, **94**, 31–69.

Glavin, T. (2006, 3 June) Shake it to the left. *Globe and Mail*, p. F7.

Glendinning, C. (1994) *My Name is Chellis and I'm in Recovery from Western Civilisation*. Boston, MA: Shambhala.

Globe and Mail (1999, 24 June) Willy Loman: the recurring nightmare. *Globe and Mail*, p. B12.

Globe and Mail (2002a, 25 June) The children's minute. *Globe and Mail*, p. A18.

Globe and Mail (2002b, 4 June) What warming means. *Globe and Mail*, p. A16.

Globe and Mail (2004a, 13 August) The soft handling of André Ouellet. *Globe and Mail*, p. A10.

Globe and Mail (2004b, 20 September) The pension trap. *Globe and Mail*, p. A12.

Globe and Mail (2005a, 18 February) The unending misery of Innu in Natuashish. *Globe and Mail*, p. A14.

Globe and Mail (2005b, 24 June) Blair to EU: wake up. *Globe and Mail*, p. A14.

Globe and Mail (2005c, 11 August) Will the U.S. respect this softwood ruling? *Globe and Mail*, p. A14.

Globe and Mail (2005d, 23 August) U.S. televangelist calls for assassination of Chavez. *Globe and Mail*. Retrieved 26 August 2005, from http://www.theglobeandmail.com/servlet/story/RTGAM.20050823.wrobertc0823/BNStory/International

Globe and Mail (2005e, 2 November) University report card. *Globe and Mail*, Section U (special section of newspaper).

Globe and Mail (2005f, 3 November) It's no answer to throw money at aboriginal ills. *Globe and Mail*, p. A16.

Globe and Mail (2006a, 28 March) How to retain workers without a big amnesty. *Globe and Mail*, p. A14.

Globe and Mail (2006b, 19 October) It's alarming how many aboriginals are in prison. *Globe and Mail*, p. A14.

Globe and Mail (2006c, 31 October) University report card. *Globe and Mail* (special magazine supplement).

Globe and Mail (2007a, 14 February) Workplace ethics 101. *Globe and Mail*, p. C5.

Globe and Mail (2007b, 16 October) University report card. *Globe and Mail* (special magazine supplement).

Gmel, G., Rehm, J., and Room, R. (2004) Contrasting individual level and aggregate level studies in alcohol research? Combining them is the answer. *Addiction Research and Theory*, **12**, 1–10.

Goenka, S. N. (1987) *The Discourse Summaries: Talks from a Ten-day Course in Vipassana Meditation.* Condensed by William Hart. Seattle, WA: Vipassana Research Publications.

Goenka, S. N. (1991) *Discourses from Ten-day Vipassana Course* (11 videotapes). Pariyatti, 867 Larmon Rd, Onalaska, WA, USA, 98570–0534. (Available only to Vipassana students.)

Gold, M. S. (1984) *800-COCAINE.* New York, NY: Bantam Books.

Goldman, A. (1981) *Elvis.* New York, NY: McGraw-Hill.

Goldstein, A. (1979) Heroin maintenance: a medical view. A conversation between a physician and a politician. *Journal of Drug Issues*, **9**, 341–347.

Golub, P. S. (2005a, July) Le grand tournant de Washington: Mondialisation, Acte II. *Le Monde diplomatique*, pp. **1**, 20–21.

Golub, P. S. (2005b, July) Dieu, la nation et l'armée, une sainte trinitée. *Le Monde diplomatique*, pp. 20–21.

Gosline, A. (2007, 26 February) Bored to death: chronically bored people exhibit higher risk-taking behavior. *Scientific American.com*. Retrieved 5 April 2007, from http://www.sciam.com/article.cfm?articleID=000A57A9-E7F2–99DF-3F76DB3012DC4FB2andpageNumber=2andcatID=4

Gossop, M. and Keaney, F. (2004) Research note—prescribing diamorphine for medical conditions: a very British practice. *Journal of Drug Issues*, **34**, 441–449.

Gossop, M., Darke, S., Griffiths, P., Hando, J., Powis, B., Hall, W., and Strang, J. (1995) The Severity of Dependence Scale (SDS): psychometric properties of the SDS in English and Australian samples of heroin, cocaine and amphetamine users. *Addiction*, **90**, 607–614.

Gould, E. (2006–2007, December–January) Ralph's last laugh: interprovincial trade deal ties the hands of government. *Briarpatch Magazine*, pp. 4–9. Retrieved 2 February 2007, from http://briarpatchmagazine.com/news/?p=366

Gould, J. E. (2007, 12 March) Drug war in Columbia going up in smoke. *Globe and Mail*, p. 10.

Gould, S. J. (1977) *Ontogeny and Phylogeny*. Harvard, MA: Harvard University Press.

Gove, M. (2003, 8 January) The hatred of America is the socialism of fools. *Times*, p. 16. Retrieved from www.timesonline.co.uk/article/0,,482–536072,00.html

Government of Canada (1864) Temperance Act. *Statutes of the Province of Canada*, 1864, Chapter 18.

Government of Canada (1878) Canada Temperance Act. *Statutes of Canada*, 1878, Chapter 16.

Government of Canada (2007) *Bill C-47: an act respecting the protection of marks related to the Olympic Games and the Paralympic Games and protection against certain misleading business associations and making a related amendment to the Trade-marks act*. Retrieved 6 October 2007, from http://www2.parl.gc.ca/HousePublications/Publication.aspx?Docid=3044596andfile=4

Governments of British Columbia and Alberta (2006, April) *Trade, investment and labour mobility agreement between British Columbia and Alberta*. Retrieved 2 February 2007, from http://www.ecdev.gov.bc.ca/ProgramsAndServices/Trade/Joint_Trade_Agreement_April_20 06.pdf

Goytisolo, J. and Grass, G. (1999, November) Que peut la littérature? *Le Monde diplomatique*, pp. 28–29.

Granfield, R. (2004) Addiction and modernity: a comment on a global theory of addiction. In P. Rosenqvist, J. Blomqvist, A. Koski-Jännes, and L. Öjesjö (eds), *Addiction and Life Course*, pp. 29–34. Helsinki, Finland: Nordic Council for Alcohol and Drug Research.

Granfield, R. and Cloud, W. (1999) *Coming Clean: Overcoming Addiction Without Treatment*. New York, NY: New York University Press.

Granfield, R. and Cloud, W. (2002, October) *The social process of exiting addiction: Recovery capital and the implications for treatment providers*. Paper presented at the conference on Addiction in the Life Course Perspective of the Kettil Bruun Society/Nordic Council for Alcohol and Drug Research, Stockholm, Sweden.

Gray, J. (1998) *False Dawn: the Delusions of Global Capitalism*. London, UK: Granta Publications.

Greater Vancouver Gateway Council (2003, July) *Economic Impact Analysis of Investment in a Major Commercial Transportation System for the Greater Vancouver Region*. Vancouver, BC: published by the author.

Greenfield, D. (1999) *Virtual Addiction: Help for Netheads, Cyber Freaks, and Those Who Love Them*. Oakland, CA: New Harbinger Publications.

Gresswell, D. M. and Hollin, C. R. (1997) Addictions and multiple murder: a behavioural perspective. In J. E. Hodge, M. McMurran, and C. R. Hollin (eds), *Addicted to Crime?*, pp. 140–165. West Sussex, UK: John Wiley & Sons.

Grimmer, T. (2006, 1 March) Despite the socialist language, capitalists like Beijing's new rural focus. *Globe and Mail*, p. B10.

Grinspoon, L. and Hedblom, P. (1975) *The Speed Culture: Amphetamine Use and Abuse in America*. Cambridge, MA: Harvard University Press.

Gross, B. (1980) *Friendly Fascism: the New Face of Power in America*. Montreal, QC: Black Rose Books.

Gurstein, P. and Small, D. (2005) From housing to home: reflexive management for those deemed hard to house. *Housing Studies*, 20, 717–735.

Gusfield, J. R. (1963) *Symbolic Crusade: Status Politics and the American Temperance Movement.* Urbana, IL: University of Illinois Press.

Gutstein, D. (2005, 28 January) Senate comes to scrutinize big media in BC: what's it like to live in Canada's media concentration capital? *Tyee.* Retrieved 22 March 2005, from http://sb4.nearlyfree.org/Mediacheck/2005/01/28/SenateScrutinizeBigMediaBC/

Gzoski, P. (2006) How to quit smoking in fifty years or less. In L. Crozier and P. Lane (eds), *Addicted: Notes from the Belly of the beast,* 2nd edn, pp. 61–81. Vancouver, BC: Greystone.

Hadaway, P., Beyerstein, B. L., and Kimball, M. (1986) Addiction as an adaptive response: is smoking a functional behavior? *Journal of Drug Issues*, 16, 371–390.

Haden, M. (2006) The evolution of the four pillars: acknowledging the harms of drug prohibition. *International Journal of Drug Policy*, 17, 124–126.

Hafner, K. (2004, 27 May) For some, the blogging never stops. *New York Times*, pp. E1, E7.

Haig-Brown, C. (1988) *Resistance and Renewal: Surviving the Indian Residential School.* Vancouver, BC: Tillacum.

Halimi, S. (2002, January) Quand la droite américaine pensait l'impensable: Des idées désormais jugées 'naturelles'. *Le Monde diplomatique*, pp. 20–21.

Halimi, S. (2005, October) L'éternal quête du modèle étranger. *Le Monde diplomatique*, pp. 8–9.

Halimi, S. (2006, November) Rituel démocratique et société de castes. *Le Monde diplomatique*, pp. 1, 20–21.

Hallowell, G. A. (1985) Prohibition. In J. H. Marsh (ed.), *The Canadian Encyclopedia*, vol. 3, p. 1491. Edmonton, AB: Hurtig.

Hammersley, R. and Ditton, J. (1994) Cocaine careers in a sample of Scottish users. *Addiction Research*, 2, 51–69.

Hammersley, R. and Reid, M. (2002) Why the pervasive addiction myth is still believed. *Addiction Research and Theory*, 10, 7–30.

Hammerton, J. A. (1929) *Barrie: the Story of a Genius.* New York, NY: Dodd, Mead, and Co.

Hando, J. and Hall, W. (1997) Patterns of amphetamine use in Australia. In H. Klee (ed.), *Amphetamine Misuse: International Perspectives on Current Trends*, pp. 81–110. Amsterdam: Harwood Academic Publishers.

Hänninen, V. and Koski-Jännes, A. (2004) Stories of attempts to recover from addiction. In P. Rosenqvist, J. Blomqvist, A. Koski-Jännes, and L. Öjesjö (eds), *Addiction and Life Course*, pp. 231–246. Helsinki, Finland: Nordic Council for Alcohol and Drug Research.

Hardin, G. (1968, 13 December) The tragedy of the commons. *Science*, 162, 1243–1248.

Harding, K. (2003, 18 June) No safety in numbers: although disability claims are down, psychological problems in the workplace have become 'a growth industry'. *Globe and Mail*, pp. C1, C5.

Harding, K. (2005, 6 May) Premiers tackle crystal meth 'curse': Western leaders call on Ottawa to join them in all-out war against highly addictive drug. *Globe and Mail*, pp. S1, S3.

Hardy, Q. (2003, 10 November) Inside dope: Canada's dirty, well-lit marijuana trade is rich, expanding … and unstoppable. *Forbes Magazine*, 172, 146–154.

Harmon, A. (2003, 25 August) Finding comfort with strangers with an online diet journal. *New York Times*, pp. A1, A10.

Harribey, J.-M. (2004, July) Dévelopement ne rime pas forcément avec croissance. *Le Monde diplomatique*, pp. 18–19.

Harris, C. (1994) Voices of disaster: smallpox around the Strait of Georgia in 1782. *Ethnohistory*, **41**, 591–626.

Harris, C. (1997–1998) Social power and cultural change in pre-colonial British Columbia. *BC Studies*, **115–116**, 45–82.

Harris, L. (2003, 15 January) Marx without the realism: the intellectual roots of America-bashing. *Opinion Journal from the Wall Street Journal Editorial Page*. Retrieved from http://www.opinionjournal.com/extra/?id=110002911

Harris, L. (2006) The magic circle. *alt.theatre: Cultural Diversity and the Stage*, **4**, 9–10, 15.

Hatterer, L. J. (1980) *The Pleasure Addicts: the Addictive pRocess—Food, Sex, Drugs, Alcohol, Work, and More.* South Brunswick, NJ: A. S. Barnes.

Hawken, P. (2007) *Blessed Unrest: How the Largest Movement in the World Came into Being.* New York, NY: Viking.

Hawthorn, T. (2003, 8 November) The real-life James Bond? *Globe and Mail*, p. F11.

Hawthorn, T. (2005, 4 May) Nothing funny about crystal meth: drug is becoming a scourge in Victoria. *Globe and Mail*, pp. S1, S3.

Health and Welfare Canada (1984) *Cancer Pain: a Monograph on the Management of Cancer Pain.* Ottawa, ON: Health and Welfare Canada.

Healy, D. (1997) *The Anti-depressant Era.* Cambridge, MA: Harvard University Press.

Healy, D. (2003) *Let Them Eat Prozac.* Toronto, ON: Lorimer.

Heath, D. B. (1987) A decade of development in the anthropological study of alcohol use: 1970–1980. In M. Douglas (ed.), *Constructive Drinking: Perspectives on Drink from Anthropology*, pp. 16–69. New York, NY: Cambridge University Press.

Heath, J. (2001) *The Efficient Society: Why Canada is as Close to Utopia as it Gets.* Toronto, ON: Penguin, Viking.

Hecksher, D. (2004) The individual narrative as a maintenance strategy. In P. Rosenqvist, J. Blomqvist, A. Koski-Jännes, and L. Öjesjö (eds), *Addiction and Life Course*, pp. 247–266. Helsinki, Finland: Nordic Council for Alcohol and Drug Research.

Heilbroner, R. L. (1961) *The Worldly Philosophers: the Life, Times, and Ideas of the Great Economic Thinkers* (rev. edn). New York, NY: Simon and Schuster.

Helzer, J. E., Robins, L. N. and Davis, D. H. (1976) Antecedents of narcotic use and addiction. A study of 898 Vietnam veterans. *Drug and Alcohol Dependence*, **1**, 183–190.

Henderson, H. (2005, February) L'imposture: Prix Nobel d'èconomie. *Le Monde diplomatique*, p. 28.

Henningfield, J. E., Cohen, C., and Slade, J. D. (1991) Is nicotine more addicting than cocaine? *British Journal of Addiction* **86**, 565–569.

Herman, A. (2001) *How the Scots Invented the Modern World.* New York, NY: Crown.

Hermann, E. and Chomsky, N. (1988) *Manufacturing Consent: the Political Economy of the Mass Media.* New York, NY: Pantheon.

Hersh, S. M. (2004, 24 May) The gray zone: how a secret Pentagon program came to Abu Ghraib. *New Yorker*, **80**, pp. 38–44.

Hersh, S. M. (2007, September–October) It will all fall down: a conversation with Seymour Hersh. *Adbusters*, **73**, 74–77.

Hickman, M., Macleod, J., and De Angelis, D. (2006) Harm reduction interventions in injection drug use. *Lancet*, **367**, 1830–1834.

Hickman, T. M. (2004) 'Mania Americana': narcotic addiction and modernity in the United States, 1870–1920. *Journal of American History*, **90** (electronic version). Retrieved 5 February 2006, from http://www.historycooperative.org.proxy.lib.sfu.ca/journals/joh/90.4/hickman.html

Hill, C. (1958) *Puritanism and Revolution: the English Revolution of the 17th Century.* New York, NY: Schocken.

Hill, C. (1973) *The World Turned Upside Down: Radical Ideas During the English Revolution.* New York, NY: Viking Books.

Hill, G. (2007, Spring) BC treaty monster grows three heads. *Conexión Latina/Latin American Connexions*, pp. 5, 7.

Hill, J. (2006, 16 November) While you were sleeping, your government sold your democracy. *Island Tides*, pp. 2, 5, 7.

Hirsch, T. (2005, 5 December) Calagary's boom: not all boats are rising. *Globe and Mail*, p. A21.

Hobsbawm, E. J. (1962) *The Age of Revolution: 1789–1848.* Cleveland, OH: World Publishing.

Hobsbawm, E. J. (1994) *Age of Extremes: the Short Twentieth Century, 1914–1991.* London, UK: Michael Joseph.

Hochschild, A. (2005) *Bury the Chains: Prophets and Rebels in the Fight to Free an Empire's Slaves.* Boston, MA: Houghton Mifflin.

Hodge, J. E., McMurran, M., and Hollin, C. R. (eds) (1997) *Addicted to Crime?* West Sussex, UK: John Wiley & Sons.

Hodgson, M. (1987) *Indian Communities Develop Futuristic Addictions Treatment and Health Approach.* Edmonton, AB: Necchi Institute on Alcohol and Drug Education.

Hoffman, B. (2003, June) The logic of suicide terrorism. *Atlantic Monthly*, **291**. Retrieved from http://www.theatlantic.com/doc/200306/hoffman

Hoffman, P. (1998) *The Man Who Loved Only Numbers: the Story of Paul Erdös and the Search for Mathematical Truth.* New York, NY: Hyperion.

Holm, B. and Reid, B. (1975) *Indian Art of the Northwest Coast.* Houston, TX: Rice University Institute for the Arts.

Holy Bible, Authorized (King James) Version (1956) Toronto, ON: Gideons International. (Original work published 1611.)

Holy Bible, New International Version (1984) Toronto, ON: International Bible Society.

Holy Bible, New Living Translation (1996) Wheaton, IL: Tyndale House.

Homer-Dixon, T. (2004, 16 February) Cold truths about global warming: winter-bound skeptics scoff at climate change. But they won't like what it's doing to us, Europe and the Gulf Stream … *Globe and Mail*, p. A13.

Homer-Dixon, T. (2005, 30 July) The rich get richer, the poor get squat. [Review of the book *Worlds Apart: Measuring International and Global Inequality.*] *Globe and Mail*, p. D3.

Homer-Dixon, T. (2006) *The Upside of Down: Catastrophe, Creativity, and the Renewal of Civilisation.* Toronto, ON: Knopf.

Horowitz, T. (1999) *Confederates in the Attic. Dispatches from the Unfinished Civil War.* New York, NY: Vintage Books.

Houpt, S. (2004, 7 January) If you can make it here … Sixteen eager contestants are vying to apprentice with flashy Manhattan real-estate mogul Donald Trump in a new show … *Globe and Mail*, p. R1.

Hourcade, B. (2004, February) Le réveil de l'Iran. *Le Monde diplomatique*, pp. 12, 13.

Howe, J. W. (1862, February) The battle hymn of the republic. *The Atlantic Monthly*, **9** (front cover).

Howlett, K. (2005, 9 September) Working-age adults falling through Canada's safety net. *Globe and Mail*, p. A5.

Howlett, K., Blackwell, R., and Waldie, P. (2004, 15 September) Behind Hollinger's web of related-party deals. *Globe and Mail*, p. B3.

Huang, R. (2001, 24 January) Work hard, burn out, drop out. *Globe and Mail*, p. B15.

Hughes, R. (1987) *The Fatal Shore: the Epic of Australia's Founding*. New York, NY: Knopf.

Hume, D. (1888) *A Treatise of Human Nature*. London, UK: Oxford University Press. (Original work published 1739.)

Hume, M. (2004a, 2 January) Derelict store key to renewal: Woodward's at core of new proposals for revitalizing impoverished area. *Globe and Mail*, p. A10.

Hume, M. (2004b, 23 March) BC salmon: Something's not fishy. *Globe and Mail*, p. A15.

Hume, M. (2004c, 2 April) Judge gives first insight into BC police raid. *Globe and Mail*, p. A9.

Hume, M. (2005a, 4 April) Biologist's research hooks DFO—but is it too late? *Globe and Mail*, pp. S1, S2.

Hume, M. (2005b, 24 May) Enlisting addicts for study proves difficult. *Globe and Mail*, pp. S1, S2.

Hume, M. (2005c, 29 July) 'Hot spot' fish areas being depleted. *Globe and Mail*, p. A7.

Hume, M. (2006a, 7 December) A home is where the hope is. *Globe and Mail*, pp. S1, S3.

Hume, M. (2006b, 18 December) No will? No way for social housing. *Globe and Mail*, pp. S1, S2.

Hume, S. (2003a, 29 March) Will salmon go the way of the buffalo? *Vancouver Sun*, pp. B4, B5.

Hume, S. (2003b, 2 August) Mr BC. *Vancouver Sun*, pp. C1, C4.

Hunt, L. G. and Chambers, C. D. (1976) *The Heroin Epidemics: a Study of Heroin Use in the United States, 1965–1973*. New York, NY: Spectrum.

Hunter, J. (2007, 22 August) NDP torn over Tsawwassen treaty. *Globe and Mail*, pp. S1, S2.

Huntington, S. (1996) *The Clash of Civilisations: Remaking of the World Order*. New York, NY: Touchstone.

Hurley, A. and Nikiforuk, A. (2005, 29 July) Don't drain on our parade: water stress in the Missouri, Mississippi and Colorado river basins will affect every single person living around the Great Lakes. *Globe and Mail*, p. A13.

Hurley, D. L. (1991) Women, alcohol and incest: an analytical review. *Journal of Studies on Alcohol*, **52**, 253–268.

Hurtig, M. (2004) *Rushing to Armageddon: the Shocking Truth About Canada, Missile Defence, and Star Wars*. Toronto, ON: McClelland & Stewart.

Hurtig, M. (2005, 2 August) *At a critical moment in human history so bizarre as to be beyond belief*. Keynote address at the Conference of the Association of World Citizens, San Francisco, CA.

Ibbitson, J. (2002a, 4 June) U.S. catches up with global warming. *Globe and Mail*, p. A13.

Ibbitson, J. (2002b, 10 June) Read Dubya's lips: there's no global warming. *Globe and Mail*, p. A15.

Ibbitson, J. (2004, 30 April) PM hopes to extricate Canada from UN box. *Globe and Mail*, p. A4.

Ibbitson, J. (2006, 1 March) Klein's revolution gives Harper a tough choice. *Globe and Mail*, pp. 1, 5.

Ignatieff, M. (2000) *The Rights Revolution*. Toronto, ON: Anansi.

Illouz, E. (2007) *Cold Intimacies: the Making of Emotional Capitalism*. Cambridge, UK: Polity.

Immen, W. (2004, 28 April) Workplace privacy gets day in court. *Globe and Mail*, pp. C1, C7.

Immen, W. (2005, 5 January) Trends to watch in the year ahead. *Globe and Mail*, pp. C1, C7.

Immen, W. (2006, 24 May) Fostering good karma a touchy subject. *Globe and Mail*, pp. C1, C8.

Inciardi, J. A. (1992) *The War on Drugs II*. Mountain View, CA: Mayfield.

Indian and Northern Affairs Canada (2004) *Fact Sheet: the Nisga'a Treaty*. Ottawa, ON: published by the author. Retrieved 13 June 2007, from http://www.ainc-inac.gc.ca/pr/info/nit_e.html

Industry Canada (2007a, 2 March) *Canada's new government moves to protect the Vancouver 2010 Olympic and Paralympic Winter Games brand* [press release]. Ottawa, ON: published by the author. Retrieved 10 April 2007, from http://www.ic.gc.ca/cmb/welcomeic.nsf/ICPagesEPrint/85256A5D006B9720852572920059A745

Industry Canada (2007b, 22 June) *Bill C-47 receives Royal Assent—Canada's new government passes legislation to ensure 2010 Winter Games are a success for Vancouver and for athletes* [press release]. Ottawa, ON: published by the author. Retrieved 1 July 2007, from http://www.ic.gc.ca/cmb/welcomeic.nsf/af913527c10aeb6a852564820068dc6c/85256a5d006b972085257302006e5ae9

Intelm, H. (2006) *How to solve every Sudoku puzzle—learn everything about Sudoku*. St Louis, MO: Geostar Publishing and Services LLC. Retrieved 17 March 2006, from http://www.howtosolveeverysudokupuzzle.com/bgr1.php

International Atomic Energy Agency (2005) *Energy and Environment Data Reference Bank*. Vienna, Austria: published by the author. Retrieved 12 January 2006, from http://www.iaea.org/inisnkm/nkm/aws/eedrb/

International Narcotics Control Board (2004) *Report of the INCB for 2003*. Vienna, Austria: published by the author.

Islam, F. (2001, 11 March) Soros: tax my speculation profits. *Guardian*, p. 2.

Island Tides (2007a, 22 March–4 April) Liberals block TILMA debate. *Island Tides*, p. 1.

Island Tides (2007b, 7 December) Schmeisers honoured with 'Right Livelihood' award. *Island Tides*, pp. 1–2.

Issachar, I. (2001, 14 September) The question is: TV or not TV: It's not only that I love Shakespeare, booze and religion less, but that I love television more. *Globe and Mail*, p. A16.

Jack, I. (2006, 11 February) Wishful thinking. *Guardian Unlimited*. Retrieved 13 June 2007, from http://books.guardian.co.uk/review/story/0,,1706258,00.htm

Jacobs, D. F. (1986) A general theory of addiction: a new theoretical model. *Journal of Gambling Behavior*, **2**, 15–31.

Jacobs, J. (1961) *The Death and Life of Great American Cities*. New York, NY: Vintage Press.

Jacobs, J. (2000) *The Nature of Economies*. Toronto, ON: Random House Canada.

Jacobsson, I. (2002) *Advertising ban and children: children have the right to safe zones*. Stockholm, Sweden: Swedish Institute. Retrieved 3 January 2003, from http://www.sweden.se/templates/cs/Article____3143.aspx

Jacquard, A. (2004, May) Finitude de notre domaine. *Le Monde diplomatique*, p. 28.

Jaffe, J. (1985) Drug addiction and drug abuse. In A. G. Gilman, L. S. Goodman, T. W. Rall, and F. Murad (eds), *Goodman and Gilman's the Pharmacological Basis of Therapeutics*, 7th edn, pp. 532–581. New York, NY: Macmillan Publishing.

Jaffe, J. (1990) Drug addiction and drug abuse. In A. G. Gilman, T. W. Rall, A. S. Nies, and P. Taylor (eds), *Goodman and Gilman's the Pharmacological Basis of Therapeutics*, 8th edn, pp. 522–573. New York, NY: Pergamon.

Jaffe, J. (1999) Conversation with Jerome H. Jaffe: journal interview 45. *Addiction*, **94**, 13–30.

Jaffrelot, C. (2004, January) L'Inde rétive au libéralisme total. *Le Monde diplomatique*, pp. 24–25.

James, W. (1981) *Pragmatism*. Indianapolis, IN: Hackett. (Original work published 1907.)

Jang, B. (2003, 12 November) BC gas firm's rules to ease. *Globe and Mail*, pp. B1, B7.

Janzen, W. (1990) *Limits on Liberty: the Experience of Mennonite, Hutterite, and Doukhobor Communities in Canada*. Toronto, ON: University of Toronto Press.

Jarvie, J. (2005, 28 August) Strategizing a Christian coup d'etat: a group of believers wants to establish scriptures-based government one city and county at a time. *Los Angeles Times*. Retrieved 28 August 2005, from http://www.commondreams.org/headlines05/0828-03.htm

Jason, L. A. and Kobayashi, R. B. (1995) Community building: our next frontier. *Journal of Primary Prevention*, **15**, 195–208.

Jenkins, S. (2006, 26 November) The really tough way to control drugs is to license them. *Sunday Times*. Retrieved from http://www.timesonline.co.uk/tol/comment/columnists/simon_jenkins/article650435.ece

Jensen, D. (2006) *Endgame*, vol. 1. *The End of Civilization*. New York, NY: Steven Stones.

Jewitt, J. (1988) *A Journal Kept at Nootka Sound*. Fairfield, WA: Ye Galleon Press. (Original work published 1824.)

Jilek, W. (1981) Anomic depression, alcoholism, and culture-congenial Indian response. *Journal of Studies on Alcohol*, **42** (Suppl. 9), 159–170.

Jiménez, M. (2004, 24 September) Mickey Mao's alliance with China's communists. *Globe and Mail*, pp. A1, A8.

Johansen, E. (2005, 4 April) To save the world: protecting the environment is fine in theory, too much trouble in practice. We're making all the wrong choices. *Vancouver Sun*, p. A11.

Johnson, C. (2004, 23 July) Council approves 600 slots for Hastings Racecourse. *Vancouver Sun*, pp. A1, A10.

Johnson, J. (2003, 8 November) In praise of the quickie. *Globe and Mail*, pp. L1, L2.

Johnston, H. (2005, 18 January) *The early history of Simon Fraser University*. Public lecture to Simon Fraser University Retirees Association, Burnaby, BC, Canada.

Jones, D. (2005, 29 October) 'In a few decades, there will be no fish': overfishing will have serious consequences for many people, prize-winning scientist says. *Globe and Mail*, pp. S1, S2.

Jong-Fast, M. (2006) Junkie grows up. In L. Crozier and P. Lane (eds), *Addicted: Notes from the Belly of the Beast*, 2nd edn, pp. 37–45. Vancouver, BC: Greystone Books.

Jonnes, J. (2002) Hip to be high: heroin and popular culture in the 20th century. In D. F. Musto (ed.), *One Hundred Years of Heroin*, pp. 227–236. Westport, CT: Auburn House.

Jünger, G. F. (2000) The rise of the new nationalism: Leipzig [extract]. In M. Perry, M. Berg, and J. Krukones (eds), *Sources of Twentieth-century Europe*, pp. 154–157. Boston, MA: Houghton Mifflin. (Original work published 1925.)

Kahn, F. R. (2004) Hard times recalled: the child labour controversy in Pakistan's soccer ball industry. In F. Bird, E. Raufflet, and J. Smucker (eds), *International Business and the Dilemmas of Development*, pp. 132–155. London, UK: Palgrave Macmillan.

Kahn, F. R. (2005, 14–16 October) *Transnational activism and the commodification of space*. Paper presented at the 10th International Conference of the Karl Polanyi Institute, Istanbul, Turkey.

Kaletsky, A. (2003, 1 May) Capitalism is humanity's most benign creation. *Times*. Retrieved 18 January 2007, from http://www.freerepublic.com/focus/f-news/903369/posts

Kapica, J. (2003, 11 December) Copyright litigation is threatening innovation. *Globe and Mail*, p. B13.

Kaplan, E. H. and Wieder, H. (1974) *Drugs Don't Take People, People Take Drugs*. Secaucus, NJ: Lyle Stuart.

Kaplan, J. (1983) *The Hardest Drug: Heroin and Public Policy*. Chicago, IL: University of Chicago Press.

Kawachi, I., Kennedy, B. P., and Lochner, K. (1997, November–December) Long live community: social capital as public health. *American Prospect*, **8**, 56–59.

Keenan, G. (2003, 18 June) Ford plans SUVs for Oakville. *Globe and Mail*, p. B1.

Kendall, P. (2004, September) *Public health (sensible) responses to opioid and other injection drug use*. Paper presented at the Moving Forward: Improving Treatment for Heroin Addiction meeting, Vancouver, BC, Canada.

Kenny, M. G. (1994) *The Perfect Law of Liberty: Elias Smith and the Providential History of America*. Washington, DC: Smithsonian Institution Press.

Kerr, T., Tyndall, M., Li, K., Montaner, J., and Wood, E. (2005a) Safer injection facility use and syringe sharing in injection drug users. *Lancet*, **366**, 316–318.

Kerr, T., Marsh, D., Li, K., Montaner, J., and Wood, E. (2005b) Factors associated with methadone maintenance therapy use among a cohort of polysubstance using injection drug users in Vancouver. *Drug and Alcohol Dependence*, **80**, 329–335.

Kershaw, S. (2005, 1 December) Caught in a web? Net addiction on the increase. *Globe and Mail*, p. A14.

Kessler, D. (2001) *A Question of Intent*. New York, NY: Public Affairs.

Kew, J. E.M. (1990) History of coastal British Columbia since 1846. In W. C. Sturtevant (Series ed.) and W. Suttles (Vol. ed.), *Handbook of North American Indians*: vol. 7. *Northwest Coast*, pp. 159–169. Washington, DC: Smithsonian Institution.

Keyder, V. B. (2005, 14–16 October) *Intellectual property: commodification and its discontents*. Paper presented at the 10th International Conference of the Karl Polanyi Institute, Istanbul, Turkey.

Khantzian, E. J. (1974) Opiate addiction: a critique of theory and some implications for treatment. *American Journal of Psychotherapy*, **28**, 59–70.

Khantzian, E. J. (1985) The self-medication hypothesis of addictive disorders: focus on heroin and cocaine dependence. *American Journal of Psychiatry*, **142**, 1259–1264.

Khantzian, E. J. and Khantzian, N. J. (1984) Cocaine addiction: is there a psychological predisposition? *Psychiatric Annals*, **14**, 753–759.

Khantzian, E. J., Mack, J. E., and Schatzberg, A. F. (1974) Heroin use as an attempt to cope: clinical observations. *American Journal of Psychiatry*, **131**, 160–164.

Khurana, R. (2002, 3 July) False prophets, lost prophets: the cult of charisma. *Globe and Mail*, p. A11.

Kiefer, O. (1934) *Sexual Life in Ancient Rome*. London, UK: Abbey Library.

Kielholz, P. and Ladewig, D. (1977) Abuse of non-narcotic analgesics. In W. R. Martin (ed.), *Drug Addiction* I: *Morphine, sedative/hypnotic and alcohol dependence*, pp. 667–672. Berlin: Springer-Verlag.

Killinger, B. (1991) *Workaholics: the Respectable Addicts—a Family Survival Guide*. Toronto, ON: Key Porter.

Kingwell, M. (2006, June) The American gigantic. *Walrus*, pp. 64–73.

Kirkey, S. (2007, 10 September) Obesity can be a mental illness, expert says. *Vancouver Sun*, pp. A1, A2.

Klee, H. (1997) A typology of amphetamine users in the United Kingdom. In H. Klee (ed.), *Amphetamine Misuse: International Perspectives on Current Trends*, pp. 35–68. Amsterdam: Harwood Academic Publishers.

Klein, N. (2000) *No Logo: Taking Aim at the Brand Bullies*. Toronto, ON: Random House of Canada.

Klein, N. (2004, September) Baghdad year zero. *Harper's Magazine*, pp. 42–53.

Klein, N. (2007) *The Shock Doctrine: the Rise of Disaster Capitalism*. Toronto, ON: Knopf Canada.

Klinenberg, E. (2003, April) Dix maîtres pour les médias américains. *Le Monde diplomatique*, p. 26.

Klinenberg, E. (2005, September) Le groupe Sinclair, empire de la télévision conservatrice aux Etats-Unis. *Le Monde diplomatique*, pp. 24–25.

Klingemann, H., Sobel, L., Barker, J., *et al.* (2001) *Promoting Self-change from Problem Substance Use. Practical Implications for Policy, Prevention, and Treatment*. Dordrecht, The Netherlands: Kluwer.

Kobler, J. (1973) *Ardent Spirits: the Rise and Fall of Prohibition*. New York, NY: Putnam.

Koch, A. and Peden, W. (1944) *The Life and Selected Writings of Thomas Jefferson*. New York, NY: Random House.

Kogawa, J. (2003) *The Rain Ascends*. Toronto, ON: Penguin Canada.

Kolata, G. (2004, 23 December) Trying to sort out drug risks, benefits. *Globe and Mail*, p. A15.

Kolko, G. (2006, October) Une économie d'aprentis sorciers. *Le Monde diplomatique*, pp. 1, 14–15.

Kolesnikoff, J. (2000) Understanding violent behavior: the 'Sons of Freedom' case. In A. Donskov, J. Woodsworth, and C. Gaffield (eds), *The Doukhobor Centenary in Canada: a Multi-disciplinary Perspective on their Unity and Diversity*, pp. 114–128. Ottawa, ON: Slavic Research Group, University of Ottawa.

Konrad, R. (2003, 15 August) Tech workers caught in a bind: U.S. computer experts forced to train lower cost foreign replacements. *Globe and Mail*, p. C2.

Koring, P. (2004a, 16 January) Bush renews effort to fund faith-based programs: U.S. President calls 'miracle of salvation' means toward solving nation's social ills. *Globe and Mail*, p. A9.

Koring, P. (2004b, 3 May) Outrage over abuse has U.S., U.K. scrambling: officials deny problem is widespread, but Amnesty cites 'patterns of torture.' *Globe and Mail*, p. A8.

Kort, M. (1996) *The Soviet Colossus: History and Aftermath*, 4th edn. Armonk, NY: M. E. Sharpe.

Koski-Jännes, A. (1998) Turning points in addiction careers: five case studies. *Journal of Substance Misuse*, **3**, 226–233.

Kowal, N. (1999) What is the issue? Pseudoaddiction or undertreatment of pain. *Nursing Economics*, **17**, 348–349.

Kristianasen, W. (2004, February) 'Tehran Avenue'. *Le Monde diplomatique*, p. 13.

Kropotkin, P. (1972) *Mutual Aid: a Factor of Evolution*, 3rd edn. London, UK: Penguin Books. (Original work published 1914.)

Krugman, P. (2005, 17 June) What's the matter with Ohio? *New York Times*, p. A23.

Krugman, P. (2007, 15 October) Gore derangement syndrome. *New York Times*, p. 21.

Kubey, R. and Csikszentmihalyi, M. (2002, February) Television addiction is no metaphor. *Scientific American*, pp. 74–80.

Kuhn, T. S. (1970) *The Structure Of Scientific Revolutions*, 2nd edn (enlarged). Chicago, IL: University of Chicago Press.

Kushner, H. I. and Sterk, C. E. (2005) The limits of social capital: Durkheim, suicide, and social cohesion. *American Journal of Public Health*, **95**, 1139–1143.

Lackner, C. (2004, 27 July) Small is scary: The Village is yet another tale of terror in a little town. Just what makes them so frightening? *Globe and Mail*, pp. R1, R5.

LaHaye, T. and Jenkins, J. B. (1995) *Left Behind: a Novel of the Earth's Last Days*. Wheaton, IL: Tyndale House.

Land, E. H. (1971) Addiction as a necessity and an opportunity. *Science*, **171**, 151–153.

Lane, P. (2001) Counting the bones. In L. Crozier and P. Lane (eds), *Addicted: Notes From the Belly of the Beast*, pp. 1–15. Vancouver, BC: Greystone Books.

Lane, P. (2004) *There is a Season: a Memoir*. Toronto, ON: McClelland & Stewart.

Langreth, R. and Harper, M. (2006, 8 May) Pill pushers: how the drug industry abandoned science for salesmanship. *Forbes*, pp. 94–102.

Lansens, L. (2003) *Rush Home Road*. Toronto, ON: Vintage Canada.

Lansing, S. (1991) *Priests and Programmers: Technologies of Power in the Engineered Landscape of Bali*. Princeton, NJ: Princeton University Press.

Lapham, L. (2003, July) Une grande lumière est apparue au président. *Le Monde diplomatique*, p. 32.

Larousserie, D. (2005, October) Einstein, un traître pour le FBI. [Review of the book *Einstein, un Traître Pour le FBI*.] *Le Monde diplomatique*, p. 30.

Larsen, B. (2007, 27 October) Teachers demand more busses: students arrive late to class because of huge lineups for SFU busses. *Burnaby Now*, p. 11.

Lasch, C. (1991) *The Culture of Narcissism: American Life in an Age of Diminishing Expectations*, 2nd edn. New York, NY: Norton.

Latouche, S. (2003, November) Pour une société de décroissance. *Le Monde diplomatique*, pp. 18–19.

Latte, A. (2006, 2 February) *Globalization and the indigenous subject: contested construction of Mapuche identity in Chile*. Unpublished guest lecture at Simon Fraser University, Burnaby, BC, Canada.

Lau, E. (2001) More and more. In L. Crozier and P. Lane (eds), *Addicted: Notes from the Belly of the Beast*, pp. 71–84. Vancouver, BC: Greystone Books.

Laurance, J. (2006, 2 June) Heroin: the solution? *Independent* (online edition). Retrieved 4 June 2006, from http://news.independent.co.uk/uk/legal/article623415.ece

Laurance, J. (2007, 20 November) Britain's first 'shooting galleries' hailed a success. *Independent*, p.6.

Leahey, T. H. (2001) *A History of Modern Psychology*, 3rd edn. Englewood Cliffs, NJ: Prentice-Hall.

Lecky, W. E. H. (1911) *A History of European Morals from Augustus to Charlemagne*, 3rd edn (revised). New York, NY: Longmans, Green & Co..

Ledain, G. (1973) *Final Report of the Commission of Inquiry into the Non-medical Use of Drugs*. Ottawa, ON: Information Canada.

Lee, J. (2004, 24 February) Premiers in town, breathing fire: equalisation cuts fuel anger, threats on health spending. *Vancouver Sun*, pp. A1, A2.

Lee, J. (2007, 6 January) Child care advocates decry cuts. *Vancouver Sun*, p. A5.

Leech, G. (2004, 12 November) Plan Colombia benefits US oil companies. *Colombia Journal Online*. Retrieved 25 November 2004, from http://www.colombiajournal.org/colombia198.htm

Leidl, P. (2007) *Vancouver: prosperity and poverty make for uneasy bedfellows in world's most 'liveable' city*. New York, NY: UNFPA: United Nations Population Fund. Retrieved 30 June 2007, from http://www.unfpa.org/swp/2007/presskit/docs/vancouver_feature_eng.doc

Lemoine, M. (2000, May) En Colombie, une nation, deux etats. *Le Monde diplomatique*, pp. 18–19.

Lemoine, M. (2001, January) Culture illicites, narcotrafic, et guerre en Colombie. *Le Monde diplomatique*, pp. 18–19.

Lemoine, M. (2005, June) Lignes de fracture en Amérique latine. *Le Monde diplomatique*, pp. 23–24.

Lenin, N. (1966) *L'Imperialisme, Stade Supreme du Capitalisme*. Peking, China: Editions en Langues Étrangères. (Original work published 1916.)

Lenin, N. (1970) *Karl Marx*. Peking, China: Editions en Langues Étrangères. (Original work published 1918.)

Leshner, A. I. (1997, 3 October) Addiction is a brain disease, and it matters. *Science*, **278**, 45–47.

LeSourd, S. (2002) *The Compulsive Woman*. Lake May, FL: Creation House Press.

Lettieri, D. J., Sayers, M., and Pearson, M. W. (eds) (1980) *Theories on Drug Abuse: Selected Contemporary Perspectives*. National Institute on Drug Abuse Research Monograph 30. (DSS Publication No. ADM 80-967). Washington, DC: US Government Printing Office.

LeVert, S. and McClain, G. (1998) *The Complete Idiot's Guide to Breaking Bad Habits*. New York, NY: Alpha Books.

Levine, H. G. (1978) The discovery of addiction: changing conceptions of habitual drunkenness in America. *Journal of Studies on Alcohol*, **39**, 143–174.

Levine, H. G. (1984) The alcohol problem in America: from temperance to alcoholism. *British Journal of Addiction*, **79**, 109–119.

Levy, A. (2000, December) Face à la drogue, le 'modèle suisse'. *Le Monde diplomatique*, p. 15.

Lew, R. (2000, December) L'empire du Milieu dans la tanière du tigre: quand la Chine courtise l'OMC. *Le Monde diplomatique*, pp. 16–17.

Lewin, M. (2001, December) La Russie face à son passé sociétique. *Le Monde diplomatique*, pp. 8–9.

Lewis, C. T. and Short, C. (1879) *A Latin Dictionary: Founded on Andrews' Edition of Freund's Latin Dictionary*. Oxford: Oxford University Press.

Lewis, J., Polanyi, K., and Kitchin, D. K. (eds) (1935) *Christianity and the Social Revolution*. London, UK: Victor Gollancz.

Lewis, N. A. (2004, 30 November) Red Cross accuses U.S. military of torture at Guantanamo Bay. *Globe and Mail*, p. A17.

Lewis, N. A. and Johnston, D. (2004, 21 December) U.S. military abused detainees, memos say. *Globe and Mail*, p. A14.

Lewis, S. R. (2003, 2 May) Will you thrive as the ranks thin out? *Globe and Mail*, p. C1.

Libby, R. T. (2005, 6 June) Treating doctors as drug dealers: the DEA's war on prescription painkillers. *Policy Analysis*, **545**. (Occasional paper of the Cato Institute, Washington, DC).

Lieberman, M. A. and Snowden, L. R. (1993) Problems in assessing prevalence and membership in self-help group participants. *Journal of Applied Behavioral Science*, **29**, 166–180.

Lifton, R. J. (1986) *The Nazi Doctors: Medical Killing and the Psychology of Genocide*. New York, NY: Basic Books.

Lim, L. (2004, 15 December) China's deadly fix for modern pressures. *BBC News*. Retrieved 15 December 2004, from http://newsvote.bbc.co.uk/mpapps/pagetools/print/news.bbc.co.uk/2/hi/asia-pacific/4085049.stm

Lindesmith, A. R. (1968) *Addiction and Opiates*, 2nd edn. New York, NY: Aldine.

Linhart, D. (2002, June) Travail en miettes, citoyen déboussolés. *Le Monde diplomatique*, pp. 4–5.

Lippman, A. (2005, 6 August) Big pharma: it's enough to make you sick. [Review of the book *Selling Sickness: How the World's Biggest Pharmaceutical Companies are Turning Us All into Patients.*] Globe and Mail, pp. D8, D9.

Livable Region Coalition (2004, October) *Will freeway expansion kill the livable region? Questions about the BC Government's Port Mann and Highway 1 proposal for the Vancouver Region.* Livable Region Coalition, Vancouver, BC, Canada. Retrieved 19 February 2007, from www.livableregion.ca/pdf/LRC_Final_1.pdf

Loewen, J. W. (1999) *Lies Across America: What Our Historic Sites Get Wrong.* New York, NY: New Press.

London, W. D. (1986) Handedness and alcoholism: a family history of left-handedness. *Alcoholism, Clinical and Experimental Research*, **10**, 357.

Lordon, F. (2003) *Et la Vertue Sauvera le Monde: Après la Débâcle Financière, le Salut par l'Éthique'?* Paris: Raisons d'Agir.

Lordon, F. (2004, March) Comment la finance a tué Moulinex: un cas d'école. *Le Monde diplomatique*, pp. 1, 22–23.

Lowe, G. (2004, 14 May) The yin and yang of change. The key to a better workplace: achieve a balance between the structural and cultural forces at play. *Globe and Mail*, p. C1.

Lowinger, P. (1977) The solution to narcotic addiction in the People's Republic of China. *American Journal of Drug and Alcohol Abuse*, **4**, 165–178.

Lowman, C., Hunt, W. A., Litten, R. Z., and Drummond, D. C. (2000) Research perspectives on alcohol craving: an overview. *Addiction*, **95** (Suppl. 2), S45–S54.

Luciw, R. (2007, 14 February) What's love got to do with it? At work, lots. *Globe and Mail*, pp. C1, C2.

Luthar, S. S. (2003) The culture of affluence: psychological costs of material wealth. *Child Development*, **74**, 1581–1593.

MacDonald, A.-M. (2003) *The Way the Crow Flies.* Toronto, ON: Knopf Canada.

Macdonald, B. (1992) *Vancouver: a Visual History.* Vancouver, BC: Talonbooks.

MacDonald, G. and Little, B. (2001, 29 September) The cash crash. *Globe and Mail*, pp. F1, F10.

MacGregor, R. (2004, 29 December) Two worlds about to collide in the new Saskatchewan. *Globe and Mail*, p. A4.

Macinnes, A. I. (1998) Scottish Gaeldom from clanship to commercial landlordism, *c.* 1600–*c.* 1850. In A. I. Macinnes, S. M. Foster, and R. K. Macinnes (eds), *Scottish Power Centres from the Early Middle Ages to the Twentieth Century*, pp. 162–190. Glasgow, UK: Cruithne Press.

Mackail, D. (1941) *The Story of J. M. B.* London, UK: Peter Davies.

MacKenzie, A. (1883) *History of the Highland Clearances.* Edinburgh, UK: Mercat.

MacKinnon, M. (2006, 3 October) No longer pushing democracy, U.S. turns back to Arab autocrats. *Globe and Mail*, p. A12.

Maclean's (2004, 15 November) University rankings'04 [special issue]. *Maclean's*, **117**.

MacLeod, A. (1999) *No Great Mischief.* Toronto, ON: McClelland & Stewart.

MacPherson, D. (2000) A framework for action: a four-pillar approach to drug problems in Vancouver. Vancouver, BC: City of Vancouver.

MacPherson, D. (2001) A framework for action: a four-pillar approach to drug problems in Vancouver (rev. edn). Vancouver, BC: City of Vancouver.

MacPherson, D., Mulla, Z., Richardson, L., and Beer, T. (2005) *Preventing Harm from Psychoactive Substance Use.* Vancouver, BC: City of Vancouver.

Mahoney, J. (2004a, 20 February) Klein issues medicare threat: Alberta willing to violate Health Act if changes aren't made to control costs. *Globe and Mail*, pp. A1, A2.

Mahoney, J. (2004b, 6 December) 'Married with children' preferred: study says even those who don't live in one still favour the traditional nuclear family. *Globe and Mail*, p. A8.

Mahoney, J. (2005a, 12 February) Sexurbia. *Globe and Mail*, pp. F1, F6.

Mahoney, J. (2005b, 23 March) Visible majority by 2017: demographic balance in Toronto, Vancouver will tip within 12 years, Statscan says. *Globe and Mail*, pp. A1, A7.

Mahoney, J. (2005c, 13 August) Designer vaginas: the latest in sexual plastic surgery. *Globe and Mail*, pp. A1, A8.

Makin, K. (2005, 9 July) What really happened to the Inuit sled dogs. *Globe and Mail*, p. A12.

Makkai, T. and McAllister, I. (1998) *Patterns of Drug Use in Australia, 1985–1995*. Canberra, Australia: Australian Government Publishing Service.

Malhotra-Singh, A. (2002, 4 November) New Dior fragrance: Scent of addiction. *San Francisco Examiner*. Retrieved from http://www.examiner.com/news

Mallick, H. (2004, 24 April) I pledge allegiance to my paycheque. *Globe and Mail*, p. F2.

Mallick, H. (2005, 10 September) The brand that didn't deliver. *Globe and Mail*, p. F2.

Mangin, M. (2000, December) Inquiétante vague de chômage. *Le Monde diplomatique*, pp. 16–17.

Manuel, A. (2007, Spring) The BC treaty process: Canada's conflict of interest. *Conexión Latina/Latin American Connexions*, p. 4.

Mao Tse Tung (1966a) Rapport sur l'enquete menee dans le Hounan a propos du mouvement paysan. In Commission pour l'Edition des Oeuvres choisies de MaoTsé-toung de Comité central du Parti communiste chinois (ed.), *Oeuvres Choisies de Mao Tsé-toung*, vol. 1, 2nd edn, pp. 21–33. Peking, China: Editions en Langues Étrangères. (Original work published 1927.)

Mao Tse Tung (1966b) L'elimination des conceptions erronées dans le parti. In Commission pour l'Edition des Oeuvres choisies de MaoTsé-toung de Comité central du Parti communiste chinois (ed.), *Oeuvres Choisies de Mao Tsé-toung*, vol. 1, 2nd edn, pp. 115–126. Peking, China: Editions en Langues Étrangères. (Original work published 1929.)

Mao Tse Tung (1966c) De la practique. In Commission pour l'Edition des Oeuvres choisies de MaoTsé-toung de Comité central du Parti communiste chinois (ed.), *Oeuvres Choisies de Mao Tsé-toung*, vol. 1, 2nd edn, p. 329. Peking, China: Editions en Langues Étrangères. (Original work published 1937.)

Mao Tse Tung (1966d) Causerie pour les rédacteurs du *Quotidien du Chansi-Soueiyuan*. In Commission pour l'Edition des Oeuvres choisies de MaoTsé-toung de Comité central du Parti communiste chinois (ed.), *Oeuvres Choisies de Mao Tsé-toung*, vol. 4, 2nd edn, pp. 253–258. Peking, China: Editions en Langues Étrangères. (Original work published 1948.)

Marcia, J. E. (1966) Development and validation of ego-identity status. *Journal of Personality and Social Psychology*, **3**, 551–558.

Marcia, J. E. (1989) Identity diffusion differentiated. In M. A. Luszcz and T. Nettelbeck (eds), *Psychological Development: Perspectives Across the Lifespan*, pp. 289–294. Amsterdam: Elsevier Science Publishers (North Holland).

Marie, V. (2007, July) *The Shadows Project Final Evaluation Report*. Unpublished report by Victoria Marie, MarieCo Research Services, Vancouver, BC.

Marín, G. (1991) Ignacio Martín-Baró, S. J. (1942–1989): obituary. *American Psychologist*, **46**, 532.

Marlatt, G. A. (1985a) Coping and substance abuse: implications for research, prevention, and treatment. In S. Shiffman and T. A. Well (eds), *Coping and Substance Use*, pp. 367–386. Orlando, FL: Academic Press.

Marlatt, G. A. (1985b) Relapse prevention: theoretical rationale and overview of the model. In G. A. Marlatt and J. R. Gordon (eds), *Relapse Prevention*, pp. 3–67. New York, NY. Guilford.

Marlatt, G. A. (1985c) Situational determinants of relapse and skill-training interventions. In G. A. Marlatt and J. R. Gordon (eds), *Relapse Prevention*, pp. 71–127. New York, NY: Guilford.

Marsa, L. (1997) *Prescriptions for Profits*. New York, NY: Scribner.

Martin, L. (2004, 29 July) Patriot game, media shame. *Globe and Mail*, p. A14.

Martin, S. (2003, 26 August) Virtuoso of inebriation: in close to 20 novels, David Adams Richards has created a rich cast of outsiders, many of whom struggle with addiction … *Globe and Mail*, pp. R1, R5.

Martin, S. T. (2001, 29 July) US vs. them: US policy not limited to borders. *St Petersburg Times Online*. Retrieved 17 September 2005, from http://www.sptimes.com/News/072901/news_pf/Worldandnation/US_policy_not_limited.shtml

Martín-Baró, I. (1994) *Writings for a Liberation Psychology*. Cambridge, MA: Harvard University Press.

Maruani, M. (2003, June) Ravages cachés du sous-emploi. *Le Monde diplomatique*, pp. 4–5.

Marx, K. (1978) Le 18-Brumaire de Louis Bonaparte, 2nd edn. In Institute du Marxisme-Léninisme (ed.), *Karl Marx et Friedrich Engels: Oeuvres Choisies*, vol. 1, pp. 414–585. Moscow, USSR: Editions du Progrès. (Original work published 1869.)

Marx, K. and Engels, F. (1948) *Manifesto of the Communist Party: Authorized English translation*. New York, NY: International Publishers. (Original work published 1848.)

Maschino, M. T. (2002, October) Les nouveaux réactionnaires: intellectuels médiatiques. *Le Monde diplomatique*, pp. 1, 28–29.

Maslow, A. H. (1973) Self-actualizing people: a study of psychological health. In R. J. Lowry (ed.), *Dominance, Self-esteem, Self-actualization: Germinal Papers of A. H. Maslow*, pp. 177–201. Monterey, CA: Brooks/Cole. (Original work published 1950.)

Mason, G. (2006, 24 August) Insight on Insite from across the pond. *Globe and Mail*, pp. S1, S2.

Mason, G. (2007, 13 March) A vote where lists are secret. *Globe and Mail*, p. A9.

Matas, R. (2000, 25 July) Squamish support land-claims settlement: $92.5-million deal ends Kitsilano Point claim. *Globe and Mail*, pp. A1, A5.

Matas, R. (2004, 5 October) Doukhobors to receive no apology from BC. *Globe and Mail*, p. A8.

Matas, R. (2005a, 9 February) Throne speech sees healthier, wealthier BC. *Globe and Mail*, p. A7.

Matas, R. (2005b, 3 August) Pot raids unrelated to Emery, police say. *Globe and Mail*, pp. S1, S3.

Maté, G. (2000) Scattered minds: a new look at the origins and healing of attention deficit disorder. Toronto, ON: Vintage Canada.

Maté, G. (2005a) Decoding the hype: looking for genetic cures for disease lets us sidestep the need to tackle the social and environmental causes. *Globeandmail.com*. Retrieved 27 August 2005, from http://www.scatteredminds.com/press/globe1.htm

Maté, G. (2005b) It's no fix, but it's the best we can do for addicts. *CannabisLink.ca*. Retrieved 27 August 2005, from http://www.mapinc.org/newstcl/v05/n237/a08.html

Maté, G. (2008) *In the Realm of Hungry Ghosts: Close Encounters with Addiction*. Toronto, ON: Knopf Canada

Mathieson, R. (2000) *The Survival of the Unfittest: the Highland Clearances and the End of Isolation*. Edinburgh, UK: John Donald.

Mattelart, A. (2003, December) Jeter les bases d'une information ethique. *Le Monde diplomatique*, p. 32.

Mattison, J. B. (1894) Morphinism in medical men. *Journal of the American Medical Association*, **23**, 187–188.

May, P. A. (1982) Substance abuse and American Indians: prevalence and susceptibility. *International Journal of the Addictions*, **17**, 1185–1209.

Mayr, E. (1982) The growth of biological thought: diversity, evolution, and inheritance. Cambridge, MA: Harvard University Press.

Mays, J. B. (1999) *In the Jaws of Black Dogs: a Memoir of Depression*. New York, NY: HarperCollins.

McAndrew, C. and Edgerton, R. B. (1969) *Drunken Comportment: a Social Explanation*. Chicago, IL: Aldine.

McArthur, K. and Pitts, G. (2003, 1 February) Fliers, airlines love their point programs: fliers getting hooked on free trips. *Globe and Mail*, pp. B2, B5.

McAuliffe, W. E. (1975) A second look at first effects: the subjective effects of opiates on nonaddicts. *Journal of Drug Issues*, **5**, 369–399.

McCarthy, S. (2004a, 14 September) Pension crisis fears deepen as US Air seeks to skip contributions. *Globe and Mail*, pp. B1, B8.

McCarthy, S. (2004b, 15 October) 'These guys are incorrigible fact-twisters'. *Globe and Mail*, p. A16.

McCarthy, S. (2005a, 12 May) UAL pension ploy could start a trend: obligation dumping may save struggling companies, but cost workers, taxpayers. *Globe and Mail*, p. B11.

McCarthy, S. (2005b, 10 October) GM braces for fallout from Delphi. *Globe and Mail*, pp. B1, B4.

McCormick, R. M. (2000) Aboriginal traditions in the treatment of substance abuse. *Canadian Journal of Counseling*, **34**, 25–32.

McCoy, C. B., McCoy, H. V., Lai, S. H., Yu, Z. N., Wang, X. R., and Meng, J. (2001) Reawakening the dragon: changing patterns of opiate use in Asia, with particular emphasis on China's Yunnan Province. *Substance Use and Misuse*, **36**, 49–69.

McDonald, R. A. J. and Barman, J. (1986) *Vancouver Past: Essays in Social History*. Vancouver, BC: University of British Columbia Press.

McFadden, J. (1987) Is guilt soluble in alcohol: an ego analytic view. *Journal of Drug Issues*, **17**, 171–186.

McFarland, J. (2003, 8 October) SEC's small step for shareholders. *Globe and Mail*, p. B2.

McFarland, J. (2004, 3 July) BCE, MTS settle bitter legal feud out of court. *Globe and Mail*, p. B2.

McFeat, T. (ed.) (1966) *Indians of the North Pacific Coast*. Toronto: McClelland & Stewart.

McGlothlin, W. H. and Anglin, M. D. (1981) Shutting off methadone: costs and benefits. *Archives of General Psychiatry*, **38**, 885–892.

McInnis, S. (2003, 5 April) Do you take VISA to love and cherish? *Globe and Mail*, p. D17.

McIntyre, J. W. R. and Houston, C. S. (1999) Smallpox and its control in Canada. *Canadian Medical Association Journal*, **161**, 1543–1546.

McKeganey, N. (2006) The lure and the loss of harm reduction in U.K. drug policy and practice. *Addiction Research and Therapy*, **14**, 557–588.

McKenna, B. (2002a, 8 February) Enron debacle should resurrect campaign finance reform. *Globe and Mail*, p. B10.

McKenna, B. (2002b, 9 September) Furor rages over IPO spinning practices. *Globe and Mail*, pp. B1, B10.

McKenna, B. (2003, 24 October) U.S. sting nabs illegal Wal-Mart workers. *Globe and Mail*, pp. B1, B8.

McKenna, B. (2004a, 16 January) Enron holds key to wider world of corporate sleaze. *Globe and Mail*, p. B6.

McKenna, B. (2004b, 30 April) U.S. pushes Canada to exploit terror laws: enforcement powers haven't been used, State Department says. *Globe and Mail*, p. A8.

McKenna, B. (2004c, 17 December) 'Swamp fox' congressman joining powerful drug lobby. *Globe and Mail*, pp. B8.

McKenna, P. (2004, 31 July) America and the 'savages'. [Review of the book *The American Empire and the Fourth World*.] *Globe and Mail*, p. D4.

McKibben, B. (2005, August) The Christian paradox: how a faithful nation gets Jesus wrong. *Harpers*, **311**, 31–37.

McKibben, B. (2007) *The Wealth of Communities and the Durable Future*. New York, NY: Times Books.

McKitrick, E. (ed.) (1963) *Slavery Defended: the Views of the Old South*. Englewood Cliffs, NJ: Prentice-Hall.

McLaren, L. (2006, 21 January) No bucks for Botox? Get credit. *Globe and Mail*, pp. L1, L7.

McLaughlin, J. P. (2006, 24 October) This festival has heart: third annual: music dance theatre heals broken lives. *Province*, p. C6.

McLaughlin, T. (2007, 1 July) Hillbilly heroin and the Wall Street boom: bankers are buckling under the strain. *Calgary Herald*, p. E3.

McLellan, A. T. and Weisner, C. (1996) Achieving the public health and safety potential of substance abuse treatments: implications for patient referral, 'treatment matching', and outcome evaluation. In W. K. Bickel and R. J. DeGrandpre (eds), *Drug Policy and Human Nature: Psychological Perspectives on the Prevention, Management, and Treatment of Illicit Drug Abuse*, pp. 127–154. New York, NY: Plenum.

McLellan, A. T., Lewis, D. C., O'Brien, C. P., and Kleber, H. D. (2000) Drug dependence, a chronic medical illness: implications for treatment, insurance, and outcomes evaluation. *Journal of the American Medical Association*, **284**, 1689–1695.

McLeod, T. H. and McLeod, I. (1987) *Tommy Douglas: the Road to Jerusalem*. Edmonton, AB: Hurtig.

McMullen, B. and Rohrbach, A. (2003) *Distance Education in Remote Aboriginal Communities: Barriers, Learning Styles, and Best Practices.* Prince George, British Columbia: College of New Caledonia Press.

McMurtry, J. (1998) *Unequal Freedoms*. Toronto, ON: Garamond Press.

McNeil, D. G. (2007, 10 September) Drugs banned, many of world's poor suffer pain. *New York Times*, p. A1.

McQuaig, L. (2001) *All You Can Eat: Greed, Lust, and the New Capitalism*. Toronto, ON: Penguin Canada.

McSweeney, T. and Turnbull, P. J. (2007) *Exploring User Perceptions of Occasional and Controlled Heroin Use: a Follow-up Study*. York, UK: Joseph Rountree Foundation.

McWilliams, G. (2002, 28 May) Gateway gets tougher: firm turns to methods of arch-rival Dell. *Globe and Mail*, p. B10.

Meier, B. (2007, 11 May) Narcotic maker guilty of deceit over marketing. *New York Times.* Retrieved 10 July 2007, from http://www.nytimes.com/2007/05/11/business/ 11drug.html?pagewanted=1andei=5070anden=9e67660274de57a3andex=1183953600

Mello, N. K. and Mendelson, J. H. (1971) A quantitative analysis of drinking patterns of alcoholics. *Archives of General Psychiatry,* **25**, 527–539.

Mello, N. K. and Mendelson, J. H. (1972) Drinking patterns during work-contingent and noncontingent alcohol acquisition. *Psychosomatic Medicine,* **34**, 139–164.

Menzies, P. (2006, Autumn) Fighting firewater fiction: dispelling myths of aboriginal alcohol use. *CrossCurrents,* **10**, 12–13.

Merton, R. K. (1957) *Social Theory and Social Structure.* New York, NY: Free Press.

Merton, T. (2000) Introduction. In *The City of God* by St Augustine, p. xvxx. Toronto, ON: Random House. (Original work published 1950.)

Meyer, R. E. (1996) The disease called addiction: emerging evidence in a 200-year debate. *Lancet,* **347**, 162–166.

Mickleburgh, R. (2003a, 29 July) Native fishery declared invalid: BC judge rules commercial angling discriminates against non-natives. *Globe and Mail,* pp. A1, A6.

Mickleburgh, R. (2003b, 23 September) Father who killed family collapses. *Globe and Mail,* pp. A1, A7.

Mickleburgh, R. (2003c, 24 September) Father killed children, wrote letters. *Globe and Mail,* p. A5.

Mickleburgh, R. (2003d, 26 September) Narcissism drove father's killing rage, court hears. *Globe and Mail,* p. A13.

Mickleburgh, R. (2003e, 2 October) Man who killed children found guilty of murder: Handel's mental-disorder defense fails. *Globe and Mail,* pp. A1, A5.

Mickleburgh, R. (2005, 30 July) Leading marijuana activist arrested: 'Prince of Pot' faces extradition for Internet sales to U.S. customers. *Globe and Mail,* pp. S1, S3.

Mickleburgh, R. (2006a, 16 February) CMS vote tips debate Day's way on private health care: entrepreneur hails BC Throne Speech. *Globe and Mail,* pp. S1, S3.

Mickleburgh, R. (2006b, 26 October) BC teacher was 'addicted' to teen sex. *Vancouver Sun,* pp. A1, A10.

Mickleburgh, R. and Galloway, G. (2007, 15 January) Storm brews over drug strategy. *Globe and Mail,* pp. A1, A5.

Mickleburgh, R. and Giroday, G. (2004, 5 August) Young men turning Viagra into lifestyle drug. *Globe and Mail,* pp. A1, A6.

Mijuskovic, B. (1988) Loneliness and adolescent alcoholism. *Adolescence,* **23**, 503–516.

Milgram, S. (1963) Behavioral study of obedience. *Journal of Abnormal and Social Psychology,* **67**, 371–378.

Miller, A. (1981) *The Drama of the Gifted Child: the Search for the True Self.* New York, NY: Basic Books.

Miller, S. A., II. (2002, 31 March) Death of a game addict: ill Hudson man took own life after long hours on Web. *Milwaukee Journal Sentinel.* Retrieved from www.jsonline.com/news/State/mar02/31536.asp

Miller, W. R. (1989) Increasing motivation for change: effective alternatives. In R. K. Hester and W. R. Miller (eds), *Handbook of Alcoholism Treatment Approaches,* pp. 67–80. New York, NY: Pergamon Press.

Miller, W. R. (1998) Researching the spiritual dimensions of alcohol and other drug problems. *Addiction,* **93**, 979–990.

Miller, W. R. (2000) Rediscovering fire: small interventions, large effects. *Psychology of Addictive Behaviors*, **14**, 6–18.

Miller, W. R. (2004) The phenomenon of quantum change. *Journal of Clinical Psychology: In Session*, **60**, 453–460.

Miller, W. R. and Hester, R. K. (1995) Treatment for alcohol problems: toward an informed eclecticism. In R. K. Hester and W. R. Miller (eds), *Handbook of Alcoholism Treatment Approaches: Effective Alternatives*, 2nd edn, pp. 1–11. Needham Heights, MA: Allyn & Bacon.

Miller, W. R. and Meyers, R. J. (with Hiller-Sturmhöfel, S.) (1999) The community-reinforcement approach. *Addiction Research and Health*, **23**, 116–121.

Miller, W. R., Brown, J. M., Simpson, *et al.* (1995) What works? A methodological analysis of the alcohol treatment outcome literature. In R. K. Hester and W. R. Miller (eds), *Handbook of Alcoholism Treatments and Approaches: Effective Alternatives*, 2nd edn, pp. 12–44. Needham Heights, MA: Allyn & Bacon.

Miller, W. R., Zweben, J., and Johnson, W. R. (2005) Evidence based treatment: why, what, where, when, and how? *Journal of Substance Abuse Treatment*, **29**, 267–276.

Milner, B. (2003a, 24 November) Trade actions reveal Bush's secret. *Globe and Mail*, p. B2.

Milner, B. (2003b, 8 December) Latest Boeing scandal likely to claim more casualties. *Globe and Mail*, p. B2.

Ministry of Small Business and Economic Development and Ministry of Transportation (2005, March) *British Columbia Ports Strategy*. Victoria, BC: published by the author.

Mingo, J., Armstrong, B., and Dodge, A. (1985) *The Couch Potato Guide to Life*. New York, NY: Avon Books.

Mitchell, A. (2002, 25 June) Earth faces supply crisis study finds. *Globe and Mail*, A9.

Mitchell, A. (2004, 31 January) Unglued: what is it with so many children today? Sullen and surly, they ignore their elders and live to be with their peers … *Globe and Mail*, pp. F1, F6.

Mittelstaedt, M. (2007a, 31 January) The fallout of global warming: 1,000 years. *Globe and Mail*, pp. A1, A14.

Mittelstaedt, M. (2007b, 20 February) A climate-change message dressed in green pinstripes. *Globe and Mail*, p. A3.

Mittelstaedt, M., Galloway, G., and Laghi, B. (2007, 1 February) Harper puts green machine in motion. *Globe and Mail*, pp. A1, A4.

Moane, G. (2003) Bridging the personal and the political: practices for a liberation psychology. *American Journal of Community Psychology*, **31**, 91–101.

Modern Drunkard Magazine Online (n.d.) *You're a drunk*. Retrieved from http://moderndrunkardmagazine.com/md_youre_a_drunk.htm

Monbiot, G. (2006, 21 March) Who really belongs to another age bushmen or the House of Lords. *Guardian Unlimited*. Retrieved 21 March 2006, from http://www.guardian.co.uk

Mooers, A. (2004, 20 December) Now the news hits home: when the local pulp mill closed, it was not just another headline. *Maclean's*, **117**, 56.

Moore, D. (2003, 26 December) Old ghosts haunt Davis Inlet residents' new town: substance abuse abounds, and bootleggers charge $300 for a 40-ounce bottle of liquor. *Globe and Mail*, p. A14.

Moore, T. (1992) *Care of the Soul: a Guide for Cultivating Depth and Sacredness in Everyday Life*. New York, NY: Harper Perennial.

More, T. (1965) *Utopia* (P. Turner, trans.). London, UK: Penguin. (Original work published 1516).

Morgan, B. (1994) *Waiting for Time*. St John's, NL: Breakwater Books.

Morgan, J. P. and Zimmer, L. (1997a) The social pharmacology of smokable cocaine: not all it's cracked up to be. In C. Reinarman and H. G. Levine (eds), *Crack in America: Demon Drugs and Social Justice*, pp. 131–170. Berkeley, CA: University of California Press.

Morgan, J. P. and Zimmer, L. (1997b) Animal self-administration of cocaine: misinterpretation, misrepresentation, and invalid extrapolation to humans. In P. G. Erickson, D. M. Riley, Y. W. Cheung, and P. A. O'Hare (eds), *Harm Reduction: a New Direction for Drug Policies and Programs*, pp. 265–289. Toronto, ON: University of Toronto Press.

Morris, A. J. and Sayre, J. (2004) *The Worlds of Economics*. Vancouver, BC: McInnes Creek Press. Available at http://www.sfu.ca/~allen/mcinnescreekpress.html

Morton, A. and Routledge, R. D. (2006) Fulton's condition factor: is it a valid measure of sea lice impact on juvenile salmon? *North American Journal of Fisheries Management*, **26**, 56–62.

Moses, B. (1999, 17 May) Workers wish for happy hours again. *Globe and Mail*, p. M1.

Moses, B. (2001, 22 May) I am not a brand. *Globe and Mail*, p. B13.

Moses, B. (2004, 9 January) Setting the pace in 2004. *Globe and Mail*, p. C1.

Motluk, A. (2004, 11 September) Is there a pill for greed? [Review of the book *The Truth About Drug Companies: How They Deceive Us and What To Do About It.*] Globe and Mail, p. D4.

Mrosovsky, N. and Sherry, D. F. (1980) Animal anorexias. *Science*, **207**, 837–842.

Mugford, S. (1995) Recreational cocaine use in three Australian cities. *Addiction Research*, **2**, 95–108.

Murphy, E. (1973) *The Black Candle*. Toronto, ON: Coles. (Original work published 1922.)

Murphy, J., Laird, N. M., Monson, R. R., Sobol, A. M., and Leighton, A. H. (2000) A 40-year perspective on the prevalence of depression: the Stirling County Study. *Archives of General Psychiatry*, **57**, 209–215.

Murphy, R. (2004, 4 September) Conrad's double toil and trouble. *Globe and Mail*, p. A15.

Murray, G. F. (1988) The road to regulation: patent medicines in Canada in historical perspective. In J. C. Blackwell and P. G. Erickson (eds), *Illicit Drugs in Canada: a Risky Business*, pp. 72–87. Scarborough, ON: Nelson Canada.

Musto, D. F. (1987) *The American Disease: Origins of Narcotic Control* (expanded edn). New York, NY: Oxford University Press.

Musto, D. F. (2002) The origins of heroin. In D. F. Musto (ed.), *One Hundred Years of Heroin*, pp. xiii–xvii. Westport, CT: Auburn House.

Mydang, S. (2007, 24 September) Monks' protest is challenging Burmese junta. *New York Times*,

National Institute on Drug Abuse (2002, Summer/Fall) Global drug use and NIDA. *NIDA INVEST Newsletter*, pp. 1–2.

Neeson, J. M. (1993) Commoners: common right, enclosure and social change in England, 1700–1820. Cambridge, UK: Cambridge University Press.

Nernberger, J. I. and Bierut, L. J. (2007, April) Seeking the connections: alcoholism and our genes. *Scientific American*, **296**, 46–53.

Neve, M. (2005, 1 January) Historical keywords: Addiction. *Lancet*, **365**, 21.

New American Bible (2002) Washington, DC: United States Conference of Catholic Bishops. Available at http://www.usccb.org/nab/bible/index.htm

New York Times (2005, 17 June) Lobbying from within. *New York Times*, p. A22.

Newcomb, M. D. and Harlow, L. L. (1986) Life events and substance use among adolescents: mediating effects of perceived loss of control and meaningfulness in life. *Journal of Personality and Social Psychology*, **51**, 564–577.

Newcomb, M. D., Maddahian, E., and Bentler, P. M. (1986) Risk factors for drug use among adolescents: concurrent and longitudinal analyses. *American Journal of Public Health*, **76**, 525–531.

Newland, M. (2007, 11 June) Why England is rotting. *Maclean's*, **120**, 24–29.

Newman, K. (2006, 15 September) The roots of rampage: school shooters have spent years trying to be accepted by peer groups that reject them, says Princeton University sociologist … *Globe and Mail*, p. A17.

Newman, P. C. (1959) *Flame of Power: Intimate Profiles of Canada's Greatest Businessmen*. Don Mills, ON: Longman Canada.

Newman, P. C. (1985) *Company of Adventurers*, vol. 1. Markham, ON: Penguin Viking.

Newman, P. C. (1991) *Company of Adventurers*, vol. 3. *Merchant Princes*. Toronto, ON: Penguin Viking.

Nickson, E. (2007, 21 April) In the name of the father, son, and shopping channel. *Globe and Mail*, p. A17.

Nikonoff, J. (2004, May) Altermondialistes tout terrain. *Le Monde diplomatique*, pp. 22–23.

Noble, D. F. (1997) *The Religion of Technology: the Divinity of Man and the Spirit of Invention*. New York, NY: Knopf.

Nolen, S. (2005, 5 September) Why Africa's the real deal: forget your notions about Africa … there are excellent business opportunities here … *Globe and Mail*, pp. B1, B5.

Nolen, S. (2006, 6 May) Last Bushmen of Klahari fight to go home. *Globe and Mail*, p. A13.

Nordt, C. and Stohler, R. (2006) Incidence of heroin use in Zurich, Switzerland: a treatment case register approach. *Lancet*, **367**, 1830–1834.

Normand, F. (1995, September) La troublante ascension de l'Opus Dei. *Le Monde diplomatique*, pp. 1, 22, 23.

Norris, M. L., Boydell, K. M., Pinkas, L. and Katzman, D. (2006) Ana and the Internet: a review of pro-anorexia websites. *International Journal of Eating Disorders*, **39**, 443–447.

Oberg, K. (1966) Crime and punishment in Tlingit society. In T. McFeat (ed.), *Indians of the North Pacific Coast*, pp. 209–222. Toronto: McClelland & Stewart. (Reprinted from *American Anthropologist*, **36**, 145–156, 1934).

Oborne, P. (2002, 24 August) Who inspired Thatcher's most damaging remark? Tony Blair's favourite guru. *Spectator*, p. 9.

O'Brian, A. (2004a, 9 February) Vancouver: world's most liveable city. *Vancouver Sun*, pp. A1, A2.

O'Brien, C. P. (2001) Drug addiction and drug abuse. In J. G. Hardman and L. E. Limbird (eds), *Goodman and Gilman's The Pharmacological Basis of Therapeutics*, 10th edn, pp. 621–642. New York, NY: McGraw-Hill.

O'Connor, N. (2005, 21 August) East siders won't give up on garden. *Courier*, p. 12.

Öjesjö, L. (2004) Turnings in alcoholism: a thematic analysis of life histories from the Lundby alcohol subset. In P. Rosenqvist, J. Blomqvist, A. Koski-Jännes and L. Öjesjö (eds), *Addiction and Life Course*, pp. 267–274. Helsinki, Finland: Nordic Council for Alcohol and Drug Research.

O'Kiely, E. (1996) *The Arts and our Town: the Community Arts Council of Vancouver 1946–1996*. Vancouver, BC: The Community Arts Council.

Olsen, S. (2005) *Just Ask Us: a Conversation with First Nations Teenage Moms*. Winlaw, BC: Sono Nis Press.

O'Meara, M. (2004) *New Culture, New Right: Anti-liberalism in Postmodern Europe*. Bloomington, IN: 1stBooks.

On-Line Gamers Anonymous (2007) On-Line Gamers Anonymous. Retrieved 7 November 2006, from http://www.olganonboard.org

Orford, J. (1985) *Excessive Appetites: a Psychological View of Addictions.* Chichester, UK: Wiley.

Orford, J. (2001a) *Excessive Appetites: a Psychological View of Addictions,* 2nd edn. Chichester, UK: Wiley.

Orford, J. (2001b) Addiction as an excessive appetite. *Addiction,* **96,** 15–33.

Orford, J., Templeton, L., Copello, A., Velleman, R., and Bradbury, C. (2000) Worrying for drinkers in the family: an interview study with Aboriginal Australians in urban areas and remote communities in the Northern Territory. Darwin, Australia: Territory Health Service, Living with Alcohol Program, Northern Territory Government, Australia.

Osborne, D. (2005) *Suicide Tuesday: Gay Men and the Crystal Meth Scare.* New York, NY: Carroll & Graf.

Ospina, H. C. (2003, April) Les paramilitaires au coeur du terrorisme d'Etat colombien: un mariage de convenance sanguinaire. *Le Monde diplomatique,* pp. 10–11.

Ospina, H. C. (2004, November) Les acteurs cachés du conflit colombien. *Le Monde diplomatique,* pp. 26–27.

Oswald, I. (1969) 'Personal view'. *British Medical Journal,* **3,** 438.

Otis, J. (2006, 16 April) Coca crop jumps despite U.S. aid. *Houston Chronicle.* Retrieved 22 April 2006, from http://www.chron.com/disp/story.msp/headline/world/3796474.html

Oxford English Dictionary (1933), 1st edn. Oxford, UK: Clarendon Press.

Oxford English Dictionary (1989), 2nd edn. Oxford, UK: Clarendon Press.

Oziewicz, E. (2004, 13 May) Shroud lifting on global gulag set up to fight 'war on terror': secret detention centres come to light as groups probe human-rights violations. *Globe and Mail,* p. A12.

Oziewicz, E. (2005, 4 November) Treatment of prisoners 'a disgrace', Carter says. *Globe and Mail,* pp. A1, A10.

Oziewicz, E. (2006a, 25 January) Europeans likely aware of torture report: Swiss official says evidence suggests that governments knew about U.S. 'outsourcing'. *Globe and Mail,* p. A15.

Oziewicz, E. (2006b, 5 December) The rich really do own the world. *Globe and Mail,* pp. A10, A11.

Pagels, E. (1995) *The Origin of Satan.* New York, NY: Random House.

Pannekoek, F. (1979, Spring) Corruption at Moose. *Beaver,* pp. 4–11.

Papineau, E. (2005) Pathological gambling in Montreal's Chinese community: an anthropological perspective. *Journal of Gambling Studies,* **21,** 157–178.

Paris, R. and Bradley, C. L. (2001) The challenge of adversity: three narratives of alcohol dependence, recovery, and adult development. *Qualitative Health Research,* **11,** 647–667.

Partridge, J. (2001, 19 October) Terrorist funding search extends to pensions. *Globe and Mail,* pp. B1, B4.

Partridge, J. (2005, 23 August) Savings gap seen as a threat to growth in Canada: companies said saving too much, households too little. *Globe and Mail,* p. B4.

Partridge, J. (2007, 31 October) Burned by the trust tax, couple turn to NAFTA. *Globe and Mail,* p. B1.

Pasco, R. (2005, 12 July) Let's turn garbage into gold: indigenous communities are tired of being dumped on—now literally. The Ashcroft proposal will not succeed. *Vancouver Sun,* p. A11.

Pattison, E. M., Sobell, M. B., and Sobell, L. C. (1977) *Emerging Concepts of Alcohol Dependence.* New York, NY: Springer.

Payne, F. E. (1993) Addiction as besetting sin. *Journal of Biblical Ethics in Medicine*, 7, 96–99.

Payne, M. (1989) *The Most Respectable Place in the Territory: Everyday Life in Hudson's Bay Company Service, York Factory, 1788 to 1870*. Ottawa, ON: Minister of Public Works and Government Service Canada.

Pearson, J. (1995) *Painfully Rich: J. Paul Getty and his Heirs*. London, UK: Macmillan.

Peele, S. (1976) Addiction is a social disease. *Addictions* (Addiction Research Foundation of Ontario), 23, 2–21. Retrieved 9 August 2005, from http://www.peele.net/lib/sociald.html

Peele, S. (1985) The meaning of addiction: compulsive experience and its interpretation. Lexington, MA: Lexington Books.

Peele, S. (1987) A moral vision of addiction: how people's values determine whether they become and remain addicts. *Journal of Drug Issues*, 17, 187–215.

Peele, S. (ed.) (1988) *Visions of Addiction: Major Contemporary Perspectives on Addiction and Alcoholism*. Lexington, MA: Lexington Books.

Peele, S. (1989) *The Diseasing of America: Addiction Treatment Out of Control*. Lexington, MA: Lexington Books.

Peele, S. and Brodsky, A. (1975) *Love and Addiction*. New York, NY: Taplinger.

Peele, S. and Butler, P. (2006, 12 April) Addictive personality. *Society Guardian*. Retrieved 12 April 2006, from http://society.guardian.co.uk/interview/story/0,,1751588,00.html

Peele, S., Brodsky, A., and Arnold, M. (1991) The truth about addiction and recovery: the life process program for outgrowing destructive habits. New York, NY: Simon and Schuster.

Penfield, W. (1969) Halsted of Johns Hopkins. *Journal of the American Medical Association*, 210, 2214–2218.

Pennebaker, J. W. (1997) *Opening Up: the Healing Power of Expressing Emotions* (rev. edn). New York, NY: Guilford Press.

Perkins, B. (1991) *Fatal Attractions: Overcoming our Secret Addictions*. Eugene, OR: Harvest House.

Perkins, J. (2004) *Confessions of an Economic Hit Man*. San Francisco, CA: Berrett-Koehler.

Perrine, D. M. (1996) *The Chemistry of Mind-altering Drugs*. Washington, DC: American Chemical Society.

Pert, C. (1997) *Molecules of Emotion: Why You Feel the Way You Feel*. New York, NY: Scribner.

Pethick, D. (1984) *Vancouver, the Pioneer Years 1774–1886*. Langley, BC: Sunfire Publications.

Petrie, B. (1985) *Failure to replicate an environmental effect of morphine hydrochloride consumption: a possible pharmacogenetic link*. Unpublished doctoral dissertation, Simon Fraser University, Burnaby, BC, Canada.

PHS Community Services Society (2005) *An Overview*. Vancouver, BC: published by the author.

Picard, A. (2002, 18 February) Fat weighs in as risk to health worldwide. *Globe and Mail*, p. A12.

Picard, A. (2004a, 13 January) Obesity now killing one in 10, study says. *Globe and Mail*, p. A10.

Picard, A. (2004b, 3 June) Our elderly are adrift in a sea of drugs. *Globe and Mail*, p. A15.

Picard, A. (2004c, 30 December) How can we improve medical reporting? Let me count the ways. *Globe and Mail*, p. A11.

Picard, A. (2005a, 6 January) Canada has a gambling problem. *Globe and Mail*, p. A13.

Picard, A. (2005b, 29 June) Obesity rates vary across ethnicities, study finds. *Globe and Mail*, p. A11.

Picard, A. (2005c, 19 August) Letting the health-care genie out of the bottle. *Globe and Mail*, p. A5.

Picard, A. (2005d, 8 September) 'New' drugs too often offer little new: breakthrough drugs are rare. Most newcomers driving up costs are just me-too marketing darlings. *Globe and Mail*, p. A21.

Picard, A. (2005e, 13 September) New anti-psychotic drugs worrying, study finds. *Globe and Mail*, p. A13.

Picard, A. (2005f, 3 November) Native health care is a sickening disgrace. *Globe and Mail*, p. A15.

Picard, A. (2005g, 10 November) Refugees in their own land. *Globe and Mail*, p. A14.

Picard, A. (2006, 16 March) Governments' gaming addictions are shameful. *Globe and Mail*, p. A13.

Pieiller, E. (2007, March) Les facettes de l'individu empêptré dans l'individualisme. *Le Monde diplomatique*, pp. 26–27.

Pinker, S. (2005, 3 August) Fix burnout factors before blaming boss. *Globe and Mail*, p. C2.

Pitts, G. (2003, 31 December) Stench of scandals lingers: aroma wafting from Italy is the now familiar scent of corporate rot that shows no sign of abating. *Globe and Mail*, pp. B1, B3.

Pitts, G. (2006, 29 May) Industrial evolution. *Globe and Mail*, pp. B1, B4.

Placonouris, G. (1998) *Crystal Children*. Vancouver, BC: Drug Book Press.

Plant, M. and Plant, M. (2006) *Binge Britain: Alcohol and the National Response*. Oxford, UK: Oxford University Press.

Plato (1930) *The Republic* (P. Shorey, trans.). Cambridge, MA: Harvard University Press. (Original work published *c.* 360 BC.)

Plato (1941) Phaedo. In L. Cooper (trans.) *Plato on the Trial and Death of Socrates*, pp. 111–192. Ithaca, NY: Cornell University Press. (Original work published *c.* 388 BC.)

Plato (1956) Protagoras. In W. K.C. Guthrie (trans.), *Protagoras and Meno*, pp. 27–100. London, UK: Penguin. (Original work published *c.* 388 BC.)

Plato (1967) Apology of Socrates. In L. Cooper (trans.) *Plato on the Trial and Death of Socrates*, pp. 49–77. Ithaca, NY: Cornell University Press. (Original work published *c.* 387 BC.)

Plato (1987) *The Republic*, 2nd edn (translated with an introduction by D. Lee). Harmondsworth, UK: Penguin Classics. Copyright © H. D. P. Lee, 1953, 1974, 1987. (Original work published *c.* 360 BC.)

Plato (2005) *The Symposium* (C. Gill, trans.). London, UK: Penguin Books. (Original work published *c.* 385 BC.)

Polanyi, K. (1935) The essence of fascism. In J. Lewis, K. Polanyi and D. K. Kitchin (eds), *Christianity and the Social Revolution*, pp. 359–394. London, UK: Victor Gollancz.

Polanyi, K. (1944) *The Great Transformation: the Political and Economic Origins of our Times*. Boston, MA: Beacon.

Polanyi, K. (1957) Aristotle discovers the economy. In K. Polanyi, C. N. Arensberg, and H. W. Pearson (eds), *Trade and Market in the Early Empires*, pp. 64–94. Glencoe, IL: The Free Press.

Polanyi, K., Arensberg, C. N., and Pearson, H. W. (eds) (1957) *Trade and Market in the Early Empires*. Glencoe, IL: The Free Press.

Polanyi, M. (2006, 3 November) God, man and the good old USA. [Review of the books *Religion Gone Bad: the Hidden Dangers of the Christian Right*; *Theocons: Secular America Under Siege*; *God and Country: How Evangelicals have Become America's New Mainstream*;

Believers: a Journey into Evangelical America; and *The Left Hand of God: Taking Our Country Back from the Religious Right.*] *Globe and Mail*, p. D8.

Poole, N. and Isaac, B. (2001) *Apprehensions: Barriers to Treatment for Substance Using Mothers.* Vancouver, BC: Centre of Excellence for Women's Health.

Poole, N. and Urquhart, C. (2007, January) *Harm reduction counselling with pregnant substance-using women: how are we doing it?* Paper presented at the Conference of the Association of Substance Abuse Programs of BC, Richmond, BC, Canada.

Porter-Williamson, K., Heffernan, E. and von Gunten, C. F. (2003) Pseudoaddiction. *Journal of Palliative Medicine*, **6**, 937–939.

Posner, M. (2003, 20 December) Lord, He's hot: talk about resurrecting your career. Name the arts genre and Jesus was there in 2003. *Globe and Mail*, pp. R1, R6.

Potvin, K. (2005a, 31 August) Democracy shines on little East End garden. *Vancouver Courier*, p. 11.

Potvin, K. (2005b, 1–14 September) One small victory for a park … and one giant leap for democracy, activism, and organisation. *Republic of East Vancouver*, pp. 1, 8.

Poupeau, F. (2004, June) Altermondialistes de tous les pays … *Le Monde diplomatique*, p. 2.

Prebble, J. (1963) *The Highland Clearances.* London, UK: Penguin Books.

Prebble, J. (1966) *Glencoe.* London, UK: Penguin Books.

Prebble, J. (1971) The lion in the north: a personal view of Scotland's history. Harmondsworth, UK: Penguin Books.

Press Association (2007, 8 March) Illegal drugs can be harmless, report says. *Guardian Unlimited.* Retrieved 9 March 2007, from http://www.guardian.co.uk/drugs/Story/ 0,,2029072,00.html?gusrc=rssandfeed=1

Preston, G. (2006, 18 August) Beggars, drug dealers kill convention. *Vancouver Sun*, p. A1.

Priest, A. (2002, 28 March) Fitness addicts. *Georgia Straight*, pp. 17, 19–20.

Priest, A. (2003, 13–20 November) Middle class addicts. *Georgia Straight*, pp. 21–28.

Priest, A. (2005, 15 August) The staggering price of survival: patients wondering why the cancer drug thalidomide costs so much. *Globe and Mail*, pp. A1, A7.

Primm, B. J. and Bath, P. E. (1973) Pseudoheroinism. *International Journal of the Addictions*, **8**, 231–242.

Pryor, W. (2003) *The Survival of the Coolest: an Addiction Memoir.* Bath, UK: Clear Press.

Puder, G. (1998, 21 April) Recovering our honour: why policing must reject the 'War on Drugs'. Paper presented at the Sensible Solutions to the Urban Drug Problem Conference of The Fraser Institute, Vancouver, BC, Canada.

Putnam, R. D. (1993, March) The prosperous community: social capital and public life. *American Prospect Online.* Retrieved 25 May 2006, from http://www.prospect.org/web/ page.ww?section=rootandname=ViewPrintandarticleId=5175

Putnam, R. D. (2000) Bowling alone: the collapse and revival of American community. New York, NY: Simon & Shuster.

Pynn, L. (2003, 17 May) Remote, rural but far from tranquil: native communities have the highest crime rates in the province. *Vancouver Sun*, p. B6.

Rabinor, J. R. (2002) *A Starving Madness: Tales of Hunger, Hope, and Healing in Psychoanalysis.* Carlsbad, CA: Gürze Books.

Radford, T. (2004, 13 March) CO_2 levels threaten Amazon rain forest. *Globe and Mail*, p. A13.

Radford, T. (2005, 30 March) Living beyond our environmental means: human pressure degrading Earth, says report backed by 1,360 scientists. *Globe and Mail*, pp. A3.

Raimbeau, C. (2005, September) En Argentine, occuper, résister, produire. *Le Monde diplomatique*, p. 10.

Ramirez, A. (2004, 8 October) Life with layoffs: the new normal. *Globe and Mail*, p. C1.

Ramonet, I. (1994, January) La pensée unique. *Le Monde diplomatique*, p. 1.

Ramonet, I. (1997, December) Désarmer les marchés. *Le Monde diplomatique*, p. 1.

Ramonet, I. (2000) *Propagande silencieuse: masses, télévision, cinéma*. Paris: Galilée.

Ramonet, I. (2002, May) La peste. *Le Monde diplomatique*, p. 1.

Ramonet, I. (2004a, June) Images et bourreaux. *Le Monde diplomatique*, p. 1.

Ramonet, I. (2004b, August) Chine mégapuissance. *Le Monde diplomatique*, p. 1.

Ramonet, I. (2005, June) Espoirs. *Le Monde diplomatique*, p. 1.

Ramonet, I. (2006a, April) Malade, la France? *Le Monde diplomatique*, p. 1.

Ramonet, I. (2006b, September) Un nouvel état du monde. *Le Monde diplomatique*, pp. 1, 14–15.

Ramonet, I. (2006–2007, December–January) Age d'or. *Manière de voir*, **90**, 4–5.

Ramonet, I. (2007, January–February) Le marché contre l'Etat. *Manière de voir*, **91**, 4–5.

Ramsey, M. (2003, 30 September) 46% of Lower Mainland adults born outside Canada: number is twice the national average. *Vancouver Sun*, pp. A1, A5.

Rand, A. (1957) *Atlas Shrugged*. New York, NY: Random House.

Rayner, A. D.M. (2007, May) *From oppressive freedom to freedom from oppression: the natural re-inclusion of the dislocated self*. Retrieved 23 October 2007, from http://people.bath.ac.uk/bssadmr/inclusionality/Dislocatedself.htm

Raynes-Goldie, K. (2004, 9 August) Apathy and irony: for many young people, caring about the world's problems can be both too painful and seemingly futile. Here's how we cope. *Globe and Mail*, p. A12.

Reguly, E. (2003, 19 November) Black owes much more to Hollinger International. *Globe and Mail*, p. B2.

Reguly, E. (2004, 6 March) Stewart gets just deserts as investors' trust betrayed. *Globe and Mail*, p. B2.

Reguly, E. (2007, 27 April) A peek into the pages of KKR's playbook. *Globe and Mail*, p. B8.

Reid, M., McCook, V., and Seymour, G. (2006, 8 December) *Uk'oodahade kwadihi dawa: read so you'll understand*. Paper presented at the Aboriginal Education Conference, Vancouver, BC, Canada.

Reinarman, C. and Levine, H. G. (1997) *Crack in America: Demon Drugs and Social Justice*. Berkeley, CA: University of California Press.

Reinarman, C., Cohen, P. D.A., and Kaal, H. L. (2004) The limited relevance of drug policy: cannabis in Amsterdam and San Francisco. *American Journal of Public Health*, **94**, 836–842.

Reinstate Third-Party Appeals (2007) *Reinstate third-party appeals in the city of Vancouver*. Published by the author. Retrieved 1 November 2007, from http://www.reinstatethird-partyappeals.org/salsbury.html

Reith, G. (2004) Consumption and its discontents: addiction, identity and the problems of freedom. *British Journal of Sociology*, **55**, 283–300.

Renzetti, E. (2005a, 29 January) Hurl, Britannia: with a rash of brawls, vomiting and urination in city streets, binge drinking among young English people, especially women, is becoming what Tony Blair called 'the new British disease'. *Globe and Mail*, pp. F4, F5.

Renzetti, E. (2005b, 30 August) The hungry food addict. [Review of the book *The Hungry Years: Confessions of a Food Addict*.] *Globe and Mail*, pp. R1, R2.

Republic of East Vancouver (2004, 8 January) Best of 2003! Say what? *Republic of East Vancouver*, p. 1.

Reuter, P. and Stevens, A. (2007) *An Analysis of UK Drug Policy: a Monograph Prepared for the UK Drug Policy Commission*. London, UK: UK Drug Policy Commission.

Reuters (2007) Experts oppose video game addiction designation. *c|net news.com*. Retrieved 22 July 2007, from http://www.news.com/Experts+oppose+video+game+addiction+designation/2100–1043_3–6192969.html?tag=item

Reynolds, C. (2006, 16 January) Videogame widows: men who love online games, and the women who hate them. *Maclean's*, **119**, 42.

Reynolds, N. (2005, 6 July) Protectionism, the sequel: scary as the original. *Globe and Mail*, p. B2.

Reynolds, N. (2006a, 17 February) Don't worry: the U.S. deficit will fix itself. *Globe and Mail*, p. B2.

Reynolds, N. (2006b, 8 November) Economists take Darwin to heart. *Globe and Mail*, p. B2.

Reynolds, N. (2007, 12 January) Iraq economy roars, despite woes. *Globe and Mail*, p. B2.

Rhoads, C. and Moffett, S. (2004, 13 February) Overseas spending weak. *Globe and Mail*, p. B11. [Reprinted from C. Rhoads and S. Moffett (2004, 13 February) A global journey reports: closed pocketbooks abroad imperil recovery, *Wall Street Journal*, p. A9.]

Richard, A. J., Bell, D. C., and Carlson, J. W. (2000) Individual religiosity, moral community, and drug user treatment. *Journal of the Scientific Study of Religion*, **39**, 240–246.

Richards, D. A. (2001) Drinking. In L. Crozier and P. Lane (eds), *Addicted: Notes from the belly of the Beast*, pp. 105–121. Vancouver, BC: Greystone Books.

Richardson, B. (2005) There's no place like home: five Canadian writes tell why they love their neighbourhoods: Vancouver, among old ghosts. *Reader's Digest Canaada*. Retrieved 20 July 2007, from http://www.readersdigest.ca/mag/2005/07/no_place_like_home.php

Richer, S. (2004, 4 December) I scream for iPod: how long can an iPod addict stay stalled at only 3,058 songs? *Globe and Mail*, pp. R1, R6.

Ricks, F., Charlesworth, J., Bellefeuille, G. and Field, A. (1999) *All Together Now: Creating a Social Capital Mosaic*. Victoria, BC: Frances Ricks and the Vanier Institute of the Family.

Rivière, P. (2003, July) Mobilisation contre le SARS, inaction contre le sida. *Le Monde diplomatique*, p. 27.

Robbeson, D. (2004, 28 February) Addiction: confessions of an on-line gambler. *Globe and Mail*, p. F7.

Robert, A.-C. (2005, June) De la rébellion à la reconstruction. *Le Monde diplomatique*, pp. **22**, 23.

Robert, A.-C. (2006, May) Occident contre Occident. *Le Monde diplomatique*, p. 3.

Roberts, P. W. (2005, 10 September) The flagging empire. *Globe and Mail*, pp. F1, F4–5.

Robertson, G. (2007, 9 November) Vancouver papers shed staff. *Globe and Mail*, p. S3.

Robins, L. N. and Murphy, G. E. (1967) Drug use in a normal population of young Negro men. *American Journal of Public Health*, **57**, 1580–1596.

Robins, L. N., Helzer, J. E., and Davis, D. H. (1975) Narcotic use in Southeast Asia and afterwards. *Archives of General Psychiatry*, **32**, 955–961.

Robinson, S. (2001, 8 June) Douse the angst, eco-freaks. *Globe and Mail*, p. A13.

Robinson, T. E. (2004, 13 August) Addicted rats. *Science*, **305**, 951–953.

Robinson, T. E. and Berridge, K. C. (2001) Incentive sensitisation and addiction. *Addiction*, **96**, 103–114.

Rochon, L. (2003, 14 May) Uncle Sam's city plan. *Globe and Mail*, p. R3.

Rogers, C. R. (1957) The necessary and sufficient conditions for therapeutic personality change. *Journal of Consulting Psychology*, **21**, 95–103.

Rohter, L. (2007, 7 May) As Pope heads to Brazil, a rival theology persists. *New York Times*, p. 1.

Rolles, S., Kushlick, D., and Jay, M. (2004) *After the War on Drugs, Options For Control*. Bristol, UK: Transform Drug Policy Foundation.

Romero, S. (2006, 3 December) Venezuela's economic boom buoys Chávez's campaign. *New York Times*, p. 8.

Room, R. (1998) Alcohol and drug disorders in the international Classification of Diseases: a shifting kaleidoscope. *Drug and Alcohol Review*, **17**, 305–317.

Room, R. (2003, 20–21 November) *Thinking about strategies to prevent substance misuse*. Paper presented at the Conference on Visioning a Future for Prevention: a Local Perspective, Vancouver, BC, Canada.

Rose, A. (2000) *Spirit Dance at Maziadin: Chief Joseph Gosnell and the Nisga'a Treaty*. Madiera Park, BC: Harbour Publishing.

Rose, N. (1985) *The Psychological Complex: Psychology, Politics and Society in England, 1869–1939*. London, UK: Routledge and Kegan Paul.

Rosenblum, A., Joseph, H., Fong, C., Kipnis, S., Cleland, C., and Portenoy, R. K. (2003) Prevalence and characteristics of chronic pain among chemically dependent patients in methadone maintenance and residential treatment facilities. *Journal of the American Medical Association*, **289**, 2370–1278.

Rorty, R. (1979) *Philosophy and the Mirror of Nature*. Princeton, NJ: Princeton University Press.

Roskies, E. and Lazarus, R. S. (1980) Coping theory and the teaching of coping skills. In P. O. Davidson and S. M. Davidson (eds), *Behavioral Medicine: Changing Health Lifestyles*, pp. 38–69. New York, NY: Brunner/Mazel.

Ross, S. and Deveau, A. (1992) *The Acadians of Nova Scotia: Past and Present*. Halifax, NS: Nimbus.

Roth, C. (1964) *The Spanish Inquisition*. New York, NY: Oxford University Press. (Original work published 1937.)

Roux, A. (2006, August) Mao, de la légende à la magie noire: biographie ou vengence? *Le Monde diplomatique*, p. 27

Roy, O. (2002, April) L'islam au pied de la lettre: retour illusoire aux origines. *Le Monde diplomatique*, p. 3l.

Royal Society for the Encouragement of Arts, Manufactures and Commerce (2007) *The Report of the RSA Commission on Illegal Drugs, Communities and Public Policy: Executive Summary*. London, UK: published by the author.

Rubin, H. (2007, 15 September) Ayn Rand's literature of capitalism. *New York Times*, pp. B1, B8. Retrieved 24 October 2007, from http://www.nytimes.com/2007/09/15/business/15atlas.html

Rufin, J.-C. (2004, August) Vulnérable Mongolie. *Le Monde diplomatique*, pp. 14–15.

Rush, B. (1790) *Inquiry into the Effects of Spiritous Liquors on the Human Body: to Which is Added a Moral and Physical Thermometer*. Boston, MA: Thomas and Andrews.

Sader, E. (2003, November) Retrouvailles Nord-Sud. *Le Monde diplomatique*, p. 16.

Sader, E. (2005, January) Rendez-vous manqué avec le mouvement social brésilien: une troisième voie de plus en plus contestée. *Le Monde diplomatique*, pp. 8–9.

St Augustine (1963) *Confessions of St Augustine* (R. Warner, trans.). New York, NY: Mentor-Omega. Copyright © 1963 by Rex Warner, renewed © 1991 by F. C. Warner. (Original work published 397 AD.)

St Augustine (2000) *The City of God* (M. Dods, trans.). Toronto, ON: Random House. (Original work published 426 AD.)

Sakamoto, K. (2004) *One Hundred Million Hearts*. Toronto, ON: Vintage Canada.

Salutin, R. (2002, 8 February) Misdirection, anti-magic and Enron. *Globe and Mail*, p. A13.

Samson, C. (2003) *A Way of Life that Does Not Exist: Canada and the Extinguishment of the Innu*. London, UK: Verso.

Samson, C. (2004) The disease over native North American drinking: experiences of the Innu of northern Labrador. In R. Coomber and N. South (eds), *Drug Use and Cultural Contexts Beyond the WEST*, pp. 137–157. London, UK: Free Association Books.

Sanger, D. E. and Forero, J. (2004, 23 November) Bush, in Colombia, promises more aid. *New York Times*, p. A3.

Sapir, J. (2006, July) La concurrence, un mythe. *Le Monde diplomatique*, p. 3.

Saramago, J. (2004, August) Que reste-t-il de la démocratie? *Le Monde diplomatique*, p. 20.

Sarason, S. B. (1974) The psychological sense of community: prospects for community psychology. San Francisco, CA: Jossey-Bass.

Sartre, J.-P. (1969) *Nausea* (L. Alexander, trans.). Norwalk, CT: New Directions. (Original work published 1938.)

Sassen, S. (2000, November) Mais pouquoi émigrent-ils? *Le Monde diplomatique*, pp. 4–5.

Saul, J. R. (1995) *The Unconscious Civilisation*. Concord, ON: Anansi Press.

Saul, J. R. (2004, March) The collapse of globalism: and the rebirth of nationalism. *Harper's Magazine*, **308**, 33–43.

Saul, J. R. (2005) *The Collapse of Globalism: and the Reinvention of the World*. Toronto, ON: Viking Canada.

Saunders, D. (2003, 24 October) Raids on Wal-Mart expose dark side of U.S. economy. *Globe and Mail*, pp. A1, A14.

Saunders, J. (2003a, 8 September) Wheat dispute goes against the grain. Analysis: latest figures show that farmers in poorer countries can't get an even break. *Globe and Mail*, pp. B1, B7.

Saunders, J. (2003b, 14 October) IT jobs contracted from far and wide: North American companies are saving money by 'offshoring'. *Globe and Mail*, p. B1.

Saunders, J. (2004, 1 September) Perle said to have put 'his own interests' ahead of shareholders. *Globe and Mail*, p. B5.

Save the Children (2000) *Milestone Reached: Partners Working so that Children Won't Have To*. (public document). Islamabad, Pakistan: Partners of the Sialkot Child Labour Project.

Schachter, H. (2003, 30 April) Anderson account: debit the client. *Globe and Mail*, p. C5.

Schachter, R. (1999, 16 June) Time to relax, regroup, and reflect on legacy statements. *Globe and Mail*, p. M1.

Schachter, S. (1982) Recidivism and self-cure of smoking and obesity. *American Psychologist*, **37**, 436–444.

Schaler, J. A. (2000) *Addiction is a Choice*. Chicago, IL: Open Court.

Schanberg, S. H. (1996, June) Six cents an hour. *Life*, **19**, 38–46.

Schechter, M. T., Strathdee, S. A., Cornelisse, P. G.A., *et al.* (1999) Do needle exchange programmes increase the spread of HIV among injection drug users? An investigation of the Vancouver outbreak. *AIDS*, **13**, F45–F51.

Schenk, S., Lacelle, G., Gorman, K., and Amit, Z. (1987) Cocaine self-administration in rats influenced by environmental conditions: implications for the etiology of drug abuse. *Neuroscience Letters*, **81**, 227–231.

Schellenberg, B. (2006, 9 June) I want a new vice, something a bit unusual. *Globe and Mail*, p. A18.

Schick, S. (2007, 22 February) How to fight the battle against e-mail addiction. *Globe and Mail*, p. B13.

Schiller, D. (2003, July) Télécommunications, les échecs d'un révolution. *Le Monde diplomatique*, pp. 28–29.

Schiller, D. (2005, February) Esclaves du portable: illusoire liberté, immense marché. *Le Monde diplomatique*, pp. 1, 22–23.

Schivelbusch, W. (1992) *Tastes of Paradise*. New York, NY: Pantheon.

Schroeder, M. (2003, 1 May) Financial job shift grows: U.S. firms plan to move 500,000 positions. *Globe and Mail*, p. B15.

Schug, S. A., Merry, A. F., and Acland, R. H. (1991) Treatment principles for the use of opioids in pain of nonmalignant origin. *Drugs*, **42**, 228–239.

Schuman, M. (2004, 14 May) Abu Ghraib: the rule, not the exception. *Globe and Mail*, p. A15.

Schwartz, A. (2006, May) Le règne des livres sans qualité. *Le Monde diplomatique*, p. 30.

Schwartz, B. (2004) *The Paradox of Choice: Why More is Less*. New York, NY: HarperCollins.

Scofield, H. (2006, 28 April) Invest in higher education to get innovative ideas flowing. *Globe and Mail*, p. B7.

Scott, J. (2006, 3 October) In governor's race, group pushes to make lower-priced housing a state issue. *New York Times on the Web*. Retrieved 20 December 2006, from http://www.housingfirst.net/n2006_10_03_nyt.html

Séguin, R. (2006, 19 December) Troubled waters. *Globe and Mail*, pp. A8, A9

Seltzer, M. (1998) Serial killers: death and life in America's wounded culture. New York, NY: Routledge.

Selye, H. (1946) The general adaptation syndrome and the diseases of adaptation. *Journal of Chemical Endocrinology*, **6**, 117–231.

Selye, H. (1976) *The Stress of Life* (rev. edn). New York, NY: McGraw-Hill.

Sennett, R. (1999) The corrosion of character: the personal consequences of work in the new capitalism. New York, NY: Norton.

Shaffer, H., Stein, S. A., Gambino, B., and Cummings, T. N. (1989) *Compulsive Gambling: Theory, Research, and Practice*. Lexington, MA: Lexington Press.

Shaham, Y., Alvares, K., Nespor, S., and Grunberg, N. E. (1992) Effect of stress on oral morphine and fentanyl self-administration in rats. *Pharmacology, Biochemistry, and Behavior*, **41**, 615–619.

Shalai-Esa, A. (2006, 1 May) U.S. auditor warns of crisis unless pension issue resolved. *Globe and Mail*, p. B11.

Shakespeare, W. (1984) The life of King Henry the Fifth. In *The Complete Plays of William Shakespeare*, pp. 429–457. New York, NY: Chatham River Press. (Original work published *c*. 1600.)

Shedler, J. and Block, J. (1990) Adolescent drug use and psychological health: a longitudinal inquiry. *American Psychologist*, **45**, 612–630.

Shelton, C. P. (2003) *Counselling events that aid and impede the self-disclosures of adult male clients: a critical incident investigation*. Unpublished master's thesis, University of British Columbia, Vancouver, BC, Canada.

Shepard, P. (1982) *Nature and Madness*. San Francisco, CA: Sierra Club Books.

Shewan, D. and Dalgarno, P. (2005) Low levels of negative health and social outcomes among non-treatment heroin users in Glasgow (Scotland): evidence for controlled heroin use? *British Journal of Health Psychology*, **10**, 33–48.

Shewan, D., Dalgarno, P., Marshall, A., *et al.* (1998) Patterns of heroin use among a non-treatment sample in Glasgow (Scotland). *Addiction Research*, **6**, 215–234.

Shewan, D., Dalgarno, P., and Reith, G. (2000) Perceived risk and risk reduction among ecstasy users: the role of drug, set, and setting. *International Journal of Drug Policy*, **10**, 431–453.

Shields, S. (2007, 20 April) Long road to a treaty. *The Tyee*. Retrieved 22 April 2007, from http://thetyee.ca/News/2007/04/20/NewRelationship/

Shimo, A. (2006, 8 July) Forums promoting anorexia pose health risk, study warns. *Globe and Mail*, p. A9.

Shimo, A. (2007, 13 January) Flirting with disaster. *Globe and Mail*, pp. F1, F6, F7.

Siegel, M. (2007, 28 August) New Orleans still facing a psychiatric emergency: two years after Katrina. *Globe and Mail*, p. A15.

Siegel, S. (n.d.) *The Effects of Opiates on Addicts*. Unpublished manuscript. (Summarized in Alexander, 1990, Chapter 4.)

Siegrist, J. (2000) Place, social exchange and health: proposed sociological framework. *Social Science and Medicine*, **51**, 1283–1293.

Silver, G. and Aldrich, M. (1979) *The Dope Chronicles: 1850–1950*. New York, NY: Harper and Row.

Simmons, R. (2002) *Odd Girl Out: the Hidden Culture of Aggression in Girls*. New York, NY: Harcourt.

Simpson, C. and Madhani, A. (2005, 9 October) U.S. cash fuels human trade. *Chicago Tribune*. Retrieved 30 October 2005, from http://www.chicagotribune.com/news/specials/chi-nepal-cash-story,1,6641346.story?page=2andcset=trueandctrack=1andcoll=chi-news-hed

Simpson, J. (2003, 10 December) The Americans' lumber clout flouts free trade. *Globe and Mail*, p. A19.

Simpson, J. (2004a, 7 February) Be scared. Be very, very scared. *Globe and Mail*, p. A19.

Simpson, J. (2004b, 30 April) The big issues: security, security, and security. *Globe and Mail*, p. A15.

Simpson, J. (2005, 5 October) The feds starved the CBC, and they won't feed it in the future. *Globe and Mail*, p. A21.

Sinaï, A. (2004, February) Le Sud se divise sur le front climatique: coup de chaleur sur la planète. *Le Monde diplomatique*, pp. 24–25.

Sinaï, A. (2006, January) Climat: un prise de conscience limitée. *Le Monde diplomatique*, p. 23.

Single, E., Christie, P., and Ali, R. (2000) The impact of cannabis decriminalisation in Australia and the United States. *Journal of Public Health Policy*, **21**, 157–186.

Slater, L. (1998) *Prozac Diary*. London, UK: Penguin.

Slater, L. (2004) *Opening Skinner's Box: Great Psychological Experiments of the Twentieth Century*. New York, NY: Norton.

Slater, L. (2007, July) Beyond the valley of the dolls. *Elle*, pp. 120, 122–124, 193–195.

Slater, P. (1976) *The Pursuit of Loneliness* (rev. edn). Boston, MA: Beacon Press.

Slater, P. (1980) *Wealth Addiction*. New York, NY: Dutton.

Small, D. (2007) Fools rush in where angels fear to tread: playing God with Vancouver's Supervised Injection Facility in the political borderland. *International Journal of Drug Policy*, **18**, 18–26.

Smart, R. and Ogborne, A. C. (1996) *Northern Spirits: a Social History of Alcohol in Canada*, 2nd edn. Toronto, ON: Addiction Research Foundation.

Smith, Adam (1991) *An Inquiry into the Nature and Causes of the Wealth of Nations*. New York, NY: Knopf. (Original work published 1776.)

Smith, Alisa (2004, 27 October) Why are U.S. drug cops in Vancouver? Despite slams from a Supreme Court judge and civil liberties advocates, America's DEA calls BC home. *Tyee*. Retrieved from http://www.thetyee.ca/News/current/ WhyUSDrugCopVan.htm

Smith, C. (2006a, 30 March) Universities fight for corporate secrecy. *Georgia Straight*. Retrieved 5 April 2006, from http://www.straight.com/content.cfm?id=16956

Smith, C. (2006b, 7–14 December) Sullivan bullish on 'disorder'. *Georgia Straight*. p. 13.

Smith, C. S. (2005, 2 December) French court rejects pedophilia convictions. *New York Times*, p. A12.

Smith, D. (2001, 26 September) U.S. stimulus could total $100-billion. *Globe and Mail*, p. B9.

Smith, D. (2004, 4 September) Pushing the environmental envelope, or else … *Globe and Mail*, p. D11.

Smith, D. E. and Gay, G. R. (eds) (1972) *It's So Good Don't Even Try It Once: Heroin in Perspective*. Englewood Cliffs, NJ: Prentice-Hall.

Smith, G. (2003, 13 December) Prairies rife with addicts to gambling, study finds. *Globe and Mail*, p. A5.

Smith, G. (2004a, 18 May) Many health-care questions unanswered, Romanow says. *Globe and Mail*, p. A4.

Smith, G. (2004b, 4 December) Swinging at the shadows: the curse of crystal meth. *Globe and Mail*, pp. A1, A7, A8.

Smith, G. M. and Beecher, H. K. (1959) Measurement of 'mental clouding' and other subjective effects of morphine. *Journal of Pharmacology and Experimental Therapeutics*, **126**, 50–62.

Smith, G. M. and Beecher, H. K. (1962a) Subjective effects of heroin and morphine in normal subjects. *Journal of Pharmacology and Experimental Therapeutics*, **136**, 47–52.

Smith, G. M. and Beecher, H. K. (1962b) Objective evidence of mental effects of heroin, morphine, and placebo in normal subjects. *Journal of Pharmacology and Experimental Therapeutics*, **136**, 53–58.

Smith, J. E., Meyers, R. J., and Miller, W. R. (2001) The community reinforcement approach to the treatment of substance use disorders. *American Journal on Addictions*, **10** (Suppl. 1), 51–59.

Smith, N. and Derkson, J. (2002) Urban regeneration: gentrification as global urban strategy. In R. Shier (ed.), *Stan Douglas: Every Building on 100 West Hastings*, pp. 62–92. Vancouver, BC: Contemporary Art Gallery/Arsenal Pulp Press.

Smythe, D. W. (1981) *Dependency Road: Communications, Capitalism, Consciousness, and Canada*. Norwood, NJ: Ablex.

Snyder, D. (2003, 1 February) Car slaves: great wheels, but he lives with mom. *Globe and Mail*, p. L2.

Sober, E. and Wilson, D. S. (1998) *Unto Others: the Evolution and Psychology of Unselfish Behavior*. Cambridge, MA: Harvard University Press.

Sogge, D. (2004, September) Une nécessaire réforme de l'aide internationale. *Le Monde diplomatique*, p. 10.

Sommers, J. and Blomley, N. (2002) 'The worst block in Vancouver.' In R. Shier (ed.), *Stan Douglas: Every Building on 100 West Hastings*, pp. 18–58. Vancouver, BC: Contemporary Art Gallery/Arsenal Pulp Press.

Somers, J., Goldner, E. M., Waraich, P. and Hsu, L. (2004) Prevalence studies of substance-related disorders: a systematic review of the literature. *Canadian Journal of Psychiatry*, **49**, 159–169.

Sonnedecker, G. (1962) Emergence of the concept of opiate addiction. 1. *Journal Mondial de Pharmacie*, **5**, 275–290.

Sonnedecker, G. (1963) Emergence of the concept of opiate addiction. 2. *Journal Mondial de Pharmacie*, **6**, 27–34.

Soros, G. (1997) The capitalist threat. *Atlantic Monthly*, pp. 45–48.

Spalding, A., Scow, A., and Gait, D. (2006) *Secret of the Dance*. Victoria, BC: Orca Book Publishers.

Spears, T. (2003, 12 March) Eating's as addictive as taking drugs, researchers find: overeaters may be trying to stimulate the brain's pleasure circuits. *Vancouver Sun*, p. A3.

Sprague, J. (2002, 25 June) It won't flow forever. *Globe and Mail*, p. A19.

Sproat, G. M. (1987) *The Nootka: Scenes and Studies of Savage Life*. Victoria, BC: Sono Nis Press. (Original work published 1868.)

Stalin, J. (1974) *Les problemes economiques du socialisme en U.R.S.S.* Pekin, China: Editions en Langues Étrangères. (Original work published 1952.)

Staniforth, M. (1967) Marcus Aurelius Antoninus. In P. Edwards (ed.), *The Encyclopedia of Philosophy*, vol. 5, pp. 156–157. New York, NY: Macmillan.

Stanton, M. D., Todd, T. C., and associates. (1982) *The Family Therapy of Drug Abuse and Addiction*. New York, NY: Guilford.

Stanton, T. (2005, 14–16 October) *Religious institutions and social reform: Karl Polanyi's 'The Great Transformation and Evangelical Revivalism'*. Paper presented at the 10th International Conference of the Karl Polanyi Institute, Istanbul, Turkey.

Starr, P. (1982) *The Social Transformation of American Medicine: the Rise of a Sovereign Profession and the Making of a Vast Industry*. New York, NY: Basic Books.

Steel, A. and Trieu, L. (1997, 25 February) It's junkie chic: Calvin rankles drug foes, kids say oh, ho hum. *Kansas City Star*, p. 1.

Steinmann, A. (2004) *Preventing Problematic Substance Use: Interview and Focus Group Report*. Vancouver, BC: Vancouver Coastal Health Authority.

Stiglitz, J. E. (2002) *Globalisation and its Discontents*. New York, NY: W. W. Norton.

Stiglitz, J. E. (2006, 28 December) John Kenneth Galbraith understood capitalism as lived—not as theorized. *Christian Science Monitor*, p. 9.

Stimson, G. V. (2007) 'Harm reduction—coming of age': a local movement with global impact. *International Journal of Drug Policy*, **18**, 67–69.

Stolaroff, M. J. (1997) *The Secret Chief: Conversations with a Pioneer of the Underground Psychedelic Therapy Movement*. Charlotte, NC: Multidisciplinary Association for Psychedelic Studies.

Stone, I. F. (1988) *The Trial of Socrates*. Boston, MA: Little, Brown.

Strange, W. G. (1977) *Job loss: a psychosocial study of worker reactions to a plant closing in a company town in South Appalachia*. Unpublished doctoral dissertation, Cornell University, Ithaca, NY.

Strathdee, S. A., Patrick, D. M., Currie, S. L., *et al.* (1997) Needle exchange is not enough: lessons from the Vancouver injecting drug use study. *AIDS*, **11**, F59–F65.

Strauss, J. (2005, 31 October) Running from the shadows of despair. *Globe and Mail*, pp. A1, A8.

Strauss, S. (2003, 12 July) Are you bitter? Soon there may be a pill to swallow. *Globe and Mail*, p. F9.

Suetonius (Gaius Suetonius Tranquillus) (1957) *The Twelve Caesars* (R. Graves, trans.). Harmondsworth, UK: Penguin. (Original work published *c*. 100 AD.)

Sullivan, P. (2003, 25 November) Vancouver is no. 2, with a bullet. *Globe and Mail* (Western edn), p. A19.

Sullivan, S. G. and Wu, Z. (2007) Rapid scale up of harm reduction in China. *International Journal of Drug Policy*, **18**, 118–128.

Sullum, J. (2003) *Saying Yes: in Defense of Drug Use*. New York, NY: Jeremy P. Tarcher/Putnam.

Sutherland, J. (2004, 26 March) Jimmy has the last laugh. *Globe and Mail*, pp. 38–48.

Sutherland, J. (2005, 7–13 January) Addicted to addiction. *Guardian Weekly*, p. 16.

Suttles, W. (1983) Productivity and its constraints: a Coast Salish case. In R. L. Carlson (ed.), *Indian art traditions of the Northwest Coast*, pp. 67–88. Burnaby, BC: Simon Fraser University, Department of Archaeology, Publication Number 13.

Suzuki, D. and Dressel, H. (2002) *Good News for a Change: How Everyday People are Helping the Planet*. Vancouver, BC: Greystone Books.

Suzuki, D. and McConnell, A. (1997) *The Sacred Balance: Rediscovering our Place in Nature*. Vancouver, BC: Douglas and McIntyre.

Svensson, B. (1996) Pundare, jonkare och andra-med narkotikan som följeslagare. Stockholm: Carlssons.

Sweanor, D., Alcabes, P. and Drucker, E. (2007) Tobacco harm reduction: how rational policy could transform a pandemic. *International Journal of Drug Policy*, **18**, 70–74.

Sweatman, M. (2001) *When Alice Lay Down with Peter*. Toronto, ON: Vintage Canada.

Symons, D. (1979) *The Evolution of Human Sexuality*. New York, NY: Oxford University Press.

Szalavitz, M. (2007, January) The trouble with troubled teen programs. *Reason Magazine*. Retrieved 17 April 2007, from http://www.reason.com/news/show/117088.html

Szasz, T. (1975) *Ceremonial Chemistry: the Ritual Persecution of Drugs, Addicts, and Pushers*. Garden City, NJ: Anchor Press.

Tapscott, D. (2002, 13 November) Stop the brain drain: mental illness is seen by some as the new 'global crisis'. So why aren't companies protecting their best assets—workers' minds, Don Tapscott asks. *Globe and Mail*, pp. C1, C9.

Tapscott, D. and Williams, A. D. (2006, 28 December) Life game a signpost for future. *Globe and Mail*, p. B2.

Tapscott, D. and Williams, A. D. (2007, 2 January) Mass collaboration unleashes 'Us' power. *Globe and Mail*, p. B2.

Tarter, R. E. and Edwards, K. I. (1987) Vulnerability to alcohol and drug abuse. a behavior-genetic view. *Journal of Drug Issues*, **17**, 67–81.

Tarter, R. E., Alterman, A. I., and Edwards, K. I. (1985) Vulnerability to alcoholism in men: a behavior-genetic perspective. *Journal of Studies on Alcohol*, **46**, 329–356.

Tawney, R. H. (1947) *Religion and the Rise of Capitalism*. New York, NY: Mentor Books. (Originally published 1926.)

Taylor, C. (1991) *The Malaise of Modernity*. Toronto, ON: Anansi.

Taylor, P. (2005) Scientists find sixth taste bud—for fat. *Globe and Mail*, p. A13.

Tennant, P. (1990) *Aboriginal People and Politics: the Indian Land Question in British Columbia, 1849–1989*. Vancouver, BC: University of British Columbia Press.

Terras, C. (2004, January) Sous la pression des Eglises. *Le Monde diplomatique*, pp. 8–9.

Thank Ha, T. (2004, 12 November) Man's suicide attempt a wakeup call about gambling, widow warns. *Globe and Mail*, p. A8.

Theodore, T. and Bisetty, K. (2004, 22 September) Clarkson tours Eastside amid howls of protestors. *Vancouver Sun*, pp. A1, A2.

Thomas, L. (2003, 17 August) Wall Street's harsh new reality. *New York Times*, pp. A1, A7.

Thompson, W. P. L. (1987) *History of Orkney*. Edinburgh, UK: Mercat.

Thompson, W. P. L. (1993) Sober and tractable? The Hudson's Bay Men in their Orkney context. *Scottish Local History*, **28**, 22–24.

Thorsell, W. (2002, 10 June) Risk it all on one turn of pitch-and-toss. *Globe and Mail*, p. A15.

Thorsen, T. (2005, 6 July) China opens game-addiction clinic. *GameSpot News*. Retrieved 22 July 2007, from http://www.gamespot.com/news/6128654.html?tag=result;title;2

Ticoll, D. (2003, 4 December) Social networking hottest net trend. *Globe and Mail*, p. B11.

Ticoll, D. (2005, 30 April) Flatism will get you everywhere. [Review of the book *The World is Flat: a Brief History of the Twenty-first Century*.] *Globe and Mail*, p. D14.

Tierney, J. (2005, 9 August) Debunking the drug war. *New York Times*, p. A19.

Tillich, P. (1948) *The Shaking of the Foundations*. New York, NY: Scribner.

Tillich, P. (1952) *The Courage to Be*. Glasgow, UK: Collins.

Time (2003) Chinese junk: China's heroin problem: a special report. *Time Asia Website*. Retrieved from http://www.time.com/time/asia/covers/1101020520/cover4.html

Times-Colonist (2006, 13 December) U.S. shows us what not to do. *Times-Colonist*, p. A14.

Timmer, S. G., Veroff, J., and Colton, M. E. (1985) Life stress, helplessness, and the use of alcohol and drugs to cope: an analysis of national survey data. In S. Shiffman and T. A. Wills (eds), *Coping and Substance Abuse*, pp. 171–198. Orlando, FL: Academic Press.

Timson, J. (2003, 1 February) How shall we reward thy loyalty? *Globe and Mail*, p. B2.

Todes, D. P. (1987) Darwin's Malthusian metaphor and Russian evolutionary thought, 1859–1917. *Isis*, **78**, 537–551.

Toussaint, E. and Millet, D. (2007, June) Banque du sud contre banque mondiale. *Le Monde diplomatique*, p. 4.

Toynbee, A. J. (1948) *Civilisation on Trial*. New York, NY: Oxford University Press.

Trace, M. and Runciman, R. (2005, 3 March) An overdose of morality: American strong-arm tactics threaten to scupper successful UN harm reduction drug programmes. *Guardian Unlimited*. Retrieved 29 January 2007, from http://www.guardian.co.uk/aids/story/0,7369,1429315,00.html

Traves, J. (2006, 18 January) CEO seeks same: the meeting's over. Now what? A new breed of matchmaking service is helping lonely executives find plane pals, dinner mates—or even their next big deal. *Globe and Mail*, p. R10.

Treaster, J. B. (1992, 22 July) Executive's secret study with heroin's powerful grip. *New York Times*, pp. A1, B4.

Trebach, A. S. (1982) *The Heroin Solution*. New Haven, CT: Yale University Press.

Trebach, A. S. (1987) *The Great Drug War: and Radical Proposals That Could Make America Safe Again*. New York, NY: Macmillan.

Tremblay, S. (1999) Illicit drugs and crime in Canada. *Juristat: Canadian Centre for Justice Statistics*, **19**, 1–13 (Statistics Canada, catalogue no. 85-002-XIE).

Tsou, J. Y. (2003) A role for reason in science. *Dialogue: Canadian Philosophical Review*, **42**, 573–598.

Tuchman, B. W. (1966) *The Proud Tower: a Portrait of the World Before the War, 1890–1914.* New York, NY: Macmillan.

Tuck, S. (2003, 2 May) Major gap opens in talks with Daimler Chrysler. *Globe and Mail*, p. B3.

Tuck, S. (2004, 13 March) Ottawa plans to scatter seed money for startups: venture capital program aimed at getting promising research to market. *Globe and Mail*, pp. B1, B6.

Tucker, M. B. (1985) Coping and drug use among heroin-addicted women and men. In S. Shiffman and T. A. Wills (eds), *Coping and Substance Abuse*, pp. 147–170. Orlando, FL: Academic Press.

Tupper, K. W. (2002) Entheogens and existential intelligence: the use of plant teachers as cognitive tools. *Canadian Journal of Education*, **27**, 499–515.

Tuttle, C. B. (1985) Drug management of pain in cancer patients. *Canadian Medical Association Journal*, **132**, 121–133.

Ubelacker, S. (2005a, 16 August) Are parents getting children hooked? Research points to chemical accumulating in saliva of young. *Globe and Mail*, p. A13.

Ubelacker, S. (2005b, 22 September) Panel rejects U.S.-style registry for acne drug. *Globe and Mail*, p. A23.

Uchitelle, L. (2006, 26 November) Here come the economic populists. *New York Times*, Section 4, pp. 1, 4.

Union of BC Indian Chiefs (2002) *Fish Farms: Zero Tolerance: Indian Salmon Don't Do Drugs.* Vancouver, BC: published by the author. Retrieved from http://www.ubcic.bc.ca/UBCICPaper.htm

Union of Concerned Scientists (2004) *Scientific Integrity in Policymaking: an Investigation into the Bush Administration's Misuse of Science.* Cambridge, MA: published by the author. Retrieved from http://www.ucsusa.org/publications/report.cfm?publicationID=730

United Nations Population Fund (2007) *State of World Population 2007: Unleashing the Potential of Urban Growth.* New York, NY: published by the author. Retrieved 30 June 2007, from http://www.unfpa.org/swp/2007/presskit/pdf/sowp2007_eng.pdf

Vaillant, G. E. (1977) *Adaptation to Life.* Boston, MA: Little, Brown.

Vaillant, G. E. (1983) *The Natural History of Alcoholism: Causes, Patterns, and Paths to Recovery.* Cambridge, MA: Harvard University Press.

Valpy, M. (2004a, 31 January) Virtually hooked: the threat of cybersex. *Globe and Mail*, p. F7.

Valpy, M. (2004b, 6 August) U.S. on dangerous course, expert warns. *Globe and Mail*, p. A6.

Valpy, M. (2004c, 7 August) Suicide bombing gaining new converts, expert says: militants see no other solutions to despair. *Globe and Mail*, p. A6.

Valpy, M. (2005, 15 July) Four bombers' profiles called typical. *Globe and Mail*, p. A9.

Vancouver Sun (2005, 26 December) Shop till you drop: it's a moral alternative. *Vancouver Sun*, p. A20.

Vancouver Sun (2007, 24 January) Alternative treatments give addicts a chance. *Vancouver Sun*, p. A12.

Van den Brink, R. (2005, June) Les raisons des Néerlandais. *Le Monde diplomatique*. p. 20.

Vanier, J. (1998) *Becoming Human.* Toronto, ON: Anansi.

Vasagar, J. (2005, 3 August) The hungry reality of free-market Niger. *Globe and Mail*, p. A3.

Vega, W. A., Kolody, B., Aguilar-Gaxiola, S., Alderete, E., Catalano, R., and Caraveo-Anduaga, J. (1998) Lifetime prevalence of DSM-III-R psychiatric disorders among urban and rural Mexican Americans in California. *Archives of General Psychiatry*, **55**, 771–778.

Vega, W. A., Zimmerman, R. S., Warheit, G. J., and Gil, A. G. (2003) Acculturation, stress and Latino adolescent drug use. In A. Maney (ed.), *Socioeconomic Conditions, Stress and Mental Disorders: Toward a New Synthesis of Research and Public Policy*, Chapter 9. Rockville, MD: NIMH. Retrieved 29 January 2007, from www.mhsip.org/pdfs/Vega.pdf

Velásquez, G. (2003, July) Hold-up sur le médicament: le profit contre la santé. *Le Monde diplomatique*, pp. 1, 26–27.

Veltmeyer, H. (2005, 14–16 October) *Neoliberal globalisation and the peasantry: political dynamics of social choice in Latin America*. Paper presented at the 10th International Conference of the Karl Polanyi Institute, Istanbul, Turkey.

Vermond, K. (2003, 28 June) Motion sickness: it's called dromomania—the compulsion to travel—and the afflicted are said to be constantly running away from the fear of being alone. *Globe and Mail*, pp. T1, T4.

Vidal, D., Linden, P., and Wuttke, B. (2004, August) Les Allemands de l'Est saisis par l'Ostalgie. *Le Monde diplomatique*, pp. 6–7.

Vigna, A. (2006, July) Les charletans du tourisme vert. *Le Monde diplomatique*. pp. 14–15.

Vlastos, G. (1992) *Socrates: Ironist and Moral Philosopher*. Cambridge, UK: Cambridge University Press.

Volkow, N. D. (2005) Confronting the rise in abuse of prescription drugs. *NIDA Notes: National Institute of Drug Abuse*, **19**, 3.

von Hayek, F. A. (1944) *The Road to Serfdom*. Chicago, IL: University of Chicago Press.

von Sydow, K., Lieb, R., Pfister, H., Höfler, M., and Wittchen, H.-U. (2002) What predicts innocent use of cannabis and progression to abuse and dependence? A 4-year prospective examination of risk factors in a community sample of adolescents and young adults. *Drug and Alcohol Dependence*, **68**, 49–64.

Walker, M. B. (1992) *The Psychology of Gambling*. Oxford, UK: Butterworth-Heinemann.

Walling, S. (2007a, 30 April) *Negotiating collaborative creation: we're all in this together*. Paper presented at Canadian Community Play Exchange, Toronto, ON, Canada.

Walling, S. (2007b) *Vancouver Moving Theatre: mandate and history*. Unpublished paper available from the author.

Walton, K. and Roberts, B. W. (2004) On the relationship between substance abuse and personality traits: abstainers are not maladjusted. *Journal of Research in Personality*, **38**, 515–535.

Warburton, H., Turnbull, P. J., and Hough, M. (2005) *Occasional and Controlled Heroin Use: Not a Problem?* York, UK: Joseph Rowntree Foundation. Available at http://www.jrf.org.uk/bookshop/details.asp?pubID=747

Warde, I. (2002, March) Surexploitation joyeuse aux Etats-Unis. *Le Monde diplomatique*, p. 27.

Warde, I. (2004, May) Irak, l'eldorado perdu. *Le Monde diplomatique*, pp. 1, 12, 13.

Warner, Jessica (1992) Before there was 'alcoholism'. Lessons from the medieval experience with alcohol. *Contemporary Drug Problems*, **19**, 409–429.

Warner, Jessica (1994) 'Resolv'd to drink no more': addiction as a preindustrial construct. *Journal of Studies on Alcohol*, **55**, 685–691.

Warner, Jessica (2002) *Craze: Gin and Debauchery in an Age of Reason*. New York, NY: Four Walls Eight Windows.

Warner, Judith (2005, 27 November) Kids gone wild. *New York Times*, Section 4, pp. 1, 4.

Warrior Publications (n.d.) *Gunboats and genocide*. Retrieved 2 April 2007, from http://itwillbethundering.resist.ca/warrior_publications/gunboatsandgenocide.html

Washton, A. M. (1989) *Treatment, Recovery, and Relapse Protection*. New York, NY: W. W. Norton.

Wasserman, J. (2007, 23 April) People shine in shadows: production vividly evokes addiction issues. *Vancouver Province*, p. B2.

Wayne, L. (2005, 8 June) Report faults Air Force in proposed Boeing deal. *New York Times*, p. C4.

Weber, M. (1958) *The Protestant Ethic and the Spirit of Capitalism*. New York, NY: Scribner. (Original work published 1920.)

Webster's International Dictionary of the English Language (1902) Springfield, MA: G. and C. Merriam Company.

Wegert, T. (2005, 21 July) The web cookie is crumbling—and marketers feel the fallout. *Globe and Mail*, p. B9.

Weil, R. (1996) Red cat, white cat: China and the contradictions of 'market socialism'. New York, NY: Monthly Review Press.

Weiner, T. (2005, 8 June) Arms fiascos leads to alarm inside Pentagon. *New York Times*, pp. A1, C4.

Weissman, D. E. and Haddox, J. D. (1989) Opioid pseudoaddiction—an iatrogenic syndrome. *Pain*, **36**, 363–366.

Weissman, R. (2007, 30 August) The benchmarks Iraq is meeting—and one it thankfully is not. Washington, DC: Multinational Monitor Editor's Blog. Retrieved 31 August 2007, from http://www.multinationalmonitor.org/editorsblog/index.php?/archives/62-The-Benchmarks-Iraq-Is-Meeting-And-One-It-Thankfully-Is-Not.html#extended

Weissmann, G. (2007) The experimental pathology of stress: from Hans Selye to Paris Hilton. *FASEB Journal*, **21**, 2635–2638.

Wente, M. (2004, 17 February) Earth to parent: not all kids are equal. *Globe and Mail*, p. A15.

Wente, M. (2005, 22 October) Needling the habit. *Globe and Mail*, A23.

West, R. (2001) Theories of addiction. *Addiction*, **96**, 3–13.

West, S. L. and O'Neal, K. K. (2004) Project D.A.R.E. outcome effectiveness revisited. *American Journal of Public Health*, **94**, 1027–1029.

Westermeyer, J. (1982) *Poppies, Pipes, and People: Opium and its Use in Laos*. Berkeley, CA: University of California Press.

Western Canada Wilderness Committee (2002) Wild fish need wild rivers and oceans. *Western Canada Wilderness Committee Educational Report*, *21*. Retrieved from http://www.wildernesscommittee.org/campaigns/marine/policy/fish_farms/reports/Vo121No05

Wheatley, M. (2005, 23 November) *Letting go of hope*. Retrieved 13 March 2006, from http://www.truthout.org/docs_2005/1123050.shtml

White, I. D., Hoskin, P. J., Hanks, G. W. and Bliss, J. M. (1991) Analgesics in cancer pain: current practice and beliefs. *British Journal of Cancer*, **63**, 271–274.

White House (2004) *National Drug Control Strategy: FY 2005 Budget Summary*. Washington, DC: Office of National Drug Control Policy.

Whyte, M. (2007, 18 March) The secret life of self-help books: Ask. Believe. Receive. Or not … *Toronto Star*. Retrieved 22 April 2007, from http://www.thestar.com/article/193263

Wibberly, C. (2005) Boomerang ads. *Drug and Alcohol Findings*, **14**, 22–25. Retrieved 7 February 2006, from http://www.drugandalcoholfindings.org.uk/Boomerang.pdf

Wiebe, J., Single, E., and Falkowski-Ham, A. (2001) *Measuring Gambling and Problem Gambling in Ontario*. Ottawa, ON: Canadian Centre on Substance Abuse and Responsible Gambling Council (Ontario). Available at http://www.responsiblegambling.org/articles/CPGI_report-Dec4.pdf

Wilber, K. (1996) *A Brief History of Everything*. Boston, MA: Shambhala.

Wilber, K. (2000) *A Brief History of Everything*, 2nd edn. Boston, MA: Shambhala.

Wilcocks, P. (2007, 30 August) Electoral boundaries show STV can work for B.C. *Times-Colonist*, p. A10.

Wild, T. C., el-Guebaly, N., Fischer, B., *et al.* (2005) Comorbid depression among untreated illicit opiate users: results from a multisite Canadian study. *Canadian Journal of Psychiatry*, **50**, 512–518.

Willcocks, P. (2004, 9 October) We should be sorry about the Doukhobor children and we should say so. *Vancouver Sun*, p. C7.

Williams, G. (2007, September–October) The resistible rise of Rupert Murdoch. *Adbusters*, **73**, 22.

Williams, J. (2007) *50 Facts that Should Change the World* (revised and updated edn). Cambridge, UK: Icon Books.

Williamson, N. (2003, 28 April) Diva of distress: singer 'addicted to turmoil and chaos'. *Globe and Mail*, p. R3.

Wilson, D. S. (2002) *Darwin's Cathedral: Evolution, Religion, and the Nature of Society*. Chicago, IL: University of Chicago Press.

Wilson, D. S. and Sober, E. (1994) Reintroducing group selection to the human behavioral sciences. *Behavioral and Brain Sciences*, **17**, 585–654.

Wilson, M., Joffe, R. T., and Wilkerson, B. (with Bastable, C.) (2000) The unheralded business crisis in Canada. Depression at work. An information paper for business, incorporating '12 Steps to a Business Plan to Defeat Depression'. Toronto, ON: Global Business and Economic Roundtable on Addiction and Mental Health. Available at http://mentalhealth roundtable.ca/aug_round_pdfs/Roundtable%20report_Jul20.pdf

Winchester, S. (2003) *The Meaning of Everything: the Story of the Oxford English Dictionary*. Oxford, UK: Oxford University Press.

Winick, C. (1962) Maturing out of narcotic addiction. *Bulletin on Narcotics*, **14**, 1–7.

Wong, J. (1996) *Red China Blues: My Long March from Mao to Now*. New York, NY: Anchor Books.

Wong, J. (2003, 12 July) Party animals: Jan Wong examines the bizarre ritual that now passes for celebration among better-off young teens. Its key features: too much alcohol, too little parental scrutiny and far, far too many strangers bent on wanton destruction. *Globe and Mail*, pp. F1, F8.

Wong, J. and Mills, C. (2005, 15 July) Jamaica's despair is fertile soil for Islam. *Globe and Mail*, p. A9.

Wong, L. (1990) Critical analysis of drug war alternatives: the need for a shift in personal and social values. *Journal of Drug Issues*, **20**, 679–688.

Wood, E., Tyndall, M. W., Spittal, P. M., *et al.* (2003) Impact of supply-side policies for control of illicit drugs in the face of the AIDS and overdose epidemics: investigation of a massive heroin seizure. *Canadian Medical Association Journal*, **168**, 165–169.

Wood, E., Kerr, T., Small, W., *et al.* (2004a) Changes in public order after the opening of a medically supervised safer injecting facility for illicit injection drug users. *Canadian Medical Association Journal*, **171**, 731–734.

Wood, E., Spittal, P. M., Small, W., *et al.* (2004b) Displacement of Canada's largest public illicit drug market in response to a police crackdown. *Canadian Medical Association Journal*, **170**, 1551–1556.

Wood, E., Kerr, T., Stoltz, J., *et al.* (2005) Prevalence and correlates of hepatitis C infection among users of North America's first medically supervised safe injection facility. *Public Health*, **119**, 1111–1115.

Wood, E. M. (1999) *The Origins of Capitalism*. New York, NY: Monthly Review Press.

Woodcock, G. (1977) *Peoples of the Coast: the Indians of the Pacific Northwest*. Edmonton, AB: Hurtig.

Woodman, M. (1982) *Addiction to Perfection: the Still Unravished Bride*. Toronto, ON: Inner City.

Woods, A. (2006, 6 November) Ottawa ignores support for injection sites: Harper government froze new sites even though own poll showed backing for them. *Vancouver Sun*. p. A1.

Woods, J. H. (1978) Behavioral pharmacology of drug self-administration. In M. A. Lipton, A. DiMascio, and K. F. Killam (eds), *Psychopharmacology: a Generation of Progress*, pp. 595–607. New York, NY: Raven.

Woodward, B. (1984) *Wired: the Short Life and Fast Times of John Belushi*. New York, NY: Simon & Shuster.

Woodward, J. (2005, 26 August) Vancouver heroin death toll rises to six in six days. *Globe and Mail*, pp. S1, S2.

Woodward, J. (2006, 8 March) SFU to create for-profit college. *Globe and Mail*, pp. S1, S3.

WorldNetDaily.com (2005, 22 August) *Robertson: time to assassinate Chavez*. Retrieved 8 October 2005, from http://worldnetdaily.com/news/article.asp?ARTICLE_ID=45916

World Health Organization (2007) *International statistical classification of diseases and related health problems 10th revision, version for 2007*. Retrieved 15 July 2007, from http://www.who.int/classifications/apps/icd/icd10online/

World Social Forum (2006) *World social forum charter of principles*. Retrieved 6 June 2006, from http://www.forumsocialmundial.org.br/main.php?id_menu=4andcd_language=2

Wright, A. (1976) *J. M. Barrie*. Edinburgh, UK: Ramsay Head Press.

Wright, J. (2003) *There Must be More Than This: Finding More Life, Love, and Meaning by Overcoming your Soft Addictions*. London, UK: Bantam Books.

Wright, R. T. (1998) *Barkerville, Williams Creek, Cariboo*, 2nd edn. Williams Lake, BC: Winter Quarters Press.

Wrightson, K. (2000) *Earthly Necessities: Economic Lives in Early Modern Britain*. New Haven, CT: Yale University Press.

Wurmser, L. (1978) *The Hidden Dimension: Psychodynamics in Compulsive Drug Use*. New York, NY: Jason Aronson.

Xinhua News Agency (2003, 6 March) Drugs pose a challenge. *ShanghaiDaily.com*. Retrieved 9 February 2007, from http://english.eastday.com/epublish/gb/paper1/834/class000100004/hwz117247.htm

Yahne, C. E., Miller, W. R., Irvin-Vitela, L., and Tonigan, J. S. (2002) Magdalena pilot project: mmotivational outreach to substance abusing women street workers. *Journal of Substance Abuse Treatment*, **23**, 49–53.

Yahya, F. (1978) *Zionist Relations with Nazi Germany*. Beirut, Lebanon: Palestine Research Centre.

Yakabuski, K. (2004, 22 September) What's in a brand name? Profit. *Globe and Mail*, p. B2.

Yalnizyan, A. (2005, 14–16 October) *De-commodification and re-commodification—thoughts on the shifting economics of health care*. Presentation to the 10th International Karl Polanyi Conference, Istanbul, Turkey.

Yamane, Y. (2007, 21 March) *Asia/online addicts get a dose of medicine from the military.* Retrieved 30 March 2007, from http://www.asahi.com/english/Herald-asahi/TKY200703210051.html

Yeary, J. (1982) Incest and chemical dependency. *Journal of Psychoactive Drugs,* **14**, 133–135.

Yi-Mak, K. and Harrison, L. (2001) Globalisation, cultural change, and the modern drug epidemics: the case of Hong Kong. *Health Risk and Society,* **3**, 39–57.

York, A. (2003) *Mercy.* Toronto, ON: Vintage Canada.

York, G. (2003a, 11 January) Couching tiger. *Globe and Mail,* pp. F4-F5.

York, G. (2003b, 4 December) Urban renewal takes its toll in Beijing. *Globe and Mail,* p. A14.

York, G. (2004a, 21 February) Jesus challenging Marx for soul of China: millions turning to Christianity even as Beijing cracks down on secret worship. *Globe and Mail,* p. A3.

York, G. (2004b, 23 October) Behind the boom: a struggle for identity and rumblings of revolt. *Globe and Mail,* pp. A3, A10–A11.

York, G. (2005a, 15 February) China wages losing war against gambling. *Globe and Mail,* p. A13.

York, G. (2005b, 5 July) Obesity equals affluence in modern China. *Globe and Mail,* p. A10.

York, G. (2005c, 13 July) 69 million Communists urged to toe the line. *Globe and Mail,* p. A3.

York, G. (2005d, 20 August) Invasion of the gold snatchers. Thousands of impoverished Mongolians illegally dig for specks of precious metal to eke out a subsistence. *Globe and Mail,* pp. F4, F5.

York, G. (2005e, 22 August) Road rash of the Mongolian hinterland. *Globe and Mail,* pp. A1, A9.

York, G. (2006, 9 February) China frets over its expanding income gap. *Globe and Mail,* pp. A1, A16.

Young, K. S. (2004) Internet addiction: a new clinical phenomenon and its consequences. *American Behavioral Scientist,* **48**, 402–415.

Your Media (2007, 21 July) *Watchdogs, advocates, and independent media.* Retrieved 21 July 2007, from http://www.yourmedia.ca/internetwork.shtml

Zernike, K. (2004, 14 May) Accused soldier paints scene of eager mayhem. *New York Times,* pp. A1, A10.

Zhou, Y. (2000) Nationalism, identity, and state-building: the antidrug crusade in the People's Republic, 1949–1952. In T. Brook and B. T. Wakabayashi (eds), *Opium Regimes: China, Britain, and Japan, 1839–1952,* pp. 380–403. Berkeley, CA: University of California Press.

Zhukovsky, D. S., Walsh, D. and Doona, M. (2000) The relative potency between high dose oral oxycodone and intravenous morphine: a case illustration. *Archives of Internal Medicine,* **160**, 853–860.

Zinberg, N. E. (1984) *Drug, Set, and Setting: the Basis for Controlled Intoxicant Use.* New Haven, CT: Yale University Press.

Zinberg, N. E. and Lewis, D. C. (1964) Narcotic usage. I. A spectrum of a difficult medical problem. *New England Journal of Medicine,* **270**, 989–993.

Zinberg, N. E., Harding, W. M., and Apsler, R. (1978) What is drug abuse? *Journal of Drug Issues,* **8**, 9–35.

Zinn, H. (1980) *A People's History of the United States.* New York, NY: HarperCollins.

Index